Molecular Neuroscience

Molecular Neuroscience

Editor: Colton Easton

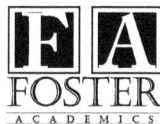

FA FOSTER
A C A D E M I C S

www.fosteracademics.com

www.fosteracademics.com

FA
FOSTER
A C A D E M I C S

Cataloging-in-Publication Data

Molecular neuroscience / edited by Colton Easton.
      p. cm.
Includes bibliographical references and index.
ISBN 978-1-63242-845-5
1. Neurosciences. 2. Molecular neurobiology. I. Easton, Colton.
RC332 .M65 2019
616.8--dc23

Foster Academics,
118-35 Queens Blvd., Suite 400,
Forest Hills, NY 11375, USA

ISBN 978-1-63242-845-5 (Hardback)

Contents

Preface

Molecular neuroscience is a subfield of neuroscience. It focuses on the examination of the concepts in molecular biology in relation to the nervous system. The communication between neurons usually takes place with the help of chemical transmission across gaps between the cells, known as synapses. The topics that are covered under this discipline include molecular neuroanatomy, the molecular basis for neuroplasticity and the effects of genetics and epigenetics on neuronal development. It also focuses on the molecular mechanisms of neurodegenerative diseases. Some of the common neurodegenerative diseases include Alzheimer's disease, Parkinson's disease and Huntington's disease. The transmitted chemicals, called neurotransmitters, are responsible in the regulation of a significant fraction of vital body functions. The ever-growing need of advanced technology is the reason that has fueled the research in the field of molecular neuroscience in recent times. It strives to provide a fair idea about this discipline and to help develop a better understanding of the latest advances within this field. As this field is emerging at a rapid pace, the contents of this book will help the readers understand the modern concepts and applications of the subject.

This book is a comprehensive compilation of works of different researchers from varied parts of the world. It includes valuable experiences of the researchers with the sole objective of providing the readers (learners) with a proper knowledge of the concerned field. This book will be beneficial in evoking inspiration and enhancing the knowledge of the interested readers.

In the end, I would like to extend my heartiest thanks to the authors who worked with great determination on their chapters. I also appreciate the publisher's support in the course of the book. I would also like to deeply acknowledge my family who stood by me as a source of inspiration during the project.

Editor

A T-type channel-calmodulin complex triggers αCaMKII activation

Hadhimulya Asmara[1,4], Ileana Micu[2,4], Arsalan P. Rizwan[1,4], Giriraj Sahu[1,4], Brett A. Simms[1,4], Fang-Xiong Zhang[3,5], Jordan D. T. Engbers[1,4], Peter K. Stys[2,4], Gerald W. Zamponi[3,4,5] and Ray W. Turner[1,3,4,6*]

Abstract

Calmodulin (CaM) is an important signaling molecule that regulates a vast array of cellular functions by activating second messengers involved in cell function and plasticity. Low voltage-activated calcium channels of the Cav3 family have the important role of mediating low threshold calcium influx, but were not believed to interact with CaM. We find a constitutive association between CaM and the Cav3.1 channel at rest that is lost through an activity-dependent and Cav3.1 calcium-dependent CaM dissociation. Moreover, Cav3 calcium influx is sufficient to activate αCaMKII in the cytoplasm in a manner that depends on an intact Cav3.1 C-terminus needed to support the CaM interaction. Our findings thus establish that T-type channel calcium influx invokes a novel dynamic interaction between CaM and Cav3.1 channels to trigger a signaling cascade that leads to αCaMKII activation.

Keywords: Calmodulin, Cav3.1, T-type channel, αCaMKII, Hippocampus, Purkinje cell, Cerebellum

Introduction

Calcium channels mediate a wide range of cellular functions that involve activation of calcium-dependent enzymes that can shape neuronal output [1]. Members of the Cav3 calcium channel family are designed to regulate calcium entry in the subthreshold voltage range to control action potential generation [2–4] and transmitter release [5–8]. Dysregulated Cav3 channels contribute to pathologies such as epilepsy, chronic pain, and ataxia [1, 9–11]. It has been well established that high voltage-activated (HVA) calcium channels interact with the calcium sensing protein calmodulin (CaM) to regulate channel function [12–14]. Moreover, calcium entry through HVA calcium channels can trigger a second messenger cascade by which CaM activates Ca^{2+}/CaM-dependent protein kinase II (CaMKII) that can modify cell activity and long-term plasticity [15–19]. In contrast, the Cav3 channel family is reported to lack CaM binding consensus motifs that would permit calcium-dependent interactions with CaM [20, 21] and there are no reports of Cav3 calcium influx triggering a signaling cascade for CaMKII activation. The available data then suggest that activation of CaM-CaMKII signaling by voltage-dependent calcium channels is restricted to HVA calcium channels that open in response to large membrane depolarizations.

We now report that under resting conditions, CaM constitutively associates with the C-terminus of Cav3.1, as revealed in both a heterologous expression system and rodent brain. In response to Cav3.1-mediated calcium influx the Cav3.1-CaM association is lost, accompanied by phosphorylation of αCaMKII in both a heterologous expression system and neurons in hippocampus and cerebellum. These results are important in providing the first evidence of a role for Cav3.1 channels in triggering αCaMKII as a second messenger involved in mediating a host of cellular functions.

Methods

Animal care and tissue dissection

Sprague-Dawley rats and C57/BL/6 mice were obtained from Charles River and maintained according to guidelines of the Canadian Council for Animal Care, and euthanized according to Standard Operating Procedures defined by the University of Calgary Animal Resource Center. All chemicals were obtained from Sigma (Oakville, ON, Canada) unless otherwise indicated. Animals at P19–40 were anaesthetized by isoflurane inhalation until unresponsive to ear

* Correspondence: rwturner@ucalgary.ca
[1]Department of Cell Biology and Anatomy, University of Calgary, Calgary, AB T2N 4N1, Canada
[3]Department of Physiology and Pharmacology, University of Calgary, AB T2N 4N1, Canada
Full list of author information is available at the end of the article

pinch and the brain dissected out in the presence of ice cold sucrose-cutting solution composed of (in mM): 215 sucrose, 25 $NaHCO_3$, 20 D-glucose, 2.5 KCl, 1.25 NaH_2PO_4 and 3 $MgCl_2$ preoxygenated by carbogen (95% O_2, 5% CO_2) gas [22]. For coimmunoprecipitations brain tissue was transferred to a lysis buffer medium comprised of (in mM): 150 NaCl, 50 Tris pH 7.5, 0.5% sodium-decholic acid, 1% NP-40, 2.5 EGTA, 0–3 $CaCl_2$, and 1 tablet complete protease inhibitor cocktail (EDTA free) in 10 ml, and stored at 4 °C. A separate set of experiments prepared brain tissue to create homogenates in different buffered levels of calcium concentration according to Lai et al. [23]. For tissue slice histochemistry sagittal cerebellar tissue slices of 150 µm thickness were prepared from P30-P40 male rats by Vibratome in ice-cold sucrose-cutting solution as above. For tissue destined for recordings, slices were incubated at 37 °C in artificial cerebrospinal fluid (aCSF) composed of (mM): 125 NaCl, 1.0 KCl, 1.5 $CaCl_2$, 1.5 $MgCl_2$, 25 $NaHCO_3$, and 25 D-glucose bubbled with carbogen gas, with a subset exposed to aCSF containing 50 mM [K]o for 10 min prior to immediate removal and fixation for immunolabel processing. Calcium influx was restricted to Cav3 calcium channels throughout by cutting tissue slices and maintaining tissue in aCSF containing 30 µM Cd^{2+}, 1 µM TTX, 10 µM DNQX and 25 µM or 100 µM DL-AP5.

Low-density cultures of hippocampal neurons were prepared from P0-P1 pups of C57/BL/6 mice initially anesthetized by placing on ice for 5–10 min. Dissected hippocampi were dissociated by papain treatment and trituration and plated on poly-L-lysine and laminin-coated glass coverslips in 24 well culture dishes at a density of 3500–5300 cells/cm^2. After plating, cells were allowed to grow on coverslips for 10 days in medium composed of (in mM): free neurobasal medium (BME), 1% B-27 supplement, 5% FBS, 0.6% glucose, 1 Na-Pyruvate, 2 L-glutamine, 10 HEPES, 1% Pen-strep. All cell culture chemicals were obtained from Life Technologies (Burlington, ON, Canada).

Molecular biology

Wild-type human Cav3.1b cDNA was donated by T. Snutch (Vancouver, BC, Canada) (GenBank accession number AF134986.1), HA-Cav3.1 and Kir2.1 cDNA from E. Bourinet (Institut de Génomique Fonctionnelle, Montpellier, FR), and CaM cDNAs by J. Adelman (Vollum Institute, OR, USA). GFP-Cav3.1 and GFP-αCaMKII were subcloned into a GFP mammalian vector (pCMV6-AN-GFP) (OriGene Technologies, Rockville, MD, USA) and mKate-CaM prepared from a pmKate2-N mammalian expression vector (Axxora, Farmingdale, NY, USA). CaMKIIN was amplified from a mouse hippocampal cDNA library (RIKEN) and cloned into the pcDNA3.1 vector (Addgene, Cambridge, MA, USA) [24]. To create a deletion of the C-terminus, PCR with specific primers was performed on Cav3.1 outside of the C-terminus region, followed by sequencing and subcloning into the pCMV6-AN-GFP vector (OriGene Technologies, Rockville, MD, USA) or the pcDNA3.1 vector (Addgene, Cambridge, MA, USA) and sequenced for final confirmation. The GFP and mKate tags were attached to the N-terminal regions of target proteins. To create the Cav3.1 pore mutant, a single point mutation PCR was performed on E354K in the pore region with the primer sequences: 5′-ACAGGTCGTTGAGCCGC-3′, followed by sequencing and subcloning into the pcDNA3.1 vector (Addgene, Cambridge, MA, USA) and sequenced for final confirmation.

Transient transfection

cDNA constructs were transiently transfected into tsA-201 cells using the calcium phosphate method [25]. Coimmunoprecipitation experiments used 5 µg cDNA for each of Cav3.1, HA-Cav3.1, CaM, CaM1234, and GFP-Cav3.1 lacking the C-terminus (GFP-Cav3.1ΔCT). FRET studies used 1 µg cDNA of GFP-Cav3.1 and mKate-CaM, and live cell imaging experiments and immunocytochemistry used 1 µg Cav3.1 or Cav3.1ΔCT or Cav3.1 pore mutant, 1 µg CaM, and 0.7 µg GFP-αCaMKII. tsA-201 were also transfected with 0.3 µg Kir2.1 cDNA where indicated. Transfected cells were incubated at 37 °C (5% CO_2) for 24 h and then transferred to a 30 °C incubator (5% CO_2) for 48–72 h prior to imaging studies or incubated at 30 °C for 48 h before being lysed using a buffered calcium concentration buffer for coimmunoprecipitations.

Coimmunoprecipitation assays

tsA-201 cells transiently transfected with Cav3.1 or Cav3.1ΔCT and either CaM or CaM1234 were lysed in a buffer containing (in mM): 150 NaCl, 50 Tris, 2.5 EGTA, 0.5% sodium-decholic acid, 1% NP-40, 0–3 $CaCl_2$, pH 7.5. The nominal level of free calcium in solutions was calculated using Maxchelator software (http://max chelator.stanford.edu/CaEGTA-NIST.htm) to conduct coimmunoprecipitations in the presence of different levels of free calcium concentration ranging from 0 to 1 mM (see [23]). Brain tissue was prepared in cell lysis buffer using a hand held glass homogenizer. Lysates from tsA-201 cells were centrifuged at 13,000 rpm for 1 min at 4 °C and supernatants were transferred to new tubes. Solubilized proteins were incubated with 1 µg of rabbit anti-Cav3.1 antibody (1:1000) corresponding to amino acid residues of the I-II linker of rat $Ca_V3.1$ [22], or with anti-CaM antibody (1:1000; Millipore, Etobicoke, ON, Canada) and 30 µl of Protein G beads (Life Technologies, Burlington, ON, Canada) while rotating overnight at 4 °C. Coimmunoprecipitates were washed three times with phosphate buffered saline (PBS) in (mM): 137 NaCl, 2.7 KCl, 1 Na_2HPO_4, 1.8 KH_2PO_4, pH 7.4 reconstituted in an equal volume of 2X loading buffer (in mM): 100 Tris, 100

2-mercaptoethanol, 4% SDS, 0.02% bromophenol blue, 20% glycerol, pH 6.8 and incubated at 100 °C for 5 min. Eluted samples were loaded on 6–10% Tris-glycine gel and resolved using SDS-PAGE. Samples were transferred to 0.2 μm PVDF membrane (Millipore, Etobicoke, ON, Canada) and Western blot analysis performed using a mouse monoclonal anti-CaM antibody (1:1000; Millipore, Etobicoke, ON, Canada) or a mouse monoclonal anti-Hemagglutinin (HA) antibody (0.4 μg; Roche, Mississauga, ON, Canada). Secondary antibodies were conjugated to horseradish peroxidase (HRP; 1:5000; Molecular Probes, Eugene, OR, USA) and reacted with ECL solution (Life Technologies, Burlington, ON, Canada).

GST-pull down assay

To prepare the GST-C-terminus of Cav3.1, we transformed Cav3.1 C-terminus GST fusion protein plasmids into BL21 and induced the expression of recombinant proteins by 0.5 mM isopropyl-β-D-1-thiogalactopyranoside. GST fusion proteins were purified from bacteria using glutathione-Sepharose 4B beads (Life Technologies, Burlington, ON, Canada) according to the protocol recommended by the manufacturer. The GST tag was then cleaved using Precision Protease (Life Technologies, Burlington, ON, Canada). Complete cleavage of the fusion protein was verified using Western blotting. The recombinant Cav3.1 C-terminus peptides were then applied to CaM sepharose beads and incubated overnight. The CaM sepharose beads were washed three times with PBS, reconstituted in equal volume of loading buffer (100 mM Tris, 4% SDS, 0.02% bromophenol blue, 20% glycerol, 100 mM 2-mercaptoethanol, pH 6.8) and incubated at 100 °C for 5 min. Eluted samples were loaded on a 6–10% Tris-glycine gel and resolved using SDS-PAGE. Samples were transferred to 0.2 μm PDVF membrane (Millipore, Etobicoke, ON, Canada) and western blot analysis was performed using a goat anti-Cav3.1 antibody targeted to the C-terminus region of the channel (1:1000; Santa Cruz, Dallas, TX, USA). The secondary antibody used was a goat antibody conjugated to HRP (1:5000; Molecular Probes, Eugene, OR, USA) and reacted with ECL solution (Life Technologies, Burlington, ON, Canada).

Western blot

Cerebellar tissue slices lysates of 150 μm thickness were incubated for 10 min in any of three conditions: low $[K]_o$ (1 mM), high $[K]_o$ (50 mM), or high $[K]_o$ with mibefradil (1 μM) and Ni^{2+} (300 μM). Homogenates were then made in the same solutions using a hand held glass homogenizer. Eluted lysates were loaded on 6–10% Tris-glycine gel and resolved using SDS-PAGE. Samples were transferred to 0.2 μm PVDF membrane (Millipore, Etobicoke, ON, Canada) and Western blot analysis

performed using a monoclonal mouse anti-αCAMKII (1:1000; Santa Cruz, Dallas, TX, USA) or a polyclonal rabbit anti-p-αCAMKII (Thr286) (1:1000; Santa Cruz, Dallas, TX, USA). The secondary antibodies used were the appropriate mouse or rabbit antibodies conjugated to HRP (1:5000; Molecular Probes, Eugene, OR, USA) and reacted with ECL solution (Life Technologies, Burlington, ON, Canada).

Live cell fluorescence spectral confocal imaging

Cultured tsA-201 cells were transiently transfected with GFP-Cav3.1 and mKate-CaM constructs for FRET imaging. Cells were seeded onto poly-L-lysine coated 35 mm plates. Cells were then incubated for 24 h at 37 °C and 5% CO_2, washed and replaced with colorless imaging medium (in mM): 148 NaCl, 3 KCl, 10 HEPES, 0 or 3 $CaCl_2$, 8 glucose, 1 $MgCl_2$, pH 7.3 at 25 °C. Cultured cells were examined with a Nikon Eclipse C1si spectral confocal laser-scanning microscope with a 40×/1.3NA oil immersion objective. For FRET imaging GFP-Cav3.1 was excited at 457 nm and mKate-CaM at 561 nm. Emission spectra of GFP and mKate were recorded between 400 nm to 750 nm. The FRET signal was measured every 10 s for 450 s.

To separate the fluorescence signals of GFP and mKate spectral images were linearly unmixed using ImageTrak software (P.K. Stys, http://www.ucalgary.ca/styslab/image trak) [26], collapsing a 32 channel spectral image into a two channel image representing the integrated intensities of GFP and mKATE fluorescence emissions. The FRET response was quantified as follows: at each time point, the mean pixel intensity of each fluorophore from the linearly unmixed image within specific cellular ROIs representing the cell cytoplasm was first calculated. The mean mKate intensity was divided by the mean GFP intensity to yield a ratio. Changes over time were expressed as a % change vs. this ratio at time 0. Expressed in mathematical terms:

$$\Delta R(t) = \frac{F_{mKate}(t)}{F_{GFP}(t)} - \frac{F_{mKate}(0)}{F_{GFP}(0)} \times 100\%$$

Where:

- $\Delta R(t)$ is the % change of mKate:GFP intensity ratio as a function of time (positive values mean an increase in mKate emission relative to GFP, implying greater FRET and therefore closer physical proximity of the two fluorescent proteins).
- $F_{mKate}(t)$ and $F_{GFP}(t)$ are the mean fluorescence intensities of the two fluorophores as a function of time
- $F_{mKate}(0)$ and $F_{GFP}(0)$ are the mean fluorescence intensities of the two fluorophores at time 0

For tests using GFP-αCaMKII expression tsA-201 cells were placed in colorless imaging medium comprised of (in mM): 148 NaCl, 1 or 50 KCl, 10 HEPES, 3 $CaCl_2$, 8 Glucose, 1 $MgCl_2$, pH 7.4 at 25 °C. For tests using GFP-αCaMKII transfection of hippocampal cultures, cells were transferred to aCSF containing 30 μM Cd^{2+}, 1 μM TTX, 10 μM DNQX and 25 μM or 100 μM DL-AP5. The GFP-αCaMKII was excited at 457 nm and fluorescence signal in the cytoplasmic and nuclear compartment of cells was measured (ImageTrak). Images were recorded every 5 or 10 s for 250 or 400 s in control (1 mM [K]o) and test media (50 mM [K]o), and in the case of Fig. 4a, b, returned to aCSF containing low [K]o. The aggregation was calculated as the change in pixel variance of GFP fluorescence (ΔSD) presented as a percentage change from control variance (SD0G) to quantify the degree of GFP-αCaMKII aggregation (ΔSD/SD0G (%)) (Figs. 4 and 6; Additional file 5: Figure S5). Alternatively, GFP-αCaMKII aggregation was calculated as the mean fluorescence intensity change (ΔF) presented as a change from control mean (F0) (Figs. 5 and 7; Additional file 8: Figure S8).

Immunohistochemistry

Tests for phosphorylation of GFP-αCaMKII and phosphorylation of αCaMKII were conducted on cultured tsA-201 cells transiently transfected with cDNA, mouse hippocampal cell cultures, and rat cerebellar tissue slices maintained as above and exposed to control or test conditions (1 mM or 50 mM [K]o). Cultured cells and tissues were then quickly washed in PBS and fixed by exposure to 4% paraformaldehyde (pH 7.4) at room temperature for 1 h and overnight at 4 °C. The cells or tissue were transferred to a working solution of 3% normal donkey or horse serum (Jackson Immuno-Research, West Grove, PA, USA), 0.2% TWEEN and 2% dimethylsulphoxide in phosphate buffer (PB). Primary antibodies were reacted for 48 h at 4 °C and washed in working solution 3 X 15 min and secondary antibodies for 4 h at room temperature. Primary antibodies corresponded to a monoclonal mouse anti-p-αCAMKII (Thr286) (1:500; Life Technologies, Burlington, ON, Canada). Secondary antibodies (1:1000) were the appropriate AlexaFluor-488 or −594 conjugated rabbit IgGs (Molecular Probes, Eugene, OR, USA). After washing in PB, sections were mounted on gel-coated slides, coverslipped with anti-fade medium and stored at −20 °C. Controls consisted of omitting the primary antibodies.

Modeling

A single compartment model of Cav3 T-type calcium channels was modified from data originally presented in Engbers et al. [27]. The model had three conductances including Cav3, HCN and a leak current. Cav3 current was based on recordings from rat cerebellar Purkinje cells, and assigned the parameters of Va −30 mV, ka −4.6, λ_{act}

3 msec; V_h: −68 mV, k_h: 6.8, λ_{inact} 12 msec; E_{Ca} = 40 mV; single channel conductance 9 pS. Parameters for I_H were Vh −80 mV, k 3, λ_{act} 200 ms; E_H = −20 mV. E_{leak} = −77 mV. Calcium diffusion was modeled using 10 hemispherical compartments with radii of 20–200 nm (20 nm increments) using a calcium diffusion coefficient of 220 μm^2/ msec. Simulations were run with custom made scripts in Matlab r2016a [27].

Statistical analysis

Statistical analysis was performed using Igor software (Wavemetrics, Lake Oswego, OR, USA) or IBM SPSS Statistics 20 Software (Armonk, NY, USA). The homogeneity of variances was assessed with Levene's and Bartlett's tests. Statistical significance was determined using a paired or unpaired Student's t-test, one-way analysis of variance (ANOVA), or with the non-parametric multiple comparison Dunn-Holland-Wolfe and Mann-Whitney Wilcoxon tests as appropriate. Statistical significance was set at $p < 0.05$ with * $p < 0.05$, ** $p < 0.01$, ns, not significant. The average values are presented either as mean ± SEM or SD as indicated.

Results

Cav3.1 coimmunoprecipitates with CaM in a calcium-dependent manner

We tested the potential for Cav3.1 and CaM to physically associate using coimmunoprecipitation, first performed in the presence of a buffered calcium concentration of 100 nM to simulate resting conditions of intracellular calcium (see Methods). All results for coimmunoprecipitations reflect data from 3 separate experiments. We found that Cav3.1 coimmunoprecipitated with CaM from rat brain lysate (Fig. 1a), indicating that CaM and Cav3.1 channels are part of a protein complex. To better define the underlying molecular determinants, we coexpressed cDNAs for CaM and Cav3.1 channels in tsA-201 cells and again were able to coimmunoprecipitate Cav3.1 and CaM (Fig. 1b). The interaction of CaM with Cav1.2 (L-type) calcium channels is known to involve the C-terminus [12]. To determine the potential involvement of the Cav3.1 C-terminus we coexpressed CaM and a Cav3.1 mutant construct lacking the C-terminus (Cav3.1ΔCT), and found no coimmunoprecipitation (Fig. 1c), indicating that the C-terminus is an essential element in a Cav3.1-CaM channel complex. To better define if the association between Cav3.1 and CaM was direct or indirect we used a binding assay involving purified CaM and internal segments of the Cav3.1 channel. This analysis revealed interactions between CaM and the Cav3.1 C-terminus, a result consistent with a direct protein-protein interaction (Fig. 1d).

It is known that at resting levels of calcium Cav1.2 channels are preassociated with ApoCaM and that an increase in the internal concentration of calcium leads

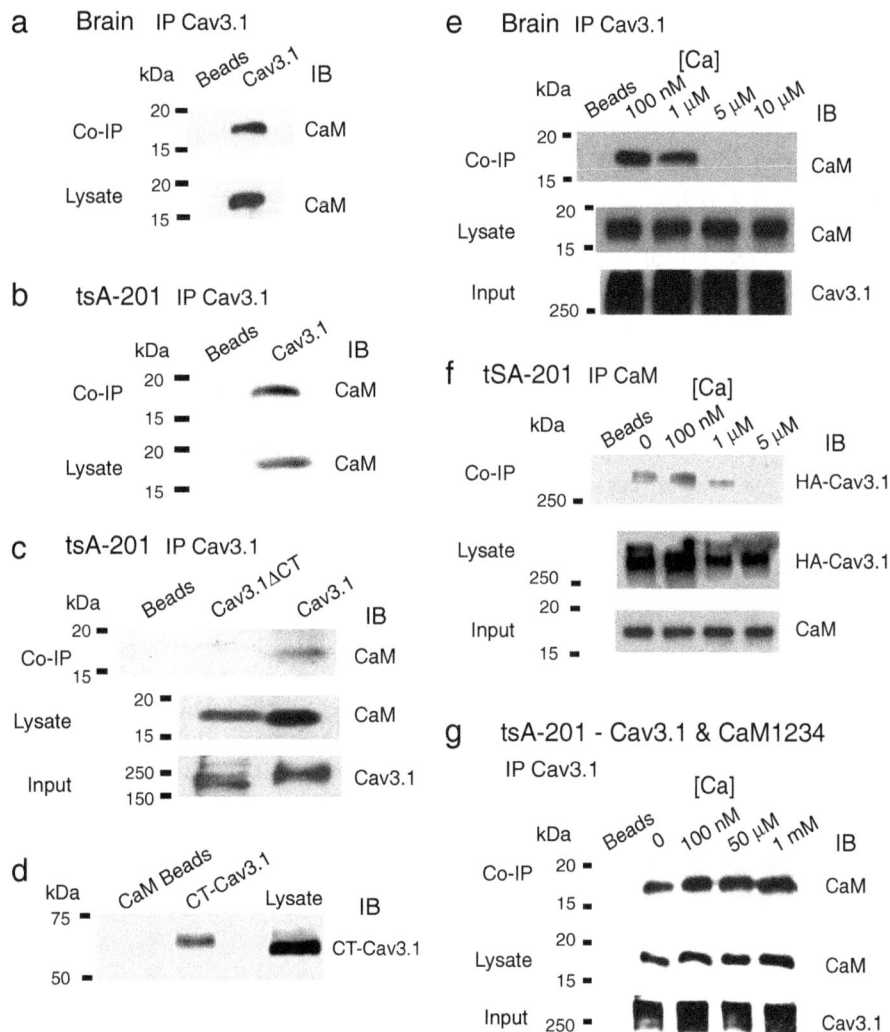

Fig. 1 Cav3.1 channels exhibit a calcium-dependent association with CaM. Biochemical analysis of binding interactions between Cav3.1 and CaM using the indicated antibodies to immunoprecipitate (IP) or immunoblot (IB). The experiments are representative of at least 3 repetitions. Input lanes reflect controls to verify the efficiency of the IP step should IB antibodies fail to reveal co-IPs. **a, b** Cav3.1 channels co-IP with CaM from rat brain lysate (**a**) and homogenates of tsA-201 cells coexpressing Cav3.1 and CaM (**b**). Co-IPs were conducted in the presence of 100 nM calcium. **c** The Cav3.1-CaM co-IP is lost for a construct lacking the Cav3.1 C-terminus (Cav3.1ΔCT). Co-IPs were conducted in the presence of 100 nM calcium. **d** A GST-pull down experiment between the C-terminus of Cav3.1 (CT-Cav3.1) onto CaM beads. GST-CT-Cav3.1 was grown in bacteria, and the GST tag subsequently cleaved off as the GST non specifically bound to CaM beads. CaM beads were instead incubated with purified recombinant Cav3.1 C-terminal peptides in the presence of 100 nM calcium and the sample eluted and run on a Western blot. The blot was probed with an antibody targeting the Cav3.1 C-terminus. **e, f** Co-IP tests conducted in the indicated calcium concentrations reveal that Cav3.1 associates with CaM only below 5 μM calcium. Co-IPs were conducted from rat brain lysates (**e**) or from homogenates of tsA-201 cell expressing HA-Cav3.1 and CaM (**f**). In (**f**) an HA antibody was used to immunoblot the HA-Cav3.1 conjugate. **g** Co-IPs from lysates of tsA-201 cells coexpressing Cav3.1 and the CaM EF-hand mutant CaM1234 reveals that CaM1234 and Cav3.1 interact in the presence of 0–1 mM calcium

to an increase in CaM binding affinity for the channel and a structural rearrangement of the CaM channel complex [13, 28–30]. To test the relative calcium dependence of the association between Cav3.1 and CaM, we immunoprecipitated Cav3.1 in the presence of specific levels of buffered calcium [23]. In this way we could test for potential constitutive binding of CaM in nominally zero calcium, near resting levels of calcium in neurons (100 nM), and in progressively higher but physiological

levels of calcium [31]. CaM coimmunoprecipitated with Cav3.1 at 0 and 100 nM levels of calcium from lysates of either rat brain or tsA-201 cells expressing Cav3.1 and CaM (Fig. 1e, f) (Additional file 1: Figure S1). However, the Cav3.1-CaM coimmunoprecipitation was lost in the presence of 5 μM or greater calcium concentrations in both rat brain and tsA-201 cells (Fig. 1e, f; Additional file 1: Figure S1). To test if the loss of a Cav3.1-CaM association reflects a calcium-dependent interaction with CaM we coexpressed in tsA-201 cells Cav3.1 and the calcium binding deficient CaM mutant CaM1234, and found that CaM1234 coimmunoprecipitated with Cav3.1 for all concentrations of calcium tested (Fig. 1g).

These results indicate that the Cav3.1-CaM association occurs preferentially in low or resting levels of calcium, suggesting that Cav3.1 channels are constitutively associated with CaM. In contrast, there is a calcium-dependent dissociation of CaM from the Cav3.1 channel, revealing a process that is distinctly different from that reported between HVA calcium channels and CaM.

Dynamics of Cav3.1 and CaM interactions revealed by FRET

To test the dynamics of the association between Cav3.1 and CaM in an intact cellular environment, we conducted FRET experiments in tsA-201 cells. For this we created constructs of a Cav3.1 channel with GFP attached to the N-terminus as a donor fluorophore (GFP-Cav3.1) and CaM with the red fluorophore mKate attached to its N-terminus (mKate-CaM) as an acceptor molecule. All tests on FRET were repeated in 3-5 cell culture plates to detect and assess emission from a large set of Regions of Interest (ROI). Control tests established that excitation using a 457 nm confocal laser line produced an emission profile characteristic of GFP in cells expressing only GFP-Cav3.1 (Fig. 2a), or cells expressing GFP-Cav3.1 together with a cDNA encoding the mKate

molecule alone (Fig. 2b). By comparison, excitation at 561 nm resulted in an emission profile for mKate in cells transfected with mKate-CaM (Fig. 2c) as well as in cells expressing the mKate molecule and GFP-Cav3.1 (Fig. 2d). Importantly, coexpressing cDNA for both GFP-Cav3.1 and mKate-CaM allowed a single excitation line at 457 nm to evoke a double peaked emission spectrum indicative of FRET between GFP and mKate (Fig. 2e). We could also detect single cells that exhibited only green fluorescence when excited at 457 nm and no signal upon excitation at 561 nm, revealing that FRET was only observed in cells that expressed both cDNAs (Fig. 2e). These results are important in revealing that the association between Cav3.1 and CaM under resting conditions occurs at distances that are sufficiently close to support FRET.

Given that coimmunoprecipitation experiments indicated a calcium-dependent loss of the Cav3.1-CaM band on western blots (Fig. 1e, f), we used FRET to further test the calcium dependence of the Cav3.1-CaM association in live cells (measured in all cases from defined ROIs pooled from 3 to 6 separate experiments). Under normal conditions, tsA-201 cells display a depolarized membrane potential that leads to a voltage-dependent inactivation of Cav3.1 calcium channels. To allow these cells to rest at a more hyperpolarized potential we coexpressed cDNA for the inward rectifying potassium channel Kir2.1 [32]. Coexpressing Kir2.1 cDNA (0.3 μg) with GFP-Cav3.1 and mKate-CaM promoted a resting potential of −57.2 mV ± 2.8 mV in 1 mM [K]o, and a depolarization to −24.1 mV ± 5.8 mV

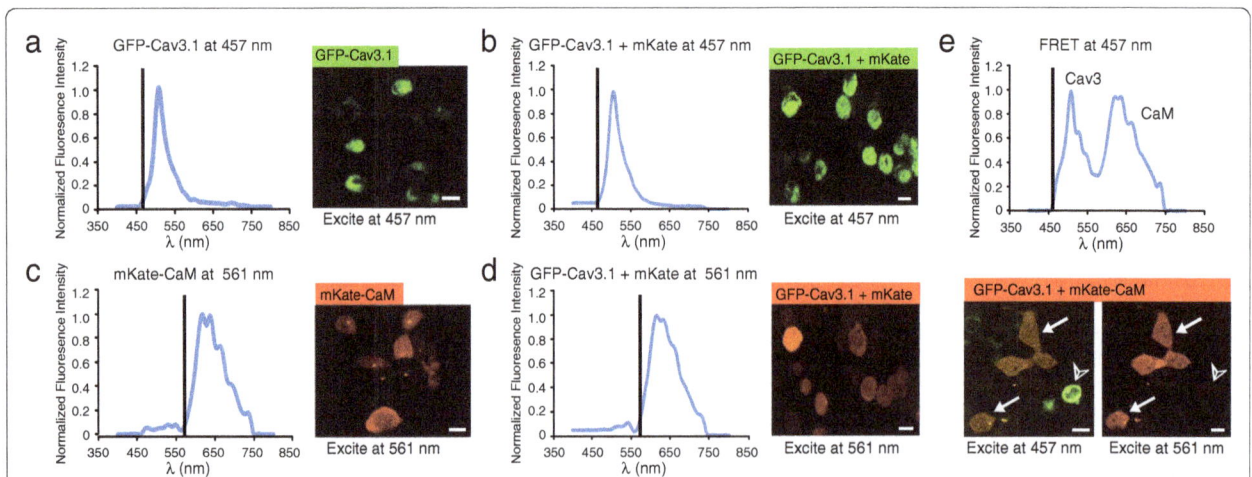

Fig. 2 Cav3.1 and CaM associate at a level that supports FRET. Fluorescence spectral confocal images of tsA-201 cells expressing constructs of GFP-Cav3.1 (donor molecule) or mKate-CaM (acceptor molecule) excited at either 457 nm or 561 nm. Plots show the excitation (*vertical line*) and the associated emission spectrum for each condition. **a, b** Applying excitation at 457 nm to cells expressing either GFP-Cav3.1 alone (**a**) or in conjunction with the mKate acceptor molecule (**b**) results in a typical GFP emission spectrum. **c, d** Applying excitation at 561 nm to cells expressing either mKate-CaM alone (**c**) or in conjunction with GFP-Cav3.1 (**d**) results in a pure mKate emission spectrum. **e** Coexpressing GFP-Cav3.1 and mKate-CaM results in a double emission profile when excitation at 457 nm promotes FRET in a subset of cells (*arrows*). A control image of the same cells excited by a 561 nm laser line at right reveals that a GFP-Cav3.1 expressing cell (*arrowhead*) that does not exhibit FRET failed to express the mKate-CaM construct. All results were derived from at least 3 separate experiments. Scale bars 10 μm

(n = 3) in the presence of 50 mM [K]o. Modeling studies of the degree of calcium accumulation near the mouth of a Cav3 calcium channel pore indicate peak values as high as 50 μM [33]. We repeated these studies for Cav3 current parameters recorded from cerebellar Purkinje cells and previously modeled with respect to activation of BK potassium channels [27]. Here the model reports an increase in predicted [Ca]i to >35 μM at 20 nm distance, and 7 μM at 40 nm distance from the channel pore (Additional file 2: Figure S2) (model parameters as described previously) [27]. This is important in validating the potential for Cav3 channels to provide the calcium necessary to promote CaM dissociation given that the coimmunoprecipitation between Cav3.1 and CaM was lost at calcium concentrations of 5 μM or more (Fig. 1e, f). Using this protocol we used the degree to which 50 mM [K]o evoked a Cav3-mediated calcium influx that could promote a loss of FRET between GFP-Cav3.1 and mKate-CaM.

Controls established that under conditions of 1.0 mM [K]o the mean level of FRET was stable over an initial 11 min period (–0.86 ± 2.63%, n = 11 ROIs) (Fig. 3a). Exposure to high [K]o then decreased FRET within 100 s (–9.1 ± 2.12%, n = 25 ROIs, p = 0.005) (Fig. 3a). To more carefully define the ability of Cav3.1-mediated calcium influx to account for the loss of FRET we substituted Cav3.1 cDNA with a GFP-Cav3.1 pore mutant that fails to conduct calcium (Fig. 3b: Additional file 3: Figure S3), and found that high [K]o exposure failed to reduce FRET under these conditions (4.55 ± 1.55%, n = 8 ROIs, p = 0.24) (Fig. 3b, c). Similarly, the loss of FRET promoted by high [K]o was blocked in the presence of the Cav3 calcium channel blockers TTA-P2 (20 μM) (Fig. 3b, c) (3.20 ± 4.86%, n = 8 ROIs, p = 0.58) or a combination of mibefradil (1 μM) and Ni^{2+} (300 μM) (–1.4 ± 1.87%, n = 25 ROIs, p = 0.99), or by 100 μM BAPTA-AM (1.2 ± 0.77%, n = 21 ROIs, p = 0.99) (Fig. 3c) (Additional file 4: Figure S4a, b). Attempts to repeat FRET measurements in dissociated hippocampal cultures were unfortunately not successful given a very low transfection efficiency of GFP-Cav3.1 and mKate-CaM. This resulted in an expression density that was too low to permit GFP excitation at 457 nm, as required to elicit mKate fluorescence as the acceptor of the GFP-mKate FRET pair. Nevertheless, the results of FRET obtained in tsA-201 cells provide strong evidence that a membrane depolarization that triggers calcium influx through Cav3.1 calcium channels is sufficient to induce a loss of FRET between GFP-Cav3.1 and mKate-CaM. The data are thus consistent with the results of coimmunoprecipitations as they indicate a constitutive association between Cav3.1 and CaM in physiologically low and nominally zero calcium conditions (BAPTA-AM), and a separation of the donor and acceptor proteins when the internal calcium concentration increased.

Cav3.1 channel-mediated calcium influx activates αCaMKII

CaM is known to activate CaMKII to act as a second messenger involved in a wide range of functions that include gene transcription to synaptic plasticity [15, 16, 19]. Given indications that calcium influx through Cav3 channels reduced the association between Cav3.1-CaM detected at rest, we explored the potential for CaM to activate CaMKII in response to a depolarizing stimulus.

Activation of GFP-αCaMKII can be detected as a change in subcellular distribution from a diffuse to an aggregated state [17, 24]. We cotransfected tsA-201 cells with Cav3.1 and/or GFP-αCaMKII to monitor the distribution of αCaMKII at rest and following depolarization-activated Cav3-mediated calcium influx. CaM was coexpressed in all cells along with Kir2.1 to maintain a hyperpolarized resting potential. The distribution of GFP-αCaMKII was quantified by measuring the change in pixel variance of GFP fluorescence detected in cytoplasmic and nuclear compartments using defined ROIs (see Methods). Cells expressing GFP-αCaMKII and Cav3.1 exhibited a predominantly uniform cytoplasmic distribution in low (1.0 mM) [K]o (Fig. 4a, c). Perfusing high (50 mM) [K]o caused the GFP-αCaMKII label to rapidly form aggregates in the cytoplasm within 50 s (p < 0.05 measured at 150 s, n = 3) (Fig. 4a, c). These results are considered physiological given that the diffuse pattern of GFP-αCaMKII distribution was stable in low (1.0 mM) [K]o (Additional file 5: Figure S5a, b) and the GFP-αCaMKII aggregates formed in high [K]o fully reversed to a diffuse distribution within 1 min upon returning to low [K]o (Fig. 4a, b), as earlier reported [17].

Our ability to visualize GFP-αCaMKII aggregate formation during live cell imaging allowed us to test calcium-dependent events that lead to αCaMKII activation. One potential source for voltage-gated calcium entry that triggers αCaMKII activation is that of Cav1.x L-type calcium channels [15]. Although HVA calcium channels were not expressed in these experiments we conducted several controls to ensure that calcium influx was restricted to Cav3.1 channels in tsA-201 cells. First, cells expressing GFP-αCaMKII without Cav3.1 coexpression did not exhibit GFP-αCaMKII aggregation (Fig. 4e, f). Second, expressing a Cav3.1 pore mutant together with GFP-αCaMKII and CaM in tsA-201 cells fully blocked the high [K]o-evoked GFP-αCaMKII aggregation (Additional file 5: Figure S5c, d), despite the ability for the Cav3.1 pore mutant to conduct calcium (Additional file 3: Figure S3). We also confirmed that calcium influx was restricted to Cav3.1 channels by blocking L-type calcium channels with 30 μM Cd^{2+} (Additional files 5 and 6: Figures S5e-h and S6), and by finding that the high [K]o-induced aggregation of GFP-αCaMKII was blocked by 1 μM mibefradil and 300 μM Ni^{2+} (Additional file 5: Figure S5g, h). High [K]o-evoked GFP-αCaMKII aggregation was further blocked

a

Low [K]o

n = 4

High [K]o

n = 5

FmKate / FGFP (% Change)

b

with Cav3.1 pore mutant

n = 5

in TTA-P2

n = 6

FmKate / FGFP (% Change)

Time (sec)

c

High K

Low K

Cav3.1PM   TTA-P2   Mib / Ni   BAPTA

FmKate / FGFP (% Change)

** ** ** * ** **

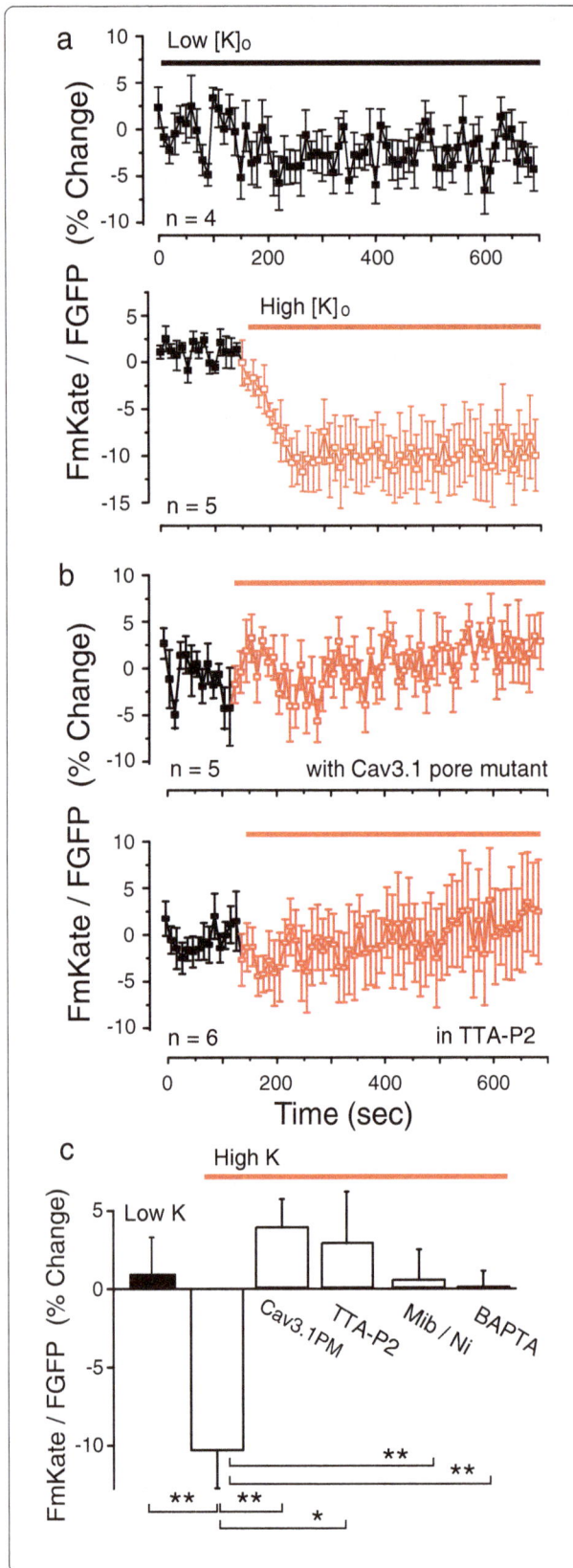

Fig. 3 The Cav3-CaM association is lost upon Cav3 channel-mediated calcium influx. **a, b** Plots of FRET over time in tsA-201 cells coexpressing GFP-Cav3.1, mKate-CaM, and Kir2.1. Cells were exposed to *Low [K]o* (1 mM) or *High [K]o* (50 mM). **a** The FRET signal is stable in low [K]o for 11 min (*upper plot*) but is lost within 50 s upon perfusion of high [K]o (*lower plot*). **b** The decrease in FRET signal in high [K]o is blocked by expressing a Cav3.1 pore mutant that does not conduct calcium (*upper plot*), or 20 μM TTA-P2 (*lower plot*). **c** Bar plots of mean measures of FRET in the indicated conditions derived from 3 to 5 plates with 8–25 ROIs at time point 140 s. Mibefradil (Mib) 1 μM, Ni^{2+} 300 μM, BAPTA-AM 100 μM. Average values are mean ± SEM. * $p < 0.05$, ** $p < 0.01$, ns, not significant

by 0.1 mM BAPTA-AM (Additional file 5: Figure S5i, j), indicating a requirement for an increase in [Ca]i subsequent to Cav3.1 channel activation. Together these data strongly suggest that all voltage-gated calcium influx that lead to αCaMKII activation in these experiments was conducted by Cav3.1 channels.

The dependence of GFP-αCaMKII aggregation upon calcium interactions with CaM was established by a loss of aggregate formation in high [K]o when CaM expression was substituted with the EF hand mutant CaM1234 (Fig. 4g, h). The activation of GFP-αCaMKII is known to require Ca^{2+}/CaM to bind to the autoregulatory domain of αCaMKII to promote autophosphorylation and self-association of the αCaMKII holoenzymes into aggregates [17, 18]. αCaMKII activity and aggregation can also be inhibited through expression of CaMKIIN, a peptide that binds to the catalytic pocket of αCaMKII [24, 34]. To test if the depolarization-induced formation of GFP-αCaMKII aggregates depended on αCaMKII phosphorylation, we expressed GFP-αCaMKII and CaMKIIN in tsA-201 cells coexpressing Cav3.1 and CaM. These tests revealed that CaMKIIN blocked formation of GFP-αCaMKII aggregates following exposure to high [K]o (Fig. 4i, j). The outcome of these tests establish that a membrane depolarization that triggers Cav3 channel-mediated calcium influx activates αCaMKII through a calcium-dependent interaction with CaM and activation of αCaMKII.

Cav3.1 calcium activation of αCaMKII depends on an intact Cav3.1 C-terminus

It is important to define if the CaM that activates αCaMKII reflects CaM dissociated from the Cav3.1 channel or from a presumed cytoplasmic source of CaM subsequent to an increase in internal calcium concentration. These two possibilities were differentiated by simultaneously imaging the effects of high [K]o exposure on GFP-αCaMKII aggregation to that of changes in [Ca]i signaled by X-rhod-1 for cells expressing either Cav3.1 or a Cav3.1ΔCT construct that lacked the C-terminus and thus the CaM binding site (cf. Fig. 1c). Importantly, the Cav3.1ΔCT construct was confirmed to form functional T-type calcium channels

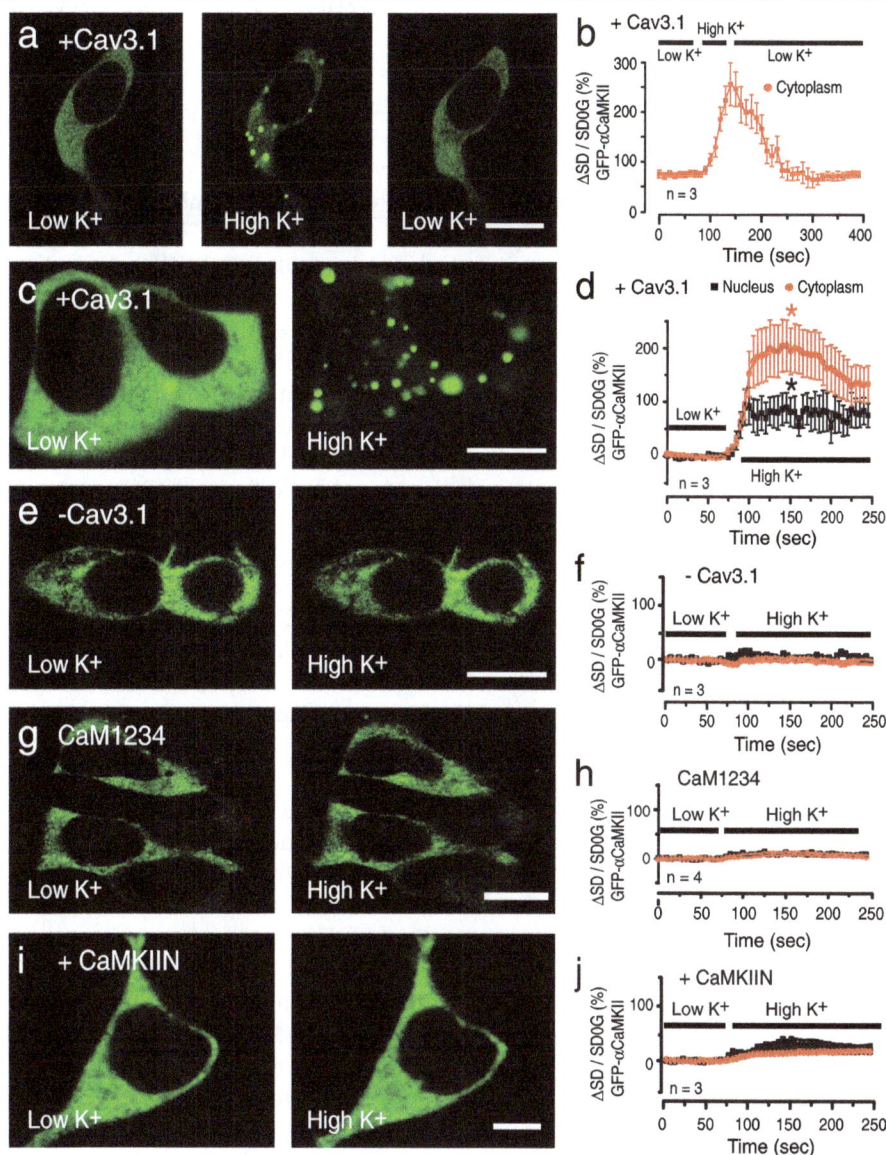

Fig. 4 Cav3 channel-mediated calcium influx leads to αCaMKII aggregation. tsA-201 cells are cotransfected with GFP-αCaMKII, CaM, Cav3.1, and Kir2.1 and exposed to low [K]o (1.0 mM) or high [K]o (50 mM). Plots of the mean pixel variance of GFP-αCaMKII fluorescence in ROIs in the cytoplasm and nuclear regions shown at *right*. **a, b** In cells coexpressing Cav3.1 GFP-αCaMKII exhibits a diffuse cytoplasmic distribution in low [K]o that changes to aggregates in high [K]o, a pattern that is fully reversible upon returning to low [K]o. **c, d** Magnified images of the distribution of GFP-αCaMKII in low [K]o and after perfusing high [K]o, with plots indicating a restriction of clusters primarily to cytoplasm and peri-nuclear regions. **e-i** Formation of GFP-αCaMKII aggregates induced by high [K]o is prevented in cells lacking Cav3.1 (**e, f**), and blocked by substitution of CaM with CaM1234 (**g, h**), or by coexpression of CaMKIIN (0.3 μg) as an inhibitor of αCaMKII phosphorylation (**i, j**). Values are mean ± SD derived from $n = 3$ plates with 12–29 ROIs. Scale bars 10 μm.* $p < 0.05$

(Additional file 7: Figure S7) that supported accumulation of intracellular calcium upon exposure to high [K]o (Fig. 5). Here we found that high [K]o-induced GFP-αCaMKII aggregation was blocked in cells expressing Cav3.1ΔCT but not Cav3.1, despite an equivalent increase in calcium fluorescence of X-rhod-1 (Fig. 5). These results are important in establishing that αCaMKII activation is mediated by Cav3.1-dependent calcium entry that requires the presence of a channel region capable of associating with CaM.

Cav3 calcium influx triggers αCaMKII phosphorylation in neurons

To determine if the Cav3.1-CaM-αCaMKII signaling cascade could be detected in neuronal populations we transiently transfected GFP-αCaMKII and Cav3.1 into dissociated cultures of hippocampal neurons. This test revealed a similar diffuse cytoplasmic distribution of GFP-αCaMKII fluorescence as found for tsA-201 cells in low levels of [K]o (Fig. 6a, b). But upon perfusion of high

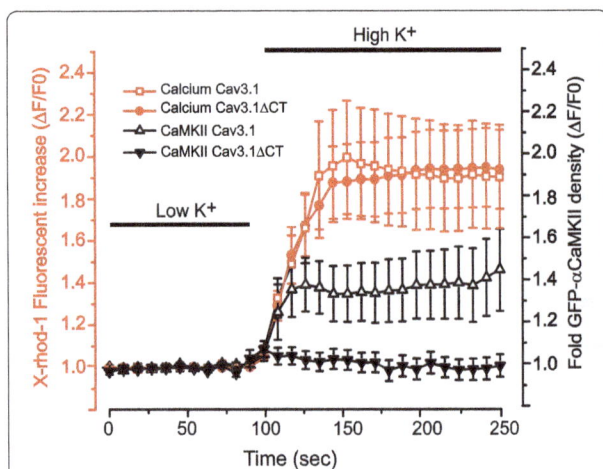

Fig. 5 Cav3.1-mediated activation of αCaMKII depends on an intact Cav3.1 C-terminus. tsA-201 cells are transfected with Cav3.1 or a Cav3.1 mutant lacking the C-terminus (Cav3.1ΔCT) to remove a site for preassociation of CaM with the Cav3.1 channel and preloaded with 2 μM X-rhod-1 to detect changes in [Ca]i. Cells are maintained at rest in low [K]o (1 mM) or exposed to 10 min of high [K]o (50 mM), with all medium containing 30 μM Cd^{2+} to block HVA calcium channels. The extent and timecourse of a shift in GFP-αCaMKII distribution from diffuse to aggregates in the cytoplasm is compared to that of a change in fluorescent intensity of X-rhod-1 relative to the mean of control baseline (ΔF/F0). High [K]o increased [Ca]i to an equivalent relative level in cells expressing either Cav3.1 or Cav3.1ΔCT but GFP-αCaMKII aggregation is blocked in cells expressing the Cav3.1ΔCT mutant. The distribution of GFP-αCaMKII is measured as density for at least 25–34 ROIs from 4 to 5 plates. Values are mean ± SEM derived from n = 4–5 plates with 25–34 ROIs

[K]o (50 mM) there was a substantial increase in the number of GFP-αCaMKII aggregates in the cytoplasm within 1.5 min (Fig. 6c, d). The aggregation of GFP-αCaMKII in high [K]o was again blocked in the presence 1 μM mibefradil/300 μM Ni^{2+} (Fig. 6e, f).

The above results are important in indicating that Cav3.1-mediated calcium influx can mediate aggregation of GFP-αCaMKII in neurons, a process that tests in tsA-201 cells indicated should involve αCaMKII phosphorylation. To visualize the activation of phosphorylated αCaMKII we used immunolabel detection for pαCaMKII in both hippocampal cell cultures and cerebellar tissue slices exposed to 10 min of high [K]o (50 mM) medium in the presence or absence of mibefradil/Ni^{2+} (Fig. 7) (Additional file 8: Figure S8). Calcium influx was restricted to Cav3 calcium channels by conducting tests in medium containing 30 μM Cd^{2+}, 10 μM DNQX, 25 μM or 100 μM DL-AP5, and 1 μM TTX, and tissues fixed for immunocytochemistry within 10 min after the high [K]o treatment. Under resting conditions of 1 mM [K]o hippocampal cell cultures and cerebellar tissue slices exhibited little if any detectable immunolabel for pαCaMKII (Fig. 7a–g). When exposed to high [K]o for 10 min hippocampal cells exhibited an increase in pαCaMKII

immunolabel that highlighted cell somata and surrounding processes (Fig. 7b, g). Exposure of cerebellar tissue slices to high [K]o revealed an increase in pαCaMKII labeling in Purkinje cell bodies (Fig. 7e, g). The high [K]o-induced increase in pαCaMKII was again blocked in the presence of 1 μM mibefradil and 300 μM Ni^{2+} for both hippocampal cultures and cerebellar tissue slices (Fig. 7c, f, g). We also found a significantly reduced level of pαCaMKII immunolabel if hippocampal cultures were pre-exposed to a peptide inhibitor specific for pαCaMKII (AIP 10 μM; n 3–4, $p < 0.01$) (Additional file 8: Figure S8).

To complement the immunolabeling tests we further examined pαCaMKII protein density in cerebellar tissue slices exposed to low [K]o or high [K]o in the presence or absence of mibefradil/Ni^{2+}-containing medium. Tissue was lysed in a medium containing the same final solution and prepared for Western blot analysis. In each case a band for pαCaMKII was detected, but the ratio of band densities (pαCaMKII/αCaMKII) was significantly greater for tissue exposed to high [K]o (n = 3; $p < 0.05$), a difference that was not present in tissues preexposed to mibefradil/Ni^{2+} (Fig. 7h).

Discussion

CaM is known to establish an association with HVA calcium channels to provide feedback regulation of channel activity or downstream activation of CaMKII. The current study is important in showing that the Cav3.1 calcium channel exhibits a novel calcium-dependent interaction with CaM that also triggers CaM-dependent activation and phosphorylation of αCaMKII. Moreover, Cav3-mediated interactions can be detected in both tsA-201 cells as well as hippocampal cerebellar neurons.

CaM association with Cav3.1 channels

The complexity and wealth of interactions that define CaM binding and modulation of HVA calcium channels have emerged over many years of work. An HVA calcium channel (e.g. Cav1.x) generally forms a pre-association with calcium free ApoCam at resting levels of internal calcium concentration, and a calcium-dependent increase in CaM binding affinity [13, 28–30]. The assays conducted here reveal that Cav3.1 channels exhibit a constitutive association with ApoCam at resting levels of calcium. The occurrence of FRET between Cav3.1 and CaM at resting levels of internal calcium confirms a close protein-protein interaction given that FRET requires two molecules to be positioned within 10–100 Å distance. CaM binding to HVA calcium channels involves at least an IQ domain on the calcium channel C-terminus, as well as an NSCaTE domain on the N-terminus [13, 35–40]. The amino acid sequence of the Cav3.1 C-terminus does not appear to present a clear IQ domain as defined for HVA channels,

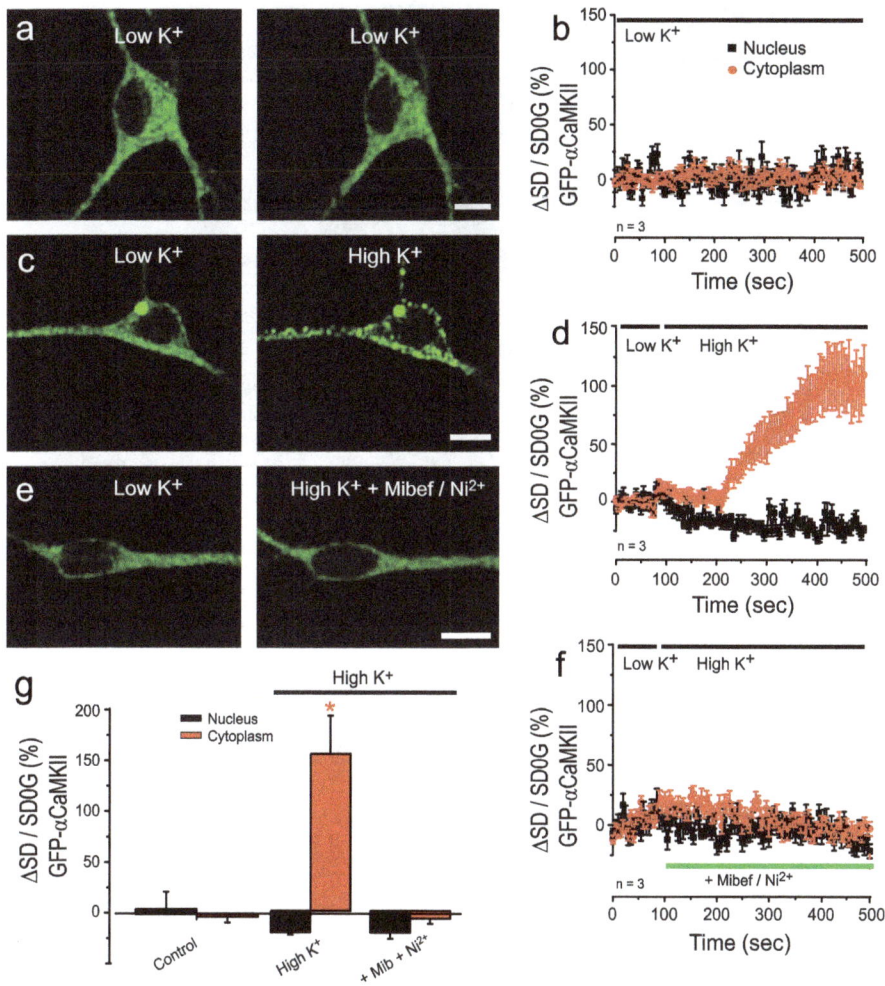

Fig. 6 GFP-αCaMKII clustering in transfected neurons. Neurons are cotransfected with GFP-αCaMKII and Cav3.1 (unlabeled) and exposed to low [K]o (1.0 mM) or high [K]o (50 mM). **a-d** A diffuse distribution of αCaMKII-GFP is stable in low [K]o over time (**a, b**), with high [K]o promoting aggregation of GFP-αCaMKII (**c, d**). **e, f** Formation of GFP-αCaMKII aggregates induced by high [K]o is blocked in the presence of mibefradil (1 μM) and Ni^{2+} (300 μM). **g** Bar plots of the mean pixel variance of GFP-αCaMKII fluorescence for the tests in (**a-f**). Values are mean ± SD derived from $n = 3$ plates with 5–10 ROIs. Scale bars 10 μm.* $p < 0.05$

nor does it exhibit a canonical CaM binding motif. Our work establishes that the Cav3.1 C-terminus is required to detect a coimmunoprecipitation between CaM and Cav3.1, with GST pull down assays supporting a direct interaction between CaM and the C-terminal region. The precise amino acid residues on the C-terminus responsible for the Cav3.1-CaM interaction remain to be determined.

The Cav3.1-CaM association is further distinguished from CaM-HVA calcium channel interactions in that membrane depolarization promotes a loss of FRET between Cav3.1 and CaM. We note that a loss of FRET could reflect a repositioning of CaM on the Cav3.1 channel, however, the loss of coIP between Cav3.1 and CaM at [Ca] greater than 1 μM indicates a physical dissociation. Moreover, Cav3.1 calcium influx proves to be sufficient to promote Cav3.1-CaM dissociation, as established

by preventing the depolarization-induced loss of FRET using Cav3 calcium channel blockers or by expressing a non calcium-conducting Cav3.1 channel pore mutant. These findings are important in revealing a dynamic interaction between Cav3.1 and CaM that is essentially opposite to that of HVA calcium channels.

αCaMKII activation

Calcium influx can activate multiple forms of CaMKII that translocate to perinuclear compartments [15, 18, 41–47], with the current work addressing αCaMKII. Activation of αCaMKII has been traced to calcium influx via specific HVA calcium channels in different cell types [15, 17, 18, 24, 44]. The current study is the first to reveal an interaction between Cav3.1 calcium influx and subsequent activation of αCaMKII. An important question is the extent to which αCaMKII is activated specifically by CaM

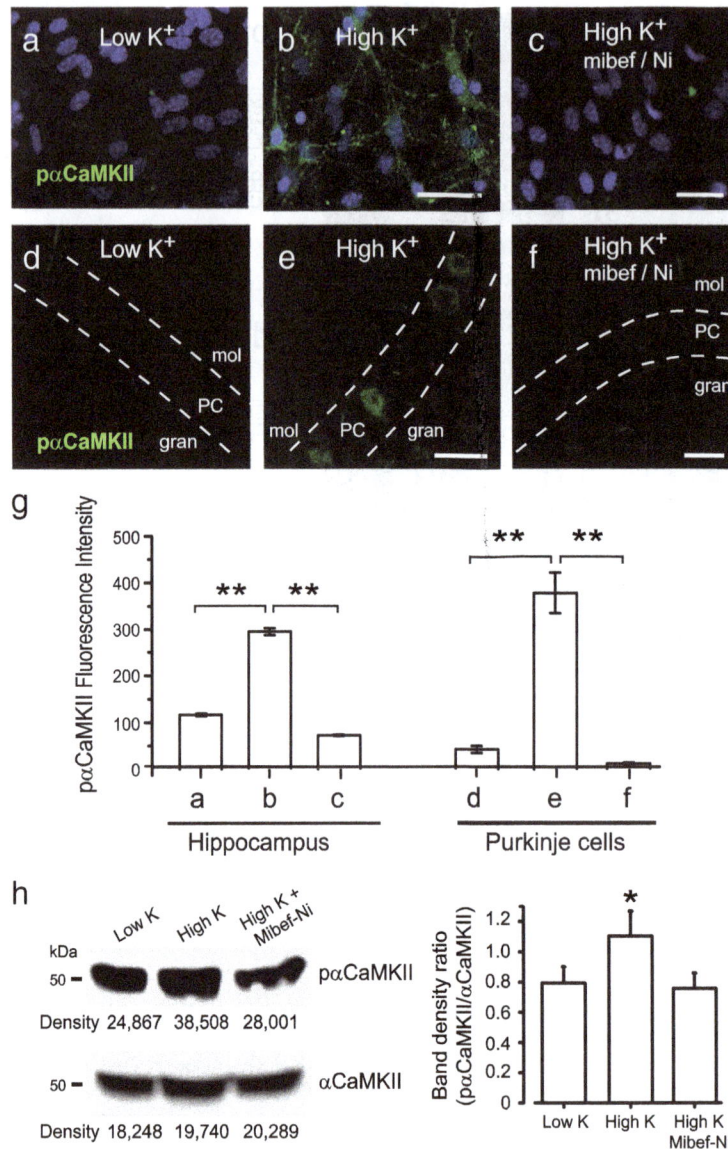

Fig. 7 Cav3 calcium influx triggers αCaMKII phosphorylation in neurons. **a-f** Confocal images of cultured mouse hippocampal cells (**a-c**), and rat cerebellar tissue slices (**d-f**). Activated αCaMKII is identified by using a phospho-αCaMKII (pαCaMKII) antibody with additional DAPI label for nuclear staining in (**a-c**). Each preparation was maintained at rest in low [K]o (1 mM) or exposed to 10 min of high [K]o (50 mM) prior to fixation within 10 min of the end of high [K]o exposure. All results were derived from at least 3 separate experiments. In all neuronal cell tests calcium influx is restricted to Cav3 channels by maintaining cells in 30 μM Cd^{2+}, 10 μM DNQX, 25 μM DL-AP5, and 1 μM TTX. **a, b** In hippocampal cell cultures high [K]o induces pαCaMKII labeling. **d, e** In cerebellar tissue slices high [K]o induces pαCaMKII labeling in Purkinje cell bodies. **c, f** High [K]o-induced labeling for pαCaMKII is blocked in both hippocampus (**c**) and cerebellum (**f**) in the presence of Cav3 channel blockers 1 μM mibefradil and 300 μM Ni^{2+}. *Dashed lines* in (**d-f**) depict the boundaries of the Purkinje cell body layer. **g** Bar plots of the mean intensity of pαCaMKII fluorescence in hippocampal cell cultures and Purkinje cells in cerebellar tissue slices for panels (**a-f**) were quantified using ImageTrak software. Scale bars 10 μm. Values are mean ± SEM derived from n = 3–4 coverslips with 30–130 ROIs. **h** Western blot analysis to test the relative density of αCaMKII and p-αCaMKII labeling in cerebellar slice lysates in low or high [K]o, with mean bar plots of the band density ratio (pαCaMKII/αCaMKII) (Image J software). The high [K]o lysate has a higher band density than either low [K]o or high [K]o in the presence of mibefradil and Ni^{2+}. Values are mean ± SEM derived from 3 separate experiments. * $p < 0.05$;** $p < 0.01$. PC, Purkinje cell layer; mol, molecular layer; gran, granule cell layer

molecules that are preassociated with Cav3.1 under resting conditions and dissociate upon channel opening, as opposed to CaM activated in the cytoplasm subsequent to a Cav3.1-mediated increase in [Ca]i. A role for CaM that dissociates from the Cav3.1 channel was supported by our finding that expression of a Cav3.1 mutant lacking the C-terminus (removing the CaM binding site) blocked depolarization-induced GFP-αCaMKII aggregation despite an equivalent elevation of [Ca]i as found with intact Cav3.1 channels (Fig. 5).

Others have shown that pH can augment calcium-dependent clustering of GFP-αCaMKII [17] so it is possible that this could contribute to our effects. But the current study establishes that calcium influx through the Cav3 channel class can initiate the steps that lead to an aggregation of GFP-αCaMKII that is fully reversible.

In neurons, synaptic stimulation induces long term changes in synaptic efficacy that involves CaMKII activation and translocation to perinuclear or synaptic regions [17, 46, 48, 49]. In this regard we found that exposure to high [K]o invoked a substantial increase in the number of GFP-αCaMKII aggregates in the cytoplasm of hippocampal neuronal cultures, and of pαCaMKII labeling in processes of cultured hippocampal neurons and in cerebellar Purkinje cell bodies. Moreover, all these effects were blocked by exposure to Cav3 channel blockers. These data verify that Cav3 channel-triggered activation of αCaMKII occurs in neuronal circuits known to exhibit long-term plasticity of synaptic function, including Cav3-mediated forms of LTP in cerebellar neurons [50, 51].

Thus, the sequence of events identified for Cav3.1-CaM-αCaMKII interactions differs from that of HVA calcium channels, revealing separate pathways to activate αCaMKII. A Cav3-initiated process is also distinct in that Cav3.1 channels can be activated over a larger voltage range than HVA calcium channels. Cav3.1-mediated activation αCaMKII may then be prominent in certain cell types or brain regions where these channels regulate cell excitability at even subthreshold potentials. However, we note that αCaMKII activation by way of Cav3.1 or HVA channel calcium influx is not mutually exclusive. Rather, we interpret these results as evidence that Cav3 calcium influx is sufficient to activate αCaMKII through a novel interaction with CaM, providing a means to complement the role for HVA calcium channels in triggering αCaMKII activation.

Additional files

Additional file 1: Figure S1. Cav3.1 channels exhibit a calcium-dependent association with CaM. **a**, **b**. Tests for coimmunoprecipitation between Cav3.1 channels and CaM from rat brain lysate (**a**) or homogenates of tsA-201 cells coexpressing Cav3.1 and CaM (**b**) in the presence of the indicated buffered levels of calcium. Cav3.1 coimmunoprecipitates with CaM in 0 and 100 nM calcium but not at 50 μM or 1 mM calcium. All results were derived from at least 3 separate experiments.

Additional file 2: Figure S2. A model of Cav3.1 channel conductance and increase in [Ca]. **a**. Plots of the voltage-dependence for activation (*blue line*) and inactivation (*orange line*) derived from steady-state voltage commands from whole-cell recordings of Cav3 current in Purkinje cells (modified from Engber et al. [27]. **b**. Calculated changes in internal calcium concentrations for a hemispherical compartment around the calcium source for a Cav3 channel with a single channel conductance of 9 pS. Voltage commands are applied from a holding potential of −75 mV in 10 mV steps to +10 mV and calcium internal concentration changes plotted for distances of 20 nm and 40 nm distance from a Cav3 channel,

leading to a peak calcium concentration of 36 μM (20 nm) and 7 μM (40 nm) for a step to − 20 mV.

Additional file 3: Figure S3. Cav3.1 channel pore mutant constructs. A single amino acid mutation of Cav3.1 creates a pore mutant that does not conduct calcium current. Shown are representative recordings and the associated I-V plot of a transient low voltage-activated current measured in the Cav3.1 mutant expressed in tsA-201 cells. Superimposed recordings and plot illustrate the records obtained in normal bathing medium and following substitution of sodium in the bathing medium by 130 NMDG.

Additional file 4: Figure S4. Block of high [K]o-mediated loss of GFP-Cav3.1 - mKate-CaM FRET. Plots of the FRET signal over time in tsA-201 cells coexpressing GFP-Cav3.1 and mKate-CaM. Values are normalized to the mean value of all fluorescence measurements in the time period. **a**, **b**. Cells were exposed to Low [K]o (1 mM) or High [K]o (50 mM). A loss of FRET encountered upon exposure to high [K]o is prevented by the Cav3 channel blockers 1 μM mibefradil and 300 μM Ni^{2+} (**a**) and in the presence of 0.1 mM BAPTA-AM (**b**). Average values are mean ± SEM.

Additional file 5: Figure S5. Activation of αCaMKII depends on Cav3.1 calcium influx and an increase in [Ca]i. The distribution of GFP-αCaMKII tested in tsA-201 cells in low [K]o (1 mM) or high [K]o (50 mM) and indicated reagents. All cells are cotransfected with CaM and Kir2.1. Plots indicate mean pixel variance of fluorescence in ROIs in cytoplasm and nuclear regions. **a**, **b**. A diffuse distribution of αCaMKII-GFP is stable in low [K]o over time. **c-h**. The aggregation of αCaMKII-GFP depends on Cav3.1-mediated calcium influx, as shown when a Cav3.1 pore mutant (Cav3.1 PM) that does not conduct calcium is expressed (**c**, **d**), the ability for high [K]o to promote aggregation in the presence of 30 μM Cd^{2+}(**e**, **f**) but not in the presence of mibefradil (1 μM) and Ni^{2+} (300 μM) (**g**, **h**). **i**, **j**. The dependence of αCaMKII-GFP aggregation induced by high [K]o exposure also depends on an increase in [Ca]i in being blocked by pre-exposure to BAPTA-AM (0.1 mM). Values are mean ± SD at 250 s derived from 3 to 4 plates with 14–19 ROIs. Scale bars 10 μm.

Additional file 6: Figure S6. Selective block of Cav1 L-type calcium channels by external Cd^{2+}. **a**, **b**. Shown are representative recordings of calcium current evoked in tsA-201 cells expressing either the Cav1.2 or Cav1.3 calcium channel isoforms (**a**) or Cav3.1 calcium channels (**b**), with associated mean I-V plots shown below. Perfusing 30 μM Cd^{2+} blocks both Cav1.2 and Cav1.3 channel isoforms (**a**) but not Cav3.1 (**b**). For Ca$_V$1.2 channel expression included 2 μg each of human- α1C-PMT2, α2δ1-PMT2 and β1B-PMT2. For Ca$_V$1.3 channel expression 2 μg each of human- α1D-GFP^{37-}, α2δ1-pcDNA and β1B-pcDNA was used. Ca$_V$1.2 and Ca$_V$1.3 expressing cells were co-transfected with 100 ng eGFPN1 for identification of transfected fluorescence cells. Average values are mean ± SEM.

Additional file 7: Figure S7. Calcium conductance of Cav3.1 channel construct lacking the C-terminus. Representative recordings and I-V plot of T-type calcium current for a Cav3.1 channel construct lacking the C terminal region (Cav3.1ΔC), removing a key site for CaM association. Average values are mean ± SEM.

Additional file 8: Figure S8. Cav3-mediated activation of αCaMKII. Bar plots of the mean fluorescence intensity of pαCaMKII in cultured hippocampal cells in low [K]o (1 mM) and following exposure to 10 min of high [K]o (50 mM) prior to fixation within 10 min of the end of high [K]o exposure. Calcium influx is restricted to Cav3 channels by maintaining cells in 30 μM Cd^{2+}, 10 μM DNQX, 100 μM DL-AP5, and 1 μM TTX. Labeling for pαCaMKII in the cytoplasm increases in high [K]o that is reduced by a peptide inhibitor specific for pαCaMKII (AIP 10 μM). Fluorescence intensity was quantified in ImageTrak software (see Methods). Values are mean ± SEM derived from $n = 3$–4 cover slips from at least 3 separate experiments with 29 ROIs. ** $p < 0.01$.

Acknowledgments

We gratefully acknowledge M. Kruskic, L. Chen, S. Hameed, J. Hameed, S. Srinivasan, W. Chen, and F. Hiess for expert technical assistance, and R. Rehak for early experimental work. This manuscript is dedicated to the memory of Dr. Shahid Hameed who left a long lasting impact on the Zamponi, Turner, and Stys labs.

Funding
This work was supported by grants from the Canadian Institutes of Health Research (R.W.T., G.W.Z., P.K.S.) and National Science and Engineering Research Council (G.W.Z.). Trainee support was provided by an Alberta Innovates - Health Solutions (AI-HS) studentship (A.P.R., B.A.S) and Postdoctoral Fellowship (F-X. Z.), and a Queen EII Scholarship (A.P.R). R.W.T., P.K.S. and G.W.Z. are AI-HS Scientists and P.K.S. and G.W.Z. hold Canada Research Chairs.

Authors' contributions
Protein biochemical and immunocytochemical tests were conducted by HA and APR, imaging by HA and IM, tissue slice experiments by APR and HA, and modeling by JDTE. cDNA constructs were prepared by HA, FZ, and BAS, PKS consulted on imaging experiments, provided reagents, and wrote the ImageTrak software, HA, IM, RWT, GWZ wrote the manuscript. RWT and GWZ supervised the study. All authors read and approved the final manuscript.

Competing interests
The authors declare that they have no competing interests.

Author details
[1]Department of Cell Biology and Anatomy, University of Calgary, Calgary, AB T2N 4N1, Canada. [2]Department of Clinical Neurosciences, University of Calgary, Calgary, AB T2N 4N1, Canada. [3]Department of Physiology and Pharmacology, University of Calgary, Calgary, AB T2N 4N1, Canada. [4]Hotchkiss Brain Institute, University of Calgary, Calgary, AB T2N 4N1, Canada. [5]Alberta Children's Hospital Research Institute, Cumming School of Medicine, University of Calgary, Calgary, AB T2N 4N1, Canada. [6]HRIC 1AA14, University of Calgary, 3330 Hospital Dr. N.W, Calgary, AB T2N 4N1, Canada.

References
1. Simms BA, Zamponi GW. Neuronal voltage-gated calcium channels: structure, function, and dysfunction. Neuron. 2014;82(1):24–45.
2. Lambert RC, Bessaih T, Crunelli V, Leresche N. The many faces of T-type calcium channels. Pflugers Arch. 2014;466(3):415–23.
3. Cribbs L. T-type calcium channel expression and function in the diseased heart. Channels (Austin). 2010;4(6):447–52.
4. Mesirca P, Torrente AG, Mangoni ME. Functional role of voltage gated Ca(2 +) channels in heart automaticity. Front Physiol. 2015;6:19.
5. Weiss N, Hameed S, Fernandez-Fernandez JM, Fablet K, Karmazinova M, Poillot C, Proft J, Chen L, Bidaud I, Monteil A, et al. A Ca(v)3.2/syntaxin-1A signaling complex controls T-type channel activity and low-threshold exocytosis. J Biol Chem. 2012;287(4):2810–8.
6. Jacus MO, Uebele VN, Renger JJ, Todorovic SM. Presynaptic Cav3.2 channels regulate excitatory neurotransmission in nociceptive dorsal horn neurons. J Neurosci. 2012;32(27):9374–82.
7. Garcia-Caballero A, Gadotti VM, Stemkowski P, Weiss N, Souza IA, Hodgkinson V, Bladen C, Chen L, Hamid J, Pizzoccaro A, et al. The deubiquitinating enzyme USP5 modulates neuropathic and inflammatory pain by enhancing Cav3.2 channel activity. Neuron. 2014;83(5):1144–58.
8. Carabelli V, Marcantoni A, Comunanza V, de Luca A, Diaz J, Borges R, Carbone E. Chronic hypoxia up-regulates alpha1H T-type channels and low-threshold catecholamine secretion in rat chromaffin cells. J Physiol. 2007; 584(Pt 1):149–65.
9. Coutelier M, Blesneac I, Monteil A, Monin ML, Ando K, Mundwiller E, Brusco A, Le Ber I, Anheim M, Castrioto A, et al. A recurrent mutation in CACNA1G alters Cav3.1 T-type Calcium-Channel conduction and causes autosomal-dominant cerebellar ataxia. Am J Hum Genet. 2015;97(5):726–37.
10. Morino H, Matsuda Y, Muguruma K, Miyamoto R, Ohsawa R, Ohtake T, Otobe R, Watanabe M, Maruyama H, Hashimoto K, et al. A mutation in the low voltage-gated calcium channel CACNA1G alters the physiological properties of the channel, causing spinocerebellar ataxia. Mol Brain. 2015;8:89.
11. Zamponi GW. Targeting voltage-gated calcium channels in neurological and psychiatric diseases. Nat Rev Drug Discov. 2016;15(1):19–34.
12. Ben-Johny M, Yue DT. Calmodulin regulation (calmodulation) of voltage-gated calcium channels. J Gen Physiol. 2014;143(6):679–92.
13. Pitt GS, Zuhlke RD, Hudmon A, Schulman H, Reuter H, Tsien RW. Molecular basis of calmodulin tethering and Ca2+–dependent inactivation of L-type Ca2+ channels. J Biol Chem. 2001;276(33):30794–802.
14. Hudmon A, Schulman H, Kim J, Maltez JM, Tsien RW, Pitt GS. CaMKII tethers to L-type Ca2+ channels, establishing a local and dedicated integrator of Ca2+ signals for facilitation. J Cell Biol. 2005;171(3):537–47.
15. Wheeler DG, Barrett CF, Groth RD, Safa P, Tsien RW. CaMKII locally encodes L-type channel activity to signal to nuclear CREB in excitation-transcription coupling. J Cell Biol. 2008;183(5):849–63.
16. Lisman J, Yasuda R, Raghavachari S. Mechanisms of CaMKII action in long-term potentiation. Nat Rev Neurosci. 2012;13(3):169–82.
17. Hudmon A, Lebel E, Roy H, Sik A, Schulman H, Waxham MN, De Koninck P. A mechanism for Ca2+/calmodulin-dependent protein kinase II clustering at synaptic and nonsynaptic sites based on self-association. J Neurosci. 2005; 25(30):6971–83.
18. Hudmon A, Schulman H. Neuronal CA2+/calmodulin-dependent protein kinase II: the role of structure and autoregulation in cellular function. Annu Rev Biochem. 2002;71:473–510.
19. Catterall WA, Leal K, Nanou E. Calcium channels and short-term synaptic plasticity. J Biol Chem. 2013;288(15):10742–9.
20. Lee JH, Daud AN, Cribbs LL, Lacerda AE, Pereverzev A, Klockner U, Schneider T, Perez-Reyes E. Cloning and expression of a novel member of the low voltage-activated T-type calcium channel family. J Neurosci. 1999;19(6):1912–21.
21. Zamponi GW. Calmodulin lobotomized: novel insights into calcium regulation of voltage-gated calcium channels. Neuron. 2003;39(6):879–81.
22. McKay BE, McRory JE, Molineux ML, Hamid J, Snutch TP, Zamponi GW, Turner RW. Ca(V)3 T-type calcium channel isoforms differentially distribute to somatic and dendritic compartments in rat central neurons. Eur J Neurosci. 2006;24(9):2581–94.
23. Lai MM, Hong JJ, Ruggiero AM, Burnett PE, Slepnev VI, De Camilli P, Snyder SH. The calcineurin-dynamin 1 complex as a calcium sensor for synaptic vesicle endocytosis. J Biol Chem. 1999;274(37):25963–6.
24. Flynn R, Labrie-Dion E, Bernier N, Colicos MA, De Koninck P, Zamponi GW. Activity-dependent subcellular cotrafficking of the small GTPase Rem2 and Ca2+/CaM-dependent protein kinase IIalpha. PLoS One. 2012;7(7):e41185.
25. Khosravani H, Altier C, Simms B, Hamming KS, Snutch TP, Mezeyova J, McRory JE, Zamponi GW. Gating effects of mutations in the Cav3.2 T-type calcium channel associated with childhood absence epilepsy. J Biol Chem. 2004;279(11):9681–4.
26. Christensen PC, Welch NC, Brideau C, Stys PK. Functional ionotropic glutamate receptors on peripheral axons and myelin. Muscle Nerve. 2016;54(3):451–9.
27. Engbers JD, Zamponi GW, Turner RW. Modeling interactions between voltage-gated Ca (2+) channels and KCa1.1 channels. Channels (Austin). 2013;7(6):524–9.
28. Ben Johny M, Yang PS, Bazzazi H, Yue DT. Dynamic switching of calmodulin interactions underlies Ca2+ regulation of CaV1.3 channels. Nat Commun. 2013;4:1717.
29. Erickson MG, Alseikhan BA, Peterson BZ, Yue DT. Preassociation of calmodulin with voltage-gated Ca(2+) channels revealed by FRET in single living cells. Neuron. 2001;31(6):973–85.
30. Erickson MG, Liang H, Mori MX, Yue DT. FRET two-hybrid mapping reveals function and location of L-type Ca2+ channel CaM preassociation. Neuron. 2003;39(1):97–107.
31. Augustine GJ, Santamaria F, Tanaka K. Local calcium signaling in neurons. Neuron. 2003;40(2):331–46.
32. Choi J, Park JH, Kwon OY, Kim S, Chung JH, Lim DS, Kim KS, Rhim H, Han YS. T-type calcium channel trigger p21ras signaling pathway to ERK in Cav3. 1-expressed HEK293 cells. Brain Res. 2005;1054(1):22–9.
33. Lacinova L, Kurejova M, Klugbauer N, Hofmann F. Gating of the expressed T-type Cav3.1 calcium channels is modulated by Ca2+. Acta Physiol (Oxf). 2006;186(4):249–60.
34. Vest RS, Davies KD, O'Leary H, Port JD, Bayer KU. Dual mechanism of a natural CaMKII inhibitor. Mol Biol Cell. 2007;18(12):5024–33.
35. Pate P, Mochca-Morales J, Wu Y, Zhang JZ, Rodney GG, Serysheva II, Williams BY, Anderson ME, Hamilton SL. Determinants for calmodulin binding on voltage-dependent Ca2+ channels. J Biol Chem. 2000;275(50):39786–92.
36. Tang W, Halling DB, Black DJ, Pate P, Zhang JZ, Pedersen S, Altschuld RA,

Hamilton SL. Apocalmodulin and Ca2+ calmodulin-binding sites on the CaV1.2 channel. Biophys J. 2003;85(3):1538–47.

37. Dick IE, Tadross MR, Liang H, Tay LH, Yang W, Yue DT. A modular switch for spatial Ca2+ selectivity in the calmodulin regulation of CaV channels. Nature. 2008;451(7180):830–4.

38. Asmara H, Minobe E, Saud ZA, Kameyama M. Interactions of calmodulin with the multiple binding sites of Cav1.2 Ca2+ channels. J Pharmacol Sci. 2010;112(4):397–404.

39. Kim J, Ghosh S, Nunziato DA, Pitt GS. Identification of the components controlling inactivation of voltage-gated Ca2+ channels. Neuron. 2004;41(5):745–54.

40. Simms BA, Souza IA, Zamponi GW. A novel calmodulin site in the Cav1.2 N-terminus regulates calcium-dependent inactivation. Pflugers Arch. 2014; 466(9):1793–803.

41. Cohen SM, Li B, Tsien RW, Ma H. Evolutionary and functional perspectives on signaling from neuronal surface to nucleus. Biochem Biophys Res Commun. 2015;460(1):88–99.

42. Ma H, Groth RD, Cohen SM, Emery JF, Li B, Hoedt E, Zhang G, Neubert TA, Tsien RW. gammaCaMKII shuttles Ca(2)(+)/CaM to the nucleus to trigger CREB phosphorylation and gene expression. Cell. 2014;159(2):281–94.

43. Deisseroth K, Heist EK, Tsien RW. Translocation of calmodulin to the nucleus supports CREB phosphorylation in hippocampal neurons. Nature. 1998; 392(6672):198–202.

44. Li B, Tadross MR, Tsien RW. Sequential ionic and conformational signaling by calcium channels drives neuronal gene expression. Science. 2016; 351(6275):863–7.

45. Wheeler DG, Groth RD, Ma H, Barrett CF, Owen SF, Safa P, Tsien RW. Ca(V)1 and Ca(V)2 channels engage distinct modes of Ca(2+) signaling to control CREB-dependent gene expression. Cell. 2012;149(5):1112–24.

46. Deisseroth K, Bito H, Tsien RW. Signaling from synapse to nucleus: postsynaptic CREB phosphorylation during multiple forms of hippocampal synaptic plasticity. Neuron. 1996;16(1):89–101.

47. Bading H, Ginty DD, Greenberg ME. Regulation of gene expression in hippocampal neurons by distinct calcium signaling pathways. Science. 1993; 260(5105):181–6.

48. Marsden KC, Shemesh A, Bayer KU, Carroll RC. Selective translocation of Ca2+/calmodulin protein kinase IIalpha (CaMKIIalpha) to inhibitory synapses. Proc Natl Acad Sci U S A. 2010;107(47):20559–64.

49. Fink CC, Meyer T. Molecular mechanisms of CaMKII activation in neuronal plasticity. Curr Opin Neurobiol. 2002;12(3):293–9.

50. Pugh JR, Raman IM. Mechanisms of potentiation of mossy fiber EPSCs in the cerebellar nuclei by coincident synaptic excitation and inhibition. J Neurosci. 2008;28(42):10549–60.

51. Ly R, Bouvier G, Schonewille M, Arabo A, Rondi-Reig L, Lena C, Casado M, De Zeeuw CI, Feltz A. T-type channel blockade impairs long-term potentiation at the parallel fiber-Purkinje cell synapse and cerebellar learning. Proc Natl Acad Sci U S A. 2013;110(50):20302–7.

2

Cannabidiol enhances morphine antinociception, diminishes NMDA-mediated seizures and reduces stroke damage via the sigma 1 receptor

María Rodríguez-Muñoz, Yara Onetti, Elsa Cortés-Montero, Javier Garzón and Pilar Sánchez-Blázquez[*] (iD)

Abstract

Cannabidiol (CBD), the major non-psychotomimetic compound present in the *Cannabis sativa* plant, exhibits therapeutic potential for various human diseases, including chronic neurodegenerative diseases, such as Alzheimer's and Parkinson's, ischemic stroke, epilepsy and other convulsive syndromes, neuropsychiatric disorders, neuropathic allodynia and certain types of cancer. CBD does not bind directly to endocannabinoid receptors 1 and 2, and despite research efforts, its specific targets remain to be fully identified. Notably, sigma 1 receptor (σ1R) antagonists inhibit glutamate *N*-methyl-D-aspartate acid receptor (NMDAR) activity and display positive effects on most of the aforesaid diseases. Thus, we investigated the effects of CBD on three animal models in which NMDAR overactivity plays a critical role: opioid analgesia attenuation, NMDA-induced convulsive syndrome and ischemic stroke. In an in vitro assay, CBD disrupted the regulatory association of σ1R with the NR1 subunit of NMDAR, an effect shared by σ1R antagonists, such as BD1063 and progesterone, and prevented by σ1R agonists, such as 4-IBP, PPCC and PRE084. The in vivo administration of CBD or BD1063 enhanced morphine-evoked supraspinal antinociception, alleviated NMDA-induced convulsive syndrome, and reduced the infarct size caused by permanent unilateral middle cerebral artery occlusion. These positive effects of CBD were reduced by the σ1R agonists PRE084 and PPCC, and absent in σ1R$^{-/-}$ mice. Thus, CBD displays antagonist-like activity toward σ1R to reduce the negative effects of NMDAR overactivity in the abovementioned experimental situations.

Keywords: Cannabidiol, Cannabinoids, Sigma 1 receptor, NMDA receptor, Neuropathology, Epilepsy, Acute pain, Stroke

Introduction

Cannabidiol (CBD), a phytocannabinoid devoid of psychoactive properties, is currently being investigated in a series of clinical trials to determine its potential for treating diseases such as epilepsy, neuropsychiatric disorders, neurodegeneration and neuropathic allodynia [1–4]. The complete pharmacology of CBD is far from understood, as multiple mechanisms of action and several pharmacological effects have been proposed. Unlike Δ^9-tetrahydrocannabinol, the main psychoactive constituent of the marijuana plant, the effects of CBD do not involve direct binding to the endocannabinoid receptors CB1 and CB2 [5, 6]; instead, CBD behaves

as a non-competitive negative allosteric modulator of CB1 receptors [7]. Allosteric modulation, in conjunction with effects not mediated by CB1 receptors, may explain the in vivo effects of this compound. Indeed, CBD at nanomolar to micromolar concentrations is reported to interact with several non-endocannabinoid signaling systems to impair the function of orphan G-protein-coupled receptor (GPR) 55 [8], the transient receptor potential of melastatin type 8 channel and, transient receptor potential of ankyrin type 1 channel [9] and to facilitate the activity of serotonin 5HT1A receptor [10] and α3 and α1 glycine receptors [11, 12].

Within this complex framework, CBD exhibits positive effects in situations in which glutamatergic signaling, particularly that mediated by *N*-methyl-D-aspartate acid receptor (NMDAR), plays a critical role. Thus, CBD exhibits antioxidant properties and protects neurons from

* Correspondence: psb@cajal.csic.es
Neuropharmacology. Department of Traslational Neuroscience, Cajal Institute, CSIC, E-28002 Madrid, Spain

glutamate-induced death but without cannabinoid receptor activation or NMDAR antagonism [13]. CBD diminishes the neural damage caused by ischemic stroke [14] and chronic diseases, including Parkinson's and Alzheimer's diseases [15–17]. CBD also shows anticonvulsant activity in many acute animal models of seizures [18, 19], and in preclinical studies, CBD is comparable to antiepileptic drugs currently used in clinical therapy [20]. CBD also modulates morphine antinociception in mice [21] and exhibits anti-allodynia effects in rodent models of neuropathy [22, 23]. Indeed, CBD prevents the onset of mechanical and thermal sensitivity induced by the taxane chemotherapeutic agent paclitaxel in a female mouse model of chemotherapy-induced peripheral neuropathy [24]. Clinical evidence suggests that CBD can be used to manage epilepsy in adults and children affected by refractory seizures and exhibits a favorable side effect profile [25].

Similar to CBD, recent work has revealed that sigma 1 receptor (σ1R) antagonism prevents GPCRs from enhancing the function of NMDARs, thereby reducing the cellular impact of excessive glutamatergic activity [26, 27]. Thus, in the aforementioned situations, σ1R ligands, particularly antagonists, exhibit potential for treating neurological diseases [28], substance abuse syndromes [29], and certain neuropsychiatric disorders [30] and may serve as adjuvants for opioid analgesia [31]. Accordingly, σ1R antagonists alleviate neuropathic allodynia and inflammatory hyperalgesia in animal models of pain involving NMDAR activation [32–34]. Additionally, σ1R ligands have been shown to enhance neuroplasticity and functional recovery following experimental stroke [35], a paradigm in which increased NMDAR activity plays a decisive role. The highly selective σ1R antagonist, S1RA, significantly reduces the cerebral infarct size and neurological deficits caused by permanent middle cerebral artery occlusion (pMCAO) [36]. Likewise, recent data suggest the involvement of σ1R in rare CNS diseases, such as Dravet syndrome [37], and the sigma ligand ANAVEX 2–73 shows potential for treating certain CNS disorders [38], including epilepsy [https://www.anavex.com/anavex-releases-promising-full-preclinical-epilepsy-data-at-antiepileptic-drug-trials-xiii-conference/].

We thus addressed whether this phytocannabinoid modulates glutamatergic NMDAR transmission via σ1R. Our study suggests that CBD displays antagonist activity toward σ1R to inhibit NMDAR function and effectively reduces its ability to dampen morphine-induced analgesia, promote NMDA-mediated convulsive syndrome and cause neuronal damage after pMCAO.

Results

CBD activity toward the σ1R-NR1 complex

To regulate NMDAR function, σ1R binds in a calcium-dependent manner to the cytosolic regulatory sequence of the NMDAR NR1 subunit but not to the NR2A subunit [27, 39]. The NMDAR NR1 subunit has only a single σ1R binding site [40], which is located on the same cytosolic region that binds calcium-activated calmodulin (CaM) to reduce the probability of calcium channel opening [41]. We have described an in vitro assay that analyzes the capacity of drugs to alter the interaction of recombinant σ1R with the regulatory cytosolic C0-C1-C2 region of the NMDAR NR1 subunit [42]. In binding assays performed using brain membranes or cells with forced σ1R expression, the affinity of ligands competing with labeled σ1R ligands is in the nM range, probably because tritiated tracers provide reliable specific signals through their binding to the most abundant low affinity state of the receptors. In the in vitro setting, σ1R antagonists at pM concentrations disrupt σ1R-NR1 associations in a concentration-dependent manner, and pM concentrations of agonists prevent the effects of the former [26, 27]. As observed for GPCRs coupled to G proteins, the affinity of σ1R when bound to target proteins increases; thus, σ1R ligands display pM instead of nM activity for σ1R-NR1 associations.

The last transmembrane region plus the cytosolic C0-C1-C2 C-terminal sequence of the NR1 subunit was covalently attached to agarose particles (see Methods). Thus, agarose-NR1 was incubated with σ1R, and after removal of the unbound σ1R, the agarose-NR1-σ1R complexes were tested to determine the effects of potential σ1R ligands. Afterwards, the extent of σ1R binding to the agarose-NR1 subunits was subsequently evaluated. The endogenous neurosteroid progesterone and the synthetic drug BD1063, both putative σ1R antagonists, exhibited ED50s of approximately 30 pM for diminishing σ1R-NR1 complex formation (Fig. 1a). Other drugs displaying antagonist activity toward σ1R, such as S1RA, fenfluramine and norfenfluramine, also showed pM activity in this in vitro setting [42]. Notably, CBD displayed a dose-dependent capacity for diminishing σ1R-NR1 associations with an ED50 of approximately 100 pM; thus, CBD behaved as a σ1R antagonist (Fig. 1a). The σ1R agonists PRE084, 4-IBP and PPCC, which did not exhibit the capacity to disrupt σ1R-NR1 complexes, antagonized the inhibitory effect of progesterone and CBD on these complexes (Fig. 1b). PPCC reduced the activity of 100 pM CBD in a concentration-dependent manner with an apparent Ki of 60 pM. In the presence of increasing concentrations of PPCC, the curves of CBD (disrupting σ1R-NR1 associations) shifted to the right (Fig. 1b). Thus, recognized σ1R antagonists and CBD diminished the interaction of σ1R with the NR1 subunit of the NMDA receptor. These data suggest that CBD does bind to σ1R to trigger its antagonist effects and disrupt σ1R-NR1 regulatory interactions.

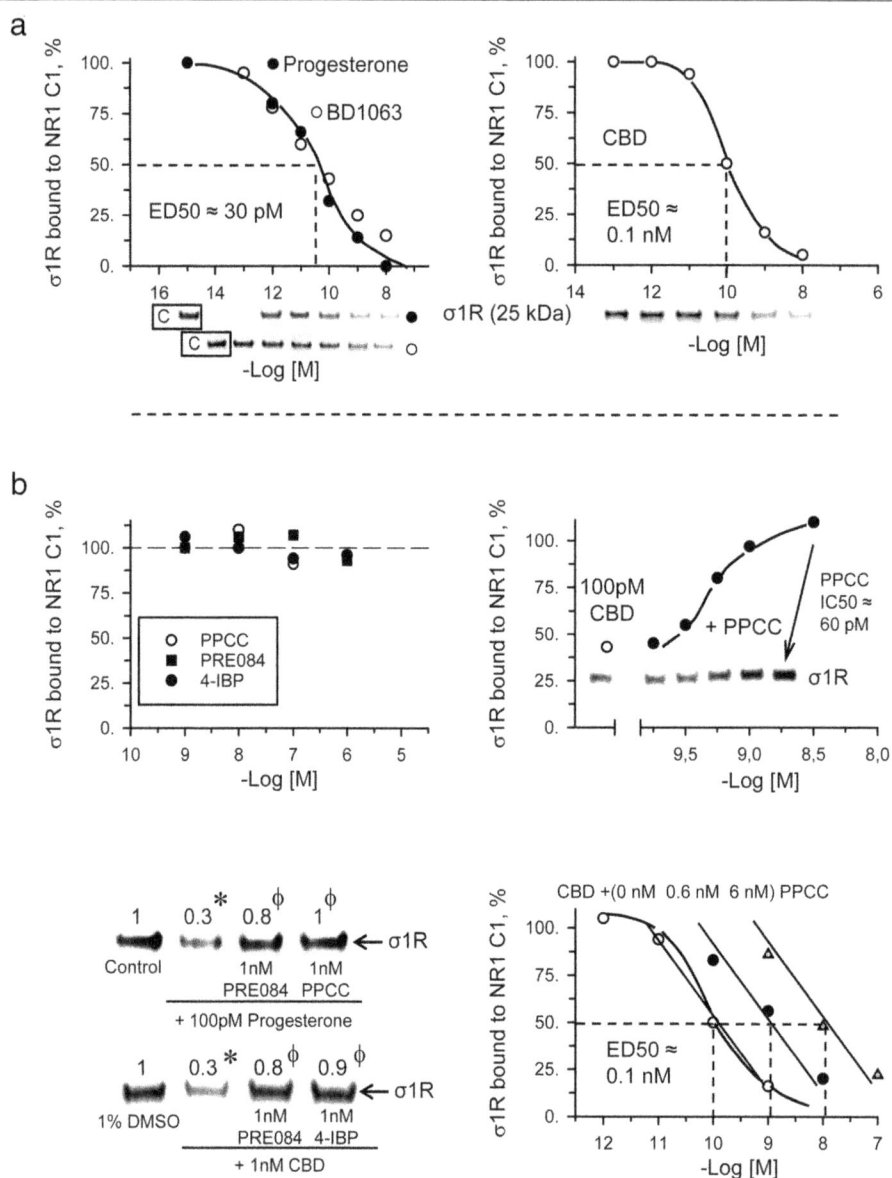

Fig. 1 CBD disrupts the association of σ1R with the NR1 subunits of NMDA receptors. In vitro assay determining ligand activity for σ1R. NHS-activated Sepharose beads covalently coupled to a sequence of the NR1 subunit containing seven residues of the transmembrane region plus C0-C1-C2 cytosolic segments were incubated with excess σ1R (1:3). Unbound σ1R was washed out, and the NR1 C1-coupled σ1R was exposed to serial concentrations of the ligands under study. σ1R that remained attached to the NR1 subunits was then evaluated by SDS-PAGE and immunoblotting. **a** Inhibitory effects of the σ1R antagonists progesterone and BD106 and of CBD on the association of σ1R with the NR1 C1 subunit. The assays were performed in the presence of 50 mM Tris-HCl (pH 7.5), 0.2% CHAPS and 2.5 mM calcium. Representative blots are shown. The ED50 values were computed using the software SigmaPlot v.14. **b** The σ1R agonists PPCC, PRE084 and 4-IBP did not alter σ1R-NR1 associations but reduced the capacity of progesterone and CBD to disrupt such associations. PPCC reduced the capacity of CBD to inhibit the binding of σ1R to NR1 subunit in a concentration-dependent manner. The assays were performed twice, and each point was duplicated. *Significant difference with respect to the control group (DMSO or saline); φ significant difference with respect to the group receiving only CBD or progesterone; ANOVA, Dunnett's multiple comparison, $p < 0.05$

CBD regulates morphine antinociception

The mu-opioid receptor in the mesencephalic periaqueductal gray matter plays the most relevant role in the antinociception produced by opioids injected by the icv route. The icv administration of all the substances studied circumvented the possibility that the drugs reached receptors beyond the brain. Subsequently, the capacity of morphine to produce supraspinal antinociception and the ability of the studied drugs to modulate this effect were studied through the warm water tail flick test.

The time-dependent antinociceptive effects of morphine, CBD, BD1063, PPCC, and combinations of these drugs were then investigated (Fig. 2). The analgesic effect of 6 nmol morphine icv peaked after 30 min reaching approximately 60% of the maximum analgesic effect measurable in this test. While CBD and the σ1R agonist PPCC did not promote antinociception in this assay, the administration of CBD (3 nmol, icv) before morphine treatment (6 nmol, icv) augmented the antinociceptive activity of the opioid (Fig. 2a). The maximum effect was observed when CBD was injected 10 min before the opioid, and this interval was used in subsequent experiments. Thus, in mice pretreated with CBD, morphine analgesia increased from $57.8 \pm 4.3\%$ to $83.4 \pm 6.1\%$ of the maximum analgesic effect.

It is known that S1RA and other σ1R antagonists administered icv at a low nmol range increase morphine analgesia in rodents, probably by the removal of a tonic constraint that this σ1R may exert over mu-opioid function [26, 27]. Indeed, pretreatment with 3 nmol BD1063 also potentiated morphine analgesia (from $55.0 \pm 4.2\%$ to $75.2 \pm 5.1\%$) (Fig. 2b). The σ1R agonist PPCC did not affect morphine antinociception but prevented CBD and BD1063 from enhancing this effect of morphine (Fig. 2a and b). The involvement of σ1R in the effects of BD1063 and CBD was ascertained using sigma receptor knockout ($\sigma1R^{-/-}$) mice. In agreement with previous reports [27], morphine yields higher analgesia in $\sigma1R^{-/-}$ mice than in their wild-type control counterparts, with an approximately 35% increase at the peak interval of 30 min post-morphine. This effect of morphine could not be altered by BD1063 or CBD in the $\sigma1R^{-/-}$ mice (Fig. 2c).

Anticonvulsant activity of CBD
Selective σ1R antagonists diminish the manifestation of the NMDA-induced convulsive syndrome [42]. Thus, the anticonvulsant activity of CBD was evaluated in an animal model in which seizures were induced by the icv administration of NMDA [43, 44]. Indeed, a dose of 1 nmol NMDA icv induced tonic convulsions in approximately 95% of the mice. With this procedure, practically all the mice exhibited a series of anomalous behaviors, such as compulsive rearing, wild running (hypermobility and circling), clonic convulsions, tonic seizures, and, in approximately 15–20% of the animals, death (Fig. 3a). The σ1R agonist PPCC did not significantly alter the behavioral effects evoked by NMDA administration. In contrast, BD1063 and CBD protected more than 50% of the mice tested from hypermobility, convulsive rearing and clonic convulsions. Moreover, tonic seizures were present in only 20% of the mice, and no mice died. Notably, the σ1R agonist PPCC counteracted the ability of CBD and BD1063 to alleviate the NMDA-induced convulsive syndrome (Fig. 3b), indicating that σ1R is necessary for CBD to produce these beneficial effects.

It has been suggested that 5HT1AR participates in CBD activity [10]. In the presence of the 5HT1AR antagonist WAY100635, CBD exhibited a reduced capacity to diminish the convulsions promoted by 1 nmol NMDA. However, WAY100635 revealed an endogenous negative control of serotonin 5HT1AR on NMDAR overactivity. Thus, WAY100635 alone enhanced wild running and tonic seizures and promoted death in mice treated with the lower dose of 0.3 nmol NMDA (Fig. 3c). Notably, the positive effects of CBD and BD1063 on diminishing NMDA-induced convulsive signs were absent when the syndrome was modeled in $\sigma1R^{-/-}$ mice (Fig. 3d).

While PPCC did not modify the latency to the first convulsive episode or its duration, CBD and BD1063 increased this latency and reduced the duration of the seizure episode. PPCC antagonized these effects of CBD and BD1063. In $\sigma1R^{-/-}$ mice, the latency, duration and intensity of the NMDA-induced seizures were not altered by the administration of CBD or BD1063 (Fig. 3e).

CBD diminished neural damage promoted by pMCAO
The administration of CBD (10 nmol, icv) 60 min post-surgery resulted in much less severe infarction. The volumetric analysis of the brain showed that neither surgery nor the icv procedure significantly changed the total brain volume (302.9 ± 13.9 mm^3 and 300.9 ± 7.9 mm^3, respectively; sham-operated mice: 299.2 ± 5.9 mm^3). However, pMCAO resulted in severe injury in mice examined 48 h after ischemia (Fig. 4). Injury was most apparent in the cerebral cortex, and the infarct volume was estimated to affect $5.4 \pm 1.2\%$ of the total brain volume. No damage was observed in the sham-operated mice. Compared with no treatment, the administration of CBD improved stroke outcomes (an approximate 75% reduction in the infarct size to $1.2 \pm 0.9\%$ of the total brain volume) after permanent cerebral ischemia. In agreement with previous reports [36], the selective σ1R antagonist BD1063 exhibited protective effects in this model. The σ1R agonist PRE084 does not alter the infarct volume promoted by pMCAO; however, PRE084 did prevent the neuroprotective effects of CBD and BD1063. As previously observed [36], $\sigma1R^{-/-}$ mice showed increased infarct volumes (up $6.73 \pm 1.8\%$ of brain volume) with respect to their wild-type ($\sigma1R^{+/+}$) controls, which were refractory to administration of either CBD or BD1063 (Fig. 4).

Discussion
The present study shows that CBD acting as an antagonist of σ1R diminishes the influence of glutamate NMDA receptors in three experimental paradigms in which this activity plays a key role, i.e., the level of morphine-evoked antinociception, the incidence of NMDA-induced convulsive activity and the extent of the neural damage caused

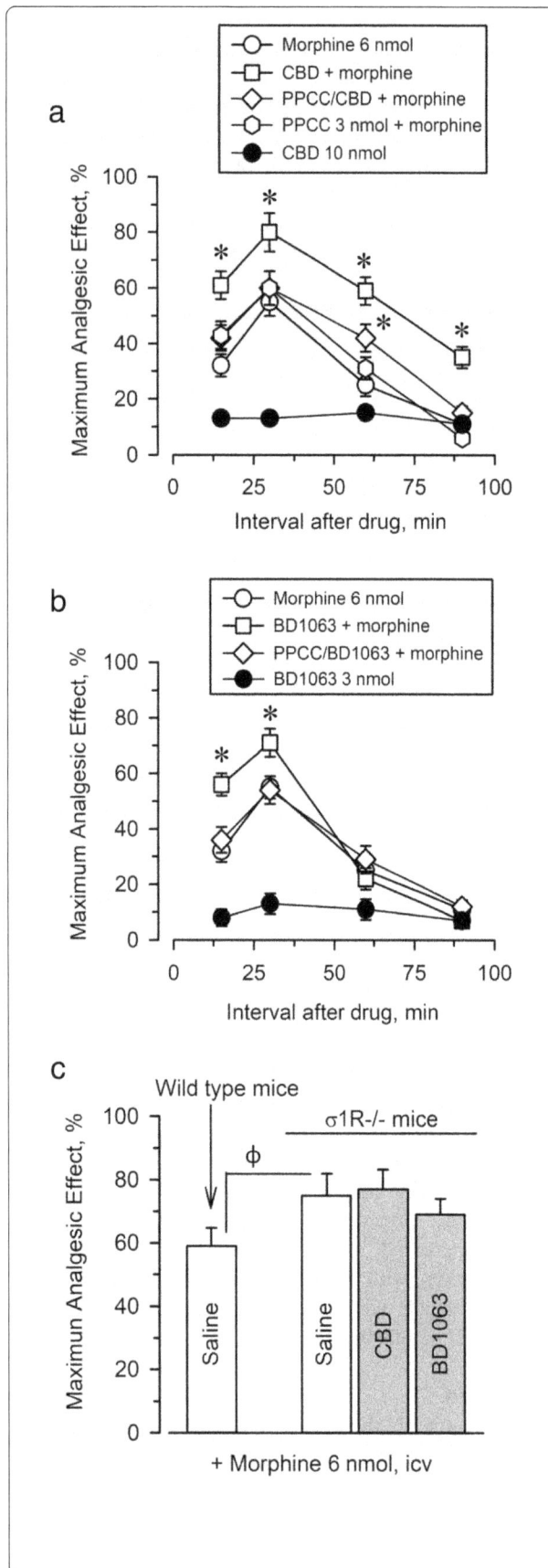

Fig. 2 Effect of CBD on morphine-induced supraspinal antinociception. Mice received 10 nmol CBD icv 10 min before 6 nmol morphine, and analgesia was evaluated with the thermal warm water (52 °C) "tail-flick" test at the indicated post-opioid intervals. Each point represents the mean ± SEM of data from eight to ten mice. **a** CBD exhibited no significant analgesic effect in this test. The analgesia produced by the combination of CBD and morphine was significantly higher than that produced by morphine alone. The σ1R agonist PPCC did not alter morphine analgesia, but icv-injection 20 min before CBD prevented the enhancement of this effect of morphine. **b** The σ1R agonist BD1063 did not produce analgesia in this test but increased morphine antinociception. This potentiation was absent when PPCC was injected icv 20 min before BD1063. **c** Morphine promotes a higher analgesic effect in σ1R$^{-/-}$ mice than in wild type control mice. In σ1R$^{-/-}$ mice, BD1063 and CBD did not modify morphine analgesia. *Significantly different from the control group receiving only 6 nmol morphine, φ significantly different from the effect of morphine in wild-type mice. ANOVA, Dunnett's multiple comparison vs control group, $p < 0.05$

by experimental ictus. These positive effects of CBD are also achieved by the direct binding of drugs to the NMDAR ionic pore to block NMDAR calcium influx (antagonists) [45–47] and by antagonists, but not agonists, of σ1R, which regulates NMDAR function [36, 48, 49]. σ1R antagonists and CBD exhibit no such control over NMDAR activity in mice lacking σ1R protein expression. This and previous observations show that CBD does not bind to the NMDAR ionic pore [13] and thus suggest that CBD displays antagonist-like activity on σ1R to counteract the negative effects of NMDAR hyperfunction in the aforementioned experimental situations.

The activity of glutamate NMDARs falls under the negative influence of some GPCRs, including CB1R [50], acetylcholine type 1 muscarinic receptor [51], serotonin 5HT1AR [52], adrenergic α1R and α2R [53], dopamine D3R and D4R [54, 55], and group III mGluR7R [56]. Among these GPCRs, 5HT1AR is a suitable candidate for mediating CBD effects [10], and in fact, the 5HT1AR antagonist WAY100635 diminished the capacity of CBD to alleviate NMDA-induced convulsive syndrome. Nevertheless, WAY100635 alone enhanced the capacity of the agonist NMDA to evoke convulsions, suggesting the endogenous inhibitory control of NMDAR activity by 5HT1AR. Certainly, WAY100635 has been described to display agonist activity toward the dopamine D4 receptor, which is negatively coupled to glutamate activity [57]. In our experimental model, WAY100635 enhanced wild running and tonic seizures and promoted death in mice treated with a lower dose of 0.3 nmol NMDA. Thus, in our convulsive model, the activity of WAY100635 toward dopamine D4 receptors can be disregarded. If CBD displays activity toward certain GPCRs to alleviate NMDA-induced convulsions, these receptors require the presence of σ1R to promote such an effect because CBD failed to do so in σ1R$^{-/-}$ mice. The σ1R agonist PPCC

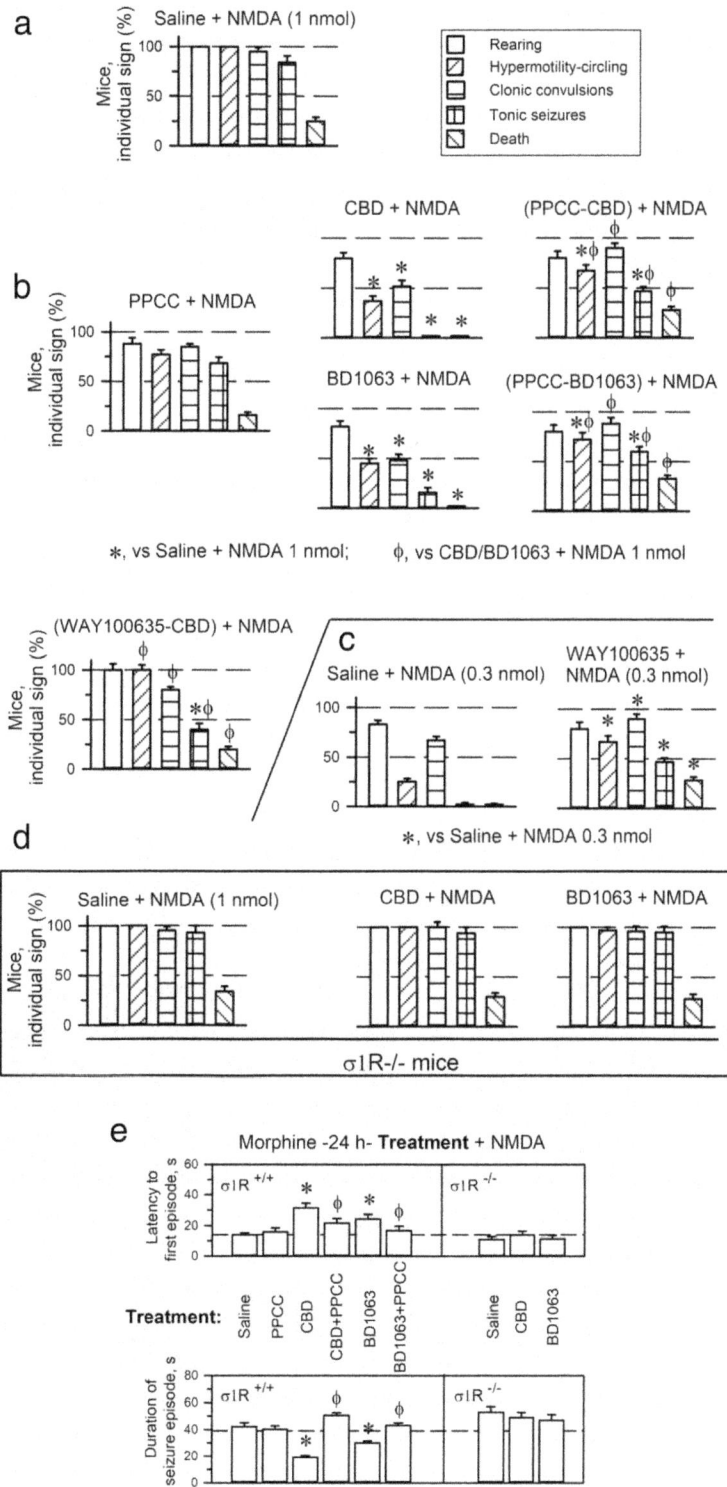

Fig. 3 (See legend on next page.)

Fig. 3 Anticonvulsant effects of CBD in a mouse model of seizures induced by NMDAR overactivation. **a** Behavioral alterations produced by the icv administration of 1 nmol NMDA to mice. Each bar indicates the percentage of mice showing the indicated sign and represents the mean ± SEM of 8 mice. **b** Effects of PPCC, CBD and BD1063 on seizures induced by NMDA. The mice received the NMDAR agonist NMDA icv (1 nmol) 30 min after the drugs (3 nmol PPCC, BD1063, CBD or 5 nmol WAY100635) and were then immediately evaluated. **c** Effect of the 5HT1AR antagonist WAY100635 on the convulsive syndrome evoked by 0.3 nmol NMDA. **d** Lack of an effect of CBD and BD1063 on seizures induced by 1 nmol NMDA in $\sigma 1R^{-/-}$ mice. **e** Effects of the treatments on the latency and duration of the seizure episodes induced by 1 nmol NMDA in wild type and $\sigma 1R^{-/-}$ mice. *Significant difference from the control group receiving NMDA and saline instead of the drugs. φ Significant difference from the corresponding NMDA-induced behavioral signs exhibited by the group receiving only CBD or BD1063, $p < 0.05$. ANOVA, Dunnett's multiple comparison vs control group, $p < 0.05$

produced no significant changes in this model but efficaciously counteracted the anticonvulsant effects of CBD. These observations suggest an essential role of $\sigma 1R$ in the negative control that CBD exerts on NMDAR activity. Indeed, in the presence of $\sigma 1R$ agonists, CBD did not exhibit the aforementioned effects, and the in vitro assays showed that CBD acts as a $\sigma 1R$ antagonist to disrupt $\sigma 1R$-NR1 complexes.

Although $\sigma 1R$ is a chaperone that regulates a series of signaling proteins in the endoplasmic reticulum in a calcium-dependent manner, this protein was discovered as a type of opioid receptor, and $\sigma 1R$ can thus be found in the cell plasma membrane [58]. In this context, $\sigma 1R$ is a regulator of NMDAR function and cooperates with histidine triad nucleotide-binding protein 1 (HINT1) to regulate NMDAR function via certain GPCRs [26]. The calcium-dependent binding of $\sigma 1R$ to NMDAR NR1 subunits that carry the cytosolic C1 segment protects the activity of NMDARs, i.e., calcium influx, from the inhibitory action of calcium-activated calmodulin $(Ca^{2+}\text{-}CaM)$. While agonists promote $\sigma 1R$ binding to the NMDAR NR1 subunit, antagonists such as CBD

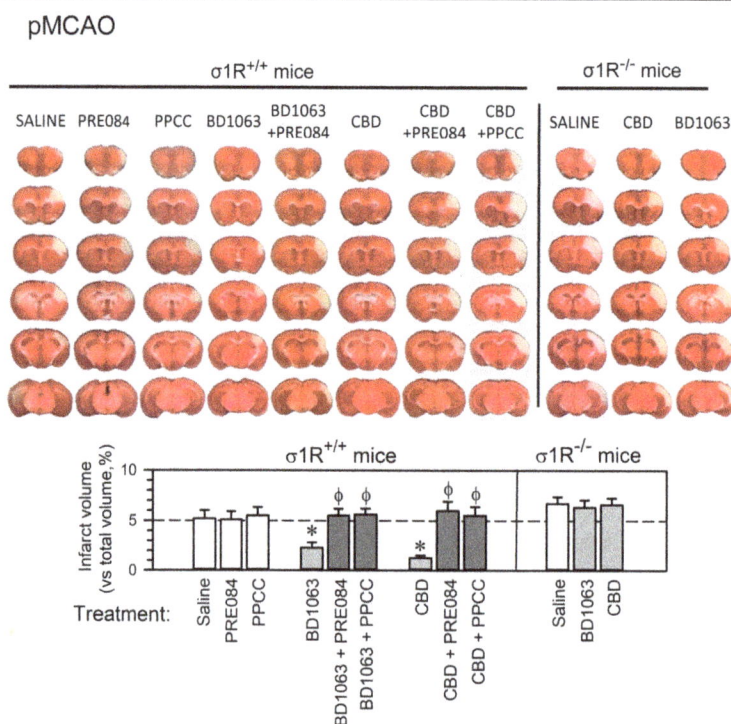

Fig. 4 CBD administration diminishes ischemic brain damage in wild-type but not $\sigma 1R^{-/-}$ mice. Upper panel, representative TTC-stained brain section images obtained from saline- and drug-treated mice (1 h after surgery) 48 h after pMCAO. White indicates infarction; red staining indicates normal tissue. Lower panel, the bar graphs quantitatively compare the infarct volume based on TTC staining from the wild type and $\sigma 1R^{-/-}$ mice treated with saline, the $\sigma 1R$ agonists PRE084 and PPCC (white bars), or the $\sigma 1R$ antagonist BD1063 and CBD (gray bars) 1 h after surgery. The groups consisted of 8 to 10 mice, and the data are presented as the mean ± SEM. *Significantly different from the saline-treated mice. φ Significantly different from mice receiving only the $\sigma 1R$ antagonist BD1063 or CBD; ANOVA, Dunnett's multiple comparison vs the corresponding control group, $p < 0.05$

disrupt these complexes to facilitate the Ca^{2+}-CaM inhibition of NMDAR function. Thus, CBD acts as a σ1R antagonist to reduce NMDAR activity.

As previously mentioned, CBD is involved in a variety of activities and may act as a sedative, anxiolytic, antipsychotic, anti-inflammatory, antioxidative, neuroprotective, anti-emetic, anticancer, antidepressant and mood-stabilizing drug, as well as have therapeutic effects on movement disorders, ischemia, diabetes, and cannabis withdrawal syndrome [30, 59–63]. Moreover, CBD exhibits anti-neuropathic effects [22, 23] and modulates morphine antinociception in mice [21]. Our data suggest that CBD acts on σ1R to alleviate the manifestation of epileptic syndrome, to protect against neural damage caused by vascular ischemia and to enhance the antinociception promoted by morphine. These findings suggest the implication of σ1R in other beneficial activities attributed to this phytocannabinoid. Indeed, σ1R is a potential target for the treatment of neuropathic pain because it interacts with and regulates NMDARs and TRPV1 calcium channels, which are key constituents of the mechanisms that modulate activity-induced sensitization in nociceptive pathways [32–34, 64]. Moreover, σ1R ligands also exhibit antidepressant, anxiolytic, neuroprotective and antioxidative effects [30, 65].

Alterations in σ1R have been consistently related to schizophrenia [66, 67]. NMDAR function is lower in this mental illness, and the negative control exerted by GPCRs, such as CB1Rs, on glutamate activity may play an essential role in the etiology of this disease [68–70]. The severity of the negative symptoms of schizophrenic patients correlates with alterations in the plasma levels of anandamide [71] and with those of neurosteroids, the putative ligands of this ligand-operated chaperone/receptor [72, 73]. Indeed, adjunct treatment with pregnenolone diminishes the negative symptoms of schizophrenia [74]. The idea that the CB1R localizes primarily in axon terminals have already been challenged [75], and a series of immunocytochemical and ultrastructural studies have demonstrated the presence of the CB1R in the somatodendritic compartment (post-synapse), both at the spinal and supraspinal levels where it co-localizes with NMDARs and PSD95 proteins. Thus, an anomalous σ1R-regulated connection between CB1R and NMDAR may contribute to the disproportionate downregulation of NMDAR activity (hypofunction), constituting a serious risk factor for the development of schizophrenia [68, 76]. In the context of negative NMDAR regulation by CB1Rs, σ1R antagonists such as CBD uncouple NMDAR function from the negative influence of GPCRs, such as CB1Rs [70, 76].

In the sub-micromolar and micromolar range, CBD affects the function of various signaling pathways. Among other targets, CBD regulates cannabinoid receptors

without displaying binding directly to them; CBD also impairs the function of the equilibrative nucleoside transporter, that of the orphan GPR55 receptor and that of the transient receptor potential of melastatin type 8 channel [8, 9]. Conversely, CBD enhances 5HT1AR, α3 and α1 glycine receptor, and transient receptor potential of ankyrin type 1 channel activity [9]. In hippocampal cultures, the CBD-mediated regulation of calcium levels is bidirectional and depends on the excitability of the cells [77]. CBD also activates the nuclear peroxisome proliferator-activated receptor γ and transient receptor potential vanilloid type 1 and 2 channels while inhibiting the cellular uptake and fatty acid amide hydrolase-catalyzed degradation of anandamide [71, 78]. CBD reduces hydroperoxide-induced oxidative damage, tissue cyclooxygenase activity, the nitric oxide production, T-cell responses, bioactive tumor necrosis factor release, and prostaglandin E2, cytokine interferon c and tumor necrosis factor production and blocks voltage-gated Na + channels [6, 77]. Whether the effects of CBD on σ1R are relevant to these activities remains to be explored. Because this exogenous cannabinoid may alter the function of a wide variety of cellular activities, the key is to determine the molecular mechanisms that are primarily implicated in a particular effect of CBD.

Our study indicates that CBD regulates the function of σ1R in at least several of the abovementioned behavioral effects. Thus, CBD's enhancement of opioid analgesia, alleviation of convulsive syndrome, protection against ischemic neural damage and anti-allodynia effects appear to involve an antagonist interaction with σ1R and the subsequent reduction of NMDAR function. This finding may help in us to understand the current pharmacology of CBD and provides new avenues for the treatment of several brain-related disorders.

Methods
Expression of recombinant proteins
The coding region of murine full-length (1–223) σ1R (AF004927), and the C-terminal region of the glutamate NMDAR NR1 subunit (NM_008169) (residues 827–938), were amplified by RT-PCR using total RNA isolated from mouse brains as the template. Specific primers containing an upstream Sgf I restriction site and a downstream Pme I restriction site were used, as described previously [27]. The PCR products were cloned downstream of the GST coding sequence and the TEV protease site. The sequenced proteins were identical to the GenBank™ sequences. The vector was introduced into E. coli BL21 (KRX #L3002, Promega, Madrid, Spain), and clones were selected on solid medium containing ampicillin. After 3 h of induction at room temperature (1 mM IPTG and 0.1% Rhamnose), the cells were collected by centrifugation, and the pellets were maintained at – 80 °C. The GST fusion proteins were purified under native conditions on GStrap

FF columns (GE#17–5130-01, Healthcare, Barcelona, Spain); when necessary, the fusion proteins retained were cleaved on the column with ProTEV protease (Promega, #V605A) and further purification was achieved by high-resolution ion exchange (Enrich Q, BioRad #780–0001) or electroelution of the corresponding gel band (GE 200, Hoefer Scientific Instruments, San Francisco, CA, USA). The sequences were confirmed through automated capillary sequencing.

Animals and drugs

Male albino CD-1 mice and homozygous ($\sigma 1R^{-/-}$) male sigma receptor knockout mice, backcrossed (N10 generation) onto a CD1 albino genetic background (ENVIGO, Milano, Italy) were used in the study. The mice were maintained at 22 °C on a diurnal 12 h light/dark cycle. Procedures involving mice adhered strictly to the guidelines of the European Community for the Care and Use of Laboratory Animals (Council Directive 86/609/EEC) and Spanish law (RD53/2013) regulating animal research. Each group consisted of eight to ten animals, which were used only once. The compounds used were as follows: morphine sulfate (mu-opiod receptor agonist, Merck, Darmstadt, Germany); NMDA (#0114); CBD (#1570); BD1063 ($\sigma 1R$ antagonist #0883); PRE084 ($\sigma 1R$ agonist #0589); (±)-PPCC oxalate ($\sigma 1R$ agonist #3870), 4-IBP ($\sigma 1R$ ligand #0748); WAY100635 maleate (5HT1A receptor antagonist #4380) were obtained from Tocris Bioscience (Bristol, UK). Progesterone ($\sigma 1R$ antagonist P7556) and pregnenolone sulfate ($\sigma 1R$ agonist P162) were obtained from Sigma-Aldrich (Spain). Test drugs were dissolved in saline except CBD and PPCC, which were prepared in a 1:1:18 (v/v/v) mixture of ethanol:Kolliphor EL (#C5135, Sigma-Aldrich): physiological saline, and injected intracerebroventricularly (icv) 30 min before NMDA administration. To facilitate selective and straightforward access to their targets, the compounds were injected (4 µL) into the lateral ventricles of mice as previously described [79]. Animals were lightly anesthetized and injections were performed with a 10 µL Hamilton syringe at a depth of 3 mm at a point of 2 mm lateral and 2 mm caudal from the bregma. The 4 µL were infused at a rate of 1 µL every 5 s. After this the needle was maintained for an additional 10 s. Mice were randomly assigned to each treatment of the selected compounds (power of 80% to detect statistically significant differences). The use of drugs, experimental design and sample size determination were approved by the Ethical Committee for Research of the CSIC (SAF2015–65420 & CAM PROEX 225/14).

Experimental protocols

In vitro interactions between recombinant proteins: Pull-down of recombinant proteins, effect of drugs on σ1R-NR1 interactions

Having demonstrated that the $\sigma 1R$ does not bind to GST (Z02039; GenScript Co., Piscataway, NJ, USA) [26],

we assessed the association of GST-free $\sigma 1Rs$ with GST-tagged NMDAR NR1 C-terminal sequence, which was immobilized through covalent attachment to NHS-activated Sepharose 4 fast flow (FF) (GE#17–0906-01; General Electric Healthcare, Spain) according to the manufacturer's instructions. The recombinant $\sigma 1R$ (100 nM) was incubated either with NHS-blocked Sepharose 4FF (negative control) or with the immobilized NR1 protein fragment in 200 µL of a buffer containing 50 mM Tris-HCl (pH 7.5) and 0.2% CHAPS in the presence of 2.5 mM of $CaCl_2$. In pilot assays, we determined that after 20 min of incubation the NR1-$\sigma 1R$ association was maximal and that, this period of time was also sufficient for the drugs to promote stable changes in their association. Thus, the samples were mixed by rotation for 20 min at RT, and $\sigma 1Rs$ bound to NR1-Sepharose 4FF were recovered by centrifugation and three cycles of washing. The agarose-attached NR1-$\sigma 1R$ complexes were incubated in the presence of increasing concentrations of the drugs under study for 20 min with rotation at room temperature in 300 µL of 50 mM Tris-HCl (pH 7.5), 2.5 mM $CaCl_2$, and 0.2% CHAPS. In this assay, $\sigma 1R$ ligands dissolved in aqueous solutions display calcium- and concentration-dependent activity in altering $\sigma 1R$-NR1 associations. If an organic solvent, such as DMSO, is required to incorporate the drug under study, i.e., CBD, DMSO must be kept below 1% in the buffer of the assay. Higher concentrations of DMSO stabilize $\sigma 1R$-NR1 associations and diminish the disruptive effects of $\sigma 1R$ antagonists. Thus, CBD was initially dissolved in 100% DMSO, and through serial dilutions, the concentrations used in the study were obtained with a final DMSO concentration of approximately 1%. Agarose pellets containing the bound proteins were obtained by centrifugation, washed thrice in the presence of 2.5 mM $CaCl_2$, and solubilized in 2× Laemmli buffer, and the content of $\sigma 1Rs$ was addressed by Western blotting.

The detached $\sigma 1Rs$ from the aforementioned procedure were resolved with SDS/polyacrylamide gel electrophoresis (PAGE) in 4–12% Bis-Tris gels (NuPAGE NP0341, Invitrogen, Thermo Fisher Scientific, Spain) with MES SDS running buffer (NuPAGE NP0002, Invitrogen) and then transferred onto 0.2 µm polyvinylidene difluoride (PVDF) membranes (162–0176; Bio-Rad, Madrid, Spain). The anti-$\sigma 1R$ (#42–3300, Invitrogen) diluted in Tris-buffered saline pH 7.7 (TBS) + 0.05% Tween 20 (TTBS) was incubated overnight at 6 °C. The primary antibody was detected using secondary antibodies conjugated to horseradish peroxidase. The western blot images showing antibody binding, were visualized by chemiluminescence (#170–5061; Bio-Rad) and recorded using a ChemiImager IS-5500 (Alpha Innotech, San Leandro, CA).

Evaluation of antinociception

The response of the animals to nociceptive stimuli was determined by the warm water (52 °C) tail-flick test as previously described [27]. The tail-flick analgesic test applies a thermal noxious stimulus to promote flicking of the mouse's tail, and opioids given by icv route increase the time elapsed between application of the stimulus and the flick. This response comprises a spinal reflex that is under facilitator drive by the brain stem nociceptive modulating network. Baseline latencies ranged from 1.5 to 2.2 s. A cut-off time of 10 s was used to minimize the risk of tissue damage. Drugs were icv injected and antinociception was assessed at different time intervals thereafter. Saline was likewise administered as a control. Antinociception was expressed as a percentage of the maximum possible effect (MPE = 100 × [test latency-baseline latency]/[cut-off time (10 s)-baseline latency]).

NMDA-induced seizures

Seizures were induced by injection of NMDA (0.3 and 1 nmol/mouse icv, in a volume of 4 μL sterile saline) as described by others [44]. The dose of 1 nmol NMDA was selected as the minimal dose that reliably induced the appearance of tonic seizures in at least 80% of treated mice. Immediately after injection animals were placed in a transparent box (20x20x30 cm) and were observed for a period of 3 min. The seizure activity consisted of a mild myoclonic phase (immobility, mouth and facial movements, tail extension, circling), rearing (violent movements of the hole body, rearing), wild running (episodes of running with explosive jumps), clonic convulsions (characterized by rigidity of the whole body including limbs flexion/extension), followed by continuous/repetitive seizure activity (tonic seizures) and, in approximately 15–20% of the animals, death. The episode typically began a few seconds after injection and evolved to its maximal intensity in less than 1 min. The results are expressed as the percentage of mice exhibiting the aforementioned signs and the mean latencies of the first body clonus.

Permanent unilateral middle cerebral artery occlusion (pMCAO) and the determination of infarct size

Focal cerebral ischemia was induced via pMCAO, as described previously [36]. Briefly, mice were anesthetized and a vertical skin incision was made between the left eye and ear under a dissection microscope. After drilling a small hole in the cranium at the level of the distal portion of the middle cerebral artery, the artery was occluded by cauterization. Flow obstruction was visually verified. Animals showing subdural haemorrhages or signs of incorrect surgery were immediately excluded from the study (< 5% in each group). The mice were returned to their cages after surgery, kept at room temperature, and allowed food and water ad libitum. Strong lesion reproducibility was observed. We exclude mice from further studies if excessive bleeding occurs during surgery, mice fail to recover from anaesthesia within 15 min, or haemorrhage was found in the brain during post-mortem examination. The investigator performing the pMCAO surgery was blinded to treatment group. To determine the infarct size 48 h after surgery, animals were euthanized and their brains were removed, after which six 1 mm-thick coronal brain slices (Brain Matrix, WPI, UK) were obtained. The sections were stained with 2,3,5-triphenyltetrazolium chloride (1% TTC, Sigma-Aldrich). Infarct volumes were calculated by sampling each side of the coronal sections with a digital camera (Nikon Coolpix 990, Tokyo, Japan). The extent of unstained infarct area (expressed in mm2) was integrated from the total area as an orthogonal projection.

Statistical analysis

The data represent the means ± SEM. The Sigmaplot/SigmaStat v.14 package (SPSS Science Software, Erkrath, Germany) was used to generate the graphs, determine parameters (interaction of drugs with σ1R-NR1 complexes), and perform the corresponding statistical analysis. The level of significance was $p < 0.05$. Data were analyzed using one-way ANOVA followed by Dunnett multiple comparisons as appropriated.

Abbreviations

5HTR: serotonin receptor; CaM: calcium-activated calmodulin; CBD: Cannabidiol; CBR: cannabinoid receptors; GPCR: G-protein-coupled receptor; HINT1: Histidine triad nucleotide-binding protein 1; NMDAR: N-methyl-D-aspartate acid receptor; NR1: NMDAR subunit 1; pMCAO: permanent middle cerebral artery occlusion; σ1R: sigma 1 receptor

Acknowledgments

We would like to thank Gabriela de Alba and Veronica Merino for their excellent technical assistance. Mice with the targeted deletion of σ1R gene were kindly provided by Dr. Manuel Merlos (Drug Discovery & Preclinical Development, Esteve, Barcelona, Spain).

Funding

This work was supported by MINECO Plan Nacional I + D + i [grant number SAF-2015-65420R].

Authors' contributions

The JGN & PSB designed the research, wrote the manuscript and provided funding. MRM, YO & ECM performed experiments and statistical analysis of data. All authors approved the final manuscript.

Competing interests

The authors declare that the research was conducted in the absence of any commercial or financial relationships that could be construed as a potential conflict of interest.

References

1. Bergamaschi MM, Queiroz RH, Zuardi AW, Crippa JA. Safety and side effects of cannabidiol, a Cannabis sativa constituent. Curr Drug Saf. 2011;6:237–49.
2. Borgelt LM, Franson KL, Nussbaum AM, Wang GS. The pharmacologic and clinical effects of medical cannabis. Pharmacotherapy. 2013;33:195–209.
3. Hill AJ, Williams CM, Whalley BJ, Stephens GJ. Phytocannabinoids as novel therapeutic agents in CNS disorders. Pharmacol Ther. 2012;133:79–97.
4. Zuardi AW. Cannabidiol: from an inactive cannabinoid to a drug with wide spectrum of action. Rev Bras Psiquiatr. 2008;30:271–80.
5. Griffin G, Atkinson PJ, Showalter VM, Martin BR, Abood ME. Evaluation of cannabinoid receptor agonists and antagonists using the guanosine-5′-O-(3-[35S]thio)-triphosphate binding assay in rat cerebellar membranes. J Pharmacol Exp Ther. 1998;285:553–60.
6. Pertwee RG. The diverse CB1 and CB2 receptor pharmacology of three plant cannabinoids: delta9-tetrahydrocannabinol, cannabidiol and delta9-tetrahydrocannabivarin. Br J Pharmacol. 2008;153:199–215.
7. Laprairie RB, Bagher AM, Kelly ME, Denovan-Wright EM. Cannabidiol is a negative allosteric modulator of the cannabinoid CB1 receptor. Br J Pharmacol. 2015;172:4790–805.
8. Ryberg E, Larsson N, Sjogren S, Hjorth S, Hermansson NO, Leonova J, et al. The orphan receptor GPR55 is a novel cannabinoid receptor. Br J Pharmacol. 2007;152:1092–101.
9. De Petrocellis L, Vellani V, Schiano-Moriello A, Marini P, Magherini PC, Orlando P, et al. Plant-derived cannabinoids modulate the activity of transient receptor potential channels of ankyrin type-1 and melastatin type-8. J Pharmacol Exp Ther. 2008;325:1007–15.
10. Russo EB, Burnett A, Hall B, Parker KK. Agonistic properties of cannabidiol at 5-HT1a receptors. Neurochem Res. 2005;30:1037–43.
11. Ahrens J, Demir R, Leuwer M, de la Roche J, Krampfl K, Foadi N, et al. The nonpsychotropic cannabinoid cannabidiol modulates and directly activates alpha-1 and alpha-1-Beta glycine receptor function. Pharmacology. 2009;83:217–22.
12. Xiong W, Cui T, Cheng K, Yang F, Chen SR, Willenbring D, et al. Cannabinoids suppress inflammatory and neuropathic pain by targeting alpha3 glycine receptors. J Exp Med. 2012;209:1121–34.
13. Hampson AJ, Grimaldi M, Axelrod J, Wink D. Cannabidiol and (−)Delta9-tetrahydrocannabinol are neuroprotective antioxidants. Proc Natl Acad Sci U S A. 1998;95:8268–73.
14. Hayakawa K, Mishima K, Fujiwara M. Therapeutic potential of non-psychotropic Cannabidiol in ischemic stroke. Pharmaceuticals (Basel). 2010;3:2197–212.
15. Fernandez-Ruiz J, Sagredo O, Pazos MR, Garcia C, Pertwee R, Mechoulam R, et al. Cannabidiol for neurodegenerative disorders: important new clinical applications for this phytocannabinoid? Br J Clin Pharmacol. 2013;75:323–33.
16. Iuvone T, Esposito G, Esposito R, Santamaria R, Di RM, Izzo AA. Neuroprotective effect of cannabidiol, a non-psychoactive component from Cannabis sativa, on beta-amyloid-induced toxicity in PC12 cells. J Neurochem. 2004;89:134–41.
17. Lastres-Becker I, Molina-Holgado F, Ramos JA, Mechoulam R, Fernandez-Ruiz J. Cannabinoids provide neuroprotection against 6-hydroxydopamine toxicity in vivo and in vitro: relevance to Parkinson's disease. Neurobiol Dis. 2005;19:96–107.
18. Perucca E. Cannabinoids in the treatment of epilepsy: hard evidence at last? J Epilepsy Res. 2017;7:61–76.
19. Leo A, Russo E, Elia M. Cannabidiol and epilepsy: rationale and therapeutic potential. Pharmacol Res. 2016;107:85–92.
20. dos Santos RG, Hallak JE, Leite JP, Zuardi AW, Crippa JA. Phytocannabinoids and epilepsy. J Clin Pharm Ther. 2015;40:135–43.
21. Neelakantan H, Tallarida RJ, Reichenbach ZW, Tuma RF, Ward SJ, Walker EA. Distinct interactions of cannabidiol and morphine in three nociceptive behavioral models in mice. Behav Pharmacol. 2015;26:304–14.
22. Costa B, Trovato AE, Comelli F, Giagnoni G, Colleoni M. The non-psychoactive cannabis constituent cannabidiol is an orally effective therapeutic agent in rat chronic inflammatory and neuropathic pain. Eur J Pharmacol. 2007;556:75–83.
23. Toth CC, Jedrzejewski NM, Ellis CL, Frey WH. Cannabinoid-mediated modulation of neuropathic pain and microglial accumulation in a model of murine type I diabetic peripheral neuropathic pain. Mol Pain. 2010;6:16.
24. Ward SJ, Ramirez MD, Neelakantan H, Walker EA. Cannabidiol prevents the development of cold and mechanical allodynia in paclitaxel-treated female C57Bl6 mice. Anesth Analg. 2011;113:947–50.
25. Hausman-Kedem M, Menascu S, Kramer U. Efficacy of CBD-enriched medical cannabis for treatment of refractory epilepsy in children and adolescents - an observational, longitudinal study. Brain and Development. 2018;40:544–51.
26. Rodríguez-Muñoz M, Cortés-Montero E, Pozo-Rodrigalvarez A, Sánchez-Blázquez P, Garzón-Niño J. The ON:OFF switch, σ1R-HINT1 protein, controls GPCR-NMDA receptor cross-regulation: implications in neurological disorders. Oncotarget. 2015;6:35458–77.
27. Rodríguez-Muñoz M, Sánchez-Blázquez P, Herrero-Labrador R, Martínez-Murillo R, Merlos M, Vela JM, et al. The σ1 receptor engages the redox-regulated HINT1 protein to bring opioid analgesia under NMDA receptor negative control. Antioxid Redox Signal. 2015;22:799–818.
28. Kourrich S, Su TP, Fujimoto M, Bonci A. The sigma-1 receptor: roles in neuronal plasticity and disease. Trends Neurosci. 2012;35:762–71.
29. Robson MJ, Noorbakhsh B, Seminerio MJ, Matsumoto RR. Sigma-1 receptors: potential targets for the treatment of substance abuse. Curr Pharm Des. 2012;18:902–19.
30. Hayashi T, Tsai SY, Mori T, Fujimoto M, Su TP. Targeting ligand-operated chaperone sigma-1 receptors in the treatment of neuropsychiatric disorders. Expert Opin Ther Targets. 2011;15:557–77.
31. Sanchez-Fernandez C, Nieto FR, Gonzalez-Cano R, Artacho-Cordon A, Romero L, Montilla-Garcia A, et al. Potentiation of morphine-induced mechanical antinociception by sigma(1) receptor inhibition: role of peripheral sigma(1) receptors. Neuropharmacology. 2013;70:348–58.
32. Kim HW, Kwon YB, Roh DH, Yoon SY, Han HJ, Kim KW, et al. Intrathecal treatment with sigma1 receptor antagonists reduces formalin-induced phosphorylation of NMDA receptor subunit 1 and the second phase of formalin test in mice. Br J Pharmacol. 2006;148:490–8.
33. Diaz JL, Zamanillo D, Corbera J, Baeyens JM, Maldonado R, Pericas MA, et al. Selective sigma-1 (sigma1) receptor antagonists: emerging target for the treatment of neuropathic pain. Cent Nerv Syst Agents Med Chem. 2009;9:172–83.
34. Romero L, Zamanillo D, Nadal X, Sanchez-Arroyos R, Rivera-Arconada I, Dordal A, et al. Pharmacological properties of S1RA, a new sigma-1 receptor antagonist that inhibits neuropathic pain and activity-induced spinal sensitization. Br J Pharmacol. 2012;166:2289–306.
35. Ruscher K, Shamloo M, Rickhag M, Ladunga I, Soriano L, Gisselsson L, et al. The sigma-1 receptor enhances brain plasticity and functional recovery after experimental stroke. Brain. 2011;134:732–46.
36. Sánchez-Blázquez P, Pozo-Rodrigalvarez A, Merlos M, Garzón J. The Sigma-1 receptor antagonist, S1RA, reduces stroke damage, ameliorates post-stroke neurological deficits and suppresses the overexpression of MMP-9. Mol Neurobiol. 2018;55:4940–51.
37. Sourbron J, Smolders I, de WP, Lagae L. Pharmacological analysis of the anti-epileptic mechanisms of Fenfluramine in scn1a mutant zebrafish. Front Pharmacol. 2017;8:191.
38. Collina S, Gaggeri R, Marra A, Bassi A, Negrinotti S, Negri F, et al. Sigma receptor modulators: a patent review. Expert Opin Ther Pat. 2013;23:597–613.
39. Martina M, Turcotte ME, Halman S, Bergeron R. The sigma-1 receptor modulates NMDA receptor synaptic transmission and plasticity via SK channels in rat hippocampus. J Physiol. 2007;578:143–57.
40. Balasuriya D, Stewart AP, Edwardson JM. The sigma-1 receptor interacts directly with GluN1 but not GluN2A in the GluN1/GluN2A NMDA receptor. J Neurosci. 2013;33:18219–24.
41. Ehlers MD, Zhang S, Bernhadt JP, Huganir RL. Inactivation of NMDA receptors by direct interaction of calmodulin with the NR1 subunit. Cell. 1996;84:745–55.
42. Rodríguez-Muñoz M, Sánchez-Blázquez P, Garzón J. Fenfluramine diminishes NMDA receptor-mediated seizures via its mixed activity at serotonin 5HT2A and type 1 sigma receptors. Oncotarget. 2018;9:23373–89.

43. Mathis C, Ungerer A. Comparative analysis of seizures induced by intracerebroventricular administration of NMDA, kainate and quisqualate in mice. Exp Brain Res. 1992;88:277–82.

44. Moreau JL, Pieri L, Prud'hon B. Convulsions induced by centrally administered NMDA in mice: effects of NMDA antagonists, benzodiazepines, minor tranquilizers and anticonvulsants. Br J Pharmacol. 1989;98:1050–4.

45. Czuczwar SJ. Glutamate receptor antagonists as potential antiepileptic drugs. Neurol Neurochir Pol. 2000;34(Suppl 8):41–6.

46. Nemmani KV, Grisel JE, Stowe JR, Smith Carliss R, Mogil JS. Modulation of morphine analgesia by site-specific N-methyl-D-aspartate receptor antagonists: dependence on sex, site of antagonism, morphine dose, and time. Pain. 2004;109:274–83.

47. Trotman M, Vermehren P, Gibson CL, Fern R. The dichotomy of memantine treatment for ischemic stroke: dose-dependent protective and detrimental effects. J Cereb Blood Flow Metab. 2015;35:230–9.

48. Kim HC, Bing G, Jhoo WK, Kim WK, Shin EJ, Im DH, et al. Metabolism to dextrorphan is not essential for dextromethorphan's anticonvulsant activity against kainate in mice. Life Sci. 2003;72:769–83.

49. Mei J, Pasternak GW. Sigma1 receptor modulation of opioid analgesia in the mouse. J Pharmacol Exp Ther. 2002;300:1070–4.

50. Sánchez-Blázquez P, Rodríguez-Muñoz M, Vicente-Sánchez A, Garzón J. Cannabinoid receptors couple to NMDA receptors to reduce the production of NO and the mobilization of zinc induced by glutamate. Antioxid Redox Signal. 2013;19:1766–82.

51. Grishin AA, Benquet P, Gerber U. Muscarinic receptor stimulation reduces NMDA responses in CA3 hippocampal pyramidal cells via Ca2+−dependent activation of tyrosine phosphatase. Neuropharmacology. 2005;49:328–37.

52. Yuen EY, Jiang Q, Chen P, Gu Z, Feng J, Yan Z. Serotonin 5-HT1A receptors regulate NMDA receptor channels through a microtubule-dependent mechanism. J Neurosci. 2005;25:5488–501.

53. Liu W, Yuen EY, Allen PB, Feng J, Greengard P, Yan Z. Adrenergic modulation of NMDA receptors in prefrontal cortex is differentially regulated by RGS proteins and spinophilin. Proc Natl Acad Sci U S A. 2006;103:18338–43.

54. Jiao H, Zhang L, Gao F, Lou D, Zhang J, Xu M. Dopamine D(1) and D(3) receptors oppositely regulate. J Neurochem. 2007;103:840–8.

55. Wang X, Zhong P, Gu Z, Yan Z. Regulation of NMDA receptors by dopamine D4 signaling in prefrontal cortex. J Neurosci. 2003;23:9852–61.

56. Gu Z, Liu W, Wei J, Yan Z. Regulation of N-methyl-D-aspartic acid (NMDA) receptors by metabotropic glutamate receptor 7. J Biol Chem. 2012;287:10265–75.

57. Rubinstein M, Cepeda C, Hurst RS, Flores-Hernandez J, Ariano MA, Falzone TL, et al. Dopamine D4 receptor-deficient mice display cortical hyperexcitability. J Neurosci. 2001;21:3756–63.

58. Su TP, Hayashi T, Maurice T, Buch S, Ruoho AE. The sigma-1 receptor chaperone as an inter-organelle signaling modulator. Trends Pharmacol Sci. 2010;31:557–66.

59. Ben AM. Cannabinoids in medicine: a review of their therapeutic potential. J Ethnopharmacol. 2006;105:1–25.

60. Crippa JA, Zuardi AW, Hallak JE. Therapeutical use of the cannabinoids in psychiatry. Rev Bras Psiquiatr. 2010;32(Suppl 1):S56–66.

61. Ghosh P, Bhattacharya SK. Anticonvulsant action of cannabis in the rat: role of brain monoamines. Psychopharmacology. 1978;59:293–7.

62. Mechoulam R, Carlini EA. Toward drugs derived from cannabis. Naturwissenschaften. 1978;65:174–9.

63. Robson PJ. Therapeutic potential of cannabinoid medicines. Drug Test Anal. 2014;6:24–30.

64. Ortiz-Renteria M, Juarez-Contreras R, Gonzalez-Ramirez R, Islas LD, Sierra-Ramirez F, Llorente I, et al. TRPV1 channels and the progesterone receptor sig-1R interact to regulate pain. Proc Natl Acad Sci U S A. 2018;115:E1657–66.

65. Pal A, Fontanilla D, Gopalakrishnan A, Chae YK, Markley JL, Ruoho AE. The sigma-1 receptor protects against cellular oxidative stress and activates antioxidant response elements. Eur J Pharmacol. 2012;682:12–20.

66. Shibuya H, Mori H, Toru M. Sigma receptors in schizophrenic cerebral cortices. Neurochem Res. 1992;17:983–90.

67. Weissman AD, Casanova MF, Kleinman JE, London ED, De Souza EB. Selective loss of cerebral cortical sigma, but not PCP binding sites in schizophrenia. Biol Psychiatry. 1991;29:41–54.

68. Rodríguez-Muñoz M, Sánchez-Blázquez P, Callado LF, Meana JJ, Garzón-Niño J. Schizophrenia and depression, two poles of endocannabinoid system deregulation. Transl Psychiatry. 2017;7:1291.

69. Marsicano G, Goodenough S, Monory K, Hermann H, Eder M, Cannich A, et al. CB1 cannabinoid receptors and on-demand defense against excitotoxicity. Science. 2003;302:84–8.

70. Rodríguez-Muñoz M, Sánchez-Blázquez P, Merlos M, Garzón-Niño J. Endocannabinoid control of glutamate NMDA receptors: the therapeutic potential and consequences of dysfunction. Oncotarget. 2016;7:55840–62.

71. Leweke FM, Piomelli D, Pahlisch F, Muhl D, Gerth CW, Hoyer C, et al. Cannabidiol enhances anandamide signaling and alleviates psychotic symptoms of schizophrenia. Transl Psychiatry. 2012;2:e94.

72. Ritsner M, Maayan R, Gibel A, Weizman A. Differences in blood pregnenolone and dehydroepiandrosterone levels between schizophrenia patients and healthy subjects. Eur Neuropsychopharmacol. 2007;17:358–65.

73. Shirayama Y, Hashimoto K, Suzuki Y, Higuchi T. Correlation of plasma neurosteroid levels to the severity of negative symptoms in male patients with schizophrenia. Schizophr Res. 2002;58:69–74.

74. Ritsner MS, Gibel A, Shleifer T, Boguslavsky I, Zayed A, Maayan R, et al. Pregnenolone and dehydroepiandrosterone as an adjunctive treatment in schizophrenia and schizoaffective disorder: an 8-week, double-blind, randomized, controlled, 2-center, parallel-group trial. J Clin Psychiatry. 2010;71:1351–62.

75. Busquets GA, Soria-Gomez E, Bellocchio L, Marsicano G. Cannabinoid receptor type-1: breaking the dogmas. F1000Res. 2016;5.

76. Sánchez-Blázquez P, Rodríguez-Muñoz M, Herrero-Labrador R, Burgueño J, Zamanillo D, Garzón J. The calcium-sensitive Sigma-1 receptor prevents cannabinoids from provoking glutamate NMDA receptor hypofunction: implications in antinociception and psychotic diseases. Int J Neuropsychopharmacol. 2014;17:1943–55.

77. Ryan D, Drysdale AJ, Lafourcade C, Pertwee RG, Platt B. Cannabidiol targets mitochondria to regulate intracellular Ca2+ levels. J Neurosci. 2009;29:2053–63.

78. De Petrocellis L, Ligresti A, Moriello AS, Allara M, Bisogno T, Petrosino S, et al. Effects of cannabinoids and cannabinoid-enriched Cannabis extracts on TRP channels and endocannabinoid metabolic enzymes. Br J Pharmacol. 2011;163:1479–94.

79. Haley TJ, MCcormick WG. Pharmacological effects produced by intracerebral injection of drugs in the conscious mouse. Br J Pharmacol Chemother. 1957;12:12–5.

3

Oxidative stress and cellular pathologies in Parkinson's disease

Lesly Puspita[1], Sun Young Chung[2] and Jae-won Shim[1]* ⓘ

Abstract

Parkinson's disease (PD) is a chronic and progressive neurodegeneration of dopamine neurons in the substantia nigra. The reason for the death of these neurons is unclear; however, studies have demonstrated the potential involvement of mitochondria, endoplasmic reticulum, α-synuclein or dopamine levels in contributing to cellular oxidative stress as well as PD symptoms. Even though those papers had separately described the individual roles of each element leading to neurodegeneration, recent publications suggest that neurodegeneration is the product of various cellular interactions. This review discusses the role of oxidative stress in mediating separate pathological events that together, ultimately result in cell death in PD. Understanding the multi-faceted relationships between these events, with oxidative stress as a common denominator underlying these processes, is needed for developing better therapeutic strategies.

Keywords: Alpha-synuclein, Dopamine neurons, Mitochondria, Oxidative stress, Parkinson's disease, Reactive oxygen species, Unfolded protein response

Introduction

Parkinson's disease (PD) is the second most common neurodegenerative disorder, characterized by serious movement disturbances such as tremor, rigidity, and bradykinesia. It is a chronic condition attributed by the selective degeneration of dopamine (DA) neurons in the midbrain substantia nigra (SN). By the time patients experience these symptoms, a portion of DA neurons that project from the SN to the striatum have already degenerated [1, 2]. Appearance of insoluble inclusions in neurons called Lewy bodies, which mainly consist of α-synuclein, is a major hallmark of this disease [1]. Based on its progressive nature, it is unlikely that the disease pathogenesis is triggered by an acute toxicity that kills cells directly. Instead, it is possible that an ongoing process such as oxidation is responsible for the gradual dysfunction that manifests across myriad cellular pathways throughout the disease trajectory.

Most PD cases are sporadic, with only about 10% associated with an inherited genetic component. Even though familial cases comprise only a minor subset of the overall PD pool, examining PD-related monogenic mutations is a valuable method of understanding disease pathogenesis and cell death which may have implications for studying the disease at large. PTEN induced putative kinase 1 (PINK1), Parkin, DJ-1, leucine-rich repeat kinase 2 (LRRK2) and α-synuclein are among the proteins which have been strongly linked to the familial forms of PD [3–7]. Of these, α-synuclein is most commonly associated with PD pathogenesis for its predominance in Lewy bodies, which develop and aggregate throughout disease progression [8, 9]. PINK1 and Parkin are involved in mitochondria-related autophagy, whereas the loss of function of these proteins leads to the accumulation of damaged mitochondria [10, 11]. DJ-1 is involved in a wide range of cellular functions, two of which include its roles as a sensor for oxidative stress and as a redox-chaperone protein [12, 13]. The physiological function of LRRK2 is less understood but neurons with mutations in this protein exhibit greater vulnerability to mitochondrial toxins [14].

Reactive oxygen species (ROS) are normally produced in the cell during mitochondrial electron transfer chain (ETC) or redox reactions and are in fact a necessary component of cellular homeostasis. As an example, several enzymes in mitogen-activated protein kinase and

---
* Correspondence: shimj@sch.ac.kr
[1]Soonchunhyang Institute of Medi-bio Science (SIMS), Soonchunhyang University, 25, Bongjeong-ro, Dongnam-gu, Cheonan-si 31151, South Korea
Full list of author information is available at the end of the article

phosphoinositide 3-kinase pathways, which are pivotal in mediating cellular responses to growth hormones and cytokines, are regulated directly by ROS [15–17]. Yet despite the importance of ROS in normal physiology, antioxidant proteins like superoxide dismutase (SOD) and glutathione (GSH) also prevent ROS levels from getting too high [18]. Failure of these antioxidants in regulating ROS levels leads to oxidative stress, which can have a variety of detrimental effects. Random oxidation of macromolecules inside the cell can damage cellular structures and even lead to cell death [19–21]. Previous publications have reported evidence of oxidative stress through the detection of oxidized DNA, lipids, and proteins in the brain tissues of both familial and sporadic PD patients [22, 23]. Since oxidative stress increases the chance of spontaneous mutations, it is possible that this can trigger mutations that make cells more vulnerable to dysfunction. Interestingly, in the SN of healthy individuals, the concentration of oxidized proteins was found to be twice that of the caudate, putamen, and the frontal cortex, indicating that susceptibility of SN to oxidative stress may contribute to the selective neuronal degeneration [24].

While many studies in the past have examined dysfunctional cellular processes in PD independently of each other, in our recent study, we sought to develop a more comprehensive understanding of the disease by examining how those processes might be interconnected [25]. Using induced pluripotent stem cell (iPSC)-derived midbrain DA neurons from patients with PINK1 or Parkin mutations, we first noted the presence of abnormal mitochondria. We also observed cytosolic α-synuclein and DA accumulation, with increased sensitivity toward oxidative stress-inducing agents, in the mutant lines [25]. Similarly, another group which had utilized LRRK2 mutant iPSC-derived neurons noted elevated expression of genes involved in oxidative stress regulation, and α-synuclein levels. Moreover, they observed cells' increased vulnerability towards H_2O_2, 6-hydroxydopamine (6-OHDA), and MG132, a proteasome inhibitor [26]. Together, these results reflect the idea that a single mutation can profoundly disrupt cellular homeostasis, implying that PD progression may be the result of a multitude of interactions between the various pathogenic phenotypes linked to cellular stress.

While oxidative stress has been thoroughly researched, advances in stem cell technology have engendered a wide range of tools with which to study and model diseases in vitro. As demonstrated by our study as well as many others, iPSCs have made it possible to study specific disease mutations using patient derived cells, which has been especially valuable in modeling neurodegenerative diseases which lack authentic animal models. Moreover, because PD is diagnosed only when the

degeneration of midbrain DA neurons has already progressed considerably, neurons from PD patient-derived iPSCs enable researchers to carefully track even minor disturbances that precede major pathogenic processes. Based on our iPSC-based findings demonstrating the contribution of oxidative stress toward triggering dysfunctional processes, this review explores how oxidative stress may play a central role in mediating disease progression (Fig. 1).

The mitochondrion is a key site of ROS production and a target of ROS-induced damage

In the inner membrane of mitochondria, electrons are transferred through a series of protein complexes via redox reactions to oxygen, the last electron acceptor. As the electrons pass, some protons are translocated by the electron carriers from the matrix to the mitochondrial intermembrane space, thereby creating a proton gradient. Protons flow back into the mitochondrial matrix following its gradient, concurrently providing energy for the ATP synthase to phosphorylate ADP into ATP. This entire process, which is a critical means of energy production, produces ROS as a major byproduct [27]. Premature electron leakage in ETC Complex I (Nicotinamide adenine dinucleotide [NADH] dehydrogenase) and Complex III (cytochrome bc1) to oxygen, is the main source of mitochondrial superoxide anions (O_2^-) [28, 29]. Production of ROS from the mitochondrial action is physiologic, but dysfunction of ETC in damaged mitochondrial causes excessive ROS production, which is quite detrimental to cells.

The involvement of mitochondria in PD pathogenesis was first brought to light after individuals consumed illicit drugs contaminated with 1-methyl-4-phenyl-1,2,3,6-tetrabydropyridine (MPTP). Symptoms resembling those present in PD were observed soon after drug intake with postmortem analyses revealing destruction of the SN [30]. Subsequent studies explained that 1-methyl-4-phenylpyridinium (MPP+), the toxic bioactive form of MPTP, undergoes oxidation by monoamine oxidase B (MAO-B) and enters the DA-producing neurons in the SN via the DA reuptake system [31]. Upon entering the cell, MPP+ inhibits the mitochondrial ETC Complex I enzyme, and NADH-ubiquinone oxidoreductase (EC 1.6.5.3), resulting in electron leakage and ROS generation in mitochondria [32]. Similarly, rotenone, a pesticide, also induces parkinsonism by inhibiting ETC Complex I. Due to its hydrophobicity, rotenone easily crosses biological membranes independently of the DA transporter and its delivery causes systemic inhibition of the mitochondrial ETC. Notably, the degeneration is specific to midbrain DA neurons, while other DA-producing neurons in the ventral tegmental area (VTA) may be relatively spared [33]. Such decline of Complex I activity and elevated intracellular

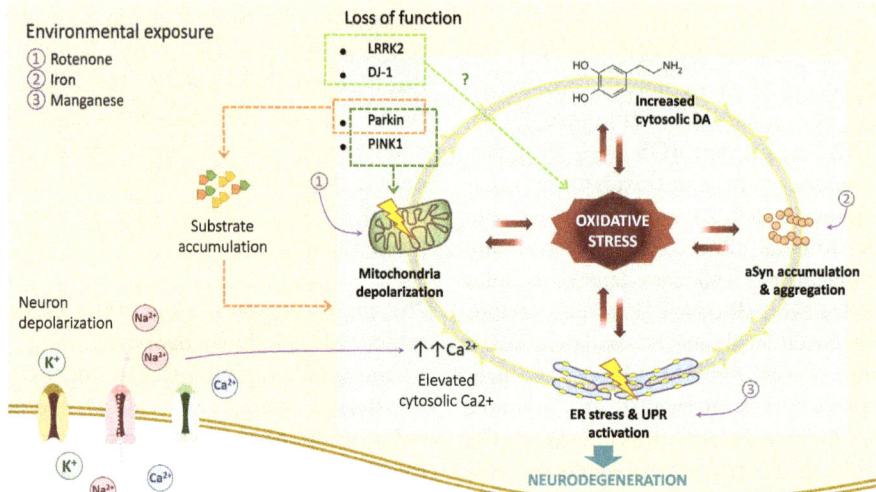

Fig. 1 Central role of chronic oxidative stress in mediating PD progression. Mitochondria depolarization, ER stress, α-synuclein accumulation and increased level of cytosolic DA are known PD phenotypes that potentially contribute to cellular oxidative stress, alone or by interacting with each other. ER regulates cytosolic calcium and thus prevents excess uptake by MCU that otherwise can stimulate ETC and ROS production in mitochondria, an essential function in neurons with intense depolarization. α-synuclein accumulation can contribute to ER stress by binding to ER chaperones and disturbing vesicle trafficking between ER and Golgi. While UPR activation also stimulate α-synuclein aggregation by unclear mechanism. Utilization of DA risks midbrain DA neurons to oxidative damage by DA metabolism. Additionally, DA has been shown to trigger α-synuclein oligomer formation and mitochondria depolarization. Altogether, these phenotypes produce oxidative environment that further amplifies the damage. Mutations that disturb the function of LRRK2, DJ-1, Parkin and PINK1 have been linked to familial cases of PD. Parkin is an E3 ubiquitin ligase and dysfunctionality of this protein results in accumulation of its substrates. Together with PINK1, Parkin is also responsible to clear up damaged mitochondria. One of DJ-1 putative role as sensor of oxidative stress may be necessary in cell protection. Single mutation in *LRRK2* resulted in increased susceptibility towards oxidative stressor, even though the mechanism is less understood. Pesticide rotenone, iron and manganese also cause cellular oxidative stress by triggering mitochondria depolarization, α-synuclein oligomerization together with ROS production and UPR activation, respectively. Long term exposure of those substances has been linked with higher risk of developing sporadic PD

ROS have been verified in the SN of the post-mortem brain of PD patients [34, 35].

Further supporting the importance of the mitochondria and its relevance in PD is the fact that PD-related genes such as *PINK1*, *PARK2* (Parkin), *DJ-1* and *LRRK2* encode proteins that regulate mitochondrial and ROS homeostasis [3, 4, 6, 7, 36]. PINK1 is a mitochondrial protein that is degraded rapidly in healthy mitochondria. In defective mitochondria, which may exhibit high levels of oxidative stress, decreased membrane potential, or the presence of misfolded proteins, the degradation of PINK1 is impeded, leading to the accumulation of PINK1 on the mitochondrial outer membrane. PINK1, which phosphorylates Parkin at Ser65, induces E3 ubiquitin ligase activity of the enzyme and its recruitment to the mitochondria. Parkin modifies proteins on the mitochondrial membrane by adding ubiquitin chains that function as signals for autophagy. The mitochondria-specific autophagy process, also known as mitophagy, ultimately results in mitochondria engulfment and degradation [10, 11] which has been demonstrated experimentally where the systemic knock-out of Parkin in mice resulted in elevated intracellular ROS levels in the VTA and a reduction in proteins involved in ETC and oxidative stress regulation [37]. In

drosophila, PINK1 null mutants exhibited reduced mitochondrial membrane potential, suboptimal ETC activity, as well as a reduction in synaptic neurotransmitter release in neural cells [38]. Moreover, accumulation of damaged mitochondria in neuronal axons, as observed in PINK1 knock-out mutants, could be a source of ROS and oxidative damage [39].

Defects in mitophagy and increased oxidative stress might also partially explain the specificity of the phenotypes in DA neurons. As shown in PINK1 null mutants that display reduced neurotransmitter release, mitochondria are critical in cells with actively firing axons [38]. In an unusual case of a woman with a homozygote recessive Parkin mutation, she remained free of PD symptoms even through her eighth decade, while her relative carrying the same mutation exhibited early onset of PD. When comparing their fibroblasts, it was found that Nip3-like protein X, which may mediate a Parkin/PINK1-independent pathway in eliminating damaged mitochondria, was highly upregulated in the asymptomatic carrier. Levels of mitochondrial membrane potential, oxygen consumption rate, and resistance capacity toward protonophore carbonyl cyanide-m-chlorophenylhydrazone (CCCP) were higher in fibroblasts derived from the asymptomatic carrier than those of the individual with PD symptoms. Although the study was conducted in fibroblasts and not midbrain DA neurons, the data strongly suggested that failure in mitochondria clearance or in other words, accumulation of defective mitochondria, was an important factor in mediating PD pathology [40]. Another protein related to a recessive form of PD, DJ-1, contains a cysteine residue (C106) that is vulnerable to oxidation during oxidative stress. Oxidation of C106 leading to the formation of cysteine-sulfinic acid has been verified using mass spectrophotometry [41] and crystal analysis of DJ-1. During oxidative stress, the oxidized DJ-1 may translocate to the outer membrane of mitochondria and it has been shown to prevent MPP + –induced cell death, the mechanism of which remains unclear [12]. In line with this finding, homozygous mutation of DJ-1 has been linked to increased mitochondrial oxidative stress in human iPSC-derived DA neurons, a feature that was accompanied by accumulation of α-synuclein and oxidized form of DA [42].

As one of the main sites of ROS production, mitochondria are particularly susceptible to oxidative stress-induced damage. Unlike nuclear DNA, mitochondrial DNA (mtDNA) are unprotected by histone proteins and therefore are easy targets of oxidation [43]. ROS production and mtDNA damage has been shown to increase with age, up to 10–20 folds higher than in nuclear DNA [44, 45]. Since most of the proteins coded by mtDNA are involved in ETC, mutations and deletions in mtDNA would likely disturb ETC and increase ROS formation, creating a vicious cycle further inflicting mitochondrial damage [46]. Another mechanism of how this cycle might work involves nitrosative stress induced by either mitochondrial toxins or mutated α-synuclein proteins. In Ryan et al., these were shown to cause sulfonation on myocyte-specific enhancer factor 2C (MEF2C). This modification inhibits MEF2C transcriptional activity and consequently, decreases expression of the target genes. One of the important genes regulated by MEF2C encodes peroxisome proliferator-activated receptor gamma coactivator 1-alpha (PGC-1a), a master regulator of mitochondria biogenesis. Therefore, failure to express PGC-1a implies dysfunction among mitochondria [47].

ER protein folding and calcium storage functions are prominent sources of ROS

The endoplasmic reticulum (ER) is the site of secretory protein production and post-translational modifications such as protein folding and glycosylation. Protein folding is a process that is greatly affected by the redox status of the ER lumen as the formation of disulfide bonds requires a highly oxidizing environment. During disulfide bond formation, electrons are transferred from the target protein to oxygen by protein disulfide isomerase and ER oxidoreductin-1, which forms ROS as byproduct [48, 49]. Quantitative analyses of protein synthesis and processing suggest that disulfide bond formation produces approximately 25% of total ROS in the ER lumen [50].

Another vital role of the ER entails regulation of intracellular calcium, involving the release or absorption of calcium to regulate its cytoplasmic concentration levels. Failure to maintain the calcium concentration in homeostasis and accumulation of misfolded proteins may lead to the activation of the unfolded protein response (UPR) [51]. UPR is a protective mechanism which is initiated by three proteins in the ER membrane: inositol-requiring enzyme 1 (IRE1), activating transcription factor (ATF) 6, and pancreatic ER kinase (PKR)-like ER kinase (PERK) which each bind to GRP78/BIP (binding immunoglobulin protein), a chaperone in the ER lumen. In the presence of misfolded proteins, BIP dissociates from the membrane proteins to bind the misfolded proteins. Dissociation from BIP activates the three membrane proteins and the following pathways. IRE1 splices the intron in X-box binding protein 1 (XBP1) RNA to produce its translationally active form. After dissociation from BIP, ATF6 is translocated from the ER to the Golgi apparatus, where it is cleaved and activated. Both XBP1 and ATF6 act as transcriptional regulators of ER chaperones and ER-associated degradation pathways, which are essential for reducing ER stress and promoting cell survival. Lastly, BIP dissociation triggers autophosphorylation of PERK into phosphorylated PERK (pPERK). Phosphorylation of initiation factor 1 subunit α (eIF2α) by p-PERK results in global attenuation of protein translation. However, the attenuation does not apply to certain PERK-downstream proteins like ATF4. Prolonged expression of ATF4 can trigger the expression of another transcription factor, C/EBP homologous protein (CHOP), and the downstream apoptotic pathway [52, 53]. Activation of the ATF4/CHOP pathway could lead to apoptosis and has thus far been suggested as a part of the neuronal apoptotic signaling pathway [54].

The ER's function in regulating calcium and the downstream events can greatly affect mitochondria. Calcium leakage from the ER into the cytosol due to ER stress can trigger excessive calcium intake by the mitochondria via mitochondrial calcium uniporter (MCU) [55–58]. ER-to-mitochondria transfer of calcium is facilitated by mitochondrial-associated membrane (MAM) which brings both organelles in close proximity [59, 60]. As visualized in human fibroblasts using green fluorescence protein-tagged ER membrane protein and the mitochondrial dye tetramethylrhodamine methyl ester, enhanced proximity of both organelles was observed in fibroblasts containing Parkin mutation compared to those of control fibroblasts [61]. As expected, calcium transfer to mitochondria was equally increased. Downregulation of Parkin substrate mitofusin 2, another MAM tethering protein [62], or exogenous expression of Parkin was shown to rescue the disturbance of calcium homeostasis in the mutant fibroblasts [61]. Moreover, it has been found that increased calcium in the mitochondria leads to the stimulation of ETC and can exacerbate ROS formation, or induce the activation of mitochondria-related apoptotic pathways [63, 64].

In PD cases, immunoreactivity of pPerk and peIF2a were observed by Hoozemans and colleagues in the SN of patients compared to those of healthy individuals [65]. Another study revealed that treatment with either MPP+ or 6-OHDA induced the changing of UPR proteins such as expression of BIP and CHOP, and phosphorylation of PERK and eIF2α, while relieving ER stress with salubrinal, a selective inhibitor of eIF2α dephosphorylation, attenuated mitochondrial toxin-induced cell death [66]. ER stress might also impact cellular oxidative stress through regulation of mitochondrial clearance. Putative ATF4 binding sites were found upstream of the transcriptional start site and in the first intron of the human $PARK2$ gene. To verify this, ER stress was triggered in SH-SY5Y, human embryonic kidney T293 cells, and mouse embryonic fibroblasts by using the ER $Ca2+$ –ATPase inhibitor thapsigargin, the N-glycosylation inhibitor tunicamycin, and inducing amino acid starvation. In all experiments, upregulation of Parkin mRNA was observed. Data from a luciferase reporter assay and chromatin immunoprecipitation provided further evidence that ATF4 functions as a transcriptional regulator of Parkin [67]. A separate study also supported this idea by showing that ATF4 protects from neuronal apoptosis by regulating the level of Parkin [68]. Altogether the studies suggest the failure in degradation of Parkin's substrates that is required during UPR activation may contribute to the neurodegeneration in PD with Parkin mutation. Nonetheless, further research is needed to determine whether ER stress is directly involved in the pathogenic mechanism of Parkin-associated PD.

Increased risk of developing sporadic PD after overexposure to manganese, copper, iron and mercury has been studied for decades [69, 70] where it has been suggested that α-synuclein, ER stress, and oxidative stress are involved in manganese toxicity in neurons. After 24 h of manganese treatment, α-synuclein oligomerization, elevated ROS, and oxidative damage of macromolecules have been observed in primary neuronal cultures. As an example, pre-treatment with GSH partially rescued the α-synuclein oligomerization and neuronal damage while H_2O_2 accelerated the process [66]. Xu et al. demonstrated that manganese treatment on rat brain slices induced expression of UPR proteins and apoptotic cell death [71]. In the rat models where α-synuclein expression was silenced by siRNA, apoptosis by manganese treatment was less pronounced. Furthermore, pPERK, pEIF2a, and ATF4 protein levels were also lower than those of wild type

(WT) rats, despite the absence of changes in pIRE1 and sXBP1, suggesting α-synuclein involvement in the UPR PERK pathway [71]. In mice with mutant A53T, interaction between α-synuclein with ER chaperones in ER lumen was observed, indicating that abnormalities in α-synuclein alone could trigger ER stress and the downstream response [72]. Activation of IRE1α/XBP1 axis of UPR was also found in iPSC-derived DA neurons obtained from patients with α-synuclein triplication. In support of this, postmortem analyses conducted in the same study verified the presence of pIRE1 together with elevated level of α-synuclein in the brain [73]. Additionally, a recent study with an animal model reported that tunicamycin, an ER stress inducer also affected the aggregation process of α-synuclein [74].

Alpha-synuclein is affected by and contributes to oxidative stress, by binding with iron and mitochondrial membrane proteins

Alpha-synuclein is a 140 kDA protein encoded by the $SNCA$ gene. As the main component of Lewy bodies, α-synuclein is a well-known player in PD pathogenesis as duplication, triplication, and point mutations in its N-terminal region (A30P, A53T and E46K) are connected to familial PD [8, 9]. A growing body of work suggests that the monomer and tetramer types are the physiological forms of α-synuclein, while oligomers and fibrils are the pathogenic forms [75, 76]. Abundance of fibril α-synuclein was detected in Lewy bodies in several studies; however, abnormal accumulation of the soluble monomer form that leads to formation of oligomers and fibrils has also been proposed as a key pathogenic event in the early stages of PD [9, 77].

Spontaneous oligomerization and fibrilization of α-synuclein have also been observed in vitro, with mutated α-synuclein oligomerizing faster than the WT form of the protein [78]. In the same study, DA treatment increased the rate of polymerization in both mutated and WT forms of α-synuclein. Evidence of α-synuclein accumulation as a signature of disease initiation was shown in Nurr1+/tyrosine hydroxylase (TH)+ neurons derived from a patient's iPSCs. Additionally, α-synuclein accumulation was observed in neurons derived from patients with PINK1 or Parkin mutations, along with abnormal mitochondrial morphology and increased sensitivity towards oxidative stress [25]. Deas et al. suggested that interactions between α-synuclein oligomers and metal ions may induce oxidative stress in human iPSC-derived neurons. Neurons with α-synuclein triplication were reported to have a higher basal level of oxidative stress. When monomer, oligomer, or fibril forms of exogenous α-synuclein were added, α-synuclein oligomers triggered oxidative stress more potently than monomers and fibrils. Neurons treated only with oligomer α-synuclein demonstrated a reduction in the level of GSH and an increase in lipid peroxidation [79]. The propensity of oligomers to induce ROS production was significantly reduced in the presence of metal chelators such as deferoxamine, indicating that α-synuclein oligomers produce superoxide radicals by binding to transition metal ions such as copper and iron [80]. In vitro incubation of α-synuclein with iron resulted in the formation of H_2O_2 and hydroxyl radicals, a finding that supported iron-rich SN neurons' selective vulnerability toward oxidative stress [81, 82]. Increased iron has also been detected in the SN of postmortem PD brains as well as living PD patients using magnetic resonance imaging [83–85]. Greater colocalization of iron and DA was found in the SN compared to those in the VTA [86], and given the ability of both substances to modify α-synuclein [81, 82], this can explain the selective vulnerability of this region.

Oxidative stress upon accumulation of α-synuclein can also be mediated by direct interaction between α-synuclein and mitochondrial membrane protein. In fact, α-synuclein has been demonstrated to disturb the translocation of nuclear-encoded mitochondrial proteins into the mitochondria by binding to translocase of the outer membrane (TOM)20 in both rotenone-treated and human α-synuclein-overexpressing animal models. The binding prevents the interaction of TOM20 with the co-receptor TOM22 and the subsequent translocation of mitochondrial-targeted proteins, which include some subunits of Complex I. As a result, mitochondrial ETC is rendered defective and intracellular oxidative stress escalates [87].

While α-synuclein toxicity can contribute in elevating cellular oxidative stress, it has also been suggested that oxidative stress can trigger the toxicity of α-synuclein. One consequence of chronic oxidative stress is lipid peroxidation of polyunsaturated fatty acids in the cell membrane, as observed in post-mortem SN [88]. A product of lipid peroxidation, 4-hyroxy-2-nonenal, prevents fibrillation of α-synuclein and supports the formation of secondary beta sheets and toxic soluble oligomers in a dose-dependent manner [89, 90]. Thus, oxidative stress can also influence α-synuclein toxicity and mediate PD pathogenesis. Incubation of α-synuclein monomers with cytochrome c/H_2O_2 led to α-synuclein aggregation in vitro by catalyzing the crosslinking of α-synuclein tyrosine residues through 3,3′-dityrosine bond formations [91, 92]. Colocalization of cytochrome c and α-synuclein has also been detected in the Lewy body of PD brains [91].

Since accumulation of α-synuclein monomers initiates the formation of aggregates, some studies have shifted their focus toward the α-synuclein degradation process. Both ubiquitin-proteasome system (UPS) and autophagy-lysosomal pathway have been linked with α-synuclein degradation [93], with more recent publications suggesting that UPS is the main α-synuclein degradation pathway under normal physiological conditions, while the lysosomal pathway is more responsive to stress or when α-synuclein is overly abundant [94, 95]. Chaperone-mediated autophagy, a subtype of lysosomal pathway, works with the help of cytosolic chaperone Hsc70 that recognizes the KFERQ peptide motif in α-synuclein [78, 95]. Then α-synuclein is delivered to a receptor in the lysosomal membrane and translocated into the lysosome, where enzymatic degradation takes place. However, in a highly oxidizing environment, the oxidized form of α-synuclein cannot be efficiently degraded, resulting in its accumulation and aggregation [78]. Its accumulation also affects vesicle trafficking between the ER and the Golgi, and reduces lysosomal degradation capacity [96–98]. Supporting this, α-synuclein had been shown to inhibit ER-Golgi transit of COPII vesicles which carries ATF6 to its activation site at the Golgi apparatus. Consequently, the protective ATF6 pathway of UPR signaling was blocked [99].

Oxidative stress and α-synuclein accumulation preceding diminished lysosomal proteolysis has also been observed in patient-derived DJ-1 mutant DA neurons [42]. Attenuation of this process results in the buildup of cargo proteins, which can trigger ER stress and activate the UPR response system, and prolonged ER stress caused by misfolded proteins has been linked to ROS production, possibly due to higher levels of protein folding activity in the ER lumen. Degradation of these misfolded proteins mitigates oxidative stress and associated cell death [96].

Elevated intracellular DA promotes oxidation and increases SN DA neurons' vulnerability towards oxidative stress

It is important to highlight that despite their relevance in PD phenotypes, α-synuclein, PINK1, Parkin, and DJ-1, are not exclusively expressed in midbrain DA neurons [3, 4, 6, 7, 36]. The specific neurodegeneration in loss of function mutants may be caused by the nature of the neurons themselves in their ability to produce and release DA, which can be highly reactive. Its metabolism can lead to the production of ROS byproducts such as hydrogen peroxide. DA synthesis involves several enzymatic reactions beginning with tyrosine hydroxylase catalyzing the hydroxylation of L-tyrosine at the phenol ring to produce L-3,4-dihydroxyphenylalanine (L-DOPA). Next, aromatic acid decarboxylase converts L-DOPA to DA. Active transport by vesicular monoamine transporter 2 (VMAT2) mediates DA storage in vesicles, an important step in protecting DA which is easily oxidized in the cytoplasm. In action potentials, DA vesicles fuse with the presynaptic membrane at the terminal button and are released into the synapse where they engage with receptors in the post-synaptic membranes. After binding, DA molecules can be reabsorbed into the cytosol via the DA transporter where it may undergo several different fates. It can be transported back into storage vesicles by VMAT2 and reused in the next axon firing, or be degraded by MAO, which leads to the production of 3,4-dihydroxyphenylacetaldehyde (DOPAL) and H_2O_2, two potent oxidizing agents [100, 101]. The enzyme aldehyde dehydrogenase turns DOPAL into the less reactive 3,4-dihydroxyphenylacetic acid (DOPAC) [101].

In the presence of iron in the cytosol, DA can be oxidized into DA-quinone (DAQ)—a highly reactive and toxic compound [102, 103]. In fact, the presence of the oxidized form of DA has been verified in iPSC-derived DA neurons containing *parkin, PINK1, LRRK2* mutations or *SNCA* triplication [42]. DAQ binds covalently with free cysteine and cysteine residues on proteins, which can drastically alter their function [104, 105]. It may also be involved in mitochondrial depolarization after DA exposure [106] and its binding to mitochondrial proteins can inhibit Complex I and IV. This was supported by the fact that treatment with quinone scavenger, GSH, reversed this effect. Proteomic analysis of isolated rat mitochondria in the same experiment revealed that mitochondrial proteins had been modified covalently by DAQ, including ubiquinol-cytochrome c reductase core protein 1 [107]. A recent study by Bondi et al. using SH-S5Y5 cells interestingly showed that DA treatment did not induce PINK and Parkin localization in the mitochondria, as CCCP treatment did. This means that despite inducing depolarization, DA did not activate the PINK1-Parkin autophagy pathway that was necessary to get rid of defective mitochondria [108]. In DJ-1 mutant human DA neurons, increased mitochondrial oxidative stress and accumulation of α-synuclein could be reversed with α-methyl-p-tyrosine, a competitive inhibitor of TH, preventing DA synthesis [42]. Accumulation of defective mitochondria by DA modification resembling mitochondria-related abnormalities were observed in several in vitro PD modeling studies involving PINK1 or Parkin mutations thus providing a basis for what may occur in sporadic cases and how the phenotypes mimic those of familial PD cases [25, 39, 40]. Moreover, a more oxidative environment due to defective mitochondria can further stimulate DA oxidation to DAQ, as indicated by increased binding of DAQ to cysteine-containing proteins in the striatum of animal models upon MPTP treatment [104]. The data altogether propose an alternate mechanism involving a positive feedback loop among PD elements that conditions the neurons into a state of chronic oxidative stress.

DA has also been shown to react and alter the function of PD related proteins, such as DJ-1, Parkin and α-synuclein [106, 109, 110]. In DA neurons, DA

modification on Parkin leads to decreased solubility, functional inactivation, and subsequent accumulation of its ubiquitin ligase E3 substrates, including Synphilin-1 and Parkin, itself [111]. Interestingly, catechol-modified Parkin was only found in the SN of normal human brain tissue, but not in other areas such as caudate-putamen, cerebellum, and adjacent red nucleus [110]. Overexpression of α-synuclein in human primary DA neurons resulted in degeneration, a phenotype that was not observed in non-DA cells nor β-synuclein-overexpressing cells. Inhibition of DA production by α-methyl-p-tyrosine, a TH inhibitor, or antioxidant vitamin E reversed the α-synuclein overexpression-induced damage, supporting the hypothesis that DA fueled-oxidative stress plays a key role in mediating α-synuclein toxicity [112]. Furthermore, another study revealed that DOPAL-induced α-synuclein oligomers damaged cellular vesicles by permeabilizing cholesterol-containing vesicular membranes and inducing leakage of DA from vesicles into the cytosol [113]. DAQ non-covalent modification on α-synuclein was also observed to stabilize the protofibril form [114].

Changes in the level of cytosolic DA during PD progression remains a controversial subject, with studies arguing for elevation or [25, 115], reduction [26] as a cause of PD-related phenotypes. This contrast may be due to the decline in cytosolic DA, a feature of PD in its later stages when neurons are no longer able to produce DA in contrast to the earlier stages when overproduction of DA may be triggered by cellular dysfunction. The idea of DA overproduction is also supported by studies reporting the role of α-synuclein in negatively regulating DA vesicle release. It was found that a 2–3-fold α-synuclein overexpression in hippocampal and ventral midbrain neurons impeded synaptic vesicle release [116] while α-synuclein knock-out mice displayed stronger release of DA upon stimulus [117]. Two potential reasons behind this could be a reduction in the number of vesicles available for release [113, 116] or inhibition of vesicle docking by α-synuclein oligomers [118]. A follow-up study demonstrated that α-synuclein oligomers prevented soluble N-ethylmaleimide-sensitive factor attachment protein receptor (SNARE) complex formation which is necessary for vesicle docking, by binding to synaptobrevin-2, a vesicle-associated membrane protein [118]. These studies collectively demonstrate synergism between α-synuclein and DA in promoting oxidative stress in DA neurons (Fig. 2).

Conclusion

The mechanism of neurodegeneration in PD still remains a controversial subject. Although PD entails a wide variety of cellular phenotypes, it is possible to decipher the events involved in the disease trajectory by studying the genetic forms of PD with the hopes of

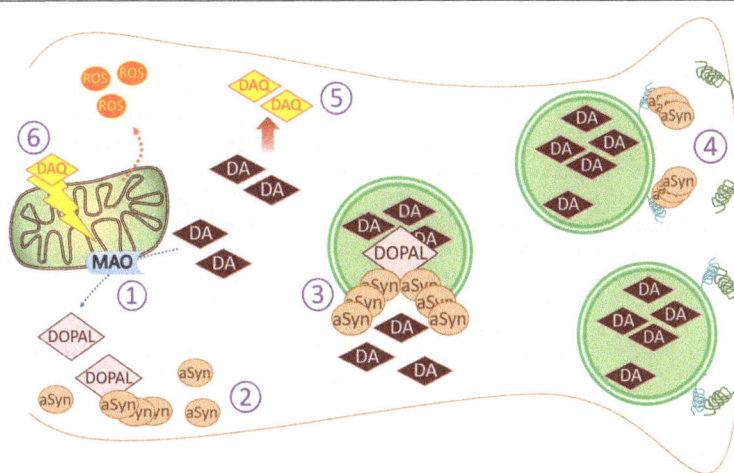

Fig. 2 Alpha-synuclein oligomers and cytosolic DA amplify each other and synergistically contribute to oxidative stress. 1) DA anabolism enzyme, MAO, turns DA into DOPAL, that later can be converted into less reactive DOPAC by another enzyme. 2) DOPAL induces α-synuclein oligomerization and prevents fibril formation. 3) DOPAL modified α-synuclein oligomers create pore-like structure in the synaptic vesicle membrane, causing DA leakage into cytosol. 4) α-synuclein oligomers are also known to negatively regulate synaptic vesicle release by preventing SNARE formation and vesicle docking. This provides more DA vesicles that can be targeted by DOPAL-α-synuclein oligomers. 5) Oxidation of cytosolic DA produces DAQ. 6) DAQ reacts with cysteine residues of mitochondrial proteins that results in mitochondria depolarization and further ROS production

extrapolating gained insights toward the sporadic, non-familial forms. Mutations in PINK1, Parkin, DJ-1, and LRRK2 result in mitochondrial perturbations and elevations in oxidative stress. Utilization of DA as a neurotransmitter renders midbrain DA neurons more prone to damage given the potential for production of oxidative and reactive byproducts in DA metabolism. Elevated ROS levels also seem to be involved in metal-exposure related toxicity suspected to cause sporadic PD. These studies hint at the idea that oxidative stress plays a central role across a variety of PD linked phenotypes. Additionally, chronic oxidative stress, beyond the load that can be adequately regulated by homeostasis, can impact macromolecules inside the cell and result in cell death [20, 119].

Considering the complexity and singularity of each PD case, a great deal of effort is required to understand general PD pathology. Collecting PD case studies is an essential step in gaining a better idea of the underlying biology and overall landscape of the disease progression. Biological events considered in this review cannot explain the full spectrum of phenotypes present in PD like pathological events that occur on an intercellular level such as neuroinflammation [120], gut microbiota homeostasis [121], or the prion-hypothesis of α-synuclein [122]; however, mounting evidence pointing to oxidative stress as a common denominator provides hope for developing a more thorough understanding that could explain the complex cellular pathologies. This review proposes intracellular oxidative stress mitigation as major path toward regenerative treatment. Treatment

with antioxidants, identification of appropriate antioxidant therapeutic candidates as well as efficient delivery methods across the blood brain barrier are major hurdles that would need to be resolved for building the groundwork for PD treatment in the context of our proposed paradigm. An additional implication is the identification of elements linked to oxidative stress as potential diagnostic targets for PD, including upregulation of lipid hydroperoxide and SOD activity, and down-regulation of antioxidant factors like sulfhydryl groups and catalase activity in the blood [123]. Advances in the area of in vitro disease modeling have illuminated novel insights regarding PD and yielded new ways of studying complex cellular phenotypes. Despite these advantages, current in vitro or even animal disease models are limited by their inability to recapitulate the disease in an aged condition, which is especially relevant to studying neurodegenerative diseases which are chronic conditions that occur late in life. This issue remains a critical challenge given that there are no definitive methods of closely mimicking the naturally aged state of cells; nevertheless, given the rapid and continued progress in the field of disease modeling particularly in the context of neurological disorders, there is hope that these strides can soon lead to the development of effective therapeutic strategies.

Abbreviations

6-OHDA: 6-hydroxydopamine; ATF: Activation transcription factor; CCCP: Carbonyl cyanide-m-chlorophenylhydrazone; CHOP: C/EBP homologous protein; DA: Dopamine; DAQ: DA-quinone; DOPAC: 3,4-dihydroxyphenylacetic acid; DOPAL: 3,4-dihydroxyphenylacetaldehyde; ER: Endoplasmic reticulum;

GSH: Glutathione; iPSC: Induced pluripotent stem cell; IRE1: Inositol-requiring enzyme 1; L-DOPA: L-3,4-dihydroxyphenylalanine; LRRK2: Leucine-rich repeat kinase 2; MAM: Mitochondrial-associated membrane; MAO-B: Monoamine oxidase B; MCU: Mitochondrial calcium uniporter; MEF2C: Myocyte-specific enhancer factor 2C; MPP + : 1-methyl-4-phenylpyridinium; MPTP: 1-methyl-4-phenyl-1,2,3,6-tetrahydropyridine; mtDNA: Mitochondrial DNA; NADH: Nicotinamide adenine dinucleotide; PERK: Pancreatic ER kinase-like ER kinase; PD: Parkinson's disease; PGC-1α: Peroxisome proliferator-activated receptor gamma coactivator 1-alpha; PINK1: PTEN induced putative kinase 1; ROS: Reactive oxygen species; SN: Substantia nigra; SNARE: Soluble N-ethylmaleimide-sensitive factor attachment protein receptor; SOD: Superoxide dismutase; TH: Tyrosine hydroxylase; TOM: Translocase of the outer membrane; UPR: Unfolded protein response; UPS: Ubiquitin-proteasome system; VMAT2: Vesicular monoamine transporter 2; VTA: Ventral tegmental area; WT: Wild type; XBP1: X-box binding protein 1

Acknowledgements
Not applicable

Funding
This work was supported by the National Research Foundation of Korea (NRF) grant (NRF-2017M3A9B4062415; NRF-2017R1A2B4003018; NRF-2016K1A4A3914725) and by the International Science and Business Belt Program (2015 K000278) funded by the Korea government (MSIP) for writing the manuscript.

Authors' contributions
LP and SJ contributed to manuscript composition as well as construction of figs. SC provided constructive suggestions and comments to improve the manuscript. All authors read and approved the final manuscript.

Competing interests
The authors declare that they have no competing interests.

Author details
[1]Soonchunhyang Institute of Medi-bio Science (SIMS), Soonchunhyang University, 25, Bongjeong-ro, Dongnam-gu, Cheonan-si 31151, South Korea. [2]Center for Stem Cell Biology, Sloan-Kettering Institute, New York, NY 10065, USA.

References

1. Bellucci A, Mercuri NB, Venneri A, Faustini G, Longhena F, Pizzi M, et al. Review: Parkinson's disease: from synaptic loss to connectome dysfunction. Neuropathol Appl Neurobiol. 2016;42:77–94.
2. Tabbal SD, Tian LL, Karimi M, Brown CA, Loftin SK, Perlmutter JS. Low nigrostriatal reserve for motor parkinsonism in nonhuman primates. Exp Neurol. 2012;237:355–62.
3. Valente EM, Abou-Sleiman PM, Caputo V, Muqit MM, Harvey K, Gispert S, et al. Hereditary early-onset Parkinson's disease caused by mutations in PINK1. Science. 2004;304:1158–60.
4. Polymeropoulos MH, Lavedan C, Leroy E, Ide SE, Dehejia A, Dutra A, et al. Mutation in the alpha-synuclein gene identified in families with Parkinson's disease. Science. 1997;276:2045–7.
5. Di Fonzo A, Rohe CF, Ferreira J, Chien HF, Vacca L, Stocchi F, et al. A frequent LRRK2 gene mutation associated with autosomal dominant Parkinson's disease. Lancet. 2005;365:412–5.
6. Nichols WC, Pankratz N, Hernandez D, Paisan-Ruiz C, Jain S, Halter CA, et al. Genetic screening for a single common LRRK2 mutation in familial Parkinson's disease. Lancet. 2005;365:410–2.
7. Bonifati V, Rizzu P, van Baren MJ, Schaap O, Breedveld GJ, Krieger E, et al. Mutations in the DJ-1 gene associated with autosomal recessive early-onset parkinsonism. Science. 2003;299:256–9.
8. Spillantini MG, Schmidt ML, Lee VM, Trojanowski JQ, Jakes R, Goedert M. Alpha-synuclein in Lewy bodies. Nature. 1997;388:839–40.
9. Bellucci Zaltieri M, Navarria L, Grigoletto J, Missale C, Spano PA. From α-synuclein to synaptic dysfunctions: new insights into the pathophysiology of Parkinson's disease. Brain Res. 2012;1476:183–202.
10. Lazarou M, Sliter DA, Kane LA, Sarraf SA, Wang C, Burman JL, et al. The ubiquitin kinase PINK1 recruits autophagy receptors to induce mitophagy. Nature. 2015;524:309–14.
11. Pickrell AM, Youle RJ. The roles of PINK1, Parkin, and mitochondrial Fidelity in Parkinson's disease. Neuron. 2015;85:257–73.
12. Canet-Avilés Wilson MA, Miller DW, Ahmad R, McLendon C, Bandyopadhyay S, Baptista MJ, Ringe D, Petsko GA, Cookson MRRM. The Parkinson's disease protein DJ-1 is neuroprotective due to cysteine-sulfinic acid-driven mitochondrial localization. Proc Natl Acad Sci U S A. 2004;101:9103–8.
13. Zondler L, Miller-Fleming L, Repici M, Gonçalves S, Tenreiro S, Rosado-Ramos R, et al. DJ-1 interactions with α-synuclein attenuate aggregation and cellular toxicity in models of Parkinson's disease. Cell Death Dis. 2014;5: e1350.
14. Cooper O, Seo H, Andrabi S, Guardia-Laguarta C, Graziotto J, Sundberg M, et al. Pharmacological rescue of mitochondrial deficits in iPSC-derived neural cells from patients with familial Parkinson's disease. Sci Transl Med. 2012;4:141ra90.
15. Ray Huang BW, Tsuji YPD. Reactive oxygen species (ROS) homeostasis and redox regulation in cellular signaling. Cell Signal. 2012;24:981–90.
16. Seo Ahn Y, Lee SR, Yeo CY, Hur KCJH. The major target of the endogenously generated reactive oxygen species in response to insulin stimulation is phosphatase and tensin homolog and not phosphoinositide-3 kinase (PI-3 kinase) in the PI-3 kinase/Akt pathway. Mol Biol Cell. 2005;16: 348–57.
17. Fujino Noguchi T, Matsuzawa A, Yamauchi S, Saitoh M, Takeda K, Ichijo HG. Thioredoxin and TRAF family proteins regulate reactive oxygen species-dependent activation of ASK1 through reciprocal modulation of the N-terminal homophilic interaction of ASK1. Mol Cell Biol. 2007;27:8152–63.
18. Indo HP, Yen HC, Nakanishi I, Matsumoto K, Tamura M, Nagano Y, et al. A mitochondrial superoxide theory for oxidative stress diseases and aging. J Clin Biochem Nutr. 2015;56:1–7.
19. Rego AC, Oliveira CR. Mitochondrial dysfunction and reactive oxygen species in excitotoxicity and apoptosis: implications for the pathogenesis of neurodegenerative diseases. Neurochem Res. 2003;28:1563–74.
20. Sies Berndt C, Jones DPH. Oxidative stress. Annu Rev Biochem. 2017;86
21. Wiseman H, Halliwell B. Damage to DNA by reactive oxygen and nitrogen species: role in inflammatory disease and progression to cancer. Biochem J. 1996;313(Pt 1):17–29.
22. Bosco DA, Fowler DM, Zhang Q, Nieva J, Powers ET, Wentworth P Jr, et al. Elevated levels of oxidized cholesterol metabolites in Lewy body disease brains accelerate alpha-synuclein fibrilization. Nat Chem Biol. 2006;2:249–53.
23. Nakabeppu Y, Tsuchimoto D, Yamaguchi H, Sakumi K. Oxidative damage in nucleic acids and Parkinson's disease. J Neurosci Res. 2007;85:919–34.
24. Floor E, Wetzel MG. Increased protein oxidation in human substantia nigra pars compacta in comparison with basal ganglia and prefrontal cortex measured with an improved dinitrophenylhydrazine assay. J Neurochem. 1998;70:268–75.
25. Chung SY, Kishinevsky S, Mazzulli JR, Graziotto J, Mrejeru A, Mosharov EV, et al. Parkin and PINK1 patient iPSC-derived midbrain dopamine neurons exhibit mitochondrial dysfunction and alpha-Synuclein accumulation. Stem Cell Reports. 2016;7:664–77.
26. Nguyen HN, Byers B, Cord B, Shcheglovitov A, Byrne J, Gujar P, et al. LRRK2 mutant iPSC-derived DA neurons demonstrate increased susceptibility to oxidative stress. Cell Stem Cell. 2011;8:267–80.
27. Loschen Azzi A, Richter C, Flohé LG. Superoxide radicals as precursors of mitochondrial hydrogen peroxide. FEBS Lett. 1974;42:68–72.

28. Drose S, Brandt U. The mechanism of mitochondrial superoxide production by the cytochrome bc1 complex. J Biol Chem. 2008;283:21649–54.

29. Kussmaul L, Hirst J. The mechanism of superoxide production by NADH: ubiquinone oxidoreductase (complex I) from bovine heart mitochondria. Proc Natl Acad Sci U S A. 2006;103:7607–12.

30. Hala Vilhelmova M, Hartmanova I, Pink WK. Chronic parkinsonism in humans due to product of meperidine-analog synthesis. Science. 1983;219:979–80.

31. Javitch JA, D'Amato RJ, Strittmatter SM, Snyder SH. Parkinsonism-inducing neurotoxin, N-methyl-4-phenyl-1,2,3,6 -tetrahydropyridine: uptake of the metabolite N-methyl-4-phenylpyridine by dopamine neurons explains selective toxicity. Proc Natl Acad Sci U S A. 1985;82:2173–7.

32. Mizuno Y, Sone N, Saitoh T. Effects of 1-methyl-4-phenyl-1,2,3,6-tetrahydropyridine and 1-methyl-4-phenylpyridinium ion on activities of the enzymes in the electron transport system in mouse brain. J Neurochem. 1987;48:1787–93.

33. Betarbet R, Sherer TB, MacKenzie G, Garcia-Osuna M, Panov AV, Greenamyre JT. Chronic systemic pesticide exposure reproduces features of Parkinson's disease. Nat Neurosci. 2000;3:1301–6.

34. Schapira AH, Cooper JM, Dexter D, Clark JB, Jenner P, Marsden CD. Mitochondrial complex I deficiency in Parkinson's disease. J Neurochem. 1990;54:823–7.

35. Parker Jr WD, Parks JK, Swerdlow RH, Complex I. Deficiency in Parkinson's disease frontal cortex. Brain Res. 2008;1189:215–8.

36. Gilks Abou-Sleiman PM, Gandhi S, Jain S, Singleton A, Lees AJ, Shaw K, Bhatia KP, Bonifati V, Quinn NP, Lynch JWP. A common LRRK2 mutation in idiopathic Parkinson's disease. Lancet. 2005;365:415–6.

37. Palacino JJ, Sagi D, Goldberg MS, Krauss S, Motz C, Wacker M, et al. Mitochondrial dysfunction and oxidative damage in parkin-deficient mice. J Biol Chem. 2004;279:18614–22.

38. Morais VA, Verstreken P, Roethig A, Smet J, Snellinx A, Vanbrabant M, et al. Parkinson's disease mutations in PINK1 result in decreased complex I activity and deficient synaptic function. EMBO Mol Med. 2009;1:99–111.

39. Wang X, Winter D, Ashrafi G, Schlehe J, Wong YL, Selkoe D, et al. PINK1 and Parkin target Miro for phosphorylation and degradation to arrest mitochondrial motility. Cell. 2011;147:893–906.

40. Koentjoro B, Park JS, Sue CM. Nix restores mitophagy and mitochondrial function to protect against PINK1/Parkin-related Parkinson's disease. Sci Rep. 2017;7:44373.

41. Kinumi Kimata J, Taira T, Ariga H, Niki ET. Cysteine-106 of DJ-1 is the most sensitive cysteine residue to hydrogen peroxide-mediated oxidation in vivo in human umbilical vein endothelial cells. Biochem Biophys Res Commun. 2004;317:722–8.

42. Burbulla LF, Song P, Mazzulli JR, Zampese E, Wong YC, Jeon S, et al. Dopamine oxidation mediates mitochondrial and lysosomal dysfunction in Parkinson's disease. Science. 2017;357:1255–61.

43. Richter Park JW, Ames BNC. Normal oxidative damage to mitochondrial and nuclear DNA is extensive. Proc Natl Acad Sci. 1988;85:6465–7.

44. Cadenas E, Davies KJ. Mitochondrial free radical generation, oxidative stress, and aging. Free Radic Biol Med. 2000;29:222–30.

45. Lee HC, Chang CM, Chi CW. Somatic mutations of mitochondrial DNA in aging and cancer progression. Ageing Res Rev. 2010;9(Suppl 1):S47–58.

46. Madamanchi NR, Runge MS. Mitochondrial dysfunction in atherosclerosis. Circ Res. 2007;100:460–73.

47. Ryan SD, Dolatabadi N, Chan SF, Zhang X, Akhtar MW, Parker J, et al. Erratum: isogenic human iPSC parkinson's model shows nitrosative stress-induced dysfunction in MEF2-PGC1α transcription. Cell. 2013;155:1652–3.

48. Pollard MG, Travers KJ, Weissman JS. Ero1p: a novel and ubiquitous protein with an essential role in oxidative protein folding in the endoplasmic reticulum. Mol Cell. 1998;1:171–82.

49. Tu BP, Weissman JS. The FAD-and O 2-dependent reaction cycle of Ero1-mediated oxidative protein folding in the endoplasmic reticulum. Mol Cell. 2002;10:983–94.

50. Princiotta MF, Finzi D, Qian SB, Gibbs J, Schuchmann S, Buttgereit F, et al. Quantitating protein synthesis, degradation, and endogenous antigen processing. Immunity. 2003;18:343–54.

51. Rao Ellerby HM, Bredesen DERV. Coupling endoplasmic reticulum stress to the cell death program. Cell Death Differ. 2004;11:372–80.

52. Han J, Kaufman RJ. The role of ER stress in lipid metabolism and lipotoxicity. J Lipid Res. 2016;57:1329–38.

53. Krebs J, Agellon LB, Michalak M. Ca(2+) homeostasis and endoplasmic reticulum (ER) stress: an integrated view of calcium signaling. Biochem Biophys Res Commun. 2015;460:114–21.

54. Galehdar Swan P, Fuerth B, Callaghan SM, Park DS, Cregan SPZ. Neuronal apoptosis induced by endoplasmic reticulum stress is regulated by ATF4–CHOP-mediated induction of the Bcl-2 homology 3-only member PUMA. J Neurosci. 2010;30:16938–48.

55. Deniaud A, Sharaf el dein O, Maillier E, Poncet D, Kroemer G, Lemaire C, et al. Endoplasmic reticulum stress induces calcium-dependent permeability transition, mitochondrial outer membrane permeabilization and apoptosis. Oncogene. 2008;27:285–99.

56. Van Coppenolle F, Vanden Abeele F, Slomianny C, Flourakis M, Hesketh J, Dewailly E, et al. Ribosome-translocon complex mediates calcium leakage from endoplasmic reticulum stores. J Cell Sci. 2004;117(Pt 18):4135–42.

57. Hammadi M, Oulidi A, Gackiere F, Katsogiannou M, Slomianny C, Roudbaraki M, et al. Modulation of ER stress and apoptosis by endoplasmic reticulum calcium leak via translocon during unfolded protein response: involvement of GRP78. FASEB J. 2013;27:1600–9.

58. De Stefani Raffaello A, Teardo E, Szabò I, Rizzuto RDA. Forty-kilodalton protein of the inner membrane is the mitochondrial calcium uniporter. Nature. 2011;476:336–40.

59. Gomez-Suaga P, Paillusson S, Stoica R, Noble W, Hanger DP, Miller CC. The ER-mitochondria tethering complex VAPB-PTPIP51 regulates autophagy. Curr Biol. 2017;27:371–85.

60. Paillusson S, Stoica R, Gomez-Suaga P, Lau DH, Mueller S, Miller T, et al. There's something wrong with my MAM; the ER-mitochondria Axis and neurodegenerative diseases. Trends Neurosci. 2016;39:146–57.

61. Gautier CA, Erpapazoglou Z, Mouton-Liger F, Muriel MP, Cormier F, Bigou S, et al. The endoplasmic reticulum-mitochondria interface is perturbed in PARK2 knockout mice and patients with PARK2 mutations. Hum Mol Genet. 2016;25:2972–84.

62. de Brito OM, Scorrano L. Mitofusin 2 tethers endoplasmic reticulum to mitochondria. Nature. 2008;456:605–10.

63. Malhotra JD, Kaufman RJ. Endoplasmic reticulum stress and oxidative stress: a vicious cycle or a double-edged sword? Antioxid Redox Signal. 2007;9:2277–93.

64. Joza N, Susin SA, Daugas E, Stanford WL, Cho SK, Li CY, et al. Essential role of the mitochondrial apoptosis-inducing factor in programmed cell death. Nature. 2001;410:549–54.

65. Hoozemans JJ, van Haastert ES, Eikelenboom P, de Vos RA, Rozemuller JM, Scheper W. Activation of the unfolded protein response in Parkinson's disease. Biochem Biophys Res Commun. 2007;354:707–11.

66. Huang Xu J, Liang M, Hong X, Suo H, Liu J, Yu M, Huang FY. RESP18 is involved in the cytotoxicity of dopaminergic neurotoxins in MN9D cells. Neurotox Res. 2013;24:164–75.

67. Bouman Schlierf A, Lutz AK, Shan J, Deinlein A, Kast J, Galehdar Z, Palmisano V, Patenge N, Berg D, Gasser TL. Parkin is transcriptionally regulated by ATF4: evidence for an interconnection between mitochondrial stress and ER stress. Cell Death Differ. 2011;18:769–82.

68. Sun X, Liu J, Crary JF, Malagelada C, Sulzer D, Greene LA, et al. ATF4 protects against neuronal death in cellular Parkinson's disease models by maintaining levels of parkin. J Neurosci. 2013;33:2398–407.

69. Gorell Johnson CC, Rybicki BA, Peterson EL, Kortsha GX, Brown GG, Richardson RJJM. Occupational exposure to manganese, copper, lead, iron, mercury and zinc and the risk of Parkinson's disease. Neurotoxicology. 1998;20:239–47.

70. Dusek P, Roos PM, Litwin T, Schneider SA, Flaten TP, Aaseth J. The neurotoxicity of iron, copper and manganese in Parkinson's and Wilson's diseases. J Trace Elem Med Biol. 2015;31:193–203.

71. Xu Wang F, Wu SW, Deng Y, Liu W, Feng S, Yang TY, Xu ZFB. Alpha-synuclein is involved in manganese-induced ER stress via PERK signal pathway in organotypic brain slice cultures. Mol Neurobiol. 2014;49:399–412.

72. Colla Coune P, Liu Y, Pletnikova O, Troncoso JC, Iwatsubo T, Schneider BL, Lee MKE. Endoplasmic reticulum stress is important for the manifestations of α-synucleinopathy in vivo. J Neurosci. 2012;32:3306–20.

73. Heman-Ackah SM, Manzano R, Hoozemans JJM, Scheper W, Flynn R, Haerty W, et al. Alpha-synuclein induces the unfolded protein response in Parkinson's disease SNCA triplication iPSC-derived neurons. Hum Mol Genet. 2017;0:1–10.

74. Cóppola-Segovia V, Cavarsan C, Maia FG, Ferraz AC, Nakao LS, Lima MM, et al. ER stress induced by Tunicamycin triggers α-Synuclein

oligomerization, dopaminergic neurons death and locomotor impairment: a new model of Parkinson's disease. Mol Neurobiol. 2017;54:5798–806.

75. Bartels T, Choi JG, DJ S. α-Synuclein occurs physiologically as a helically folded tetramer that resists aggregation. Nature. 2011;477:107–10.

76. Marques O, Outeiro TF. Alpha-synuclein: from secretion to dysfunction and death. Cell Death Dis. 2012;3:e350.

77. Volles MJ, Lansbury Jr PT. Zeroing in on the pathogenic form of alpha-synuclein and its mechanism of neurotoxicity in Parkinson's disease. Biochemistry. 2003;42:7871–8.

78. Martinez-Vicente M, Talloczy Z, Kaushik S, Massey AC, Mazzulli J, Mosharov EV, et al. Dopamine-modified alpha-synuclein blocks chaperone-mediated autophagy. J Clin Invest. 2008;118:777–88.

79. Deas E, Cremades N, Angelova PR, Ludtmann MH, Yao Z, Chen S, et al. Alpha-Synuclein oligomers interact with metal ions to induce oxidative stress and neuronal death in Parkinson's disease. Antioxid Redox Signal. 2016;24:376–91.

80. Levin J, Hogen T, Hillmer AS, Bader B, Schmidt F, Kamp F, et al. Generation of ferric iron links oxidative stress to alpha-synuclein oligomer formation. J Park Dis. 2011;1:205–16.

81. Tabner BJ, Turnbull S, El-Agnaf O, Allsop D. Production of reactive oxygen species from aggregating proteins implicated in Alzheimer's disease, Parkinson's disease and other neurodegenerative diseases. Curr Top Med Chem. 2001;1:507–17.

82. Jellen LC, Lu L, Wang X, Unger EL, Earley CJ, Allen RP, et al. Iron deficiency alters expression of dopamine-related genes in the ventral midbrain in mice. Neuroscience. 2013;252:13–23.

83. Dexter DT, Wells FR, Agid F, Agid Y, Lees AJ, Jenner P, et al. Increased nigral iron content in postmortem parkinsonian brain. Lancet. 1987;2:1219–20.

84. Michaeli S, Oz G, Sorce DJ, Garwood M, Ugurbil K, Majestic S, et al. Assessment of brain iron and neuronal integrity in patients with Parkinson's disease using novel MRI contrasts. Mov Disord. 2007;22:334–40.

85. Pyatigorskaya N, Sharman M, Corvol JC, Valabregue R, Yahia-Cherif L, Poupon F, et al. High nigral iron deposition in LRRK2 and Parkin mutation carriers using R2* relaxometry. Mov Disord. 2015;30:1077–84.

86. Hare DJ, Lei P, Ayton S, Roberts BR, Grimm R, George JL, et al. An iron-dopamine index predicts risk of parkinsonian neurodegeneration in the substantia nigra pars compacta. Chem Sci. 2014;5:2160–9.

87. Di Maio R, Barrett PJ, Hoffman EK, Barrett CW, Zharikov A, Borah A, et al. alpha-Synuclein binds to TOM20 and inhibits mitochondrial protein import in Parkinson's disease. Sci Transl Med. 2016;8:342ra78.

88. Dexter Carter CJ, Wells FR, Javoy-Agid F, Agid Y, Lees A, Jenner P, Marsden CDDT. Basal lipid peroxidation in substantia nigra is increased in Parkinson's disease. J Neurochem. 1989;52:381–9.

89. Qin Z, Hu D, Han S, Reaney SH, Di Monte DA, Fink AL. Effect of 4-hydroxy-2-nonenal modification on alpha-synuclein aggregation. J Biol Chem. 2007; 282:5862–70.

90. Bae EJ, Ho DH, Park E, Jung JW, Cho K, Hong JH, et al. Lipid peroxidation product 4-hydroxy-2-nonenal promotes seeding-capable oligomer formation and cell-to-cell transfer of alpha-synuclein. Antioxid Redox Signal. 2013;18:770–83.

91. Hashimoto Takeda A, Hsu LJ, Takenouchi T, Masliah EM. Role of cytochrome c as a stimulator of α-synuclein aggregation in Lewy body disease. J Biol Chem. 1999;274:28849–52.

92. Ruf RA, Lutz EA, Zigoneanu IG, Pielak GJ. Alpha-Synuclein conformation affects its tyrosine-dependent oxidative aggregation. Biochemistry. 2008;47: 13604–9.

93. Webb Ravikumar B, Atkins J, Skepper JN, Rubinsztein DCJL. α-Synuclein is degraded by both autophagy and the proteasome. J Biol Chem. 2003;278: 25009–13.

94. Ebrahimi-Fakhari D, Cantuti-Castelvetri I, Fan Z, Rockenstein E, Masliah E, Hyman BT, et al. Distinct roles in vivo for the ubiquitin-proteasome system and the autophagy-lysosomal pathway in the degradation of alpha-synuclein. J Neurosci. 2011;31:14508–20.

95. Majeski AE, Dice JF. Mechanisms of chaperone-mediated autophagy. Int J Biochem Cell Biol. 2004;36:2435–44.

96. Haynes CM, Titus EA, Cooper AA. Degradation of misfolded proteins prevents ER-derived oxidative stress and cell death. Mol Cell. 2004;15:767–76.

97. Cooper AA, Gitler AD, Cashikar A, Haynes CM, Hill KJ, Bhullar B, et al. Alpha-synuclein blocks ER-Golgi traffic and Rab1 rescues neuron loss in Parkinson's models. Science. 2006;313:324–8.

98. Mazzulli Zunke F, Isacson O, Studer L, Krainc DJR. α-Synuclein–induced lysosomal dysfunction occurs through disruptions in protein trafficking in human midbrain synucleinopathy models. Proc Natl Acad Sci. 2016;113: 1931–6.

99. Credle Forcelli PA, Delannoy M, Oaks AW, Permaul E, Berry DL, Duka V, Wills J, Sidhu AJJ. α-Synuclein-mediated inhibition of ATF6 processing into COPII vesicles disrupts UPR signaling in Parkinson's disease. Neurobiol Dis. 2015;76: 112–25.

100. Goldstein DS, Sullivan P, Holmes C, Miller GW, Alter S, Strong R, et al. Determinants of buildup of the toxic dopamine metabolite DOPAL in Parkinson's disease. J Neurochem. 2013;126:591–603.

101. Meiser J, Weindl D, Hiller K. Complexity of dopamine metabolism. Cell Commun Signal. 2013;11:34.

102. Graham DG. Oxidative pathways for catecholamines in the genesis of neuromelanin and cytotoxic quinones. Mol Pharmacol. 1978;14:633–43.

103. Tse DC, McCreery RL, Adams RN. Potential oxidative pathways of brain catecholamines. J Med Chem. 1976;19:37–40.

104. LaVoie MJ, Hastings TG. Dopamine quinone formation and protein modification associated with the striatal neurotoxicity of methamphetamine: evidence against a role for extracellular dopamine. J Neurosci. 1999;19: 1484–91.

105. Hastings TG, Lewis DA, Zigmond MJ. Role of oxidation in the neurotoxic effects of intrastriatal dopamine injections. Proc Natl Acad Sci U S A. 1996; 93:1956–61.

106. Van Laar VS, Mishizen AJ, Cascio M, Hastings TG. Proteomic identification of dopamine-conjugated proteins from isolated rat brain mitochondria and SH-SY5Y cells. Neurobiol Dis. 2009;34:487–500.

107. Khan FH, Sen T, Maiti AK, Jana S, Chatterjee U, Chakrabarti S. Inhibition of rat brain mitochondrial electron transport chain activity by dopamine oxidation products during extended in vitro incubation: implications for Parkinson's disease. Biochim Biophys Acta. 2005;1741:65–74.

108. Bondi Zilocchi M, Mare MG, D'Agostino G, Giovannardi S, Ambrosio S, Fasano M, Alberio TH. Dopamine induces mitochondrial depolarization without activating PINK1-mediated mitophagy. J Neurochem. 2016;136: 1231–91.

109. Conway KA, Rochet JC, Bieganski RM, Lansbury Jr PT. Kinetic stabilization of the alpha-synuclein protofibril by a dopamine-alpha-synuclein adduct. Science. 2001;294:1346–9.

110. LaVoie MJ, Ostaszewski BL, Weihofen A, Schlossmacher MG, Selkoe DJ. Dopamine covalently modifies and functionally inactivates parkin. Nat Med. 2005;11:1214–21.

111. Meng F, Yao D, Shi Y, Kabakoff J, Wu W, Reicher J, et al. Oxidation of the cysteine-rich regions of parkin perturbs its E3 ligase activity and contributes to protein aggregation. Mol Neurodegener. 2011;6:34.

112. Xu J, Kao SY, Lee FJ, Song W, Jin LW, Yankner BA. Dopamine-dependent neurotoxicity of alpha-synuclein: a mechanism for selective neurodegeneration in Parkinson disease. Nat Med. 2002;8:600–6.

113. Plotegher N, Berti G, Ferrari E, Tessari I, Zanetti M, Lunelli L, et al. DOPAL derived alpha-synuclein oligomers impair synaptic vesicles physiological function. Sci Rep. 2017;7:40699.

114. Bisaglia M, Tosatto L, Munari F, Tessari I, de Laureto PP, Mammi S, et al. Dopamine quinones interact with alpha-synuclein to form unstructured adducts. Biochem Biophys Res Commun. 2010;394:424–8.

115. Kitada T, Asakawa S, Hattori N, Matsumine H, Yamamura Y, Minoshima S, et al. Mutations in the parkin gene cause autosomal recessive juvenile parkinsonism. Nature. 1998;392:605–8.

116. Nemani VM, Lu W, Berge V, Nakamura K, Onoa B, Lee MK, et al. Increased expression of alpha-synuclein reduces neurotransmitter release by inhibiting synaptic vesicle reclustering after endocytosis. Neuron. 2010;65:66–79.

117. Abeliovich A, Schmitz Y, Farinas I, Choi-Lundberg D, Ho WH, Castillo PE, et al. Mice lacking alpha-synuclein display functional deficits in the nigrostriatal dopamine system. Neuron. 2000;25:239–52.

118. Choi BK, Choi MG, Kim JY, Yang Y, Lai Y, Kweon DH, et al. Large alpha-synuclein oligomers inhibit neuronal SNARE-mediated vesicle docking. Proc Natl Acad Sci U S A. 2013;110:4087–92.

119. Zhao J, Yu S, Zheng Y, Yang H, Zhang J. Oxidative modification and its implications for the neurodegeneration of Parkinson's disease. Mol Neurobiol. 2017;54:1404–18.

120. Ransohoff RM. How neuroinflammation contributes to neurodegeneration. Science. 2016;353:777–83.

121. Sampson TR, Debelius JW, Thron T, Janssen S, Shastri GG, Ilhan ZE, et al. Gut Microbiota Regulate Motor Deficits and Neuroinflammation in a Model of Parkinson's Disease. Cell. 2016;167:1469–1480.e12.
122. Luk KC, Kehm V, Carroll J, Zhang B, O'Brien P, Trojanowski JQ, et al. Pathological -Synuclein transmission initiates Parkinson-like neurodegeneration in nontransgenic mice. Science. 2012;338:949–53.
123. de Farias CC, Maes M, Bonifacio KL, Bortolasci CC, de Souza Nogueira A, Brinholi FF, et al. Highly specific changes in antioxidant levels and lipid peroxidation in Parkinson's disease and its progression: disease and staging biomarkers and new drug targets. Neurosci Lett. 2016;617:66–71.

4

VGLUT1 or VGLUT2 mRNA-positive neurons in spinal trigeminal nucleus provide collateral projections to both the thalamus and the parabrachial nucleus in rats

Chun-Kui Zhang[1†], Zhi-Hong Li[1†], Yu Qiao[1,2†], Ting Zhang[1], Ya-Cheng Lu[1], Tao Chen[1], Yu-Lin Dong[1], Yun-Qing Li[1*] and Jin-Lian Li[1*] [iD]

Abstract

The trigemino-thalamic (T-T) and trigemino-parabrachial (T-P) pathways are strongly implicated in the sensory-discriminative and affective/emotional aspects of orofacial pain, respectively. These T-T and T-P projection fibers originate from the spinal trigeminal nucleus (Vsp). We previously determined that many vesicular glutamate transporter (VGLUT1 and/or VGLUT2) mRNA-positive neurons were distributed in the Vsp of the adult rat, and most of these neurons sent their axons to the thalamus or cerebellum. However, whether VGLUT1 or VGLUT2 mRNA-positive projection neurons exist that send their axons to both the thalamus and the parabrachial nucleus (PBN) has not been reported. Thus, in the present study, dual retrograde tract tracing was used in combination with fluorescence in situ hybridization (FISH) for VGLUT1 or VGLUT2 mRNA to identify the existence of VGLUT1 or VGLUT2 mRNA neurons that send collateral projections to both the thalamus and the PBN. Neurons in the Vsp that send collateral projections to both the thalamus and the PBN were mainly VGLUT2 mRNA-positive, with a proportion of 90.3%, 93.0% and 85.4% in the oral (Vo), interpolar (Vi) and caudal (Vc) subnucleus of the Vsp, respectively. Moreover, approximately 34.0% of the collateral projection neurons in the Vc showed Fos immunopositivity after injection of formalin into the lip, and parts of calcitonin gene-related peptide (CGRP)-immunopositive axonal varicosities were in direct contact with the Vc collateral projection neurons. These results indicate that most collateral projection neurons in the Vsp, particularly in the Vc, which express mainly VGLUT2, may relay orofacial nociceptive information directly to the thalamus and PBN via axon collaterals.

Keywords: Vesicular glutamate transporters, Spinal trigeminal nucleus, Thalamus, Parabrachial nucleus, Collateral projection, Rat

Introduction

It is well established that the spinal trigeminal nucleus (Vsp), which contains the oral subnucleus (Vo), interpolar subnucleus (Vi) and caudal subnucleus (Vc), sends dense projection fibers not only to the thalamus [1, 2] but also the parabrachial nucleus (PBN) in the rat [3]. Previous studies have indicated that approximately 20%

of neurons in the Vc had collateral projections to the contralateral thalamus and ipsilateral PBN, and more than 90% are distributed in lamina I (marginal zone) [4]. It is reported that the neurons in lamina I of the Vc respond exclusively or maximally to noxious orofacial stimuli [5].

Glutamate is the main excitatory neurotransmitter in the central nervous system. Since the successful cloning of the vesicular glutamate transporter (VGLUT) in the late 1990s [6–9], three types of VGLUTs have been identified. Two types, VGLUT1 and VGLUT2, have been considered definitive markers for glutamatergic neurons

* Correspondence: deptanat@fmmu.edu.cn; jinlian@fmmu.edu.cn
†Equal contributors
[1]Department of Anatomy and K.K. Leung Brain Research Centre, The Fourth Military Medical University, Xi'an, People's Republic of China
Full list of author information is available at the end of the article

[6, 7, 10–14]. The different distribution patterns of the two types of VGLUTs in the central nervous system suggest that they may play different functional roles [11]. Previous reports have indicated the different distribution patterns of VGLUT1 and VGLUT2 mRNA in the principal sensory trigeminal nucleus (Vp) and Vsp of rats [15–17], in which single Vp neurons that express both VGLUT1 and VGLUT2 mRNA constituted approximately 64% of glutamatergic Vp neurons and the majority of glutamatergic T-T projection neurons in the Vp co-express VGLUT1 and VGLUT2 mRNA. A previous study [15] also showed that the glutamatergic T-T projection neurons in the Vsp mainly express VGLUT2, whereas trigemino-cerebellar projection neurons mainly express VGLUT1, which occurs most frequently in the Vi, less in the Vp, and least in the Vo. However, no single neurons that express VGLUT1 or VGLUT2 mRNA sending collateral projections to both the thalamus and PBN were reported in the Vsp, although many VGLUT1 or VGLUT2-positive axon terminals were identified in the PBN, as previously reported [14]; moreover, whether collateral projection neurons that express VGLUT1 or VGLUT2 mRNA are involved in nociceptive signal transmission has not been reported. Thus, in the present study, we primarily examined (1) which of the two main isoforms of VGLUTs may be expressed in the T-T and T-P collateral projection neurons in each of the subdivisions of the Vsp via FISH histochemistry combined with tract tracing after microinjection of a retrograde tracer (tetramethylrhodamine dextran amine, TMR) or wheat germ agglutinin-horseradish peroxidase (WGA-HRP) into the thalamic region and injection of Fluoro-Gold (FG) into the PBN region, respectively, and (2) whether the collateral projection neurons in the Vsp may be related to nociceptive signal transmission. The nociceptive neurons were confirmed by immunoreactivity for Fos, the protein product of the *c-fos* proto-oncogene, after subcutaneous injection of formalin into the upper lips [18, 19, 20]. In addition, in the Vc, the collateral projection neurons in synaptic contact with calcitonin gene related peptide (CGRP)-like immunoreactive (-LI) axon terminals were also considered nociceptive [21]. The synaptic relationship of collateral projection neuronal profiles (FG- and WGA-HRP-labeled) to axon terminals that exhibited CGRP-LI was also examined using electron microscopy.

Methods
Animals
A total of 51 adult male rats (Sprague-Dawley) that weighed between 280 and 320 g (China SH, Xi'an, People's Republic of China) were used in the current study.

Animal use and care was approved by the Animal Care and Use Committee at the Fourth Military Medical University. Of these rats, 30 rats were used for dual retrograde tract-tracing combined with FISH histochemistry or immunofluorescence histochemistry, 15 rats were used for anterograde tract-tracing combined with immunofluorescence histochemistry, and 6 rats were used for electron microscopy.

Microinjection of TMR and FG solution into the thalamus and PBN for retrograde tract-tracing
Following an intraperitoneal injection of sodium pentobarbital (40 mg/kg body weight), the anaesthetized rats were placed in a stereotaxic frame (NARISHIGE, Japan). Using a glass micropipette (internal tip diameter: 15–25 μm) that was attached to a 1 μl Hamilton microsyringe, 0.6–0.8 μl of 10% TMR (D-3308, 3000 MW; Molecular Probes, Eugene, OR, USA) dissolved in 0.1 M of citrate-NaOH (pH 3.0) was injected into the right thalamus, and 0.2 μl of 4% FG (80,014, Biotium, Hayward, CA, USA) dissolved in normal saline was injected into the left PBN. After each injection, the glass micropipette was maintained in place for 15 min. All 30 rats injected with TMR and FG were allowed to survive for 7 days. Furthermore, the rats were equally divided into two groups. While lightly anaesthetized with ethyl ether, 0.1 ml of normal saline was injected into the upper lip ipsilateral to the FG injection site of the 15 rats in the first group, whereas the rats in the second group were subcutaneously injected with 0.1 ml of 4% formalin dissolved in normal saline into the upper lip ipsilateral to the FG injection site. The animals subsequently survived for 2 h prior to euthanasia. The results of the tract tracing were obtained from 6 rats in which the tracer was injected properly into the two target areas; the remaining 24 rats were discarded because of inappropriate injection sites.

FISH histochemistry combined with FG and TMR retrograde tract tracing
The riboprobes for VGLUT1 mRNA and VGLUT2 mRNA have previously been described [22]. A cDNA fragment of VGLUT1 (nucleotides 855–1788; GenBank accession number XM_133432.2) or VGLUT2 (nucleotides 848–2044; GenBank accession number NM_080853.2) was cloned into a vector pBluescript II KS (+) (Stratagene, La Jolla, CA, USA). Using the linearized plasmids as templates, we subsequently synthesized the digoxigenin (DIG)-labeled antisense single-strand RNA probes with a DIG RNA labeling kit (Roche Diagnostic, Basel, Switzerland).

Seven days after the injection of FG and TMR, the 15 rats in the first group were re-anaesthetized intraperitoneally with an overdose of sodium pentobarbital (60 mg/kg); the rats were then transcardially perfused with 0.01 M of sodium phosphate-buffered 0.9% (w/v) saline (PBS, pH 7.3), followed by 500 ml of 4% (w/v) paraformaldehyde in 0.1 M of phosphate buffer (PB, pH 7.3). After perfusion, the brains were further postfixed in 4% paraformaldehyde for 3 days at 4 °C. Cryoprotected with 30% (w/v) sucrose in 0.1 M of PB for 2 days, the whole brains were serially cut into 20-μm-thick transverse sections using a freezing microtome (Leica CM1950; Leica, Germany).

The sections were divided into 7 series of alternate serial sections. One series of sections was directly mounted onto clean glass slides and air dried. In these sections, the location and extent of the TMR and FG injection sites, as well as the distribution of TMR- and FG-labeled neurons in the Vsp, were observed with an epifluorescence microscope (BX60; Olympus, Tokyo, Japan) under an appropriate filter for TMR (excitation 540–552 nm; emission 575–625 nm) and FG (excitation 360–370 nm; emission≥395 nm).

An additional three series of the sections were used for FISH combined with immunofluorescence histochemistry. In brief, free-floating sections were treated with 2% H_2O_2 in 0.1 M of PB for 10 min at room temperature (RT). After rinsing with 0.1 M of PB, the sections were incubated in 0.3% Triton-X100 in 0.1 M of PB at RT for 20 min and 10 min in acetylation solution, which consisted of 0.25% (v/v) acetic anhydride in 0.1 M of triethanolamine. After rinsing for 10 min twice, the sections were pre-hybridized for 1 h at 58 °C in a hybridization buffer, which contained 50% (v/v) formamide, 5 × saline sodium citrate (SSC; 1×SSC = 0.15 M of NaCl and 0.015 M of sodium citrate, pH 7.0), 2% (w/v) blocking reagent (Roche Diagnostics), 0.1% (w/v) N-lauroylsarcosine (NLS) and 0.1% (w/v) sodium dodecyl sulfate (SDS). VGLUT1 or VGLUT2 riboprobes were subsequently added into the hybridization system with a final concentration of 1 μg/ml and hybridized at 58 °C for 20 h. After two washes for 20 min at 55 °C with wash buffer, which contained 2 × SSC, 50% (v/v) formamide and 0.1% (w/v) NLS, the hybridized sections were incubated with 20 μg/ml ribonuclease A for 30 min at 37 °C in a mixture of 10 mM of Tris–HCl (pH 8.0), 1 mM of EDTA and 0.5 M of NaCl, followed by 2 washes for 20 min at 37 °C in 0.2 × SSC that contained 0.1% (w/v) NLS. The sections were subsequently incubated overnight at room temperature with a mixture of 0.5 μg/ml peroxidase-conjugated anti-digoxigenin sheep antibody (11–207–733-910; Roche Diagnostics, Basel, Switzerland), 1 μg/ml guinea pig anti-FG antibody (NM-101, Protos Biotech Corporation, NY, USA) and 1 μg/ml rabbit anti-TMR antibody (A-6397, Invitrogen, Eugene, OR, USA) in 0.1 M of Tris–HCl (pH 7.5)-buffered 0.9% (w/v) saline (TS 7.5) that contained 1% blocking reagent

(TSB). To amplify the VGLUT1 or VGLUT2 mRNA hybridization signals, we performed the biotinylated tyramine (BT)-glucose oxidase (GO) amplification method with a reaction mixture that consisted of 1.25 μM of BT, 3 μg/ml GO, 2 mg/ml β-D-glucose, and 1% bovine serum albumin (BSA) in 0.1 M of PB for 30 min. The sections were subsequently treated with a mixture of 10 μg/ml Fluorescein Avidin D (A-2001; Vector, Burlingame, CA, USA), 10 μg/ml Alexa 647-conjugated goat anti-guinea pig IgG antibody (A-21450; Invitrogen) and 10 μg/ml Alexa 594-conjugated donkey anti-rabbit antibody (A-21207; Invitrogen) in TSB for 4 h.

The FISH was also performed using the sense probe (the third and fourth series of sections); however, no hybridization signals were detected in these sections.

CGRP-immunoreactive axonal varicosities in the Vc were detected in apposition to FG- and TMR-labeled neuronal profiles by triple-immunofluorescence histochemistry

The fifth series of the sections through the Vc was incubated overnight with a mixture of 1 μg/ml guinea pig anti-FG antibody (Protos Biotech Corporation), 0.5 μg/ml rabbit anti-TMR antibody(Invitrogen), and 1 μg/ml goat anti-CGRP antibody (ab36001; Abcam) in PBS-XCD. After three washes with PBS, the sections were treated with 10 μg/ml biotinylated donkey anti-goat IgG (AP180B, Millipore, Temecula, CA, USA). The sections were then further incubated overnight with a mixture of 10 μg/ml Alexa 647-conjugated goat anti-guinea pig IgG antibody (Invitrogen), 10 μg/ml Alexa 594-conjugated donkey anti-rabbit IgG antibody (Invitrogen), and 10 μg/ml Fluorescein Avidin D (Vector) in PBS that contained 5% (v/v) normal donkey serum.

The sixth sections, which contained the Vsp of the rats injected with FG and TMR, were used to conduct the control experiments for immunofluorescence histochemistry, in which CGRP antibody was omitted. Under these conditions, no immunoreactivity for the omitted antibody was observed.

Detection of Fos immunoreactivity in Vc neurons labeled with FG and TMR by triple-immunofluorescence histochemistry

The last sections through the Vc of the rats in the first group and the sections through the Vc from the second group injected with FG, TMR, and formalin were also processed for triple-immunofluorescence histochemistry for Fos, TMR and FG. Briefly, the sections were incubated with (1) a mixture of 1 μg/ml mouse anti-Fos antibody (ab 208,942, Abcam, Cambridge, MA, USA), 1 μg/ml guinea pig anti-FG antibody (NM-101, Protos Biotech Corporation) and 0.5 μg/ml rabbit anti-TMR antibody (A-6397, Invitrogen) in PBS that contained 0.3% (v/v) Triton X-100, 0.25%

(w/v) λ-carrageenan, and 3% (v/v) donkey serum (PBS-XCD) overnight at room temperature; (2) 10 μg/ml biotinylated donkey anti-mouse IgG (AP192B, Millipore, Temecula, CA, USA); and (3) a mixture of 10 μg/ml Alexa 647-conjugated goat anti-guinea pig IgG antibody (A-21450, Invitrogen), 10 μg/ml Alexa594-conjugated donkey anti-rabbit IgG antibody (A-21207, Invitrogen), and 10 μg/ml Fluorescein Avidin D (A-2001; Vector) in PBS that contained 3% (v/v) normal donkey serum.

Another series of sections from the second group was used to conduct the control experiments for immunofluorescence histochemistry, in which the Fos antibody was omitted. Under these conditions, no immunoreactivity for the omitted antibody was observed.

Immunofluorescence histochemistry combined with biotinylated dextran amine (BDA) anterograde tract tracing

Anterograde tract tracing from the Vsp to the PBN regions was performed using BDA (D1956, Invitrogen) in 15 rats. In each rat, 0.2 μl of 2% (w/v) BDA in distilled water was injected into the Vo (5 rats), Vi (5 rats) or Vc (5 rats). After a period of 5 days, the rats injected with BDA were sacrificed. Similar to the procedure of the FG and TMR injection experiments, the brainstem of the rats was cut into transverse sections in series, and one series of sections through Vo, Vi or Vc was directly incubated with Fluorescein Avidin D to detect the location and extent of the BDA injection site.

The sections through the PBN from the rats that had a proper BDA injection site were subsequently incubated overnight at room temperature with a mixture of 1 μg/ml mouse anti-NeuN antibody (MAB377; Millipore, Billerica, MA) and 2 μg/ml guinea pig anti-VGLUT2 (135,404, Synaptic Systems, Goettingen, German) in PBS that contained PBS-XCD, followed by 6 h at RT with a mixture of 5 μg/ml Fluorescein Avidin D (Vector), 5 μg/ml Alexa 594-conjugated goat anti-guinea pig IgG antibody (A-11076, Invitrogen) and 5 μg/ml Alexa 647-conjugated donkey anti-mouse IgG antibody (A-31571, Invitrogen).

Confocal laser scanning microscopy for the immunofluorescence stained sections

After incubation, all immunofluorescence stained sections were observed under a confocal laser scanning microscope (FV1000; Olympus, Tokyo, Japan) with appropriate laser beams and filter sets for fluorescein (excitation 488 nm, emission 510–530 nm), TMR and Alexa 594 (excitation 543 nm, emission 590–615 nm) or Alexa 647 (excitation 633 nm, emission 650 nm). We captured the digital images with an FV10-ASW 1.6 from Olympus; following modifications (15–20% contrast enhancement) in Photoshop CS4 (Adobe Systems, San Jose, CA), these images were saved as TIFF files.

Cell counting and statistics

In the 3 rats in which the FG injection into the PBN and TMR injection into the thalamus were successful, the TMR- and FG-labeled cell bodies of neurons that expressed VGLUT1 or VGLUT2 mRNA were identified by FISH combined with retrograde tract tracing. For these counts, in each rat, we selected 15 sections that covered the whole rostral-caudal axis of the Vsp, 5 sections of the Vo, 5 sections of the Vi and 5 sections of the Vc. In the other 3 rats, after the TMR and FG were administered and the formalin was subcutaneously injected into the upper lip ipsilateral to the FG injection site, the TMR- or FG-labeled cell bodies of neurons that expressed Fos immunoreactivity were identified by immunohistochemistry combined with retrograde tract tracing. For these counts, in each rat, 10 sections that covered the whole rostral-caudal axis of the Vc were selected. The target areas (Vo, Vi or Vc) were subsequently photographed with a confocal laser microscope under a 10× objective, and the number of neurons double-labeled with TMR/FG, TMR/VGLUT1 mRNA, TMR/VGLUT2 mRNA, FG/VGLUT1 mRNA, or FG/VGLUT2 mRNA, and the neurons triple-labeled with TMR/FG/VGLUT1, TMR/FG/VGLUT2 or TMR/FG/Fos were counted based on these photographs. In all experiments, only cells with a clear nucleus were counted.

For statistics, the numbers of the counted cells of each rat were initially summed and then averaged among the three rats. All data are presented as the mean ± standard deviation (SD). *Student's t* test was used to determine whether the number of Fos immuno-reactive cells in the Vc of the rats after formalin injection was significantly different from that in the rats injected with normal saline. For cell counting in the Vc, the identification of each lamina of the Vc referred to the rat brain atlas by Paxinos [23] and the book "The Rat Nervous System" by Paxinos [24]. The layers consist of a marginal layer (lamina I) and substantia gelatinosa (lamina II), which together comprise the superficial laminae, and a deeper magnocellular layer (laminae III and IV; a separate lamina III is not obvious in the rat; however, it is typically included in the magnocellular layer).

Triple immune-electron microscopy showed CGRP-immunoreactive terminals in synaptic contact with WGA-HRP- and FG-labeled neuronal profiles in Vc

Six rats were injected with WGA-HRP and FG for electron microscopy. In each rat, 0.2 μl of FG was injected by pressure into the left PBN as previously described. After 4 days, the rats were re-anaesthetized with sodium pentobarbital (40 mg/kg body weight) and stereotaxically injected with 0.6 μl of 1% WGA-HRP (PL-1026, Vector) into the right thalamus of the FG injected rats. The procedures for the stereotaxic microinjection of the WGA-HRP solution were the same as described for FG. After the injection of WGA-HRP, the rats were allowed to survive for 3 days.

The rats were deeply anaesthetized and transcardially perfused with 200 ml of 4% (w/v) paraformaldehyde, 0.1% (w/v) glutaraldehyde, and 15% (v/v) saturated picric acid in 0.1 M of PB. The brainstems were serially cut into 50-μm-thick transverse sections with a Vibratome (Microslicer DTM-1000; Dosaka EM, Kyoto, Japan). The staining of WGA-HRP was processed using tetramethylbenzidine (TMB) with sodium tungstate as a stabilizer [25], and the WGA-HRP reaction products were further intensified with DAB/cobalt/H_2O_2 solution. The sections that contained the injection sites were subsequently mounted onto glass slides for the conformation of the injection site. The sections through the Vc from 3 animals with both WGA-HRP and FG injection sites restrained in the target area were selected and incubated in a mixture of 25% (w/v) sucrose and 10% (v/v) glycerol in 0.05 M of PB for 1 h. The sections were transiently frozen and thawed with liquid nitrogen. Following incubation at room temperature with 0.05 M of Tris-HCl-buffered saline (TBS; pH 7.4) that contained 20% (v/v) normal donkey serum for 1 h, the sections were processed for double immunolabeling of FG and CGRP. In brief, the sections were incubated at room temperature overnight with 1 μg/ml rabbit anti-FG antibody (A153-I, Millipore) and 1 μg/ml mouse anti-CGRP antibody (ab81887, Abcam) in TBS that contained 2% (v/v) normal donkey serum (TBS-D). After rinsing with TBS, the sections were incubated in TBS-D with 10 μg/ml 1.4-nm gold-particle-conjugated goat anti-rabbit IgG antibody (2004; Nanoprobes, Stony Brook, NY, USA) and 10 μg/ml biotin-conjugated donkey anti-mouse IgG antibody (Millipore) overnight. The sections were subsequently treated with 1% (w/v) glutaraldehyde in 0.1 M of PB (pH 7.4) for 10 min and rinsed with distilled water. An HQ Silver Kit (2012; Nanoprobes) was subsequently employed to perform silver enhancement. The sections were then incubated with a 1:50-diluted Elite ABC Kit (PK-2101, Vector) in 0.05 M of TBS for 6 h and further treated with 0.02% (w/v) 3,3-diaminobenzidine tetrahydrochloride (DAB; D5637, Sigma, St. Louis, MO, USA) and 0.3% (v/v) H_2O_2 in 0.05 M of Tris–HCl (pH 7.6) for 30 min. The sections were subsequently incubated in 1% (w/v) OsO_4 in 0.1 M of PB (pH 7.4) for 35 min and counterstained in 70% ethanol that contained 1% (w/v) uranyl acetate for 1 h. With dehydration, the sections were mounted onto silicon-coated glass slides, and 1 was embedded in epoxy resin (Durcupan; Fluka, Buchs,

Switzerland). Once the resin polymerized, section fragments that contained the superficial layer of the Vc were removed from the resin. The selected tissue fragments were further cut into 60-nm-thick sections using an ultramicrotome (Reichert-Nissei Ultracut S; Leica). The ultrathin sections were then mounted onto single-slot grids coated with pioloform membranes and detected with a JEM-1400 electron microscope (JEM, Tokyo, Japan).

Results

Both a TMR injection into the thalamus and an FG injection into the PBN were performed in 30 rats. In the sites of the TMR or FG injections into the thalamus or PBN, a dense core of the tracer was surrounded by a diffuse halo of the same. The brightest injection areas were considered to represent the injection site. When a TMR injection site was confined within the targeted area in the VPM and Po and their immediate vicinities, the TMR injection into the thalamus was considered successful. When the lateral and medial parabrachial nuclei (LPB and MPB), including the Kölliker-Fuse nucleus, were involved in an injection site, the FG injection into the PBN region was considered successful. Thus, 6 of the 30 rats were considered to be successfully injected, as the TMR and FG injection sites both involved the target area (Figs. 1, 2 and 6). Although the location and extent of the injection sites in these 3 rats (R4, R7, and R13 in TMR and FG; R18, R25, and R29 in TMR, FG, Fos) were variable, the patterns of retrograde labeling in the Vsp were relatively similar.

Dual retrograde tract tracing combined with FISH histochemistry for VGLUT1 or VGLUT2 mRNA

To examine whether Vsp neurons that express VGLUT1 or VGLUT2 mRNA may send their axon collaterals to the contralateral thalamus and ipsilateral PBN, retrograde tract tracing combined with FISH histochemistry for VGLUT1 or VGLUT2 mRNA was performed after TMR injection into the right thalamus and FG injection into the left PBN in R4, R7 and R13 (Figs. 1 and 2). Using confocal laser scanning microscopic detection, many TMR- or FG-labeled neurons were observed in the left Vsp (ipsilateral to the FG injection into the PBN; contralateral to the TMR injection into the thalamus), whereas only a small number were observed on the right side. Thus, all observations were focused on the left Vsp.

In general, the results indicated that relatively more TMR-labeled neurons were observed in the Vi (Figs. 3b and 4b), and fewer neurons were scattered within the Vo (Figs. 3a and 4a) and Vc (Figs. 3c and 4c). FG-labeled neurons were distributed in the Vo with slight dominance at the caudal levels (Figs. 3a and 4a), whereas the ventral and dorsal parts at the rostro-caudal axis of

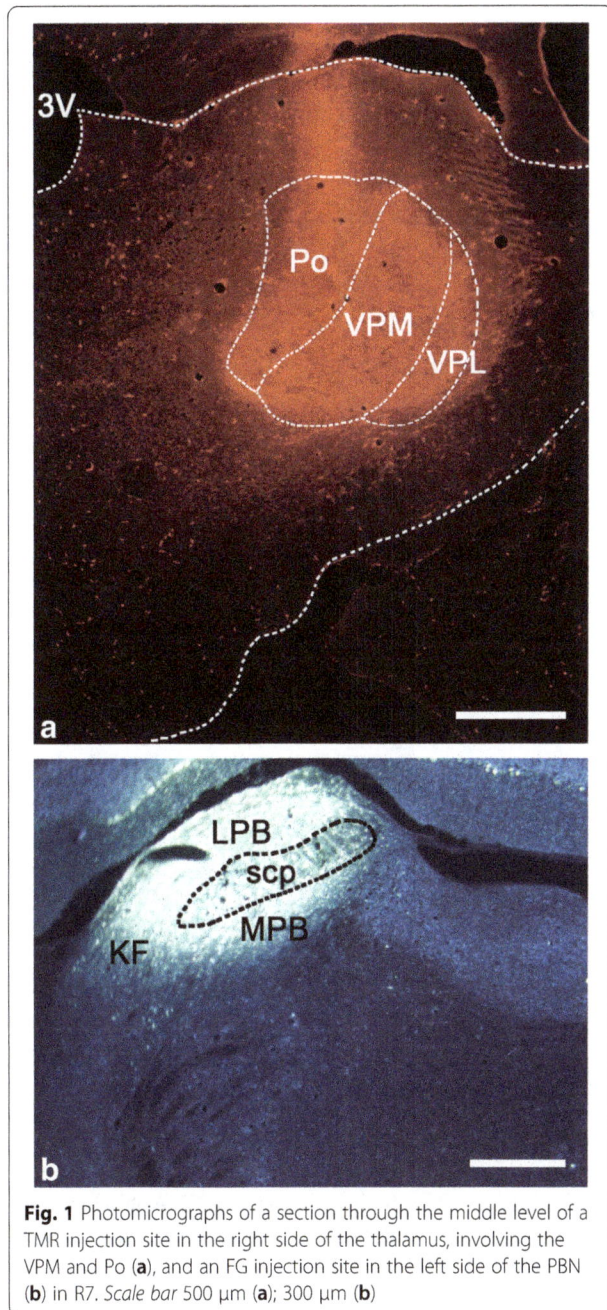

Fig. 1 Photomicrographs of a section through the middle level of a TMR injection site in the right side of the thalamus, involving the VPM and Po (**a**), and an FG injection site in the left side of the PBN (**b**) in R7. *Scale bar* 500 μm (**a**); 300 μm (**b**)

the Vi showed slight dominance at the rostral levels (Figs. 3b and 4b). In the Vc, most of the TMR-labeled neurons were located in the superficial layer (Figs. 3c and 4c). Similar to the TMR-labeled neurons, the FG-labeled neurons in the Vc were mainly distributed in the superficial layer (Fig. 3c, c2, c4; Fig. 4c, c2, c4). There was a substantial number of neuronal cells with VGLUT2 mRNA signals distributed throughout the Vsp (Fig. 3c). In contrast, neurons with VGLUT1 mRNA signals were also abundant in the Vi (Fig. 4b, b3, b4), whereas only a small number were scattered in the Vo (Fig. 4a, a3, a4) and Vc (Fig. 4c, c3, c4).

Moreover, the VGLUT1 mRNA-positive neurons were mainly distributed in the deep layer of the Vc (compare Fig. 4c with Fig. 3c).

Furthermore, cell counts were performed in the Vsp of the three rats with images obtained via confocal laser scanning microscopy (Tables 1 and 2). TMR/FG double-labeled neurons in the Vo, Vi and Vc accounted for (90.5 ± 1.8) %, (92.5 ± 1.9) % and (49.6 ± 1.0) % of the TMR-labeled cells, respectively, and (53.5 ± 2.5) %, (73.6 ± 1.2) % and (43.7 ± 1.9) % of the FG-labeled cells, respectively (Table 1). Overall, (88.2 ± 2.5) %, (92.0 ± 5.3) % and (64.5 ± 1.0) % of the TMR retrograde-labeled neurons and (6.0 ± 0.2) %, (22.2 ± 1.6) % and (0.7 ± 0.1) % of the VGLUT2 mRNA positive cells exhibited double labeling of TMR and VGLUT2 mRNA in the Vo, Vi and Vc, respectively (Table 1). Furthermore, (83.9 ± 1.6) %, (96.6 ± 1.1) % and (90.7 ± 2.9) % of the FG retrogradely labeled neurons and (9.7 ± 0.2) %, (29.2 ± 0.7) % and (1.1 ± 0.1) % of the VGLUT2 mRNA-positive cells exhibited double labeling for both FG and VGLUT2 mRNA (Table 1). TMR/FG/VGLUT2 triple-labeled neurons accounted for (81.7 ± 3.5) %, (86.0 ± 0.7) %, and (42.4 ± 0.9) % of the TMR-labeled neurons, (48.3 ± 1.7) %, (68.4 ± 0.3) % and (37.3 ± 1.6) % of the FG-labeled neurons, (5.6 ± 0.1) %, (20.7 ± 0.2) % and (0.4 ± 0.0) % of the VGLUT2 mRNA positive cells, and (90.3 ± 4.1) %, (93.0 ± 1.2) % and (85.4 ± 0.7) % of the TMR/FG double labeled neurons in the Vo, Vi and Vc (Table 1).

Moreover, (19.1 ± 2.5) %, (0.5 ± 0.4) % and (4.5 ± 2.1) % of the TMR retrogradely labeled neurons and (12.6 ± 1.9) %, (0.2 ± 0.1) % and (1.2 ± 0.6) % of the VGLUT1 mRNA positive cells exhibited dual labeling of TMR/VGLUT1 mRNA in the Vo, Vi and Vc, respectively (Table 2). Overall, (14.1 ± 2.4) %, (1.3 ± 0.7) % and (4.1 ± 2.0) % of the FG retrogradely labeled neurons and (16.1 ± 2.6) %, (0.5 ± 0.2) % and (1.2 ± 0.6) % of the VGLUT1 mRNA-positive cells were double labeled for both FG and VGLUT1 mRNA (Table 2). TMR/FG/VGLUT1 triple-labeled neurons comprised (26.8 ± 3.0) % and (1.0 ± 0.7) % of the MR-labeled neurons, (15.5 ± 2.2) % and (0.9 ± 0.6) % of the FG-labeled neurons, (17.7 ± 2.4) % and (0.3 ± 0.2) % of the VGLUT1 mRNA positive cells, and (29.9 ± 3.0) % and (2.0 ± 1.4) % of the FG/TMR double-labeled neurons in the Vo and Vc, respectively (Table 2). In the Vi, no TMR/FG/VGLUT1 triple-labeled neurons were identified; however, some neurons showed TMR/FG, TMR/VGLUT1 or FG/VGLUT1 double-labeling (Table 2).

Thus, these data indicated that the vast majority of the Vo, Vi and Vc neurons that projected both ipsilaterally to the PBN and contralaterally to the thalamus by way of axon collaterals were VGLUT2 mRNA-

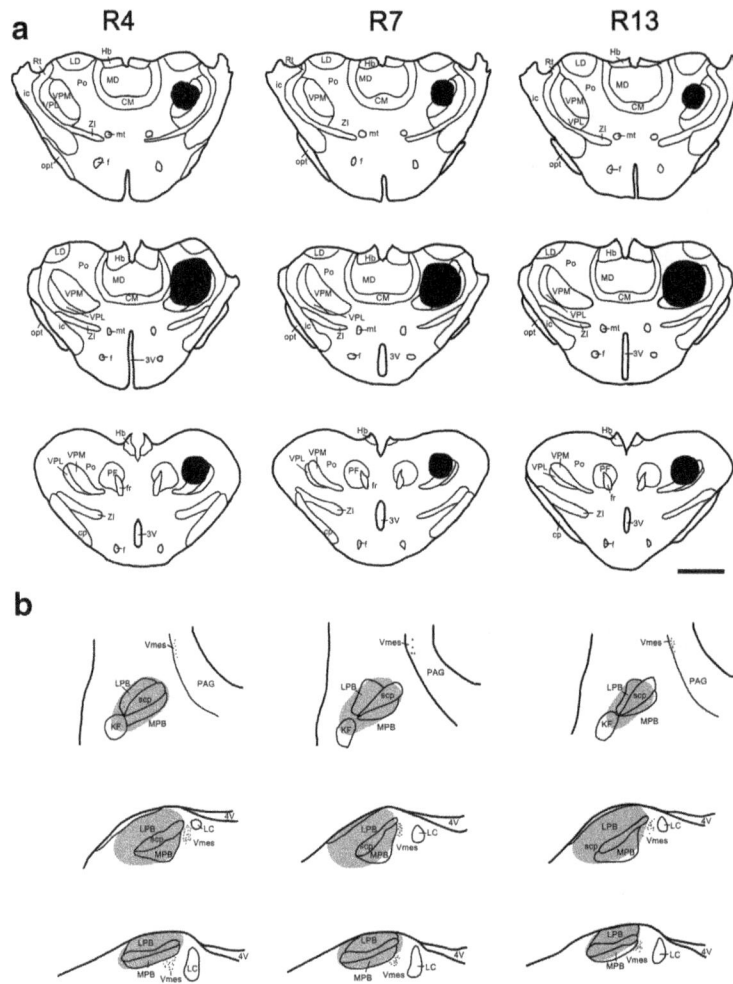

Fig. 2 Projection drawings indicate the sites of TMR injection into the thalamus and FG injection into the PBN in three rats (R4, R7, and R13). **a** Three different sections from rostral to caudal of the thalamus show the TMR injection sites confined in the VPM, the Po and their vicinities. **b** FG was injected into the left PBN, with the densest core (blackened areas) covering parts throughout the PBN and the KF. *Scale bar* 2 mm (**a**); 1 mm (**b**)

positive (Table 1), whereas a limited number expressed VGLUT1 mRNA (Table 2).

Immunofluorescence histochemistry combined with anterograde tract-tracing after BDA injection into the Vo, vi and Vc

Anterograde tract-tracing experiments combined with immunofluorescence histochemistry for VGLUT2-LI were performed in 15 rats after unilateral injection of BDA into the Vo, Vi and Vc (Fig. 5a-c); the BDA injection sites were also immunostained with NeuN. The site of the BDA injection in the rats covered nearly the complete extent of the Vo (Fig. 5a), Vi (Fig. 5b) and Vc (Fig. 5c). In these experiments, the distribution of BDA-labeled axons and terminals in the PBN was very similar (Fig. 5a1, b1, c1). Anterograde labeling was present bilaterally in the PBN and KF, with a clear ipsilateral

predominance. The highest density of BDA-labeled axon terminals was present caudally in the KF and in the ventral portion of the LPB (Fig. 5a1, b1, c1). The sections stained by triple-immunofluorescence labeling for VGLUT2/NeuN/BDA (for the rats injected with BDA to the Vo, Vi and Vc) were subsequently examined under a confocal laser scanning microscope, and the results showed that many BDA-labeled small granules in the PBN and KF showed VGLUT2 immunoreactivity (Fig. 5a2, b2, c2).

Immunoreactivities for Fos in the Vc after subcutaneous injection of formalin into the rat upper lip

To examine whether the Vc collateral projection neurons previously identified may be involved in the transmission of orofacial nociceptive information, retrograde tract tracing combined with Fos immunohistochemistry was

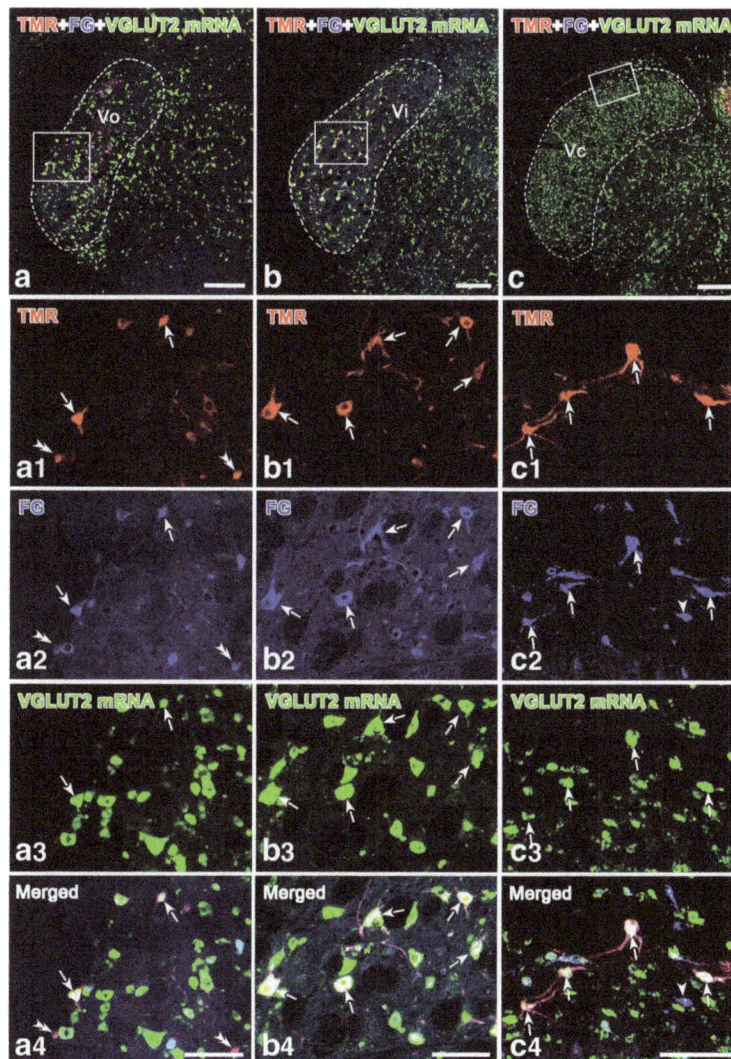

Fig. 3 Collateral projection neurons to both the thalamus and the PBN labeled with hybridization signals for VGLUT2 mRNA in the Vo (**a**, a1-a4), Vi (**b**, b1-b4) and Vc (**c**, c1-c4). Some neurons are retrogradely labeled with TMR and FG. Immunoreactivity for TMR is visualized with Alexa 594 (*red*), and immunoreactivity for FG is visualized with Alexa 647 (*blue*), whereas the VGLUT2 mRNA hybridization signals are shown with fluorescein (*green*). Images (a1-a4, b1-b4 And c1-c4) are the magnified images of the framed areas in (**a**, **b** and **c**), respectively. The *arrows* in (a1-c4) indicate the cell bodies triply labeled with TMR/FG/VGLUT2 mRNA signals (*white*); the *double arrowheads* in a1-c4 indicate the cell bodies dually labeled with TMR and FG (*purple red*); the *single arrowheads* in (a1-c4) point to cell bodies singly labeled with FG (*blue*). Scale bar 300 μm (a-c); 100 μm (a1-c4)

performed after TMR injection into the right thalamus and FG injection into the left PBN. Similar to the first group that was injected with normal saline in the upper lip, 3 rats in the second group were also considered successful, as both of the injection sites of FG and TMR were restricted in the PBN and thalamus, respectively (R18, R25, and R29, Fig. 6). The results showed that Fos-LI cell bodies in the superficial layer (laminar I and laminar II) of the left Vc in the rats injected with formalin (Fig. 7e-h) significantly increased (Fig. 8a, $P < 0.001$, 30 sections from 3 rats) compared with those in the rats injected with normal saline (Fig. 7a-d). Moreover, the percentage of FG/TMR dual-labeled neurons in the

superficial layer that showed Fos LI also significantly increased [(24.3 ± 2.8) % to (42.8 ± 3.8) %, $P < 0.001$, 30 sections from 3 rats] with the formalin injection (Fig. 8b). In detail, for the animals injected with formalin, (29.3 ± 0.4) % and (24.5 ± 1.7) % of the Fos labeled Vc neurons were identified in laminae I and II, respectively, and (46.2 ± 0.5) % was distributed in lamina III (Table 3). TMR/FG double-labeled neurons were mainly distributed in lamina I of the Vc, with (64.0 ± 4.4) % of the total double-labeled neurons in lamina I and only (15.5 ± 6.5) % and (22.1 ± 2.9) % scattered in laminae II and III, respectively. In addition, TMR/FG/Fos triple-labeled neurons were mainly distributed in lamina I of the Vc and

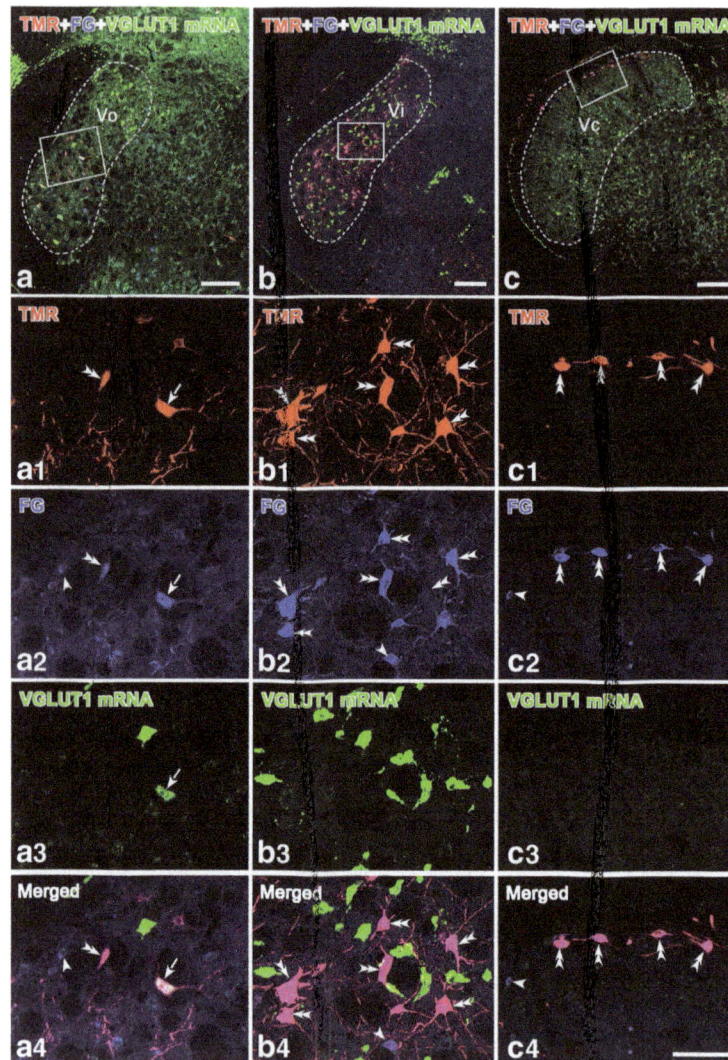

Fig. 4 Collateral projection neurons to both the thalamus and the PBN labeled with hybridization signals for VGLUT1 mRNA in the Vo (**a**, a1-a4), Vi (**b**, b1-b4) and Vc (**c**, c1-c4). Some neurons are retrogradely labeled with TMR and FG. Immunoreactivity for TMR is visualized with Alexa 594 (*red*), and immunoreactivity for FG is visualized with Alexa 647 (*blue*), whereas the VGLUT1 mRNA hybridization signals are shown with fluorescein (*green*). Images (a1-a4), (b1-b4) and (c1-c4) are the magnified images of the framed areas in (**a**), (**b**) and (**c**), respectively. The *arrows* in (a1-a4) indicate the cell bodies triply labeled with TMR/FG/VGLUT1 mRNA signals (*white*); the *double arrowheads* in (a1-c1) indicate the cell bodies dually labeled with TMR and FG (*purple red*); the *single arrowheads* in (a1-c1) point to cell bodies singly labeled with FG (*blue*). *Scale bar* 300 μm (**a-c**); 100 μm (a1-c4)

accounted for (77.8 ± 2.1) % of the total triple-labeled neurons in the Vc (Table 3).

CGRP-like immunopositive axon terminals formed close contacts or asymmetric synapses with the neuronal soma or dendrites of the collateral projections into the thalamus and LPB in Vc

To further investigate whether the Vc collateral projection neurons previously identified directly received peripheral nociceptive afferents, a triple-labeled immunofluorescence histochemical technique for CGRP, TMR and FG was used. Under a confocal laser scanning microscope, CGRP-LI was mainly observed in axonal terminals in the superficial layers of the Vc (Fig. 9a, b). No CGRP-positive products were identified in the cell bodies or dendrite profiles. Some CGRP-LI axonal terminals were observed to be in close apposition with TMR/FG double-labeled neuronal cell bodies and dendrites in laminae I and II of the Vc (Fig. 9f).

The pre-embedded triple immune-electron microscopic method was performed in three rats to further examine whether CGRP-LI axon terminals may form synaptic contacts with the PBN and thalamus collateral projection neurons in the Vc. After the WGA-HRP injection into the right thalamus and the FG injection into the left PBN, retrograde tract tracing combined with

Table 1 Number of TMR, FG and VGLUT2 mRNA-labeled neurons in the Vo, Vi, and Vc of R4, R7 and R13

	Vo	Vi	Vc
(1)TMR	92 ± 8	176 ± 9	65 ± 8
(2)FG	155 ± 9	222 ± 11	73 ± 4.5
(3)VGLUT2 mRNA	1347 ± 96	732 ± 27	6285 ± 132
(4)TMR + FG	83 ± 9	163 ± 6	32 ± 3.3
(5)[(4)/(1)] × 100	(90.5 ± 1.8)%	(92.5 ± 1.9)%	(49.6 ± 1.0)%
(6)[(4)/(2)] × 100	(53.5 ± 2.5)%	(73.6 ± 1.2)%	(43.7 ± 1.9)%
(7)TMR + VGLUT2 mRNA	81 ± 6	162 ± 18	42 ± 5
(8)[(7)/(1)] × 100	(88.2 ± 2.5)%	(92.0 ± 5.3)%	(64.5 ± 1.0)%
(9)[(7)/(3)] × 100	(6.0 ± 0.2)%	(22.2 ± 1.6)%	(0.7 ± 0.1)%
(10)FG + VGLUT2 mRNA	130 ± 10	214 ± 13	66 ± 6
(11)[(10)/(2)] × 100	(83.9 ± 1.6)%	(96.6 ± 1.1)%	(90.7 ± 2.9)%
(12)[(10)/(3)] × 100	(9.7 ± 0.2)%	(29.2 ± 0.7)%	(1.1 ± 0.1)%
(13)FG + TMR + VGLUT2 mRNA	75 ± 6	152 ± 7	27 ± 3
(14)[(13)/(1)] × 100	(81.7 ± 3.5)%	(86.0 ± 0.7)%	(42.4 ± 0.9)%
(15)[(13)/(2)] × 100	(48.3 ± 1.7)%	(68.4 ± 0.3)%	(37.3 ± 1.6)%
(16)[(13)/(3)] × 100	(5.6 ± 0.1)%	(20.7 ± 0.2)%	(0. 4 ± 0.0)%
(17)[(13)/(4)] × 100	(90.3 ± 4.1)%	(93.0 ± 1.2)%	(85.4 ± 0.7)%

TMR is injected in the right thalamus, and FG is injected into the left PBN. The cell body counts were performed for three rats on the left side. Each figure showing the number of cell bodies of one animal was the average of the three rats (5 sections from each rat). The sections were 20 μm thick. FG, TMR and VGLUT2 mRNA represent all FG-, TMR- and VGLUT2 mRNA-labeled neurons; data are shown as the mean ± standard deviation (SD)

Table 2 Number of TMR, FG and VGLUT1 mRNA-labeled neurons in the Vo, Vi, and Vc of R4, R7 and R13

	Vo	Vi	Vc
(1)TMR	90 ± 8	180 ± 10	63 ± 7
(2)FG	155 ± 9	223 ± 8	71 ± 5.3
(3)VGLUT1 mRNA	136 ± 9	634 ± 15	241 ± 12
(4)TMR + FG	81 ± 8	172 ± 12	31 ± 4.5
(5)[(4)/(1)] × 100	(89.5 ± 1.5)%	(95.1 ± 1.3)%	(49.0 ± 2.6)%
(6)[(4)/(2)] × 100	(51.8 ± 2.4)%	(77.2 ± 2.8)%	(43.2 ± 3.4)%
(7)TMR + VGLUT1 mRNA	17 ± 4	1 ± 0.8	3 ± 2
(8)[(7)/(1)] × 100	(19.1 ± 2.5)%	(0.5 ± 0.4)%	(4.5 ± 2.1)%
(9)[(7)/(3)] × 100	(12.6 ± 1.9)%	(0.2 ± 0.1)%	(1.2 ± 0.6)%
(10)FG + VGLUT1 mRNA	22 ± 4	3 ± 1	3 ± 2
(11)[10)/(2)] × 100	(14.1 ± 2.4)%	(1.3 ± 0.7)%	(4.1 ± 2.0)%
(12)[(10)/(3)] × 100	(16.1 ± 2.6)%	(0.5 ± 0.2)%	(1.2 ± 0.6)%
(13)TMR + FG + VGLUT1 mRNA	24 ± 5	0	1 ± 0
(14)[(13)/(1)] × 100	(26.8 ± 3.0)%	0	(1.0 ± 0.7)%
(15)[(13)/(2)] × 100	(15.5 ± 2.2)%	0	(0.9 ± 0.6)%
(16)[(13)/(3)] × 100	(17.7 ± 2.4)%	0	(0.3 ± 0.2)%
(17)[(13)/(4)] × 100	(29.9 ± 3.0)%	0%	(2.0 ± 1.4)%

TMR is injected into the right thalamus, and FG is injected into the left PBN. The cell body counts were performed for three rats on the left side. Each figure showing the number of cell bodies of one animal was the average of the three rats (5 sections from each rat). The sections were 20 μm thick. FG, TMR and VGLUT1 mRNA represent all FG-, TMR- and VGLUT1 mRNA-labeled neurons; data are shown as the mean ± standard deviation (SD)

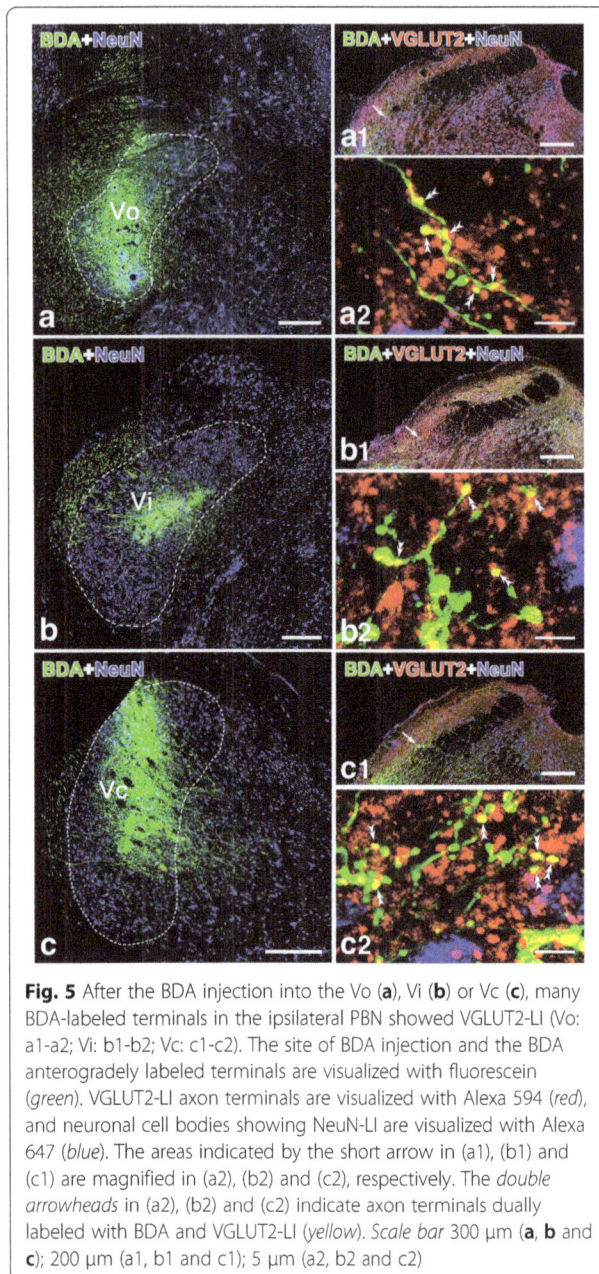

Fig. 5 After the BDA injection into the Vo (**a**), Vi (**b**) or Vc (**c**), many BDA-labeled terminals in the ipsilateral PBN showed VGLUT2-LI (Vo: a1-a2; Vi: b1-b2; Vc: c1-c2). The site of BDA injection and the BDA anterogradely labeled terminals are visualized with fluorescein (*green*). VGLUT2-LI axon terminals are visualized with Alexa 594 (*red*), and neuronal cell bodies showing NeuN-LI are visualized with Alexa 647 (*blue*). The areas indicated by the short arrow in (a1), (b1) and (c1) are magnified in (a2), (b2) and (c2), respectively. The *double arrowheads* in (a2), (b2) and (c2) indicate axon terminals dually labeled with BDA and VGLUT2-LI (*yellow*). *Scale bar* 300 μm (**a**, **b** and **c**); 200 μm (a1, b1 and c1); 5 μm (a2, b2 and c2)

large dendritic processes of neurons that projected to the VPM and Po regions of the thalamus (Fig. 10a, d, double arrowheads). Some of the cytoplasm and large dendritic processes of neurons were also labeled with silver-intensified gold particles indicating FG labeling (Fig. 10b, d, arrows), which projected to the parabrachial region. Some of the neuronal cell bodies or dendrite profiles in the superficial layer of the Vc often showed WGA-HRP/FG double-labeling (Fig. 10d). Moreover, the CGRP-LI axon terminals were often observed in asymmetric synaptic contact with dendritic profiles that were labeled retrogradely with WGA-HRP/FG (Fig. 10d), which indicates that these neurons collaterally project to the thalamus and PBN.

Discussion

It has been reported that some projection neurons in lamina I of the spinal dorsal horn [26] or medullary dorsal horn (Vc) of the rat [4] send their axons to both the thalamus and the PBN by way of axon collaterals; however, no previous study has reported the existence of these neurons in the Vo, Vi, and Vc or which VGLUTs may be expressed in the T-T and T-P collateral projection neurons in the Vsp. Thus, in the present study, retrograde tract tracing was performed to examine whether Vsp neurons may be labeled with two types of retrograde tracers that were injected into the thalamus and PBN of each rat. FISH histochemistry was further performed to examine the expression of VGLUT1 mRNA and VGLUT2 mRNA in these collaterally projecting neurons.

The results of the present study have indicated the existence of collaterally projecting neurons in the Vo, Vi and Vc, and these collateral projection neurons in the Vo, Vi and Vc exclusively expressed VGLUT2 mRNA and not VGLUT1 mRNA, with the exception of a few Vo collateral projection neurons that were VGLUT1 mRNA-positive. Moreover, the collaterally projecting neurons in the Vc may be related to the transmission of orofacial nociceptive information.

VGLUT1 and VGLUT2 mRNA-expressing neurons in Vsp send axon collaterals to both the thalamus and the PBN

It has been reported that the trigeminothalamic fibers of the rat project to the thalamus bilaterally with contralateral predominance [27, 28]. Therefore, in the present study, TMR was injected into the contralateral thalamus, and it was ensured that the injection site covered the VPM and Po. TMR-labeled neurons were distributed in all subdivisions of the contralateral Vsp (Vo, Vi, and Vc). They were most prevalent in the Vi, followed by the Vo, with the smallest in number in the Vc. These data appear to be in fairly good accordance with data previously reported in the rat [15, 29]. The TMR-labeled neurons

CGRP-like immunohistochemistry was visualized with a typical TMB reaction method for WGA-HRP and the immunogold silver method for FG, whereas CGRP-labeling was identified by the immunoperoxidase method.

In the Vc, electron-dense peroxidase reaction products (DAB reaction) that indicated CGRP labeling were identified within axon terminals, which were filled with round, black, clearly defined synaptic vesicles (Fig. 10c, d). In the superficial layer of the Vc, TMB reaction products that consisted of black crystals with high electronic densities indicating WGA-HRP labeling were identified in the cytoplasm and

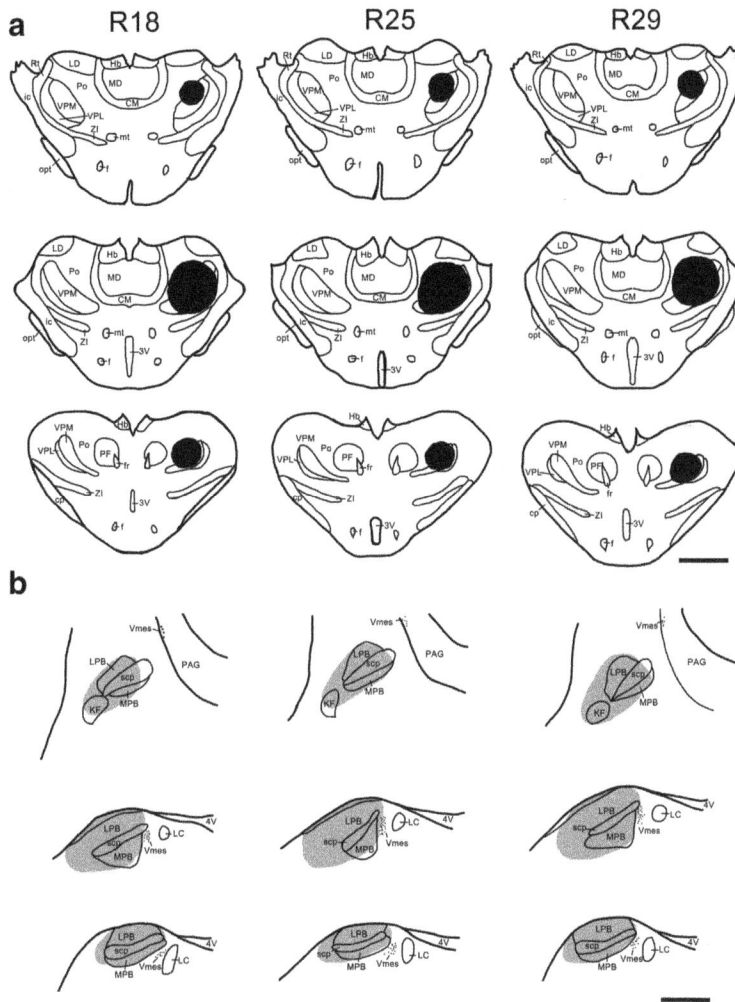

Fig. 6 Projection drawings of the sites of TMR injection into the thalamus and FG injection into the PBN in three rats (R18, R25, and R29) that received formalin injection prior to perfusion. **a** Three different sections from rostral to caudal of the thalamus show the TMR injection into the right side of the thalamus site involving the VPM, the Po and their vicinities. **b** FG was injected into the left PBN, with the densest core (blackened areas) covering parts throughout the PBN and the KF. *Scale bar* 2 mm (**a**); 1 mm (**b**)

in the Vc showed a laminar pattern, with most of the retrogradely labeled neurons in the superficial layers (laminae I and II) as previously reported [4, 30]. Previous studies regarding direct projection from the Vo to the thalamus are contradictory: studies [29, 31] have shown retrogradely labeled neurons in the Vo, whereas other studies [2, 32] have not. In the present study, we observed TMR-labeled neurons throughout the Vo, with more neurons in the ventrolateral part. This distribution pattern is similar to that reported by Guy et al. [31].

It has been established that the projection fibers from the Vc to the PBN in the rat mainly terminate in the PBN portions lateral and ventromedial to the superior cerebellar peduncle [4, 33–35]. These PBN areas of termination of projection fibers from the ipsilateral Vsp (Vo, Vi, Vc) appeared to be included in the FG injection sites in the present study. As the PBN is dorsomedial to

the Vp, the injection site was strictly limited within the PBN without contaminating the Vp, which receives direct projections from the Vsp. The FG-labeled neurons were observed in the bilateral Vsp with ipsilateral predominance. This finding is consistent with previous studies that described direct Vsp projections to the PBN with ipsilateral predominance in the rat [33, 35–37]. According to the present results, the PBN-projecting neurons were distributed among the entire Vo and Vi, whereas Vc neurons that send projections to the PBN were mainly located in the superficial layer, which is also consistent with previous studies [4, 34, 35, 38].

In the present study, following the TMR injection contralaterally into the thalamus and the FG injection ipsilaterally into the PBN, TMR/FG double-labeled neurons in the Vo, Vi and Vc were frequently encountered. Neurons dually labeled for TMR and FG were distributed in

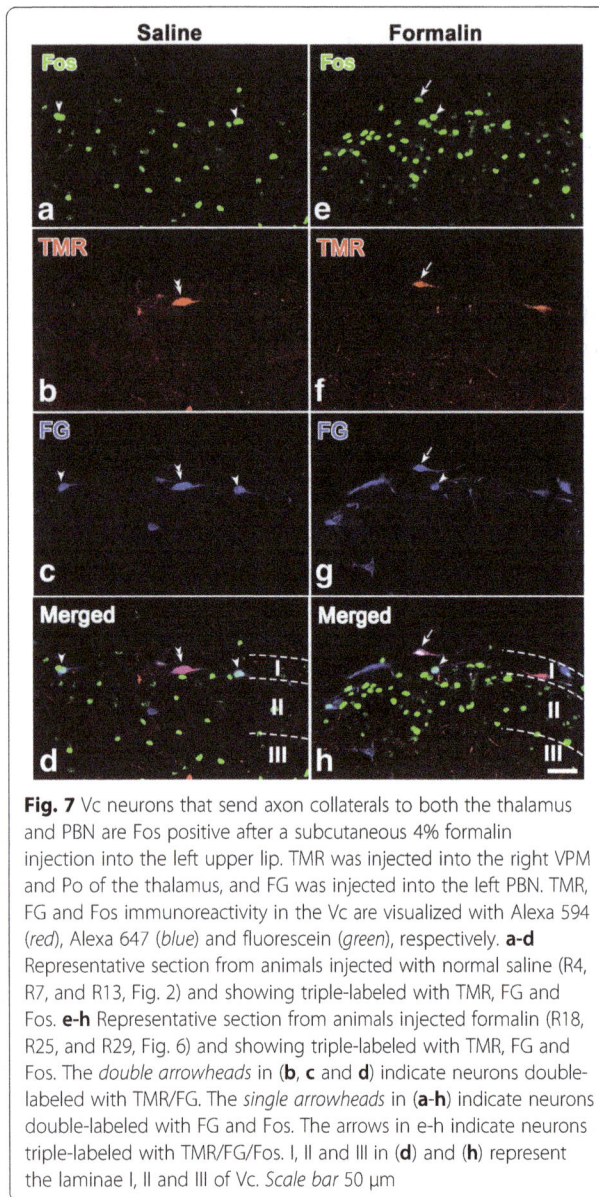

Fig. 7 Vc neurons that send axon collaterals to both the thalamus and PBN are Fos positive after a subcutaneous 4% formalin injection into the left upper lip. TMR was injected into the right VPM and Po of the thalamus, and FG was injected into the left PBN. TMR, FG and Fos immunoreactivity in the Vc are visualized with Alexa 594 (*red*), Alexa 647 (*blue*) and fluorescein (*green*), respectively. **a-d** Representative section from animals injected with normal saline (R4, R7, and R13, Fig. 2) and showing triple-labeled with TMR, FG and Fos. **e-h** Representative section from animals injected formalin (R18, R25, and R29, Fig. 6) and showing triple-labeled with TMR, FG and Fos. The *double arrowheads* in (**b**, **c** and **d**) indicate neurons double-labeled with TMR/FG. The *single arrowheads* in (**a-h**) indicate neurons double-labeled with FG and Fos. The arrows in e-h indicate neurons triple-labeled with TMR/FG/Fos. I, II and III in (**d**) and (**h**) represent the laminae I, II and III of Vc. *Scale bar* 50 μm

have further indicated the existence of neurons in the Vi and Vo that also send collateral projection to both the PBN and the thalamus; however, these collateral projection neurons have not been reported in previous studies.

In the present study, FISH histochemistry for VGLUT1 or VGLUT2 mRNA was combined with double retrograde tract tracing using TMR injected into the thalamus and FG injected into the PBN. The results indicated that most TMR/FG doubly labeled Vsp neurons express VGLUT2 mRNA (90.3% in the Vo, 93.0% in the Vi, and 85.4% in the Vc), whereas almost no TMR/FG-labeled Vi and Vc neurons express VGLUT1 mRNA (Tables 1 and 2). Dual FISH histochemistry performed in a previous study [16] also indicated that no single Vsp neurons co-express VGLUT1 and VGLUT2 mRNAs. Thus, it was assumed that glutamatergic T-T and T-P collateral projection neurons in the Vsp mainly express VGLUT2 mRNA.

Collateral projection neurons in Vc are related to the transmission of orofacial nociceptive information

The Vc is often referred to as the medullary dorsal horn and is considered to be homologous to the spinal dorsal horn both structurally and functionally [39]. The superficial laminae of the Vc contains many neurons that constitute the main relay for nociceptive primary afferents from the orofacial regions [39–41], and previous studies have indicated that substance P (SP)-containing small-diameter primary afferent fibers and CGRP-LI primary afferent fibers terminate mainly in laminae I and II [42–45]. Thus, in the present study, when some TMR/FG double-labeled soma and dendrites of neurons in laminae I and II of the Vc were in apposition to CGRP-LI terminals under the confocal laser-scanning microscope, they were assumed to receive and transmit nociceptive inputs. Furthermore, the results of the electron microscopy also indicated that CGRP-LI axon terminals (labeled with DAB reaction) formed asymmetric synapses with the soma or dendrite profiles of the TMR/FG double-labeled collateral projection neurons in the Vc. In accordance with the present data, previous studies in primates have indicated that many nociceptive neurons in the Vc receive direct primary nociceptive afferent input and send projection fibers to both the PBN and the thalamus, including the VPM and Po, by way of axon collaterals [4, 26, 46–48].

Furthermore, the nociceptive nature of Vc neurons that were retrogradely labeled with TMR and FG injected into the thalamus and PBN was identified by the expression of Fos-LI after the injection of formalin solution into the upper lip of rats. Previous studies have shown that noxious stimulation of different orofacial sites induced Fos-LI in

all subdivisions of the Vsp (Vo, Vi, and Vc); they were most prevalent in the Vi, followed by the Vo, with the smallest number in the Vc (Table 1). In the Vc, the TMR/FG double-labeled neurons were distributed in a laminar pattern, with the vast majority in lamina I. A previous study [4] also indicated that neurons in the Vc sent collateral projections to both the thalamus and the PBN, with more than 90% of the projecting neurons distributed in lamina I. Thus, the Vc neurons double-labeled with TMR/FG, which were observed in the present study, are considered to represent fairly well the Vc neurons that send their axons both ipsilaterally to the PBN and contralaterally to the thalamus by way of axon collaterals. Moreover, the results of the present study

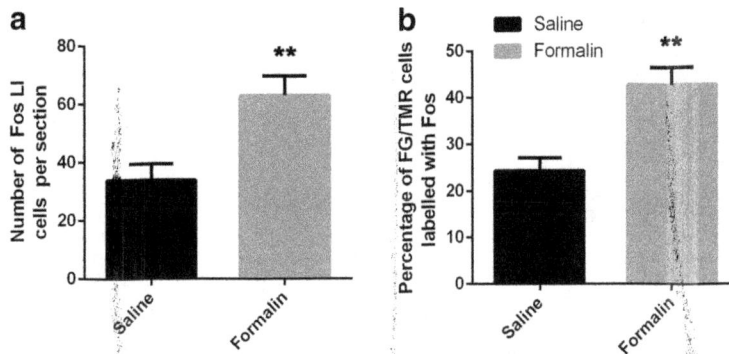

Fig. 8 Comparison of the number of Fos-like immunoreactive (LI) neuronal cells in the superficial layer (laminae I and II) of the Vc in rats injected with normal saline and rats injected with formalin. **a** Compared with rats injected with normal saline, the number of Fos-LI cells per section in the superficial layer of the Vc significantly increased after the injection of formalin into the upper lip of rats. **b** The percentage of FG/TMR double-labeled neurons in one section in the superficial layer of the Vc showed Fos-LI substantially increased in rats injected with formalin. **P < 0.001, 30 sections from 3 rats

the ipsilateral Vc, mainly in laminae I and II [18, 49–52]. Therefore, Fos-LI has often been used for the investigation of somatotopy in the trigeminal nociceptive pathways [18, 53, 54]. In the present study, after subcutaneous injection of formalin into the upper lip of rats, Fos-LI was induced in many neurons in the Vc, particularly in the superficial laminae of the dorsomedial part. This distribution pattern of Fos-LI was consistent with previous studies [18, 19, 55, 56] and appeared to be compatible with the somatotopy of the projection of the trigeminal nerve [24]. We also performed triple-labeling of TMR/FG/Fos to identify the expression of Fos-LI in TMR/FG double-labeled neurons. The neurons that supply relatively localized orofacial regions are somatotopically organized within the Vc [24]. We noxiously stimulated only the upper lip, and it may be assumed that only some of the nociceptive neurons in the Vc were activated. Thus, the present result that 34.0% of TMR/FG double-labeled neurons expressed Fos-LI may indicate that a substantial proportion of the collateral projection neurons in the Vc are activated by noxious stimulation of the orofacial region.

Functional implications of the glutamatergic collateral projection neurons in Vsp

The thalamus and PBN are two nuclei with distinctly different roles. As shown in the present results, the injection site in the thalamus covered the VPM and Po. These two thalamic relay nuclei receive their afferent input from the Vsp and project to the somatosensory cortex in a complementary pattern [15, 16, 57, 58]. Both nuclei are critical in the formation of discriminative somatic sensation of orofacial regions [39, 59, 60]. The function of the PBN is relatively complicated. It is involved not only in gustatory functions [61–63] and autonomic regulatory processes [38, 64–68] but also affective processes [69–71], particularly in the affective aspects of pain [5, 38, 72, 73]. The information conveyed by the T-P pathways likely contributes more to the affective component of the pain experience than to the discriminative somatic sensation [39, 74]. In brief, the T-T and T-P projections are related to the discriminative somatic sensation and the affective component of orofacial sensation, respectively.

In situ hybridization detection was used for VGLUT1 and VGLUT2 mRNA, which have been well

Table 3 Number of neurons labeled with FG, TMR and (or) Fos in the Vc of R18, R25 and R29

	Lamina I	Lamina II	Lamina III	Total
(1)TMR	92 ± 9 (59.3 ± 1.5)%	12 ± 3 (7.9 ± 2.5)%	51 ± 7 (33.1 ± 0.3)%	142 ± 18
(2)FG	81 ± 8 (57.5 ± 1.8)%	21 ± 4 (15.5 ± 4.0)%	39 ± 6 (27.6 ± 0.7)%	155 ± 18
(3)Fos	344 ± 18 (29.3 ± 0.4)%	287 ± 11 (24.5 ± 1.7)%	541 ± 16 (46.2 ± 0.5)%	1172 ± 46
(4)TMR + FG	29 ± 6 (64.0 ± 4.4)%	7 ± 2 (15.5 ± 6.5)%	11 ± 4 (22.1 ± 2.9)%	47 ± 12
(5)TMR + FG + Fos	13 ± 4 (77.8 ± 2.1)%	2 ± 1 (14.2 ± 7.0)%	2 ± 0 (10.4 ± 1.6)%	16 ± 5
(6)[(5)/(4)] × 100	(42.1 ± 5.8)%	(29.4 ± 3.4)%	(16.4 ± 3.1)%	(34.4 ± 2.4)%

TMR is injected into the collateral thalamus, and FG is injected into the ipsilateral PBN. The cell body counts were performed for three rats on the ipsilateral side of the FG injection site. Each figure showing the number of cell bodies of one animal was the average of the three rats (10 sections from each rat). The sections were 20 μm thick. FG, TMR and Fos represent all FG-, TMR- and Fos-labeled neurons; data are shown as the mean ± standard deviation (SD)

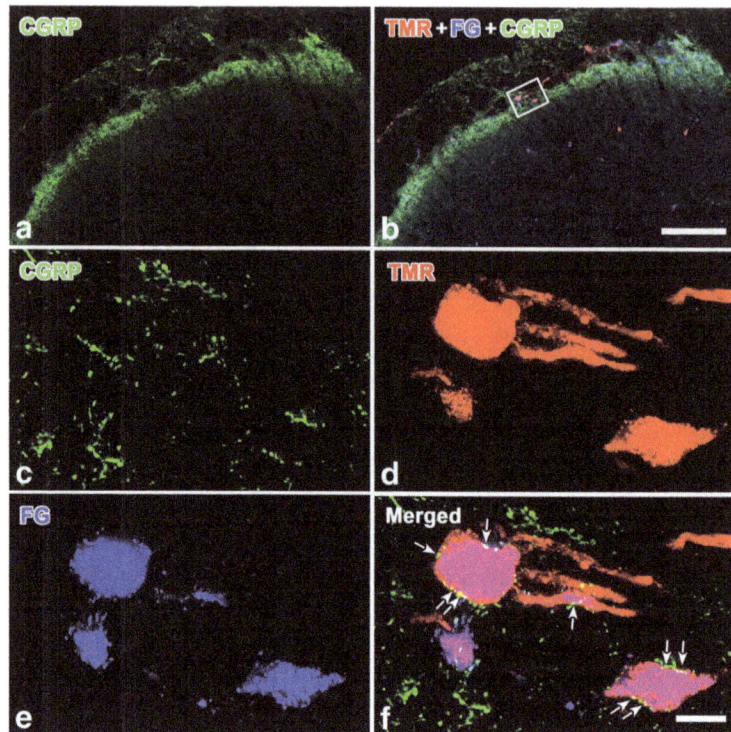

Fig. 9 CGRP-positive terminals have close contacts with collateral projection neurons in the Vc superficial layer. TMR was injected into the right VPM and Po of the thalamus, and FG was injected into the left PBN in three rats (R4, R7, and R13, Fig. 2). TMR, FG and CGRP immunoreactivity in the superficial layer of the Vc are visualized with Alexa 594 (*red*), Alexa 647 (*blue*) and fluorescein (*green*), respectively. The boxed area in (**b**) is magnified in (**c-f**). The *arrows* in f indicate that some CGRP-LI axonal terminals are in close contact with TMR/FG double-labeled cell body or dendritic profiles. *Scale bar* 200 μm (in **a** and **b**); 20 μm (in **c-f**)

established as the specific markers for glutamatergic neurons in the CNS [10–14, 75–78]. The distribution of VGLUT1 and VGLUT2 in the CNS exhibited a complementary pattern [14], which indicates that there may be a distinct functional difference between these two proteins. In the Vsp, as shown in a previous study, the distribution and projection of VGLUT1 and VGLUT2 mRNA-positive neurons are also different [17]. VGLUT1 mRNA-expressing neurons are distributed in the Vo, Vi, and Vc, and some VGLUT1 mRNA-expressing neurons in the Vi, and a few neurons in the Vo send VGLUT1-positive axon terminals to the trigeminal motor nucleus [17] and cerebellum [15]. Moreover, nearly all Vo, Vi and Vc neurons express VGLUT2 mRNA signals and send VGLUT2-positive axon terminals to the contralateral thalamus [15]. The current findings showed that Vsp neurons sending collateral projections to the thalamus and PBN mainly expressed VGLUT2 mRNA signals, which indicates that VGLUT2 and not VGLUT1 was potentially involved in the transmission of orofacial information from the Vsp to the thalamus and PBN.

The subnuclei of the Vsp (Vo, Vi, and Vc) have been indicated to be different in their functional properties:

they are related to different types of sensory information from orofacial regions [24]. Among these nuclei, the Vc has been widely investigated for its role in the transmission of orofacial nociceptive information. According to the results of the present and previous studies, Vc neurons sending collateral projections to the thalamus and PBN were mainly distributed in the superficial laminae [4, 79]. The superficial laminae of the Vc are the primary gateway for the peripheral noxious information transmitted from the orofacial region [39, 80, 81]. CGRP is regarded as a key mediator released from trigeminal ganglion neurons to the superficial laminae of the Vc after the stimulation of sensory nerve endings and is responsible for the transmission of pain sensation [82]. In the present study, we determined that CGRP-LI terminals formed asymmetric synapses with somatic or dendritic profiles of the neurons projecting collaterally to the thalamus and PBN in the superficial laminae of the Vc. The collateral projecting neurons were also activated after painful stimulation of the lip. It may be assumed from the present results that the VGLUT2-positive neurons in the superficial laminae of the Vc may receive pain information from the primary afferent fibers of the trigeminal nerve and simultaneously relay it to the thalamus and PBN.

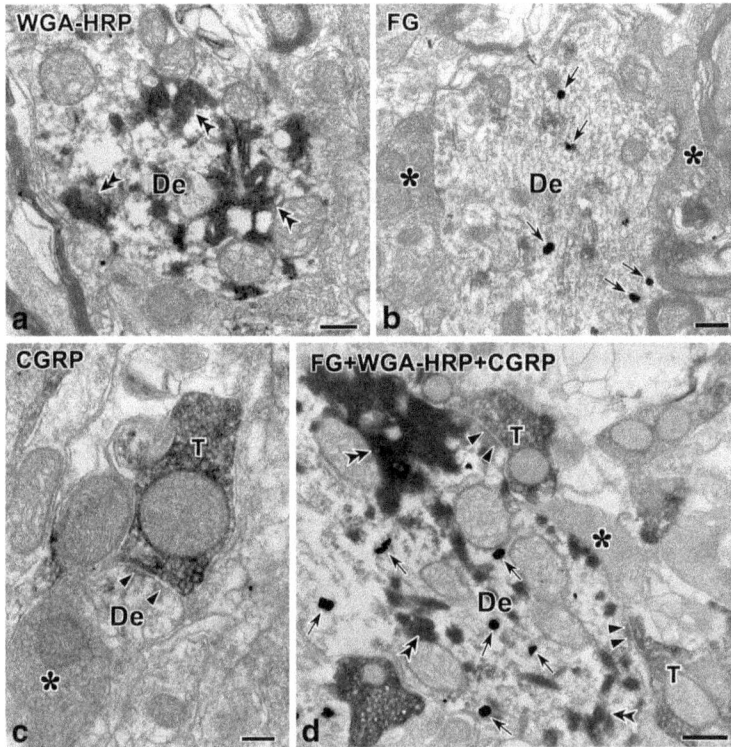

Fig. 10 Electron microphotographs of the superficial layer of the Vc after triple-labeling with WGA-HRP, FG and CGRP. Axon terminals labeled with CGRP (**c**, **d**) form asymmetric synapses (*black arrowheads*) with WGA-HRP and FG dually labeled dendritic profiles (De) in the superficial layer of the Vc after a WGA-HRP injection into the right thalamus and an FG injection into the left LPB. CGRP-LI is represented with electron-dense, amorphous products of DAB reaction (**c**, **d**). Silver-intensified gold particles produced with the immunogold-silver method indicate FG labeling (**b**, **d**; *arrows*). Electron-dense, amorphous material produced by the peroxidase reaction indicate WGA-HRP labeling (TMB reaction; **a**, **d**; *double arrowheads*). De, dendritic profiles; T, CGRP-LI axon terminals; *, CGRP-negative axon terminals. *Scale bar* 250 nm (**a**, **b**, **c** and **d**)

According to the present data, the VGLUT2-expressing neurons in the Vi and Vo also send axonal collaterals to the thalamus and PBN. Previous studies have shown that the Vi is primarily concerned with the transmission of tactile sensation and low-threshold signals from orofacial regions, and Vi neurons predominately respond to the stimulation of individual vibrissae in rats [83, 84]. Vo neurons are closely related to the transmission of orofacial propioceptive sensation [24]. Thus, it is plausible that VGLUT2-expressing neurons in the Vi or Vo may relay orofacial tactile sensation or proprioceptive sensation, respectively, to the thalamus and PBN. The T-T projection from the Vi is related to discriminative orofacial tactile sensation from the vibrissae [24]. The T-P projection from the Vi may be related to affective reactions evoked by orofacial tactile sensation from the vibrissae. Moreover, it has been reported that amputation of vibrissae may induce anxiety in rats [85]. The T-T and T-P projections from the Vo are mainly concerned with discriminative orofacial proprioceptive sensation and concomitant affective reactions, respectively [24]. Whether the discriminative sensation and affective reactions of orofacial tactile and proprioceptive sensation are transmitted by these collateral projection neurons in the Vi and Vo remains to be discovered. Our data further confirmed that trigemino-thalamic and trigemino-parabrachial collateral projection neurons were VGLUT2 mRNA-positive, which further indicates that orofacial nociceptive information uses glutamate as a neurotransmitter recruited by VGLUT2.

Conclusions

In summary, the present study indicates T-T and T-P collateral projection neurons that send their axon terminals to both the thalamus and the PBN by way of axon collaterals are mainly localized in the Vo, Vi and Vc. Glutamatergic T-T and T-P collateral projection neurons in the Vo, Vi and Vc mainly express VGLUT2 mRNA. Some T-T and T-P collateral projection neurons that express Fos-LI in the Vc are closely related to the transmission of orofacial nociceptive information after subcutaneous injection of formalin into the upper lip. Moreover, the collateral projection neurons in the Vc that formed synaptic contacts with CGRP-LI primary afferent axon terminals were also considered nociceptive.

Abbreviations

3 V: Third ventricle; 4 V: Fourth ventricle; CM: Central medial thalamic nucleus; cp: Cerebral peduncle; f: Fornix; FG: Fluoro-Gold; FISH: Fluorescence in situ hybridization; fr: Fasciculus retroflexus; Hb: Habenular nucleus; ic: Internal capsule; KF: Kölliker-Fuse nucleus; LC: Locus coeruleus; LD: Laterodorsal thalamic nucleus; LPB: Lateral parabrachial nucleus; MD: Mediodorsal thalamic nucleus; MPB: Medial parabrachial nucleus; mt: Mammillothalamic tract; opt: Optic tract; PAG: Periaqueductal gray; PBN: Parabrachial nucleus; PF: Parafascicular thalamic nucleus; Po: Posterior thalamic nuclear group; Rt: Reticular thalamic nucleus; scp: Superior cerebellar peduncle; TMR: Tetramethylrhodamine; T-P: Trigemino-parabrachial (T-P) pathways; T-T: Trigemino-thalamic pathways; Vc: Caudal subnucleus of spinal trigeminal nucleus; VGLUT: Vesicular glutamate transporter; Vi: Interpolar subnucleus of spinal trigeminal nucleus; Vmes: Trigeminal mesencephalic nucleus; Vo: Oral subnucleus of spinal trigeminal nucleus; Vp: Principal sensory trigeminal nucleus; VPL: Ventral posterolateral thalamic nucleus; VPM: Ventral posteromedial thalamic nucleus; Vsp: Spinal trigeminal nucleus; ZI: Zona incerta

Acknowledgements

Not applicable.

Funding

This work was supported by the National Natural Science Foundation of China (No. 81571074).

Authors' contributions

JLL, YQL and TC designed the experiments; CKZ conducted the experiments; TZ and YCL assisted with the immunoelectron microscopic staining; YQ assisted with cell counting and statistics; CKZ and ZHL wrote the manuscript; and JLL, YQL and YLD helped revise the manuscript. All authors read and approved the final manuscript.

Competing interests

The authors declare that they have no competing interests.

Author details

[1]Department of Anatomy and K.K. Leung Brain Research Centre, The Fourth Military Medical University, Xi'an, People's Republic of China. [2]Student Brigade, Fourth Military Medical University, Xi'an, People's Republic of China.

References

1. Erzurumlu RS, Killackey HP. Efferent connections of the brainstem trigeminal complex with the facial nucleus of the rat. J Comp Neurol. 1979;188:75–86.
2. Fukushima T, Kerr FW. Organization of trigeminothalamic tracts and other thalamic afferent systems of the brainstem in the rat: presence of gelatinosa neurons with thalamic connections. J Comp Neurol. 1979;183:169–84.
3. Yoshida A, Chen K, Moritani M, Yabuta NH, Nagase Y, Takemura M, Shigenaga Y. Organization of the descending projections from the parabrachial nucleus to the trigeminal sensory nuclear complex and spinal dorsal horn in the rat. J Comp Neurol. 1997;383:94–111.
4. Li J, Xiong K, Pang Y, Dong Y, Kaneko T, Mizuno N. Medullary dorsal horn neurons providing axons to both the parabrachial nucleus and thalamus. J Comp Neurol. 2006;498:539–51.
5. Light AR, Sedivec MJ, Casale EJ, Jones SL. Physiological and morphological characteristics of spinal neurons projecting to the parabrachial region of the cat. Somatosens Mot Res. 1993;10:309–25.
6. Ni B, Wu X, Yan GM, Wang J, Paul SM. Regional expression and cellular localization of the Na(+)-dependent inorganic phosphate cotransporter of rat brain. J Neurosci. 1995;15:5789–99.
7. Herzog E, Bellenchi GC, Gras C, Bernard V, Ravassard P, Bedet C, Gasnier B, Giros B, El Mestikawy S. The existence of a second vesicular glutamate transporter specifies subpopulations of glutamatergic neurons. J Neurosci 2001; 21:RC181.
8. Hisano S, Hoshi K, Ikeda Y, Maruyama D, Kanemoto M, Ichijo H, Kojima I, Takeda J, Nogami H. Regional expression of a gene encoding a neuron-specific Na(+)-dependent inorganic phosphate cotransporter (DNPI) in the rat forebrain. Brain Res Mol Brain Res. 2000;83:34–43.
9. Gras C, Herzog E, Bellenchi GC, Bernard V, Ravassard P, Pohl M, Gasnier B, Giros B, El Mestikawy SA. Third vesicular glutamate transporter expressed by cholinergic and serotoninergic neurons. J Neurosci. 2002;22:5442–51.
10. Fremeau RT Jr, Kam K, Qureshi T, Johnson J, Copenhagen DR, Storm-Mathisen J, Chaudhry FA, Nicoll RA, Edwards RH. Vesicular glutamate transporters 1 and 2 target to functionally distinct synaptic release sites. Science. 2004;304:1815–9.
11. Fremeau RT Jr, Troyer MD, Pahner I, Nygaard GO, Tran CH, Reimer RJ, Bellocchio EE, Fortin D, Storm-Mathisen J, Edwards RH. The expression of vesicular glutamate transporters defines two classes of excitatory synapse. Neuron. 2001;31:247–60.
12. Fremeau RT Jr, Voglmaier S, Seal RP, Edwards RH. VGLUTs define subsets of excitatory neurons and suggest novel roles for glutamate. Trends Neurosci. 2004;27:98–103.
13. Fujiyama F, Furuta T, Kaneko T. Immunocytochemical localization of candidates for vesicular glutamate transporters in the rat cerebral cortex. J Comp Neurol. 2001;435:379–87.
14. Kaneko T, Fujiyama F. Complementary distribution of vesicular glutamate transporters in the central nervous system. Neurosci Res. 2002;42:243–50.
15. Ge SN, Li ZH, Tang J, Ma Y, Hioki H, Zhang T, Lu YC, Zhang FX, Mizuno N, Kaneko T, Liu YY, Lung MS, Gao GD, Li JL. Differential expression of VGLUT1 or VGLUT2 in the trigeminothalamic or trigeminocerebellar projection neurons in the rat. Brain Struct Funct. 2014;219:211–29.
16. Ge SN, Ma YF, Hioki H, Wei YY, Kaneko T, Mizuno N, Gao GD, Li JL. Coexpression of VGLUT1 and VGLUT2 in trigeminothalamic projection neurons in the principal sensory trigeminal nucleus of the rat. J Comp Neurol. 2010;518:3149–68.
17. Pang YW, Ge SN, Nakamura KC, Li JL, Xiong KH, Kaneko T, Mizuno N. Axon terminals expressing vesicular glutamate transporter VGLUT1 or VGLUT2 within the trigeminal motor nucleus of the rat: origins and distribution patterns. J Comp Neurol. 2009;512:595–612.
18. Strassman AM, Vos BP, Mineta Y, Naderi S, Borsook D, Burstein R. Fos-like immunoreactivity in the superficial medullary dorsal horn induced by noxious and innocuous thermal stimulation of facial skin in the rat. J Neurophysiol. 1993;70:1811–21.
19. Oyamaguchi A, Abe T, Sugiyo S, Niwa H, Takemura M. Selective elimination of isolectin B4-binding trigeminal neurons enhanced formalin-induced nocifensive behavior in the upper lip of rats and c-Fos expression in the trigeminal subnucleus caudalis. Neurosci Res. 2016;103:40–7.
20. Sugiyo S, Uehashi D, Satoh F, Abe T, Yonehara N, Kobayashi M, Takemura M. Effects of systemic bicuculline or morphine on formalin-evoked pain-related behaviour and c-Fos expression in trigeminal nuclei after formalin injection into the lip or tongue in rats. Exp Brain Res. 2009;196:229–37.
21. Iyengar S, Ossipov MH, Johnson KW. The role of CGRP in peripheral and central pain mechanisms including migraine. Pain. 2017;158:543-59.
22. Nakamura K, Watakabe A, Hioki H, Fujiyama F, Tanaka Y, Yamamori T, Kaneko T. Transiently increased colocalization of vesicular glutamate transporters 1 and 2 at single axon terminals during postnatal development of mouse neocortex: a quantitative analysis with correlation coefficient. Eur J Neurosci. 2007;26:3054–67.
23. Paxinos G, Watson C. The rat brain in stereotaxic coordinates. 6th ed. Amsterdam: Elsevier Academic Press; 2007.
24. Paxinos G. The Rat Nervous System. 3rd ed. Amsterdam: Elsevier Academic Press; 2004. p. 817–51.
25. Gu Y, Chen Y, Ye L. Electron microscopical demonstration of horseradish peroxidase by use of tetramethylbenzidine as chromogen and sodium

tungstate as stabilizer (TMB-ST method): a tracing method with high sensitivity and well preserved ultrastructural tissue. J Neurosci Methods. 1992;42:1–10.

26. Hylden JL, Nahin RL, Traub RJ, Dubner R. Expansion of receptive fields of spinal lamina I projection neurons in rats with unilateral adjuvant-induced inflammation: the contribution of dorsal horn mechanisms. Pain. 1989;37:229–43.

27. Iwata K, Kenshalo DR Jr, Dubner R, Nahin RL. Diencephalic projections from the superficial and deep laminae of the medullary dorsal horn in the rat. J Comp Neurol. 1992;321:404–20.

28. Krout KE, Belzer RE, Loewy AD. Brainstem projections to midline and intralaminar thalamic nuclei of the rat. J Comp Neurol. 2002;448:53–101.

29. Kemplay S, Webster KE. A quantitative study of the projections of the gracile, cuneate and trigeminal nuclei and of the medullary reticular formation to the thalamus in the rat. Neuroscience. 1989;32:153–67.

30. Aicher SA, Hermes SM, Hegarty DM. Corneal afferents differentially target thalamic- and parabrachial-projecting neurons in spinal trigeminal nucleus caudalis. Neuroscience. 2013;232:182–93.

31. Guy N, Chalus M, Dallel R, Voisin DL. Both oral and caudal parts of the spinal trigeminal nucleus project to the somatosensory thalamus in the rat. Eur J Neurosci. 2005;21:741–54.

32. Erzurumlu RS, Bates CA, Killackey HP. Differential organization of thalamic projection cells in the brain stem trigeminal complex of the rat. Brain Res. 1980;198:427–33.

33. Cechetto DF, Standaert DG, Saper CB. Spinal and trigeminal dorsal horn projections to the parabrachial nucleus in the rat. J Comp Neurol. 1985; 240:153–60.

34. Slugg RM, Light AR. Spinal cord and trigeminal projections to the pontine parabrachial region in the rat as demonstrated with Phaseolus vulgaris leucoagglutinin. J Comp Neurol. 1994;339:49–61.

35. Feil K, Herbert H. Topographic organization of spinal and trigeminal somatosensory pathways to the rat parabrachial and Kolliker-fuse nuclei. J Comp Neurol. 1995;353:506–28.

36. Standaert DG, Watson SJ, Houghten RA, Saper CB. Opioid peptide immunoreactivity in spinal and trigeminal dorsal horn neurons projecting to the parabrachial nucleus in the rat. J Neurosci. 1986;6:1220–6.

37. Dallel R, Ricard O, Raboisson P. Organization of parabrachial projections from the spinal trigeminal nucleus oralis: an anterograde tracing study in the rat. J Comp Neurol. 2004;470:181–91.

38. Allen GV, Barbrick B, Esser MJ. Trigeminal-parabrachial connections: possible pathway for nociception-induced cardiovascular reflex responses. Brain Res. 1996;715:125–35.

39. Dubner R, Bennett GJ. Spinal and trigeminal mechanisms of nociception. Annu Rev Neurosci. 1983;6:381–418.

40. Bereiter DA, Hirata H, Hu JW. Trigeminal subnucleus caudalis: beyond homologies with the spinal dorsal horn. Pain. 2000;88:221–4.

41. Woda A. Pain in the trigeminal system: from orofacial nociception to neural network modeling. J Dent Res. 2003;82:764–8.

42. Priestley JV, Somogyi P, Cuello AC. Immunocytochemical localization of substance P in the spinal trigeminal nucleus of the rat: a light and electron microscopic study. J Comp Neurol. 1982;211:31–49.

43. Pearson JC, Jennes L. Localization of serotonin- and substance P-like immunofluorescence in the caudal spinal trigeminal nucleus of the rat. Neurosci Lett. 1988;88:151–6.

44. Li YQ, Substance P. Receptor-like immunoreactive neurons in the caudal spinal trigeminal nucleus send axons to the gelatinosus thalamic nucleus in the rat. J Hirnforsch. 1999;39:277–82.

45. Li JL, Ding YQ, Xiong KH, Li JS, Shigemoto R, Mizuno N. Substance P receptor (NK1)-immunoreactive neurons projecting to the periaqueductal gray: distribution in the spinal trigeminal nucleus and the spinal cord of the rat. Neurosci Res. 1998;30:219–25.

46. Willis WD, Westlund KN. Neuroanatomy of the pain system and of the pathways that modulate pain. J Clin Neurophysiol. 1997;14:2–31.

47. Willis WD Jr, Zhang X, Honda CN, Giesler GJ Jr. Projections from the marginal zone and deep dorsal horn to the ventrobasal nuclei of the primate thalamus. Pain. 2001;92:267–76.

48. Graziano A, Jones EG. Widespread thalamic terminations of fibers arising in the superficial medullary dorsal horn of monkeys and their relation to calbindin immunoreactivity. J Neurosci. 2004;24:248–56.

49. Sugimoto T, Hara T, Shirai H, Abe T, Ichikawa H, Sato T. C-fos induction in the subnucleus caudalis following noxious mechanical stimulation of the oral mucous membrane. Exp Neurol. 1994;129:251–6.

50. Carstens E, Saxe I, Ralph R. Brainstem neurons expressing c-Fos immunoreactivity following irritant chemical stimulation of the rat's tongue. Neuroscience. 1995;69:939–53.

51. Hathaway CB, Hu JW, Bereiter DA. Distribution of Fos-like immunoreactivity in the caudal brainstem of the rat following noxious chemical stimulation of the temporomandibular joint. J Comp Neurol. 1995;356:444–56.

52. Martinez S, Belmonte C. C-Fos expression in trigeminal nucleus neurons after chemical irritation of the cornea: reduction by selective blockade of nociceptor chemosensitivity. Exp Brain Res. 1996;109:56–62.

53. Morgan JI, Curran T. Stimulus-transcription coupling in the nervous system: involvement of the inducible proto-oncogenes fos and jun. Annu Rev Neurosci. 1991;14:421–51.

54. Adams JC. Sound stimulation induces Fos-related antigens in cells with common morphological properties throughout the auditory brainstem. J Comp Neurol. 1995;361:645–68.

55. Li JL, Kaneko T, Nomura S, Li YQ, Mizuno N. Association of serotonin-like immunoreactive axons with nociceptive projection neurons in the caudal spinal trigeminal nucleus of the rat. J Comp Neurol. 1997;384:127–41.

56. Fujisawa N, Terayama R, Yamaguchi D, Omura S, Yamashiro T, Sugimoto T. Fos protein-like immunoreactive neurons induced by electrical stimulation in the trigeminal sensory nuclear complex of rats with chronically injured peripheral nerve. Exp Brain Res. 2012;219:191–201.

57. Lu SM, Lin RC. Thalamic afferents of the rat barrel cortex: a light- and electron-microscopic study using Phaseolus vulgaris leucoagglutinin as an anterograde tracer. Somatosens Mot Res. 1993;10:1–16.

58. Diamond ME, Armstrong-James M, Ebner FF. Somatic sensory responses in the rostral sector of the posterior group (POm) and in the ventral posterior medial nucleus (VPM) of the rat thalamus. J Comp Neurol. 1992;318:462–76.

59. Rausell E, Jones EG. Chemically distinct compartments of the thalamic VPM nucleus in monkeys relay principal and spinal trigeminal pathways to different layers of the somatosensory cortex. J Neurosci. 1991;11:226–37.

60. Hartings JA, Simons DJ. Inhibition suppresses transmission of tonic vibrissa-evoked activity in the rat ventrobasal thalamus. J Neurosci. 2000;20:RC100.

61. Norgren R, Leonard CM. Taste pathways in rat brainstem. Science. 1971;173:1136–9.

62. Ogawa H, Hayama T, Ito S. Response properties of the parabrachio-thalamic taste and mechanoreceptive neurons in rats. Exp Brain Res. 1987;68:449–57.

63. Travers JB, Travers SP, Norgren R. Gustatory neural processing in the hindbrain. Annu Rev Neurosci. 1987;10:595–632.

64. Chamberlin NL, Saper CB. Topographic organization of cardiovascular responses to electrical and glutamate microstimulation of the parabrachial nucleus in the rat. J Comp Neurol. 1992;326:245–62.

65. Krukoff TL, Harris KH, Jhamandas JH. Efferent projections from the parabrachial nucleus demonstrated with the anterograde tracer Phaseolus vulgaris leucoagglutinin. Brain Res Bull. 1993;30:163–72.

66. Jhamandas JH, Petrov T, Harris KH, Vu T, Krukoff TL. Parabrachial nucleus projection to the amygdala in the rat: electrophysiological and anatomical observations. Brain Res Bull. 1996;39:115–26.

67. Fulwiler CE, Saper CB. Subnuclear organization of the efferent connections of the parabrachial nucleus in the rat. Brain Res. 1984;319: 229–59.

68. Bester H, Besson JM, Bernard JF. Organization of efferent projections from the parabrachial area to the hypothalamus: a Phaseolus vulgaris-leucoagglutinin study in the rat. J Comp Neurol. 1997;383:245–81.

69. Balaban CD, Thayer JF. Neurological bases for balance-anxiety links. J Anxiety Disord. 2001;15:53–79.

70. Petrovich GD, Swanson LW. Projections from the lateral part of the central amygdalar nucleus to the postulated fear conditioning circuit. Brain Res. 1997;763:247–54.

71. Tassoni G, Bucherelli C, Bures J. Postacquisition injection of tetrodotoxin into the parabrachial nuclei elicits partial disruption of passive avoidance reaction in rats. Behav Neural Biol. 1992;57:116–23.

72. Bernard JF, Bester H, Besson JM. Involvement of the spino-parabrachio -amygdaloid and -hypothalamic pathways in the autonomic and affective emotional aspects of pain. Prog Brain Res. 1996;107:243–55.

73. Bester H, Chapman V, Besson JM, Bernard JF. Physiological properties of the lamina I spinoparabrachial neurons in the rat. J Neurophysiol. 2000; 83:2239–59.

74. Ma W, Peschanski M. Spinal and trigeminal projections to the parabrachial nucleus in the rat: electron-microscopic evidence of a spino-ponto-amygdalian somatosensory pathway. Somatosens Res. 1988;5:247–57.

75. Takamori S, Rhee JS, Rosenmund C, Jahn R. Identification of a vesicular glutamate transporter that defines a glutamatergic phenotype in neurons. Nature. 2000;407:189–94.

76. Takamori S, Rhee JS, Rosenmund C, Jahn R. Identification of differentiation-associated brain-specific phosphate transporter as a second vesicular glutamate transporter (VGLUT2). J Neurosci. 2001;21:RC182.

77. Takamori S. VGLUTs: 'exciting' times for glutamatergic research? Neurosci Res. 2006;55:343–51.

78. Kaneko T, Fujiyama F, Hioki H. Immunohistochemical localization of candidates for vesicular glutamate transporters in the rat brain. J Comp Neurol. 2002;444:39–62.

79. Li H, Li YQ. Collateral projection of substance P receptor expressing neurons in the medullary dorsal horn to bilateral parabrachial nuclei of the rat. Brain Res Bull. 2000;53:163–9.

80. Cadden SW, Orchardson R. The neural mechanisms of oral and facial pain. Dent Update. 2001;28:359–67.

81. Sessle BJ. The neurobiology of facial and dental pain: present knowledge, future directions. J Dent Res. 1987;66:962–81.

82. Kuzawinska O, Lis K, Cessak G, Mirowska-Guzel D, Balkowiec-Iskra E. Targeting of calcitonin gene-related peptide action as a new strategy for migraine treatment. Neurol Neurochir Pol. 2016;50:463–7.

83. Jacquin MF, Golden J, Panneton WM. Structure and function of barrel 'precursor' cells in trigeminal nucleus principalis. Brain Res. 1988;471:309–14.

84. Veinante P, Deschenes M. Single- and multi-whisker channels in the ascending projections from the principal trigeminal nucleus in the rat. J Neurosci. 1999;19:5085–95.

85. Kozlovskii VL, Mosin AE, Ivakina LV. The effect of calcium channel blockers on anxiety evoked by amputation of the vibrissae in rats. Eksp Klin Farmakol. 1997;60:10–2.

5

Naked mole-rat cortical neurons are resistant to acid-induced cell death

Zoé Husson and Ewan St. John Smith[*]

Abstract

Regulation of brain pH is a critical homeostatic process and changes in brain pH modulate various ion channels and receptors and thus neuronal excitability. Tissue acidosis, resulting from hypoxia or hypercapnia, can activate various proteins and ion channels, among which acid-sensing ion channels (ASICs) a family of primarily Na$^+$ permeable ion channels, which alongside classical excitotoxicity causes neuronal death. Naked mole-rats (NMRs, *Heterocephalus glaber*) are long-lived, fossorial, eusocial rodents that display remarkable behavioral/cellular hypoxia and hypercapnia resistance. In the central nervous system, ASIC subunit expression is similar between mouse and NMR with the exception of much lower expression of ASIC4 throughout the NMR brain. However, ASIC function and neuronal sensitivity to sustained acidosis has not been examined in the NMR brain. Here, we show with whole-cell patch-clamp electrophysiology of cultured NMR and mouse cortical and hippocampal neurons that NMR neurons have smaller voltage-gated Na$^+$ channel currents and more hyperpolarized resting membrane potentials. We further demonstrate that acid-mediated currents in NMR neurons are of smaller magnitude than in mouse, and that all currents in both species are reversibly blocked by the ASIC antagonist benzamil. We further demonstrate that NMR neurons show greater resistance to acid-induced cell death than mouse neurons. In summary, NMR neurons show significant cellular resistance to acidotoxicity compared to mouse neurons, contributing factors likely to be smaller ASIC-mediated currents and reduced NaV activity.

Keywords: ASIC, Acid-induced currents, Acidotoxicity, Naked mole-rat, Hippocampus

Introduction

Acid-sensing channels (ASICs) are ion channels of the ENaC/Deg superfamily and most subunits are activated by extracellular protons [1, 2]. Six different ASIC subunits are encoded by 4 ASIC genes (ASIC1a, ASIC1b, ASIC2a, ASIC2b, ASIC3 and ASIC4), which assemble as homo- or heterotrimers [3]; neither ASIC2b nor ASIC4 form proton-sensitive homotrimers. ASICs are primarily permeable to Na$^+$, although ASIC1a homomeric channels are also Ca^{2+} permeable [2]. In the central nervous system (CNS), neurons have been shown to primarily express ASIC1a homomers and heteromers of ASIC1a/2a and ASIC1a/2b [4–8], where they have been demonstrated to have key roles in synaptic plasticity [9–11] and fear conditioning [12–14], as well as being major players in neuronal death resulting from brain ischemia [5, 15–17], and neurodegenerative diseases [18–20].

Regulation of brain pH is a highly complex and important process [21]. Brain tissue acidosis can result either from an increase in tissue partial pressure of carbon dioxide (PCO$_2$) during hypercapnia, or from the accumulation of the byproducts of anaerobic metabolism, such as lactate and protons, during hypoxia [22]. During periods of tissue acidosis, activation of ASICs by extracellular acidification is worsened by the release of allosteric modulators such as lactate [23], spermine [16] and arachidonic acid [24, 25]. In addition to the activation of the Ca^{2+} permeable ASIC1a channel [15, 16], a drop in pH also modulates the activity of numerous others ion channels, including voltage-gated ion channels [26–29] and glutamate receptors [30, 31], therefore leading to disturbance in ion homeostasis, excitotoxicity and ultimately neuronal death [5, 15, 16].

Naked mole-rats (NMRs, *Heterocephalus glaber*) are subterranean rodents belonging to the Bathyergidae African mole-rat family found in East Africa [32]. Unusually for a mammal, NMRs are eusocial [33, 34]. However, NMRs also

---
* Correspondence: es336@cam.ac.uk
Department of Pharmacology, University of Cambridge, Tennis Court Road, Cambridge CB2 1PD, UK

display a range of remarkable physiological peculiarities, which is beginning to make a significant impact on biomedical research [35]. The unusual physiology of the NMR includes: extreme longevity with no increased risk of death with ageing [36], an apparent absence of age-related neurodegenerative disorders [37, 38], resistance to cancer [39–41], insensitivity to certain noxious and irritant stimuli [42–45] and hypoxia/hypercapnia resistance resulting from altered NMDA receptor function and an ability to utilize fructose as an energy source [46–49]. It is striking that NMRs are resistant to many pathological conditions known to involve ASICs. Recordings of ASIC-mediated currents in dorsal root ganglion (DRG) sensory neurons demonstrated an increased frequency and magnitude of ASIC responses in NMR neurons compared to mouse neurons [43], with APETx2, an inhibitor of ASIC3-containing ASICs, demonstrating a key role for ASIC3, even though nmrASIC3 does not appear to form functional homotrimers [50]. Previously we mapped out ASIC expression in different NMR brain regions and observed similar expression between mouse and NMR, a key exception being much lower ASIC4 levels throughout the NMR brain [51], however, no one has yet studied the function of ASICs in NMR brain neurons.

In this study, we investigated acid-induced currents in mouse and NMR neurons using whole-cell patch clamp recording of cultured neonatal hippocampal and cortical neurons. We find that NMR neurons have ASIC-mediated currents of significantly smaller peak current amplitude than those recorded from mouse neurons and that NMR neurons are resistant to acid-induced cell death. Overall, these results suggest that the reduced acid-induced cell death in NMR neurons may be neuroprotective.

Methods
Animals
All experiments were conducted in accordance with the United Kingdom Animal (Scientific Procedures) Act 1986 Amendment Regulations 2012 under a Project License (70/7705) granted to E. St. J. S. by the Home Office; the University of Cambridge Animal Welfare Ethical Review Body also approved procedures. Breeding couples of 1 male and 2 female C57/bl6 mice were conventionally housed with nesting material and a red plastic shelter; the holding room was temperature-controlled (21 °C) and mice were on a normal 12-h light/dark cycle with food and water available ad libitum. Naked mole-rats were bred in house and maintained in a custom-made caging system with conventional mouse/rat cages connected by different lengths of tunnel. Bedding and nesting material were provided along with running wheels and chew blocks. The room was warmed to 28 °C and humidified, with a heat cable to provide extra warmth running under 2–3 cages, and red lighting (08:00–16:00) was used.

Neuronal cultures
P0-P2 mice and P0-P5 naked mole-rats were used to prepare cortical and hippocampal neuronal cultures. Multiple pups (2-4) were used to prepare a single culture. Following decapitation, heads were immediately placed in dishes containing ice-cold Hank's Balanced Salt Solution (HBSS) solution (20 mM HEPES, 30 mM glucose in HBSS, Life Technologies). Brains were removed, transferred to a new dish and the two hippocampi and cortices were isolated. Tissues were subsequently incubated in an enzymatic digestion solution: 2 mg/mL papain (Worthington Biochemical Corporation) in Hibernate-Ca^{2+} solution (Brain Bits), activated by 0.5 mM Glutamax (Life Technologies) at 37 °C for 30 min in a 5% CO_2 incubator. The digestion solution was then replaced by HBSS solution supplemented with DNAse I (250 Kunitz units/mL, Sigma Aldrich) and tissues were slowly triturated (5-7 times) using a P1000 pipette. Neuronal suspensions were filtered through a 100 μm nylon cell strainer (Corning) to remove non-dissociated pieces of tissues before centrifugation for 5 mins at 1100 rpm at room temperature. Supernatants were discarded and the pellets carefully resuspended in HBSS solution. After further centrifugation for 5 min 1100 rpm at room temperature, pellets were resuspended in MEM/HS solution: 10% heat-inactivated horse serum (Life Technologies), 2 mM glucose, 0.0025% Glutamax, and 0.2 mg/mL primocin (InVivogen). Hippocampal and cortical neurons were plated on 35 mm plastic dishes (Fisher Scientific), previously coated with 100 mg/mL poly-L-lysine (Sigma-Aldrich), rinsed with water and dried, at a density of 300,000 cells/mL (2 mL/dish). After a 4-h incubation in a 37 °C / 5% CO_2 incubator, the MEM/HS solution was removed and the dishes were flooded with Neurobasal/B27 solution (1X B27 Supplement, 0.0025% Glutamax, and 0.2 mg/mL primocin). Naked mole-rat neurons were kept at 33 °C in 5% CO_2 incubator, whereas mouse neurons were kept at 37 °C in a 5% CO_2 incubator; this is due to NMRs being cold-blooded and NMR cells do not withstand 37 °C for long periods of time [52]. Half of the medium was exchanged for fresh medium every 2-3 days until the cultures were used for experiments.

Electrophysiology
Hippocampal and cortical neurons from mouse and NMR were used for whole-cell patch-clamp recordings at 9-12 days in vitro (DIV9-12). Recordings were performed at room temperature using the following solutions: extracellular (in mM) – 140 NaCl, 4 KCl, 2 $CaCl_2$, 1 $MgCl_2$, 4 glucose, 10 HEPES, adjusted to pH 7.4 with NaOH and 300–310 mOsm with sucrose; intracellular (in mM) – 110 KCl, 10 NaCl, 1 $MgCl_2$, 1 EGTA, 10 HEPES, 2 Na_2ATP, 0.5 Na_2GTP, adjusted to pH 7.3 with KOH and to 310–315 mOsm with sucrose. Acidic extracellular solutions were made using MES (pH 5.0). Patch

pipettes were pulled (Model P-97, Flaming/Brown puller; Sutter Instruments,) from borosilicate glass capillaries (Hilgenberg GmbH) and had a resistance of 6-10 MΩ. Data were acquired using an EPC10 amplifier and Patch-master software (HEKA). Whole-cell currents were recorded at 20 kHz, pipette and membrane capacitance were compensated using Patchmaster macros, and series resistance was compensated by > 60%. Cell capacitances and resting membrane potentials were measured just after cell opening in whole-cell configuration. To study macroscopic voltage-gated currents, a standard voltage-step protocol was used whereby cells were held at – 120 mV for 200 msecs before stepping to the test potential (– 80 mV - + 65 mV in 5 mV increments) for 50 msecs, returning to the holding potential (– 60 mV) for 200 msecs between sweeps. In some experiments, tetrodotoxin (300 nM, Alomone Labs) was perfused for 30 s before repeating the voltage-step protocol. To measure neuronal acid-sensitivity, cells were exposed to the following protocol: 5 s of pH 7.4; 5-s of pH 5; and 5 s of pH 7.4. ASIC antagonists (100 µM Benzamil, Sigma) were perfused during 30 s before applying another 5 s pulse of pH 5. After 90 s wash time with pH 7.4 solution, a 5 s pulse of pH 5 was applied to check for reversal of any block observed. Current amplitude was measured in Fitmaster (HEKA) by taking the maximum peak response and subtracting the mean baseline amplitude in the preceding 50 msec (voltage-gated currents) or ~ 2.5 s (ASIC currents); current amplitude was normalized for cell size by dividing by cell capacitance. Using Igor Pro, for each individual cell that underwent the voltage-step protocol, the following equation was fitted to the normalized inward currents:

$$i(x) = \Gamma \cdot x \cdot \frac{1-e^{-\frac{x-Erev}{25mV}}}{1-e^{-\frac{x}{25mV}}} \cdot \frac{1}{\left(1-e^{\frac{x-VHalf}{slope}}\right)^3}$$

where Erev is the reversal potential; Vhalf the half-activating potential; Γ a constant and x the command potential. Similarly, a Boltzmann equation was fitted to the normalized outward currents:

$$\frac{I}{Imax} = \frac{1}{1+e^{\frac{(VHalf-Vm)}{slope}}}$$

where Vm is the membrane voltage and VHalf the voltage at half-maximal activation. To determine the inactivation time of the ASIC-mediated currents, a single exponential was fitted. Data are expressed as mean ± standard error of the mean (SEM). Using Prism (Graph-Pad), paired t-tests were used to compare the effects of ASIC antagonists on proton-gated currents within both mouse and NMR neuron datasets; unpaired t-tests were used to compare parameters, such as neuronal resting

membrane potential and capacitance and ASIC-mediated current amplitude, between mouse and NMR neuron datasets.

Acid-induced cell death assays

Mouse and NMR neurons were used to measure acid-induced cell death at DIV9-12. The pH 7.4 and pH 5 extracellular solutions used were the same as those described above for electrophysiology experiments. Neuronal cultures from both mouse and NMR were rinsed twice with 37 °C solution (pH 7.4 or pH 5) and then incubated with pH 7.4 or pH 5 solution for 2 h at 37 °C. Cultures from both conditions were then rinsed with warm pH 7.4 solution and incubated during 30 min with pH 7.4 solution containing 1.5 mM propidium iodide (PI, Sigma Aldrich) to stain necrotic cells and Hoechst 33,342 (dilution 1/2500, Sigma) to label all nuclei. Labelled cultures were imaged using an epifluorescence microscope (Olympus) equipped with a 20X objective (Olympus) and a QImaging camera. To determine the percentage of dead necrotic PI-positive cells, we used the software Fiji to count the total number of cells per field of view by counting nuclei on the Hoechst images, and subsequently counting the number of PI-positive nuclei on the PI images. One to three dishes per condition were used, and three different images per dish were taken. Data were collected from three different cultures and each culture was prepared from multiple animals. A one-way ANOVA test (Prism, GraphPad) corrected for multiple comparisons (Tukey test) was used to compare the percentage of cell death in each field of view at pH 7.4 and pH 5 in both species. Data are expressed as mean ± standard error of the mean (SEM).

Results

Basic electrophysiological properties and voltage-gated Na+ channel activity differ between NMR and mouse neurons

Electrophysiological recordings from NMR neurons have been performed in both DRG sensory neurons [43, 50] and CNS neurons [46, 47, 53]. However, neuronal activity from NMR CNS has only been recorded in brain slices, in the form of field excitatory postsynaptic potentials, and the basic electrophysiological properties of NMR neurons in hippocampal and cortical cultures have not yet been described.

We first compared the capacitance and resting membrane potential of NMR and mouse neurons from both cortical and hippocampal neuronal cultures (Fig. 1). The capacitance of NMR neurons was significantly smaller than in mouse neurons in both cortical and hippocampal cultures (cortex: 17.27 ± 1.02 pF versus 28.72 ± 2.32 pF for NMR (n = 30) and mouse (n = 24) neurons, respectively; hippocampus: 17.41 ± 1.03 pF versus 38.13 ± 3.

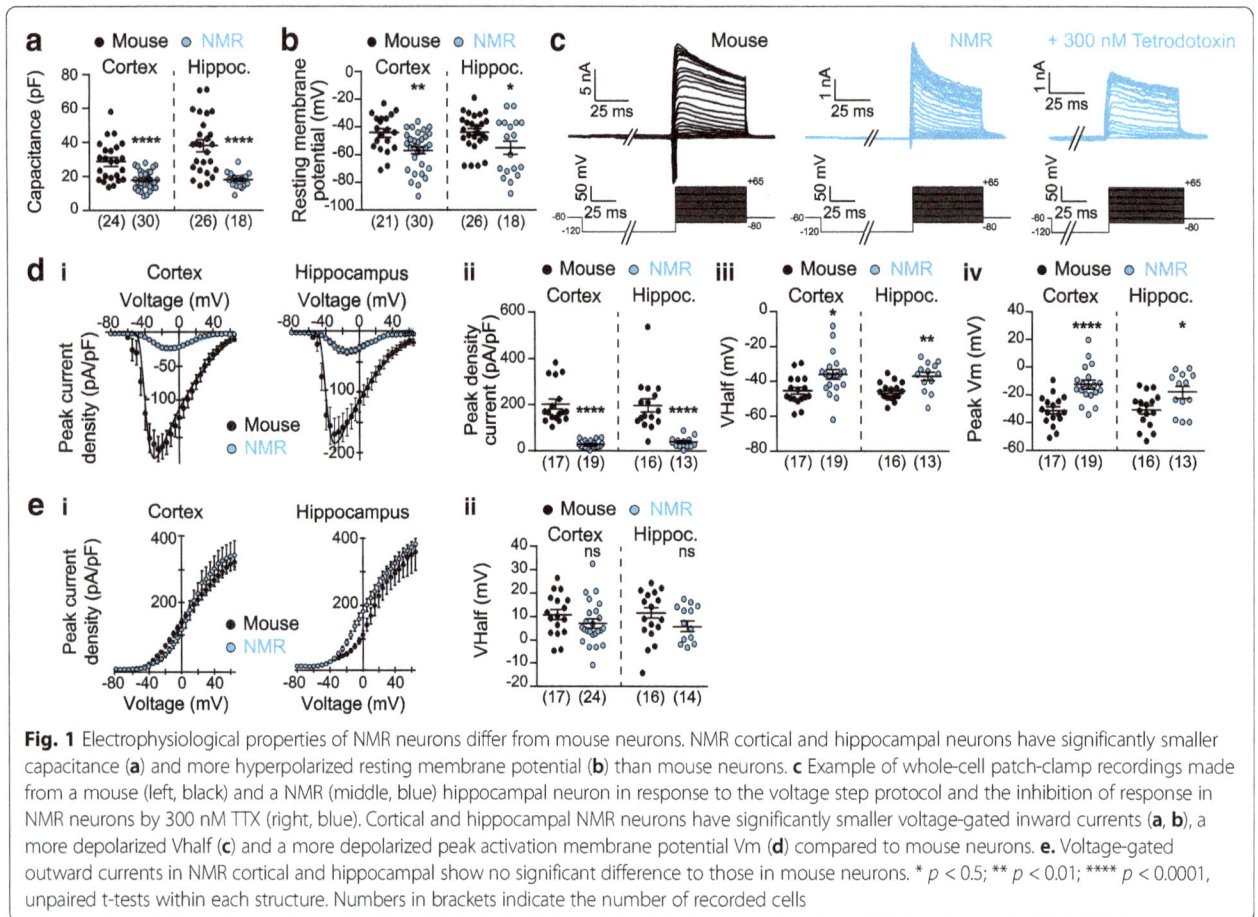

Fig. 1 Electrophysiological properties of NMR neurons differ from mouse neurons. NMR cortical and hippocampal neurons have significantly smaller capacitance (**a**) and more hyperpolarized resting membrane potential (**b**) than mouse neurons. **c** Example of whole-cell patch-clamp recordings made from a mouse (left, black) and a NMR (middle, blue) hippocampal neuron in response to the voltage step protocol and the inhibition of response in NMR neurons by 300 nM TTX (right, blue). Cortical and hippocampal NMR neurons have significantly smaller voltage-gated inward currents (**a, b**), a more depolarized Vhalf (**c**) and a more depolarized peak activation membrane potential Vm (**d**) compared to mouse neurons. **e.** Voltage-gated outward currents in NMR cortical and hippocampal show no significant difference to those in mouse neurons. * $p < 0.5$; ** $p < 0.01$; **** $p < 0.0001$, unpaired t-tests within each structure. Numbers in brackets indicate the number of recorded cells

27 pF for NMR ($n = 18$) and mouse ($n = 26$) neurons, respectively; unpaired two-sided t-tests, **** $p < 0.0001$, Fig. 1a). Resting membrane potentials were measured as soon as the whole-cell configuration was established and NMR neurons were significantly more hyperpolarized than mouse neurons, in both cortical and hippocampal cultures (cortex: -57.03 ± 2.64 mV versus -44.05 ± 2.84 mV for NMR ($n = 30$) and mouse ($n = 21$) neurons, respectively; hippocampus: -55.11 ± 4.79 mV versus -43.85 ± 2.59 mV for NMR ($n = 18$) and mouse ($n = 26$) neurons, respectively; unpaired two-sided t-tests; ** $p < 0.01$; * $p < 0.05$, Fig. 1b).

We then investigated macroscopic voltage-gated currents in NMR and mouse neurons, using a voltage-step whereby cells were held at -120 mV for 200 msecs before stepping to the test potential (-80 mV to $+65$ mV in 5 mV increments) for 50 msecs, and returning to the holding potential (-60 mV) for 200 msecs between sweeps (Fig. 1c). Both NMR and mouse neurons showed inward and outward currents (Fig. 1c-e). In some experiments, the voltage-step protocol was run twice, the second time after 300 nM tetrodotoxin (TTX) had been applied for 30 s to investigate the contribution of TTX-sensitive voltage-gated Na$^+$ channels (NaVs) to the

macroscopic voltage-gated inward currents recorded in NMR neurons (Fig. 1c, right panel). In both cortical and hippocampal NMR neurons, the voltage-gated inward currents were fully blocked by 300 nM TTX ($n = 8$ and $n = 2$ for cortical and hippocampal neurons, respectively). The fact that no inward current remained after application of 300 nM TTX indicates that only NaVs were activated with our voltage-step protocol and that there was no measurable contribution of voltage-gated Ca^{2+} channels to the inward currents recorded. Moreover, these results indicate that cortical and hippocampal NMR neurons only express TTX-sensitive NaVs.

Strikingly, NMR neurons had a significantly smaller inward peak current density in both cortical and hippocampal cultures (cortex: 28.79 ± 3.83 pA/pF versus 202.40 ± 21.35 pA/pF for NMR ($n = 19$) and mouse ($n = 17$) neurons, respectively; hippocampus: 39.00 ± 6.39 pA/pF versus 196.70 ± 28.28 pA/pF for NMR ($n = 13$) and mouse ($n = 16$) neurons, respectively; unpaired two-sided t-tests, **** $p < 0.0001$, Fig. 1d.i-ii). Additionally, the voltage of half-activation (Vhalf) and the peak inward current amplitude potential (peak Vm) were more depolarized in NMR neurons compared to mouse neurons (cortex: Vhalf: -36.12 ± 2.80 mV versus $-45.42 \pm 1.$

99 mV and peak Vm: -12.43 ± 3.02 mV versus -31.27 ± 2.61 mV for NMR ($n = 19$) and mouse ($n = 17$) neurons, respectively; hippocampus: Vhalf: -37.10 ± 2.34 mV versus -45.71 ± 1.30 mV and peak Vm: -17.62 ± 4.00 mV versus -30.68 ± 3.09 mV for NMR ($n = 13$) and mouse ($n = 16$) neurons, respectively; unpaired two-sided t-tests, **** $p < 0.0001$, ** $p < 0.01$; * $p < 0.05$, Fig. 1d.iii-iv). These results suggest that NMR neurons may be less excitable compared to mouse neurons, with more hyperpolarized resting membrane potentials and smaller voltage-gated inward currents that are activated at more depolarized potentials, i.e. a greater depolarizing stimulus is required to activate NMR voltage-gated inward currents that produce much smaller currents.

By contrast, current-voltage curves for voltage-gated outward currents were similar between NMR and mouse neurons from both cortical and hippocampal neurons (Fig. 1e.i) and Vhalfs were not significantly different (cortex: 7.13 ± 1.91 mV versus 10.77 ± 2.18 mV for NMR ($n = 24$) and mouse ($n = 17$) neurons, respectively;

hippocampus: 5.15 ± 2.50 mV versus 11.59 ± 2.26 mV for NMR ($n = 14$) and mouse ($n = 16$) neurons, respectively; unpaired two-sided t-tests, $p = 0.221$ and $p = 0.094$ for cortex and hippocampus respectively, Fig. 1e.ii).

Acid-induced currents are mediated by ASICs in both NMR and mouse neurons

The expression profile of ASIC subunits is similar in mouse and NMR brains, with the exception of lower levels of ASIC4 throughout the NMR brain [51], results suggesting that functional ASIC-mediated currents should be present in NMR as others have shown in mouse [4, 5, 7, 8, 15].

A 5 s pulse of pH 5 was applied to NMR and mouse neurons from both hippocampal and cortical neurons and rapidly activating and inactivating acid-induced responses were recorded in every cell of both species (Fig. 2a). However, the peak current density of acid-mediated responses recorded in NMR neurons was significantly smaller than in mouse neurons, in both hippocampal and cortical

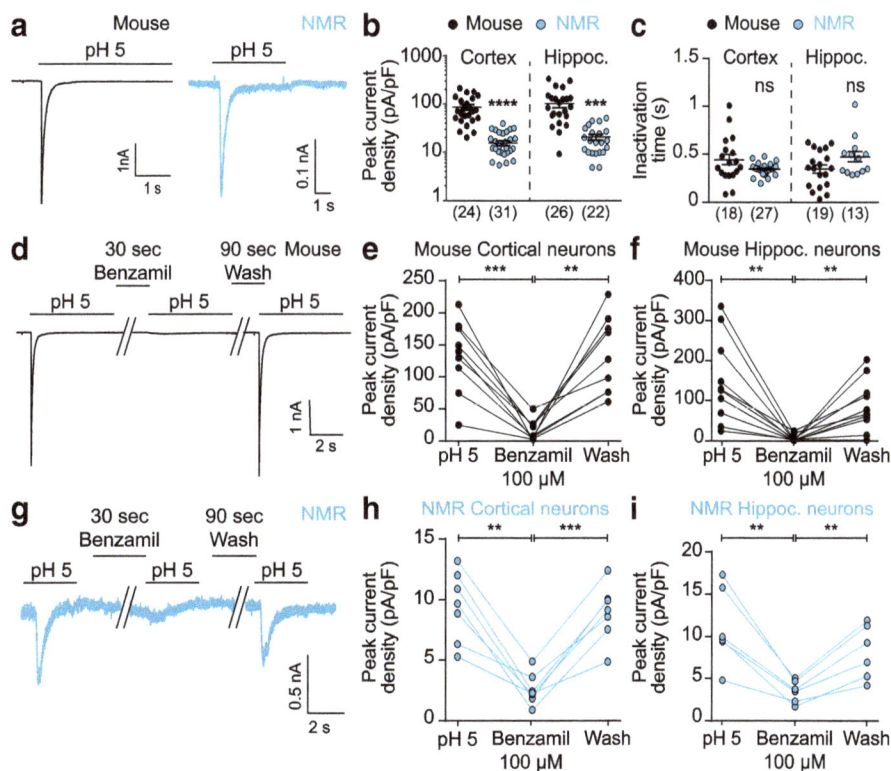

Fig. 2 ASICs mediate acid-induced currents in NMR and mouse CNS neurons. **a** Both mouse (black trace, left) and NMR (blue trace, right) neurons respond to a pH 5 solution with a transient inward current. **b** Acid-induced currents are of significantly smaller amplitude in NMR neurons compared to mouse neurons. **c** Inactivation time constants of the acid-induced responses are similar between NMR and mouse neurons. **d** Example trace of an acid-induced current elicited by a pH 5 solution and the effect of 100 μM benzamil in a mouse cortical neuron. **e**, **f** Acid-induced currents in both cortical and hippocampal mouse neurons were reversibly blocked by 100 μM benzamil ($n = 9$ and $n = 10$ cortical and hippocampal neurons, respectively). **g** Example trace of an acid-induced current evoked by a pH 5 solution in a cortical NMR neuron showing inhibition by 100 μM benzamil. **h**, **i** In both cortical ($n = 7$) and hippocampal ($n = 6$) NMR neurons, acid-induced currents were reversibly blocked by 100 μM benzamil. ** $p < 0.01$; **** $p < 0.0001$, one-way ANOVA paired tests, Tukey's multiple comparison tests. Numbers into brackets indicates the number of recorded cells

neurons (cortex: 15.41 ± 1.82 pA/pF versus 85.66 ± 10.90 pA/pF for NMR ($n = 31$) and mouse ($n = 24$) neurons, respectively; hippocampus: 20.54 ± 2.86 pA/pF versus 100.90 ± 17.68 pA/pF for NMR ($n = 22$) and mouse ($n = 26$) neurons, respectively; unpaired two-sided t-tests, **** $p < 0.0001$, *** $p < 0.001$, Fig. 2b). By contrast, the inactivation time constant of the acid-mediated currents was similar between NMR and mouse neurons (cortex: 0.35 ± 0.012 s versus 0.44 ± 0.056 s for NMR ($n = 27$) and mouse ($n = 18$) neurons, respectively, unpaired two-sided t-test, $p = 0.0516$; hippocampus: 0.47 ± 0.06 s versus 0.35 ± 0.04 s for NMR ($n = 13$) and mouse ($n = 19$) neurons, respectively; unpaired two-sided t-test, $p = 0.0861$, Fig. 2c).

The transient nature of the acid-mediated inward currents in both NMR and mouse neurons is characteristic of ASIC-mediated currents [3] and to confirm the involvement of ASICs we utilized the non-selective ASIC antagonist benzamil [54]. After a first application of pH 5 for 5 s, we applied 100 μM benzamil for 30 s before a second pH 5 pulse, then followed by a wash period of 90 s (Fig. 2d, g). In cortical and hippocampal mouse neurons, the acid-induced currents were reversibly blocked by 100 μM benzamil (cortex: pH 5: 133.60 ± 19.01 pA/pF; benzamil: 16.77 ± 5.28 pA/pF; wash: 133.80 ± 19.88 pA/pF ($n = 9$); hippocampus: pH 5: 151.00 ± 33.64 pA/pF; benzamil: 7.84 ± 2.67 pA/pF; wash: 89.26 ± 20.48 pA/pF ($n = 10$); one-way paired ANOVA test, Tukey's multiple comparison test, *** $p < 0.001$, ** $p < 0.01$, Fig. 2e-f). This result concurs with previous studies indicating that acid-evoked currents in mouse hippocampal and cortical neurons are mediated by ASICs [4, 8, 15].

Similarly, in cortical and hippocampal NMR neurons, acid-induced currents were reversibly inhibited by 100 μM benzamil (cortex: pH 5: 9.66 ± 1.09 pA/pF; benzamil: 2.78 ± 0.49 pA/pF; wash: 9.13 ± 0.89 pA/pF ($n = 7$); hippocampus: pH 5: 11.13 ± 1.88 pA/pF; benzamil: 3.50 ± 0.53 pA/pF; wash: 8.15 ± 1.30 pA/pF ($n = 6$); one-way paired ANOVA test, Tukey's multiple comparison test, *** $p < 0.001$, ** $p < 0.01$, Fig. 2h-i). This is the first demonstration of functional ASIC-mediated currents in CNS NMR neurons.

NMR neurons are resistant to acid-induced cell death

ASICs are involved in acid-induced cell death, so-called acidotoxicity, which can occur during periods of ischemia [5, 15, 16]. Because NMR neurons exhibit significantly smaller ASIC currents (Fig. 2), we hypothesized that this could be neuroprotective when neurons are in an acidic environment. We exposed neuronal cultures from mouse and NMR cortices to a pH 7.4 or a pH 5 solution for 2 h at 37 °C. Nuclei were stained by Hoechst 33,342 and necrotic (dead) neurons were labeled using propidium iodide (PI) (Fig. 3). Percentages of dead neurons were calculated by counting the number of necrotic

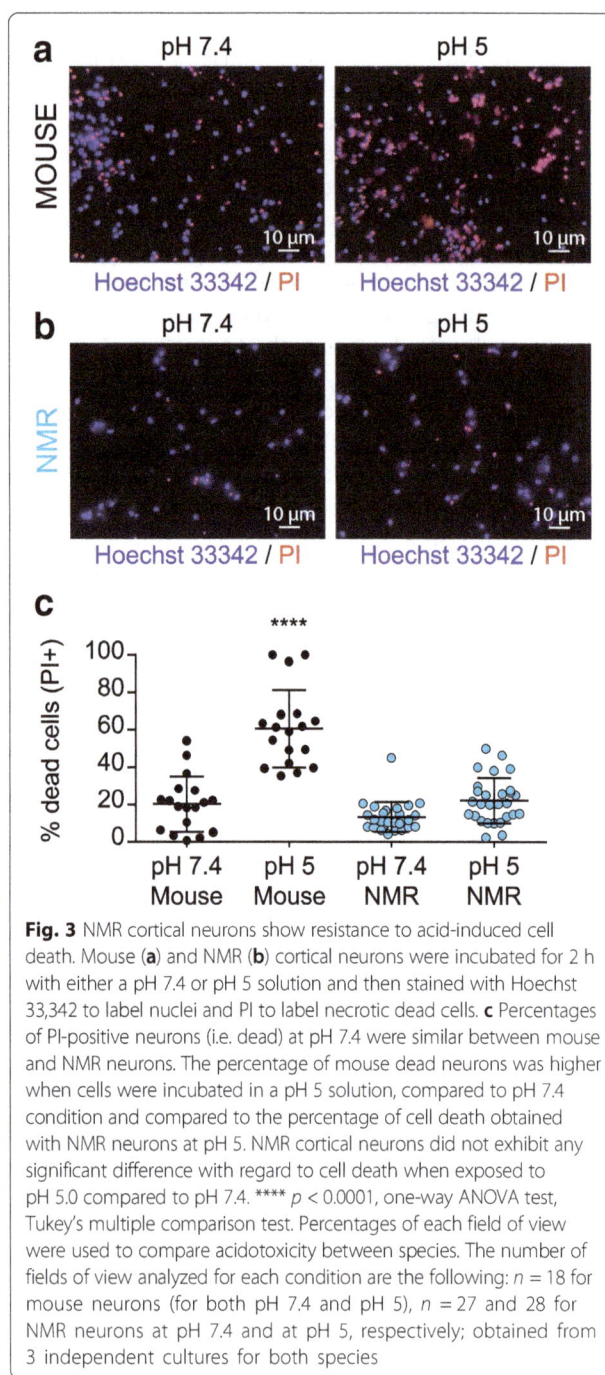

Fig. 3 NMR cortical neurons show resistance to acid-induced cell death. Mouse (**a**) and NMR (**b**) cortical neurons were incubated for 2 h with either a pH 7.4 or pH 5 solution and then stained with Hoechst 33,342 to label nuclei and PI to label necrotic dead cells. **c** Percentages of PI-positive neurons (i.e. dead) at pH 7.4 were similar between mouse and NMR neurons. The percentage of mouse dead neurons was higher when cells were incubated in a pH 5 solution, compared to pH 7.4 condition and compared to the percentage of cell death obtained with NMR neurons at pH 5. NMR cortical neurons did not exhibit any significant difference with regard to cell death when exposed to pH 5.0 compared to pH 7.4. **** $p < 0.0001$, one-way ANOVA test, Tukey's multiple comparison test. Percentages of each field of view were used to compare acidotoxicity between species. The number of fields of view analyzed for each condition are the following: $n = 18$ for mouse neurons (for both pH 7.4 and pH 5), $n = 27$ and 28 for NMR neurons at pH 7.4 and at pH 5, respectively; obtained from 3 independent cultures for both species

PI-positive cells over the total number of Hoechst 33,342-positive neurons in the field of view, and a one-way ANOVA test corrected for multiple comparisons (see *Methods*) was used to compare neuronal death at pH 5 between both species (Fig. 3c). At pH 7.4, percentages of dead cells were comparable between mouse and NMR cortical cultures (mouse - pH 7.4: $20.31 \pm 3.50\%$, $n = 18$ fields of view; NMR – pH 7.4: $13.31 \pm 1.53\%$, $n = 27$ fields of view; from 3 independent experiments), suggesting no differences in neuronal death under basal conditions between NMR and mouse cultures. When incubated for 2 h in pH 5 solution, mouse cortical neurons exhibited a significantly increased percentage of cell death compared to all other conditions (mouse – pH 5: $60.55 \pm 4.87\%$, $n = 18$ fields of view; NMR – pH 5: $22.29 \pm 2.30\%$, $n = 28$ fields of view, from 3 independent experiments, $p < 0.0001$, ****). By contrast, when NMR cortical neurons were exposed to pH 5 for 2 h, no difference in the level of cell death was observed compared to incubation at pH 7.4. Similar results were obtained using mouse and NMR hippocampal neurons (data not shown). This indicates that NMR neurons are resistant to acid-induced cell death, possibly due to their reduced ASIC currents compared to mouse neurons.

Discussion

In this study, we recorded for the first time from cultured NMR brain neurons and described their basic electrophysiological properties (Fig. 1). We showed that NMR neuronal capacitance was smaller than in mouse neurons and that the resting membrane potential of NMR neurons is more hyperpolarized than in mouse neurons. One point to consider is that neurons were recorded from blindly and so we can only broadly compare hippocampal and cortical neurons between species and cannot comment on if these differences occur in all types of neuron or specific neuronal subpopulations, such as interneurons. Although capacitance and resting membrane potential values obtained from mouse neurons were similar to those reported by others using cultured rodent neurons [55, 56], for NMR neurons however, previous data from others found their resting membrane potential to be more hyperpolarized (NMR cortical neurons: -57.03 ± 2.64 mV, NMR hippocampal neurons: -55.11 ± 4.79 mV, Fig. 1; NMR hippocampal pyramidal neurons (4 months old): -70.3 ± 6.1 mV, NMR hippocampal dentate granule cells (4 months old): -75.1 ± 3.6 mV, [53]). Explanations for differences observed in resting membrane potentials between studies are the recording conditions (in vitro vs. in vivo), the developmental stage of the animal from which neurons are obtained and the constituents of the intracellular and extracellular solutions. When comparing our study with that of Penz and colleagues, who reported more hyperpolarized resting membrane potentials, two factors that could contribute to the difference observed is that we made recordings from cultured neurons, whereas they used brain slices, and secondly, we isolated neurons from neonatal animals, whereas slice recordings were made from animals aged at least 4-months.

A standard voltage-step protocol that has been already successfully used in NMR sensory neurons to predominantly isolate NaV activity [43] was used to measure macroscopic voltage-gated current activity in mouse and NMR neurons. NaV currents recorded from mouse neurons were not different to what have been recorded in similar experimental conditions (for example, mouse cortical neurons at DIV 10-12: Vhalf: -41.62 ± 1.46 mV in [57] versus this study: -45.42 ± 1.99 mV). Similarly, inward currents recorded in NMR brain neurons were also very similar to currents recorded in NMR sensory neurons (NMR cortex: Vhalf: -36.12 ± 2.80 mV; NMR hippocampus: Vhalf: -37.10 ± 2.34 mV; NMR DRG neurons: Vhalf: from -34.2 ± 0.1 mV to -44.6 ± 0.5 mV [43]). However, NMR inward currents significantly differed from mouse currents: the peak current density was significantly smaller and the Vhalf and peak Vm values were more depolarized. These differences in NMR NaV activity likely result from differences in amino acid sequence of NaV subunits and/or differential expression of accessory subunits and warrant further investigation. We also found that addition of 300 nM TTX completely abolished all voltage-gated inward currents demonstrating an absence of TTX resistant NaV subunits in the NMR brain, this result aligns with the observation that the TTX-resistant NaV subunits, NaV1.5, NaV1.8 and NaV1.9 are not expressed in the central nervous system [58]. It should also be noted that although NMR neurons were cultured at 32 °C under hypoxic (3% O_2) conditions, recordings under normoxic, standard laboratory conditions, whereas NMRs live in a hypoxic and hypercapnic environment [59, 60], which may influence channel activity in vivo.

ASIC activity in brain neurons is now accepted as a key factor in numerous physiological and pathological conditions [61]. However, nothing is known about acid-induced responses in NMR brain neurons, which is of considerable interest considering the behavioral hypoxia/hypercapnia resistance and lack of acid-induced nocifensive behavior display by NMR that are likely adaptations to adapting to a safe, but relatively hypoxic and hypercapnic habitat [35]. Recently, we described ASIC subunit expression in the NMR CNS [62], which is similar to that in the mouse CNS, with the exception of lowered ASIC4 levels in the NMR brain. However, evidence for functional ASIC activity is lacking and is of particular interest in light of our recent finding that nmrASIC3 forms non-functional homomers [50]. Here, we find that NMR brain neurons produce ASIC-mediated currents in response to acid stimulation, in both hippocampus and cortex, as demonstrated by acid-induced responses being fully, reversibly blocked by 100 μM benzamil (Fig. 2). However, the peak current density of NMR ASIC-mediated responses was significantly reduced compared to responses recorded in mouse neurons. The reasons for such reduction in ASIC currents in NMR neurons is not known and additional research is needed to determine what underpins this different, e.g. are regulators of ASIC plasma membrane trafficking different in NMR? Is there a different developmental expression profile of ASICs between mouse and NMR? With regard to the ASIC currents themselves, they have similar inactivation kinetics in both NMR and mouse neurons (Fig. 2c), which suggests that a similar mixture of ASIC subunits are expressed, as our previous mRNA based analysis suggested [62].

Incubation with a pH 5.0 solution showed that unlike mouse neurons, NMR neurons do not undergo any significant acid-induced cell death (Fig. 3). This is the first demonstration of resistance to acid-induced neuronal death in NMR neurons. In rodent neurons, some factors shown to be protective against acid-induced neuronal injury, include lower temperature [63], pharmacological blockade or genetic deletion of ASIC activity [15] or ASIC trafficking [64], i.e. it is established that ASICs play a key role in acidotoxicity. Considering the similar prevalence of ASIC currents, we suggest that the reduced ASIC-mediated current amplitude observed in NMR neurons may be an additional neuroprotective mechanism in NMR brains, alongside the previously described increased hypoxia-inducible transcription factor (HIF1-α) expression [65] or more efficient in vivo CO_2 buffering [47]. One possible mechanism for the decreased amplitude observed is reduced ASIC plasma membrane trafficking which is known to be modulated by an extracellular acidic environment [64]. However, it is also possible that the reduced acid-induced cell death observed is not ASIC-dependent because although ASIC activation appears to play a major role in neuronal injury [61], several other molecular players are also modulated by a drop in extracellular pH, such as NaVs [27, 28] and glutamate receptors [31] and may contribute to the lowered acid-induced cell death observed, for example, here we also show that NMR neurons also have smaller NaV-mediated currents, which may also add a layer of neuroprotection.

Conclusions

In this work, we describe for the first time the basic electrophysiological properties of NMR neurons in culture and showed that the resting membrane potential of NMR neurons is more hyperpolarized, as well as the amplitude of NaVs being smaller than that of mouse neurons. We then demonstrated that acid-induced currents are present in NMR neurons and are, as in mouse, ASIC-mediated. The key result is that acid-induced cell death is virtually absent in NMR neurons, with reduced ASIC and NaV amplitudes likely contributing to this observation, and thus this is a further adaptation enabling NMR to live in a subterranean, hypercapnic/hypoxic environment.

Abbreviations

ASIC: Acid-sensing ion channel; CNS: Central nervous system; DRG: Dorsal root ganglion; NaV: Voltage-gated Na⁺ channel; NMR: Naked mole-rat; TTX: Tetrodotoxin

Acknowledgements

Thanks to all members of ESS lab for their useful discussions, and in particular to the assistant staff in the Department of Pharmacology and Animal Facility for their technical help and animal husbandry.

Funding

This work was supported by an Isaac Newton Trust Research Grant from the University of Cambridge. ZH was funded by a EMBO Long-Term Fellowship (ALTF1565-2015).

Authors' contributions

ZH and ESS designed the study. ZH performed all the experiments and analysed the data. ZH and ESS wrote the manuscript. Both authors read and approved the final manuscript.

Competing interests

The authors declare that they have no competing interests.

References

1. Gründer S, Pusch M. Biophysical properties of acid-sensing ion channels (ASICs). Neuropharmacology. 2015;94:9–18.
2. Waldmann R, Champigny G, Bassilana F, Heurteaux C, Lazdunski M. A proton-gated cation channel involved in acid-sensing. Nature. 1997;386: 173–7.
3. Hesselager M, Timmermann DB, Ahring PK. pH dependency and desensitization kinetics of Heterologously expressed combinations of acid-sensing Ion Channel subunits. J Biol Chem. 2004;279:11006–15.
4. Baron A, Waldmann R, Lazdunski M. ASIC-like, proton-activated currents in rat hippocampal neurons. J Physiol. 2002;539:485–94.
5. Sherwood TW, Lee KG, Gormley MG, Askwith CC. Heteromeric acid-sensing ion channels (ASICs) composed of ASIC2b and ASIC1a display Novel Channel properties and contribute to acidosis-induced neuronal death. J Neurosci. 2011;31:9723–34.
6. Wu L-J, Duan B, Mei Y-D, Gao J, Chen J-G, Zhuo M, et al. Characterization of acid-sensing ion channels in dorsal horn neurons of rat spinal cord. J Biol Chem. 2004;279:43716–24.
7. Gao J, Wu LJ, Xu L, Le XT. Properties of the proton-evoked currents and their modulation by CA 2+ and Zn2+ in the acutely dissociated hippocampus CA1 neurons. Brain Res. 2004;1017:197–207.
8. Askwith CC, Wemmie JA, Price MP, Rokhlina T, Welsh MJ. Acid-sensing Ion Channel 2 (ASIC2) modulates ASIC1 H+−activated currents in hippocampal neurons. J Biol Chem. 2004;279:18296–305.
9. Wemmie JA, Chen J, Askwith CC, Hruska-Hageman AM, Price MP, Nolan BC, et al. The acid-activated ion channel ASIC contributes to synaptic plasticity, learning, and memory. Neuron. 2002;34:463–77.
10. Liu MG, Li HS, Li WG, Wu YJ, Deng SN, Huang C, et al. Acid-sensing ion channel 1a contributes to hippocampal LTP inducibility through multiple mechanisms. Sci Rep. 2016;6:1–14.
11. Mango D, Braksator E, Battaglia G, Marcelli S, Mercuri NB, Feligioni M, et al. Acid-sensing ion channel 1a is required for mGlu receptor dependent long-term depression in the hippocampus. Pharmacol Res. 2017;119:12–9.

12. Vralsted VC, Price MP, Du J, Schnizler M, Wunsch AM, Ziemann AE, et al. Expressing acid-sensing ion channel 3 in the brain alters acid-evoked currents and impairs fear conditioning. Genes Brain Behav. 2011;10:444–50.

13. Taugher RJ, Lu Y, Fan R, Ghobbeh A, Kreple CJ, Faraci FM, et al. ASIC1A in neurons is critical for fear-related behaviors. Genes Brain Behav. 2017;16:745–55.

14. Wemmie JA, Coryell MW, Askwith CC, Lamani E, Leonard AS, Sigmund CD, et al. Overexpression of acid-sensing ion channel 1a in transgenic mice increases acquired fear-related behavior. Proc Natl Acad Sci. 2004;101:3621–6.

15. Xiong Z-G, Zhu X-M, Chu X-P, Minami M, Hey J, Wei W L, et al. Neuroprotection in ischemia: blocking calcium-permeable acid-sensing ion channels. Cell. 2004;118:687–98.

16. Duan B, Wang Y-Z, Yang T, Chu X-P, Yu Y, Huang Y, et al. Extracellular Spermine exacerbates ischemic neuronal injury through sensitization of ASIC1a channels to extracellular acidosis. J Neurosci. 2011;31:2101–12.

17. Gu L, Liu X, Yang Y, Luo D, Zheng X. ASICs aggravate acidosis-induced injuries during ischemic reperfusion. Neurosci Lett. 2010;479:63–8.

18. Friese MA, Craner MJ, Etzensperger R, Vergo S, Wemmie JA, Welsh MJ, et al. Acid-sensing ion channel-1 contributes to axonal degeneration in autoimmune inflammation of the central nervous system. Nature Med. 2007;13:1483–9.

19. Chu X-P, Xiong Z-G. Physiological and pathological functions of acid-sensing ion channels in the central nervous system. Curr Drug Targets. 2012;13:263–71.

20. Gonzales EB, Sumien N. Acidity and acid-sensing ion channels in the normal and Alzheimer's disease brain. J Alzheimers Dis. 2017;57:1137–44.

21. Chesler M. Regulation and modulation of pH in the brain; 2003. p. 1183–221.

22. Rehncrona S. Brain acidosis. Ann Emerg Med. 1985;14:770–6.

23. Immke DC, McCleskey EW. Lactate enhances the acid-sensing Na+ channel on ischemia-sensing neurons. Nat Neurosci. 2001;4:869–70.

24. Allen NJ, Attwell D. Modulation of ASIC channels in rat cerebellar Purkinje neurons by ischaemia-related signals. J Physiol. 2002;543:521–9.

25. Smith ES, Cadiou H, McNaughton PA. Arachidonic acid potentiates acid-sensing ion channels in rat sensory neurons by a direct action. Neuroscience. 2007;145:686–98.

26. Tombaugh GC, Somjen GG. Effects of extracellular pH on voltage-gated Na +, K+ and Ca2+ currents in isolated rat CA1 neurons. J Physiol. 1996;493: 719–32.

27. Nakamura M, Jang I-S. Acid modulation of tetrodotoxin-resistant Na+ channels in rat nociceptive neurons. Neuropharmacol. 2015;90:82–9.

28. Nakamura M, Kim DY, Jang IS. Acid modulation of tetrodotoxin-sensitive Na+ channels in large-sized trigeminal ganglion neurons. Brain Res. 2016;1651:44–52.

29. Sepulveda FV, Pablo Cid L, Teulon J, Niemeyer MI. Molecular aspects of structure, gating, and physiology of pH-sensitive background K2P and Kir K +–transport channels. Physiol Rev. 2015;95:179–217.

30. Mcdonald JW, Bhattacharyya T, Sensi SL, Lobner D, Ying HS, Canzoniero LMT, et al. Extracellular Acidity Potentiates AMPA Receptor-Mediated Cortical Neuronal Death. J Neurosci. 1998;18:6290–9.

31. Traynelis SF, Cull-Candy SG. Proton inhibition of N-methyl-D-aspartate receptors in cerebellar neurons. Lett to Nat. 1990;345:347–50.

32. Bennett NC, Faulkes CG. African mole-rats: ecology and Eusociality. Cambridge: Cambridge University Press; 2000.

33. Brett RA. The ecology of naked mole-rat colonies: burrowing, food and limiting factors. In: Sherman P, Jarvis J, Alexander R, editors. Biol. Naked Mole-Rat. Princeton: Princeton University Press; 1991. p. 137–84.

34. Jarvis JUM. Reproduction of naked mole-rats. In: Sherman P, Jarvis J, Alexander M, editors. Biol. Naked Mole-Rat. Princeton: Princeton University Press; 1991. p. 384–425.

35. Schuhmacher L, Husson Z, Smith ES. The naked mole-rat as an animal model in biomedical research: current perspectives. Open Access Anim Physiol. 2015;7:137.

36. Ruby JG, Smith M, Buffenstein R. Naked mole-rat mortality rates defy gompertzian laws by not increasing with age. Elife. 2018;7:1–18.

37. Edrey YH, Medina DX, Gaczynska M, Osmulski PA, Oddo S, Caccamo A, et al. Amyloid beta and the longest-lived rodent: the naked mole-rat as a model for natural protection from alzheimer's disease. Neurobiol Aging. 2013;34:2352–60.

38. Orr ME, Garbarino VR, Salinas A, Buffenstein R. Sustained high levels of neuroprotective, high molecular weight, phosphorylated tau in the longest-lived rodent. Neurobiol Aging. 2015;36:1496–504.

39. Seluanov A, Hine C, Azpurua J, Feigenson M, Bozzella M, Mao Z, et al. Hypersensitivity to contact inhibition provides a clue to cancer resistance of naked mole-rat. Proc Natl Acad Sci U S A. 2009;106:19352–7.

40. Tian X, Azpurua J, Hine C, Vaidya A, Myakishev-Rempel M, Ablaeva J, et al. High-molecular-mass hyaluronan mediates the cancer resistance of the naked mole rat. Nature. 2013;499:346–9.

41. Liang S, Mele J, Wu Y, Buffenstein R, Hornsby PJ. Resistance to experimental tumorigenesis in cells of a long-lived mammal, the naked mole-rat (Heterocephalus glaber). Aging Cell. 2010;9:626–35.

42. Park TJ, Lu Y, Jüttner R, Smith ESJ, Hu J, Brand A, et al. Selective inflammatory pain insensitivity in the African naked mole-rat (Heterocephalus glaber). PLoS Biol. 2008;6:0156–70.

43. Smith ESJ, Omerbašić D, Lechner SG, Anirudhan G, Lapatsina L, Lewin GR. The molecular basis of acid insensitivity in the African naked mole-rat. Science. 2011;334:1557–60.

44. Smith ESJ, Blass GRC, Lewin GR, Park TJ. Absence of histamine-induced itch in the African naked mole-rat and "rescue" by substance P. Mol Pain. 2010;6:29.

45. Lavinka PC, Brand A, Landau VJ, Wirtshafter D, Park TJ. Extreme tolerance to ammonia fumes in African naked mole-rats: animals that naturally lack neuropeptides from trigeminal chemosensory nerve fibers. J Comp Physiol A Neuroethol Sensory Neural Behav Physiol. 2009;195:419–27.

46. Larson J, Park TJ. Extreme hypoxia tolerance of naked mole-rat brain. Neuroreport. 2009;20:1634–7.

47. Park TJ, Reznick J, Peterson BL, Blass G, Omerba D, Bennett NC, et al. Fructose-driven glycolysis supports anoxia resistance in the naked mole-rat. Science. 2017;311:307–11.

48. Peterson BL, Larson J, Buffenstein R, Park TJ, Fall CP. Blunted neuronal calcium response to hypoxia in naked mole-rat hippocampus. PLoS One. 2012;7:1–8.

49. Peterson BL, Park TJ, Larson J. Adult naked mole-rat brain retains the NMDA receptor subunit GluN2D associated with hypoxia tolerance in neonatal mammals. Neurosci Lett. 2012;506:342–5.

50. Schuhmacher L-N, Callejo G, Srivats S, Smith ESJ. Naked mole-rat acid-sensing ion channel 3 forms nonfunctional homomers, but functional heteromers. J Biol Chem. 2018;293:1756–66.

51. Schuhmacher L, Smith ESJ. Expression of acid-sensing ion channels and selection of reference genes in mouse and naked mole rat. Mol Brain. 2016; 9(1):97.

52. Omerbašić D, Smith ESJ, Moroni M, Homfeld J, Eigenbrod O, Bennett NC, et al. Hypofunctional TrkA accounts for the absence of pain sensitization in the African naked mole-rat. Cell Rep. 2016;17:748–58.

53. Penz OK, Fuzik J, Kurek AB, Romanov R, Larson J, Park TJ, et al. Protracted brain development in a rodent model of extreme longevity. Sci Rep. 2015;5:11592.

54. Baron A, Lingueglia E. Pharmacology of acid-sensing ion channels – physiological and therapeutical perspectives. Neuropharmacology. 2015;94: 19–35.

55. Evans MS, Collings MA, Brewer GJ. Electrophysiology of embryonic, adult and aged rat hippocampal neurons in serum-free culture. J Neurosci Methods. 1998;79:37–46.

56. Yang J, Thio LL, Clifford DB, Zorumski CF. Electrophysiological properties of identified postnatal rat hippocampal pyramidal neurons in primary culture. Dev Brain Res. 1993;71:19–26.

57. Wang X, Zhang XG, Zhou TT, Li N, Jang CY, Xiao ZC, et al. Elevated neuronal excitability due to modulation of the voltage-gated sodium channel Nav1.6 by Aβ1-42. Front Neurosci. 2016;10:1–9.

58. Catterall WA. Voltage-gated sodium channels at 60 : structure, function and. Pathophysiology. 2012;11:2577–89.

59. Shams I, Avivi A, Nevo E. Oxygen and carbon dioxide fluctuations in burrows of subterranean blind mole rats indicate tolerance to hypoxic – hypercapnic stresses. Comp Biochem Physiol A Mol Integr Physiol. 2005;142:376–82.

60. Mcnab BK. The metabolism of fossorial rodents: a study of convergence. Ecol Soc Am. 1966;47:712–33.

61. Huang Y, Jiang N, Li J, Ji Y-H, Xiong Z-G, Zha X. Two aspects of ASIC function: synaptic plasticity and neuronal injury. Neuropharmacology. 2015;94:1–6.

62. Schuhmacher L, St E, Smith J. Expression of acid-sensing ion channels and selection of reference genes in mouse and naked mole rat. Mol Brain. 2016: 1–12.

6

Direct interaction with 14–3-3γ promotes surface expression of Best1 channel in astrocyte

Soo-Jin Oh[1,2,3], Junsung Woo[1,3], Young-Sun Lee[6], Minhee Cho[4], Eunju Kim[4], Nam-Chul Cho[2], Jae-Yong Park[6], Ae Nim Pae[2], C. Justin Lee[1,3,5*] and Eun Mi Hwang[4,5*]

Abstract

Background: Bestrophin-1 (Best1) is a calcium-activated anion channel (CAAC) that is expressed broadly in mammalian tissues including the brain. We have previously reported that Best1 is expressed in hippocampal astrocytes at the distal peri-synaptic regions, called microdomains, right next to synaptic junctions, and that it disappears from the microdomains in Alzheimer's disease mouse model. Although Best1 appears to be dynamically regulated, the mechanism of its regulation and modulation is poorly understood. It has been reported that a regulatory protein, 14-3-3 affects the surface expression of numerous membrane proteins in mammalian cells.

Methods: The protein-protein interaction between Best1 and 14-3-3γ was confirmed by yeast-two hybrid assay and BiFC method. The effect of 14-3-3γ on Best1-mediated current was measured by whole-cell patch clamp technique.

Results: We identified 14-3-3γ as novel binding partner of Best1 in astrocytes: among 7 isoforms of 14-3-3 protein, only 14-3-3γ was found to bind specifically. We determined a binding domain on the C-terminus of Best1 which is critical for an interaction with 14-3-3γ. We also revealed that interaction between Best1 and 14-3-3γ was mediated by phosphorylation of S358 in the C-terminus of Best1. We confirmed that surface expression of Best1 and Best1-mediated whole-cell current were significantly decreased after a gene-silencing of 14-3-3γ without a significant change in total Best1 expression in cultured astrocytes. Furthermore, we discovered that 14-3-3γ-shRNA reduced Best1-mediated glutamate release from hippocampal astrocyte by recording a PAR1 receptor-induced NMDA receptor-mediated current from CA1 pyramidal neurons in hippocampal slices injected with adenovirus carrying 14-3-3γ-shRNA. Finally, through a structural modeling, we found critical amino acid residues containing S358 of Best1 exhibiting binding affinities to 14-3-3γ.

Conclusions: 14-3-3γ promotes surface expression of Best1 channel in astrocytes through direct interaction.

Keywords: Astrocyte, Bestrophin-1, 14–3-3γ, Surface expression, Glutamate

Introduction

Astrocytes provide structural and trophic support to neurons as well as an active interaction with neurons. It has been reported that astrocytes can be activated by a variety of physiological and pathological stimuli which can evoke increases in intracellular Ca^{2+} in astrocytes [1, 2]. Astrocytes, in turn, elicit the release of active substances called gliotransmitters to regulate neuronal activities [3–6]. Recently, several studies have shown that hippocampal astrocytes express machinery responsible for Ca^{2+}-dependent and channel-mediated glutamate release, which is encoded by Best1 channel [7, 8]. *Bestrophin* is the gene responsible for a dominantly inherited, juvenile-onset form of macular degeneration called Best's vitelliform macular dystrophy. It has been shown to encode a functional Ca^{2+}-activated anion channel (CAAC) directly activated by submicromolar intracellular Ca^{2+} concentration in nonneuronal tissue and peripheral neurons [9]. Our previous studies indicate that Best1 has a permeability to gamma aminobutyric acid (GABA), which

* Correspondence: cjl@kist.re.kr; emhwang@kist.re.kr
[1]Center for Neuroscience, Korea Institute of Science and Technology, Seoul, Korea
[4]Center for Functional Connectomics, Korea Institute of Science and Technology, Seoul, Korea
Full list of author information is available at the end of the article

contributes majorly to the tonic form of neuronal inhibition [10]. We also demonstrated that Best1 releases glutamate, which targets and activates synaptic NMDA receptors in hippocampal CA1 pyramidal neurons [11] to modulate hippocampal synaptic plasticity [12].

This glutamate- and GABA-permeable Best1 is selectively expressed at the astrocytic microdomains adjacent to glutamatergic synapse by electron microscopy [13]. In our recent study, we observed that astrocytes around amyloid plaques in Alzheimer's disease (AD) model mouse become reactive and produce GABA [14]. Meanwhile, Best1 channel is redistributed away from microdomains to the soma and processes of reactive astrocytes, possibly switching its target from synaptic NMDA receptors to extrasynaptic GABA receptors [14]. Therefore, regulation of surface expression and channel distribution of the glutamate- and GABA-permeable Best1 probably have critical roles in astrocyte-neuron interaction and regulation of synaptic functions. Despite accumulating lines of evidence that Best1 has significant roles in synaptic functions both in physiological condition and in pathological condition of the brain [15] and its surface expression is dynamically regulated, relatively little is known about its mechanisms of regulation and modulation, especially of the regulation of surface expression.

To further explore the regulatory mechanism of the surface expression of Best1, we set forth to identify novel binding partners of Best1. The 14–3-3 proteins are a family of conserved regulatory molecules expressed in all eukaryotic organisms [16]. They have ability to bind a multitude of functionally wide array of cellular proteins. Through interaction with its effector proteins, 14–3-3 proteins participate in vital regulatory processes such as neuronal development, apoptotic cell death, cell cycle control, viral and bacterial pathogenesis and cellular activity including the subcellular localization of target proteins [17, 18]. They are abundantly expressed in the brain and have been detected in the cerebrospinal fluid (CSF) of patients with the various neurological disorders [19]. Several studies demonstrated that 14–3-3 proteins, by binding to phosphorylated motifs, promote the plasma membrane expression of integral membrane proteins such as the nicotinic acetylcholine and GABA receptors [20, 21], potassium channels [22, 23], the epithelial Na^+ channel, ENaC [24, 25] and TRPM4b channel [26]. These interactions between 14 and 3-3 proteins and various ion channels and possible role of the interaction in the pathophysiology of the brain suggest possible involvement of 14–3-3 protein in Best1 channel function. Therefore, we have employed biochemical and electrophysiological assays to investigate the potential protein-protein interaction between 14 and 3-3γ and Best1 channel. We demonstrate that 14–3-3γ promotes the surface expression of Best1 by interaction to C-terminus of Best1 in astrocytes.

Methods

Animals

Ca^{2+}/calmodulin-dependent kinase IIα promoter-driven Cre (CaMKIIα-Cre) transgenic mice purchased from Jackson Laboratory were used for cell type specific gene silencing system. For electrophysiological experiments, 7 to 8-week-old male mice were used. Animal care and handling were performed according to the directives of the Animal Care and Use Committee and institutional guidelines of KIST (Seoul, Korea).

Cell culture

HEK293T cells were cultured in Dulbecco's modified Eagle's medium (DMEM; Gibco) and COS7 cells were cultured in RPMI medium 1640 (Gibco) supplemented with 10% heat-inactivated fetal bovine serum and 1000 units ml^{-1} penicillin–streptomycin. Cultures were maintained at 37 °C in a humidified 5% CO_2-containing atmosphere. For primary culture of cortical astrocytes, P0-P3 C57BL/6 J mice were used. The cerebral cortex was dissected free of adherent meninges, minced and dissociated into single cell suspension by trituration through a Pasteur pipette. Dissociated cells were plated onto either 12 mm glass coverslips or six-well plates coated with 0.1 mg ml^{-1} poly d-lysine. Cells were grown in DMEM supplemented with 25 mM glucose, 10% heat-inactivated horse serum, 10% heat-inactivated fetal bovine serum, 2 mM glutamine and 1000 units ml^{-1} penicillin–streptomycin. Cultures were maintained at 37 °C in a humidified 5% CO_2-containing atmosphere. Astrocyte cultures prepared in this way were previously determined by glial fibrillary acidic protein (GFAP) staining to be greater than 95% astrocytes [27].

Electrophysiological recording from cultured astrocytes

In whole-cell patch clamp, patch pipettes which have 3 ~ 6 MΩ of resistance are filled with the standard intracellular solution. Current voltage curves were established by applying 100-, 200-, or 1000 ms duration voltage ramps from −100 to +100 mV. Data were acquired by an Axopatch 200A amplifier controlled by Clampex 10.2 via Digidata 1322A data acquisition system (Axon Instruments). Experiments were conducted at room temperature (20 ~ 24 °C). To activate CAAC or Best1 directly, high Ca^{2+}-containing intracellular patch pipette solution was applied to cultured astrocytes, which is comprised of 146 mM CsCl, 5 mM (Ca^{2+})-EGTA-NMDG, 2 mM $MgCl_2$, 8 mM HEPES, and 10 mM Sucrose at pH 7.3, adjusted with NMDG. For control experiments, Ca^{2+}-free intracellular solution comprised of 146 mM CsCl, 5 mM EGTA-NMDG, 2 mM $MgCl_2$, 8 mM HEPES, and 10 mM Sucrose at pH 7.3, adjusted with NMDG was used. The concentration of free $[Ca^{2+}]_i$ in the solution was determined as described [28]. The extracellular solution was comprised of 150 mM NaCl, 10 mM HEPES, 3 mM KCl, 2 mM $CaCl_2$, 2 mM $MgCl_2$, and 5.5 mM glucose at pH 7.3 with NaOH (~ 320 mOsm).

Yeast two-hybrid assay

The Best1 was ligated into pGBKT7 encoding for the GAL4 DNA binding domain (BD) and the 14–3-3γ was cloned into pGADT7 encoding for the activation domain (AD). To assess the protein–protein interaction between Best1 and 14-3-3γ, both BD/ mBest1 and AD/14–3-3γ were co-transformed into the yeast strain AH109. AH109 is unable to synthesize histidine. However, interaction between Best1 and 14–3-3γ enables the yeast to make the His3 enzyme, thereby permitting histidine biosynthesis and growth on His minimal medium.

Construction of BEST1-deletion or S358A mutants

We used full length mouse Best1 cDNA which was cloned in our previous study [7] and cDNAs of 7 isoform of 14-3-3 were kindly provided from Dr. Dukryong Kim (Gyeongsang National University). For searching the binding site between BEST1 and 14–3-3γ, 4 kinds of C-terminal deletion mutant (C1, C2, C3 and ΔC1) and 1 point mutant (S358A) were generated by EZchange™ Site-directed mutagenesis kit (Enzymonics, Korea) and confirmed by sequencing.

14–3-3γ shRNA, and virus production

The 14–3-3γ nucleotides from 544 to 564 (5′-ggacaac-tacctgatcaagaa) were selected for target region of 14–3-3γ-shRNA. For shRNA expression, 14–3-3γ shRNA was synthesized as followings: 5′-t ggacaactacctgatcaagaatt caagagattcttgatcaggtagttgtccttttttc-3′ and 5′-tcgagaaaaaa ggacaactacctgatcaagaatctcttgaattcttgatcaggtagttgtcca-3′. The annealed double stranded oligo was inserted into HpaI-XhoI restriction enzyme sites of pSicoR lentiviral vector (provided by Dr. T. Jacks; [29]) and verified by sequencing. Scrambled shRNA-containing pSicoR construct (control-shRNA) was used as control. To express shRNA with adenovirus in a Cre-dependent manner, pSicoR cassette containing U6 promoter, shRNA sequences and CMV-GFP flanked by loxP sites was transferred to pAd/CMV/V5-DEST plasmid (Invitrogen). Using these viral vectors, adenovirus was packaged at KIST Virus Facility (http://virus.kist.re.kr).

Biotinylation assay

For surface biotinylation, 14–3-3γ-shRNA or control-shRNA infected cultured astrocytes were incubated at 4 °C and washed three times with PBS. Surface expressed proteins were then biotinylated in PBS containing sulfo-NHS-SS-biotin (Pierce) for 30 min. After biotinylation, cells were washed with quenching buffer (100 mM glycine in PBS) to remove excess biotin and then washed three times with PBS. The cells were then lysed and incubated with high capacity NeutrAvidin-agarose resin (Thermo science). After three washes with lysis buffer, bound proteins are eluted by SDS sample buffer and subjected to western blot analysis.

Delivery of adenoviral vector containing 14–3-3γ-shRNA into mouse hippocampus

The adenovirus carrying 14–3-3γ-shRNA was injected into hippocampal CA1 region of CaMKIIα-Cre transgenic mouse brain. Because loxP-floxed shRNA in the adenoviral construct can be cleaved by Cre expression in the pSicoR system [29], delivering an adenoviral particle containing pSicoR-14-3-3γ-shRNA into CaMKIIα-Cre transgenic mouse brain allowed us to achieve CA1 pyramidal neuron-specific recovery of 14–3-3γ expression. After 2 weeks incubation, the mice were sacrificed for whole cell patch clamp recordings at 9 ~ 10 weeks of age. Only male mice were used in this study.

Western blotting

Gene silencing of 14–3-3γ was tested by western blotting. To observe shRNA-mediated inhibition of 14–3-3γ expression, adenovirus carrying control-shRNA or 14–3-3γ-shRNA was infected to cultured astrocytes seeded on 35 mm dishes. After 72 h incubation, cells were lysed with RIPA buffer. 40 μg of proteins were separated by SDS–PAGE using 10% gels and blotted onto PVDF membranes. The blots were incubated overnight at 4 °C with anti-14-3-3γ antibody (1:500; Abcam). The blots were then washed and incubated with horseradish peroxidase-conjugated goat anti-mouse or anti-rabbit IgG, followed by washing and detection of immunoreactivity with enhanced chemiluminescence (Amersham Biosciences). The band intensity was acquired and analyzed by ImageQuant LAS 4000 (General Electric Company).

Immunocytochemistry

The specificity of antibody (Abcam, rabbit polyclonal antibody 1:100) was tested by immunocytochemistry in cultured astrocytes in combination with 14–3-3γ-shRNA. Primary cultured astrocytes were transfected with 14–3-3γ-shRNA, grown on coverslips for additional 48 h. The cells were fixed in 4% paraformaldehyde for 30 min at room temperature, then permeabilized with PBS with 0.5% NP40 for 5 min. Non-specific binding was prevented with 1 h incubation in 2% donkey serums. Cells were incubated with the anti-14-3-3γ, and anti-GFAP (Millipore, chicken polyclonal antibody 1:500) primary antibodies for overnight at 4 °C. After washing, DyLight 488 or 649-conjugated secondary antibody (Jackson lab, 1:400) was added and incubated for 2 h at room temperature. The cells were washed and mounted, and then observed by confocal microscopy (Nikon A1). 3D reconstructions were generated from stacks of images with the confocal microscope software NIS-Elements.

Co-immunoprecipitation

Flag-14-3-3γ and GFP-Best1 were co-expressed in COS7 cells and 24 h post-transfection, extracted with buffer (50 mM Tris-HCl, pH 7.4, 150 mM NaCl, 5 mM EDTA, 1 mM PMSF, and 1% NP-40) containing a protease-inhibitor cocktail. Whole cell lysates were incubated on ice for 30 min and then cleared at 20,000 g for 20 min at 4 °C and immunoprecipitated with Flag. After 2 h incubation at 4 °C, the beads were washed four times with ice cold phosphate-buffered saline (PBS). Bound proteins were eluted with SDS sample buffer, separated on 12% SDS–PAGE gels. The blots incubated overnight at 4 °C with anti-Flag antibody (1:1000; Santa Cruz Biotechnology) or anti-GFP antibody (1:1000; Abcam). Blots were then washed and incubated with horseradish peroxidase-conjugated goat anti-mouse or anti-rabbit IgG, followed by washing and detection of immunoreactivity with enhanced chemiluminescence (Amersham Biosciences) and captured by ImageQuant LAS 4000 (General Electric Company).

Bimolecular fluorescence complementation (BiFC) experiment

Best1 WT, mutants (ΔC1, S358A) and 14–3-3γ were cloned into bimolecular fluorescence complement (pBiFC)-VN173 and pBIFC-VC155 vectors. HEK293T cells were transfected with each cloned BiFC vectors or co-transfected with cloned BiFC vectors in all possible pairewise combinations. These cells were fixed with 4% paraformaldehyde for 20 min at room temperature and washed twice with ice-cold phosphate-buffered saline (PBS). After fixation, the nuclei were stained with DAPI and mount with Dako fluorescence mounting medium. Venus fluorescence signals were observed by confocal microscopy (Nikon A1).

Ca^{2+} imaging

For Ca^{2+} imaging, cultured astrocytes were incubated with 5 μM Fura-2 AM in 1 μM pluronic acid (Invitrogen) for 30 min at room temperature and subsequently transferred to a microscope stage for imaging using extracellular solution which was comprised of 150 mM NaCl, 10 mM HEPES, 3 mM KCl, 2 mM CaCl$_2$, 2 mM MgCl$_2$, and 5.5 glucose at pH 7.3 with NaOH (~320 mOsm). Intensity images of 510 nm wavelength were taken at 340 and 380 nm excitation wavelengths, and the two resulting images were taken for ratio calculations. Imaging Workbench software (INDEC Bio-Systems) was used for acquisition of intensity images and conversion to ratios.

Electrophysiological recording from hippocampal slices

The brain from deeply anaesthetized mouse was rapidly removed and submerged in an ice-cold oxygenated artificial cerebrospinal fluid (ACSF) composed of 130 mM NaCl, 24 mM NaHCO$_3$, 3.5 mM KCl, 1.25 mM NaH$_2$PO$_4$, 1.5 mM CaCl$_2$, 1.5 mM MgCl$_2$ and 10 mM glucose saturated with 95% O$_2$ ~ 5% CO$_2$, at pH 7.4. The hemisected brain was glued onto the stage of a vibrating microtome (Leica VT1000S) and sections of 300 μm thickness were cut and stored in an incubation chamber at room temperature for about 1 h before use. Slices were placed on the stage of an upright microscope underneath a nylon restraining grid, and superfused with oxygenated ACSF composed of 130 mM NaCl, 24 mM NaHCO$_3$, 3.5 mM KCl, 1.25 mM NaH$_2$PO$_4$, 1.5 mM CaCl$_2$, 5 μM MgCl$_2$ and 10 mM glucose saturated with 95% O$_2$ ~ 5% CO$_2$, at pH 7.4.at room temperature (23 °C). The pipette solution for patching CA1 neuron contained 140 mM Cs-MeSO$_4$, 10 mM HEPES, 7 mM NaCl, 4 mM Mg-ATP and 0.3 mM Na-GTP at pH 7.3 adjusted with CsOH (~280 Osm). Visually guided whole-cell patch recordings were obtained from CA1 pyramidal neurons. 0.5 μM TTX and 20 μm bicuculline were added to the extracellular solution. Recordings were obtained using Axopatch 200A (Axon instruments) and filtered at 2 kHz. All described experimental procedures were performed in accordance with the institutional guidelines of Korea Institute of Science and Technology (KIST).

Molecular modeling

The X-ray structures of a human 14–3-3γ protein (PDB code: 3UZD) and chicken Best1 (PDB code: 4RDQ) were retrieved from PDB bank (http://www.rcsb.org). The human (accessible code: O76090) and mouse Best1 (accessible code: O88870) amino acid sequences were obtained from the UniProt database for homology modeling. The sequence alignment of hBest1 or mBest1 with cBEST crystal structure was conducted by ClustalW implemented in DiscoveryStudio program (Accelrys). The 20 homology models on each species were generated using MODELLER in DiscoveryStudio program. The homology model of Best1 was selected with low PDF total energy. In chain A of both Best1 homology models, Ser358 residue was manually converted to phospho-Ser in DiscoveryStudio program and then the eight amino acids containing pSer358 were extracted from homology models (RRApS^{358}FMGS for human; RRHpS^{358}FMGS for mouse).

14–3-3γ protein and octa-peptide of Best1 were prepared with neutralization at pH 7.4 and energy minimization by Protein Prep Wizard in Maestro program (Schrodinger LLC). The grid box was automatically generated with peptide docking mode around HDAC4 peptide bound in 14-3-3γ protein. The Best1 peptides were flexibly docked into binding site of 14-3-3γ protein by Glide-SP Peptide module in Maestro program.

Result

14–3-3γ specifically interacts with Best1

To identify potential interacting partners for Best1, we performed conventional yeast-two hybrid (Y2H) and membrane Y2H screening using cytosolic N- and C-termini and full-length Best1 as bait. Among the positive clones, we identified 14–3-3γ as a binding partner protein of Best1. The potential interaction between these two proteins was further validated by using the full-length cDNAs of Best1 and mouse 14–3-3γ. We found that Best1 and 14–3-3γ formed a positive yeast colony in membrane Y2H under TLH- (the absence of Threonine, Leucine, and Histidine in yeast media) conditions, while the empty vector did not (Fig. 1a).

The 14-3-3 proteins are a family of conserved regulatory molecules in which seven mammalian isoforms (β, γ, η, ζ, ε, τ, and σ) are highly homologous and capable of

binding to the same target. To examine the interaction between other 14-3-3 isoforms and mBest1 in a mammalian system, we constructed expression vectors for hemagglutinin (HA)-tagged 14–3-3β, γ, η, ζ, ε, τ, and σ (HA–14-3-3β, γ, η, ζ, ε, τ, and σ) and co-expressed with GFP–mBest1 in COS7 cells. We then performed co-immunoprecipitation (Co-IP) on cell lysates with an anti-HA antibody and then blotted with an anti-GFP antibody. The results showed that GFP–Best1 was associated only with HA–14-3-3γ (Fig. 1b). The association of GFP-Best1 with 14–3-3γ was reconfirmed when we used Flag-tagged 14–3-3γ (Flag–14-3-3γ) and GFP–Best1 in COS7 cells (Fig. 1c). To test whether such interactions between Best1 and 14–3-3γ can be observed in COS7 cells, we also examined the expression pattern of GFP-tagged Best1 and mCherry-tagged 14–3-3γ in these cells. We observed a strong co-localization of Best1 and 14–3-3γ proteins (in yellow color) particularly in the plasma membrane rich regions of transfected COS7 cells as indicated by an arrow (Fig. 1d). These results indicate that among seven 14–3-3 isoforms, 14–3-3γ isoform specifically interacts with Best1.

C-terminus of Best1 is critical for binding with 14–3-3γ

To investigate which part of Best1 contributes to binding with 14–3-3γ protein, we predicted the putative

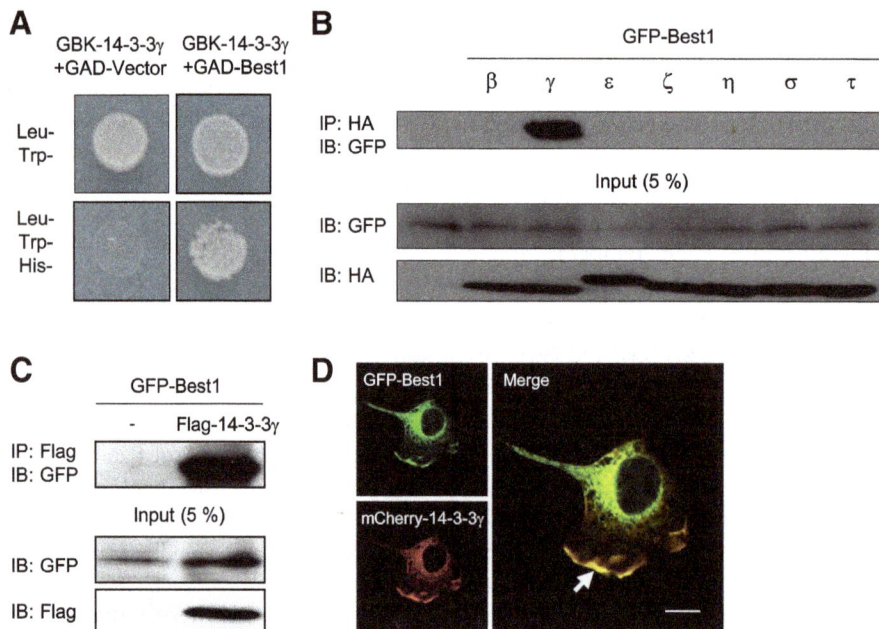

Fig. 1 14–3-3γ interacts with Best1. a Identification of 14–3-3γ as a direct binding partner of Best1 in the yeast two-hybrid system. b Co-IP of GFP-Best1 with HA-tagged 14-3-3 isoforms in COS7 cells. Whole lysate of COS7 cells was immunoprecipitated with anti-HA antibody and then analyzed by Western blot with anti-GFP antibody. 5% of the total lysate was used as input for the immunoprecipitation. c Co-IP of Flag-14-3-3γ with GFP-Best1. Whole lysate of COS7 cells was immunoprecipitated with anti-Flag antibody and then analyzed by Western blot with anti-GFP antibody. 5% of the total lysate was used as input for the immunoprecipitation. d Representative confocal image of co-localization of Best1 and 14–3-3γ. GFP-tagged Best1 and mCherry-14-3-3γ were co-transfected in COS7 cell. Scale bar, 10 μm phosphorylation sites in Best1 amino acid sequence for binding with 14–3-3γ through the web server that allows users to predict 14–3-3-binding sites in a protein of interest [http://www.compbio.dundee.ac.uk/1433pred/]. Because it was proposed that Bestrophin's C-termini are involved in protein-protein interaction [9], 14–3-3γ binding motif probably resides on the C-terminus of Best1, which is known to be a cytosolic domain according to the recently reported crystal structure of Best1 [30, 31]. To test this possibility and to determine the minimum 14–3-3γ-binding domain, we generated a series of GFP-tagged 14-3-3γ construct by subdividing Best1-C into three parts (Fig. 2a), which are Best1-C1 (292–380 amino acid residues), Best1-C2 (381–470

amino acid residues) and Best1-C3 (471–551 amino acid residues). We then performed Co-IP on cell lysates with an anti-GFP antibody and then blotted with an anti-HA antibody (Fig. 2b). We found that 14–3-3γ interacted with Best1-C1, but not with Best1-C2 or Best1-C3. It is generally accepted that a number of binding partners for 14–3-3 share a common binding determinant that mediates their contact with 14–3-3. Several reports demonstrated that phosphorylation of target protein is the primary mechanism that controls 14–3-3 binding [17]. A few conserved phosphorylation sites were suggested as consensus 14–3-3 recognition motif [22, 32, 33]. There is a putative 14–3-3γ binding motif RRHpSF which contains serine phosphorylation site (S358) within the

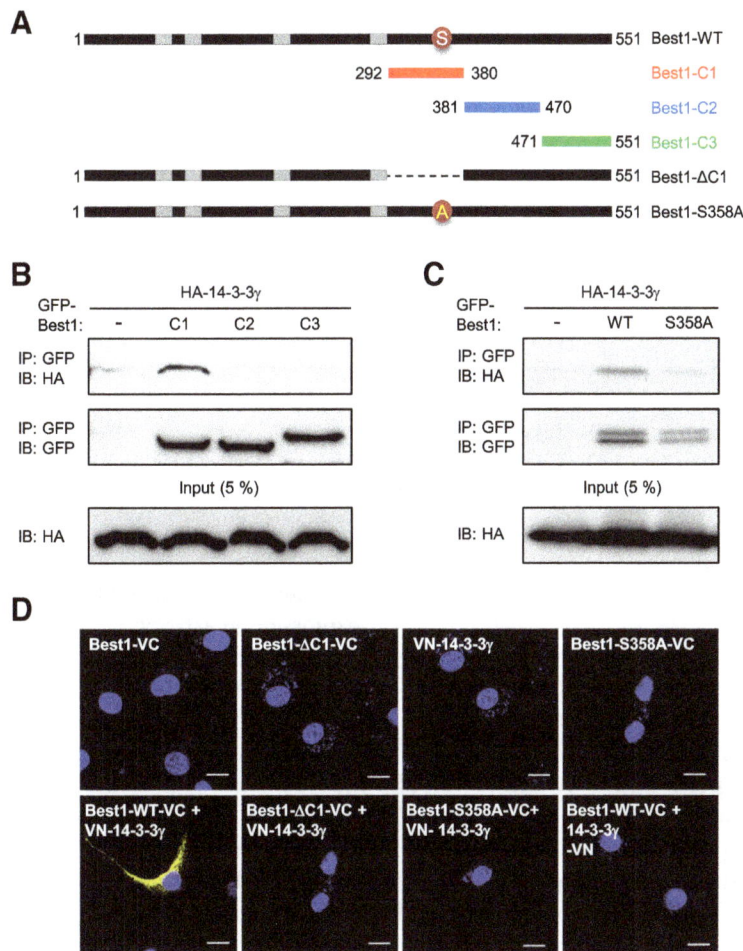

Fig. 2 C-terminus of Best1 is important for binding with 14–3-3γ. **a** Schematic diagram of full-length (Best1-WT), the first C-terminal region (292–380 amino acids, Best1-C1), the second C-terminal region (381–470 amino acids, Best1-C2), the third C-terminal region (471–551 amino acids, Best1-C3), C1 deleted mutant of Best1 (Best1-ΔC1) and S358A mutant of Best1 (Best1-S358A). **b** Co-IP of HA-14-3-3γ with GFP-Best1-C1 (C1), GFP-Best1-C2 (C2) and GFP-Best1-C3 (C3). Whole lysate of COS7 cells was immunoprecipitated with anti-HA antibody and then analyzed by Western blot with anti-GFP antibody. 5% of the total lysate was used as input for the immunoprecipitation. **c** Co-IP of HA-14-3-3γ with GFP-Best1-WT (WT) and GFP-tagged S358A mutant of Best1 (S358A). Whole lysate of COS7 cells was immunoprecipitated with anti-HA antibody and then analyzed by Western blot with anti-GFP antibody. 5% of the total lysate was used as input for the immunoprecipitation. **d** BiFC experiment with VN-14-3-3γ and Best1-VC, where N- and C-terminal halves of Venus fluorescent protein were fused to 14-3-3γ and Best1, respectively. BiFC fluorescent signals were detected by the yellow color. The fluorescent signal was detected at the plasma membrane of the cells by the yellow color. Cells only expressing both Best1-WT-VC and VN-14-3-3γ showed intense fluorescent signal (lower left panel). Scale bar, 10 μm

Best1-C1 of Best1. To test whether this S358 of Best1 is the critical residue necessary for 14–3-3γ binding, we replaced S358 of GFP-tagged Best1 to alanine (S358A). Co-IP experiment revealed a drastic reduction in binding of S358A mutant of Best1 with 14–3-3γ (Fig. 2c), suggesting that phosphorylation at S358 at Best1 is critical for the interaction with 14–3-3γ.

We then examined the interaction between Best1 and 14–3-3γ at the single-cell level by bimolecular fluorescence complementation (BiFC) assay, which allows visualization of two independent proteins in close spatial proximity [34]. We constructed Best1 and 14–3-3γ, whose N- and C- termini were fused with one complementary halves of split Venus fluorescent protein, either N-terminal half (VN) or C-terminal half (VC), and then both were transfected into HEK293T cells (Fig. 2d). Strong yellow fluorescence was detected when the split Venus halves were on complementary positions (Best1-VC and VN-14-3-3γ, Fig. 2d, lower left). In contrast, very weak or virtually no BiFC signal was detected from the cells transfected with VN-14-3-3γ and Best1-ΔC1-VC which is a C1 deletion mutant of Best1 (Fig. 2a) fused to VC (Fig. 2d, lower second). In addition, we also tested Best1-S358A-VC (Fig. 2d, lower third) and found no BiFC signal with VN-14-3-3γ. As a negative control, when Best1 or 14–3-3γ was expressed with only one half of split Venus, no BiFC fluorescence was detected (Fig. 2d, upper panels). Taken together, the C-terminal domain (292–380 amino acid residues) of Best1 is important for binding with 14–3-3γ and potential phosphorylation site S358 within this region is critical for the interaction with 14–3-3γ.

Phospho-Serine358 residue of Best1 interacts with 14–3-3γ

We carried out the peptide docking based on the molecular modeling to predict the binding mode of the putative 14–3-3γ binding motif of Best1 with 14–3-3γ (PDB: 3UZD) [35]. The putative 14–3-3γ binding motif RRApS^{358}FMG of human Best1 (hBest1) and RRHpS^{358}FMG of mBest1, identified by mutation study in Fig. 2, were well-fitted to central groove of 14–3-3γ (Fig. 3a). The interaction and orientation of hBest1 and mBest1 were stabilized by charge interactions of Arg57-Arg132-Tyr133 triad of 14–3-3γ with pSer358 of Best1, and backbone hydrogen bonding of Lys50, Asn178 and Asn229 residues (Fig. 3b, c). Hydrophobic side chains of hBest1 and mBest1 interacts with Ile222, Leu225 and Trp233 of hydrophobic groove of the 14–3-3γ. On the other side of its groove, Met360 occupied the charged region of 14–3-3γ, composed of Ser46, Lys50, and Asn178. This docking simulation provided structural binding details of putative binding motif of Best1 that

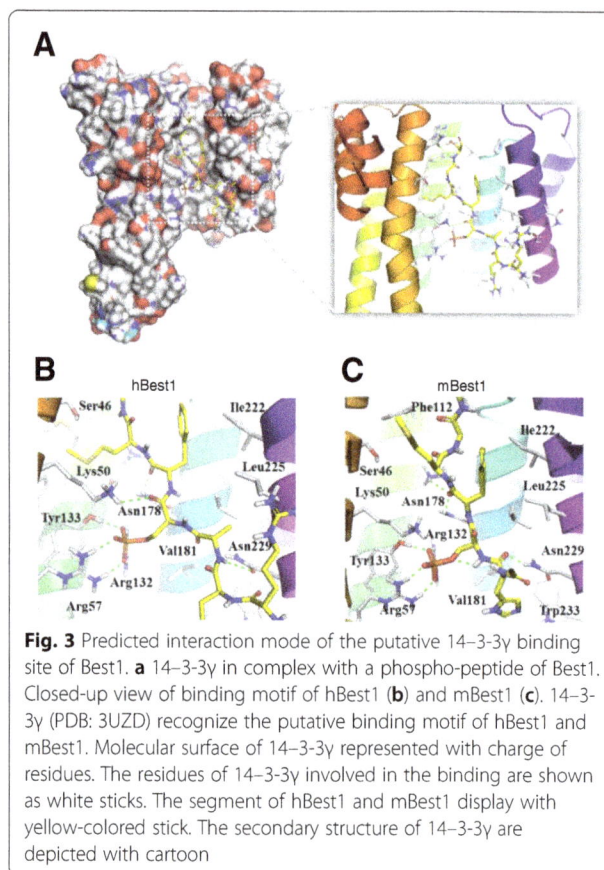

Fig. 3 Predicted interaction mode of the putative 14–3-3γ binding site of Best1. **a** 14–3-3γ in complex with a phospho-peptide of Best1. Closed-up view of binding motif of hBest1 (**b**) and mBest1 (**c**). 14–3-3γ (PDB: 3UZD) recognize the putative binding motif of hBest1 and mBest1. Molecular surface of 14–3-3γ represented with charge of residues. The residues of 14–3-3γ involved in the binding are shown as white sticks. The segment of hBest1 and mBest1 display with yellow-colored stick. The secondary structure of 14–3-3γ are depicted with cartoon

the segment containing pSer358 of Best1 is an essential for 14–3-3γ recognition and binding.

14–3-3γ-shRNA reduced the Best1 current and membrane expression in astrocyte

Astrocytes have been shown to express five isoforms of 14–3-3 by RT-PCR: β, γ, η, ξ, and ε [36]. To determine the function of 14–3-3γ in regards to Best1 in astrocyte, a 14–3-3γ-specific short hairpin RNA (shRNA, 14–3-3γ-shRNA) was designed and tested to selectively knockdown the expression of 14–3-3γ transcript. Western blot analysis showed that the expression of 14–3-3γ-shRNA resulted in about 57% knockdown of endogenous 14–3-3γ protein in cultured astrocytes (Fig. 4a). Considering that the efficiency of cell transfection with pSicoR-control-shRNA or pSicoR-14-3-3γ-shRNA was around 60%, about 90% of knockdown of 14–3-3γ expression was achieved by 14–3-3γ-shRNA. We also confirmed that cultured astrocyte transfected with pSicoR-14-3-3γ-shRNA-mCherry showed an effective knockdown of endogenous 14–3-3γ protein level (Fig. 4b) without any change of cellular morphology or size (Fig. 4c) by immunocytochemistry.

To test whether gene-silencing of 14–3-3γ affects astrocytic Best1 current, we subsequently recorded

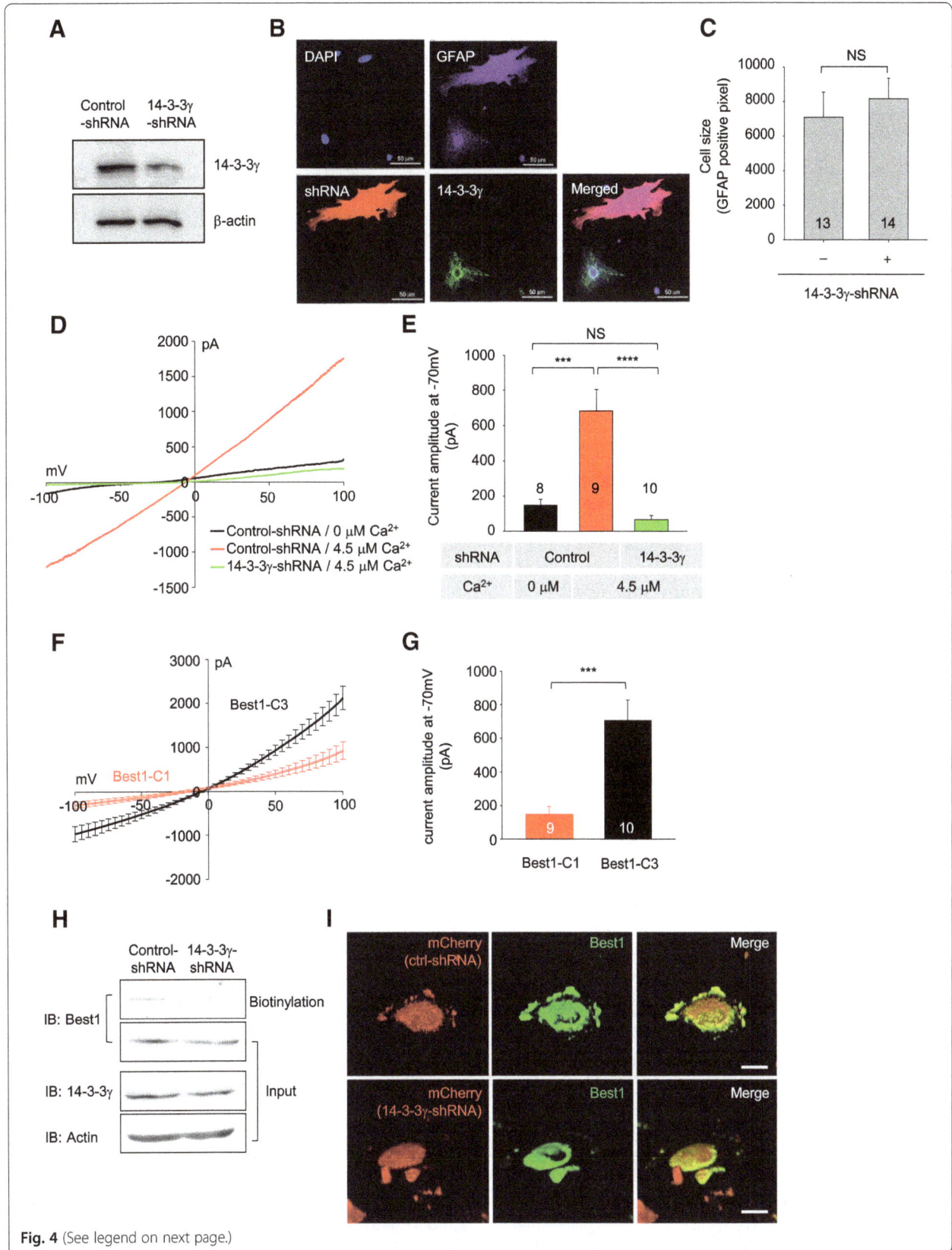

Fig. 4 (See legend on next page.)

Fig. 4 14–3-3γ -shRNA reduced the expression of 14–3-3γ and membrane expression of Best1 in astrocyte. **a** 14–3-3γ shRNA reduced the level of 14–3-3γ expression mRNA in cultured astrocytes as determined by Western blot. Cultured astrocytes were transfected with pSicoR-control-shRNA or pSicoR-14-3-3γ-shRNA and β-actin was used as an internal control. **b** Confocal immunofluorescence images of cultured astrocytes transfected with pSicoR-14-3-3γ-shRNA-mCherry. Scale bar, 50 μm. **c** Quantification of the two-dimensional cell area by counting the number of GFAP positive pixel for the experiment described in (**a**). Numbers of determinations are indicated on the bar graph. NS $p = 0.5726$ (unpaired two-tailed t test). **d** Representative I–V responses of cultured astrocyte expressing pSicoR-control-shRNA or pSicoR-14-3-3γ-shRNA under whole-cell patch-clamp configuration using 4.5 μM Ca^{2+}-containing or 0 Ca^{2+}-containing patch pipette solution. **e** Bar graph showing summary of current amplitudes (mean ± SEM). The current responses were recorded in response to a voltage ramp command (from −100 to +100 mV, 1 s duration, 0.2 Hz; V_h of −70 mV). Numbers of determinations are indicated on the bar graph. Asterisk indicates a significant difference determined by one-way ANOVA test and Tukey's multiple comparison test (****$p < 0.0001$, ***$p = 0.0001$, NS $p = 0.7227$). **f** Averaged I–V responses of cultured astrocytes expressing Best1-C1 or Best1-C3 under whole-cell patch-clamp configuration using 4.5 μM Ca^{2+}-containing patch pipette solution. **g** Bar graph showing summary of current amplitudes (mean ± SEM). The current responses were recorded in response to a voltage ramp command (from −100 to +100 mV, 1 s duration, 0.2 Hz; V_h of −70 mV). Numbers of determinations are indicated on the bar graph. Asterisk indicates a significant difference determined by unpaired two-tailed t-test (***$p < 0.001$). **h** Cell-surface biotinylation assay in cultured astrocytes. When astrocytes transiently transfected with 14-3-3γ-shRNA, surface expression of Best1 is dramatically decreased. **i** Cultured astrocytes transfected with pSicoR-control-shRNA-mCherry (upper panel) or pSicoR-14-3-3γ-shRNA-mCherry (bottom panel) were imaged by confocal microscopy using antibodies against Best1 and 3D reconstructions were generated from stacks of images. Scale bars, 20 μm

astrocytic Best1 current in control-shRNA- or 14–3-3γ-shRNA-expressing cultured astrocytes using whole-cell patch clamp recording, as previously described [37]. We directly induce an increase in conductance in astrocytes by a membrane rupture for whole-cell mode with internal solutions containing high free $[Ca^{2+}]_i$ (~ 4.5 μM). We found that Ca^{2+}-activated Best1 current in cultured astrocyte was significantly suppressed by 14–3-3γ-shRNA expression (Fig. 4d, e, current amplitude at $V_h = -70$ mV; control-shRNA-expressing astrocytes, 684 ± 121 pA, $n = 9$; 14–3-3γ-shRNA-expressing astrocytes, 67 ± 23 pA, $n = 10$; ****$p < 0.0001$ vs control-shRNA group; one-way ANOVA and Tukey's multiple comparison test). The control group astrocytes expressing control-shRNA recorded with no free $[Ca^{2+}]_i$ –containing internal solutions did not show any significant current as expected (Fig. 4d, e, current amplitude at $V_h = -70$ mV; 148 ± 34 pA, $n = 8$).

To test the functional consequence of the interaction between the C-terminus of Best1 and 14–3-3γ, we over-expressed Best1-C1 and recorded Ca^{2+}-activated Best1 current in cultured astrocytes. We found that Best1 current amplitude was significantly reduced by the over-expression of Best1-C1 in astrocytes compare to that of Best1-C3 which is not capable of interacting with 14–3-3γ (Fig. 4f, g, current amplitude at $V_h = -70$ mV; Best1-C1-expressing astrocytes, 148.7 ± 46.8 pA, $n = 9$; Best1-C3-expressing astrocytes, 705.6 ± 122.6 pA, $n = 10$; ***$p = 0.0008$ vs Best1-C1 group; unpaired two-tailed t-test). This set of results is explained by a competition between endogenous Best1 and over-expressed Best1-C1 to interact with 14–3-3γ.

14–3-3γ-shRNA could reduce surface expression of Best1 in astrocyte. To test the function of 14–3-3γ in surface expression of Best1 in astrocyte, we performed a surface biotinylation assay in cultured astrocyte. Treatment with 14–3-3γ-shRNA caused a dramatic reduction in surface expression of the endogenous Best1 channel

proteins, measured by surface biotinylation, in comparison to control-shRNA treatment, without affecting the total Best1 protein levels in astrocytes (Fig. 4h). We also examined the surface expression of Best1 by immunocytochemistry to determine the effect of 14–3-3γ shRNA on the subcellular localization of Best1 (Fig. 4i). Best1 channels were highly localized at the plasma membrane of cultured astrocytes in the presence of control-shRNA, while they were less localized at the plasma membrane in the presence of 14–3-3γ shRNA. These results demonstrate that 14–3-3γ promotes the surface expression of Best1 by interaction with C-terminus of Best1 in astrocytes.

14–3-3γ shRNA reduced Best1 mediated glutamate release from hippocampal astrocyte

We have previously demonstrated that astrocytes release glutamate upon GPCR activation via Best1 [13]. We also demonstrated that the target of Best1-mediated astrocytic glutamate is the synaptically localized, NR2A containing NMDA receptors (NMDAR) in hippocampal CA1 pyramidal neurons [11, 12]. To test whether 14–3-3γ contributes to astrocytic glutamate release via Best1, we directly measured the effects of astrocyte-specific knocking down of 14–3-3γ in vivo by introducing adenovirus carrying 14–3-3γ-shRNA into hippocampal CA1 region of CaMKIIα-Cre mice (see Methods). To induce astrocytic glutamate release, we used 30 μM TFLLR, PAR1 agonist applications to activate PAR1, which is known to be expressed mostly in CA1 hippocampal astrocytes. We applied to whole brain slices by perfusion and recorded TFLLR-induced whole cell current at −60 mV from CA1 pyramidal neuron in hippocampal slices prepared from adenovirus-injected mouse brain in the presence of tetrodotoxin (TTX) and Bicuculline. Compared to the control-shRNA, 14–3-3γ-shRNA markedly reduced

TFLLR-induced astrocytic glutamate release via Best1 (Fig. 5a, b, current amplitude at V_h of −60 mV; control-shRNA-expressing astrocytes, 7.7 ± 1.0 pA, $n = 10$; 14–3-3γ-shRNA-expressing astrocytes, 3.0 ± 1.7 pA, $n = 9$; *$p = 0.0413$ vs control-shRNA group; one-way ANOVA test). As we have shown in previous studies [4, 13], astrocytic PAR-1 mediated glutamate release induced by TFLLR was APV sensitive (data not shown). 14–3-3γ-shRNA-expressing cultured hippocampal astrocytes did not show any difference in TFLLR-induced Ca^{2+} increase compared to control-shRNA-expressing astrocytes (Fig. 5c, d). These results demonstrate that 14–3-3γ can regulate the surface expression of Best1 in vivo.

Discussion

We have identified strong interaction between Best1 and 14–3-3γ and the interaction is γ isoform specific among seven 14–3-3 isoforms. Using truncated Best1 and Best1 mutant, we have shown that 292–380 amino acids of the C-terminus contribute to the interaction between the channel and the 14–3-3γ and Ser358 residue of Best1 is critical for this interaction. The binding motif was further narrowed down by molecular modeling to be RRApS[358]FMG of hBest1 and RRHpS[358]FMG of mBest1. The most striking finding was that gene-silencing of 14–3-3γ expression in astrocytes disrupted (i) the expression of Best1 functional current in cultured astrocytes, (ii)

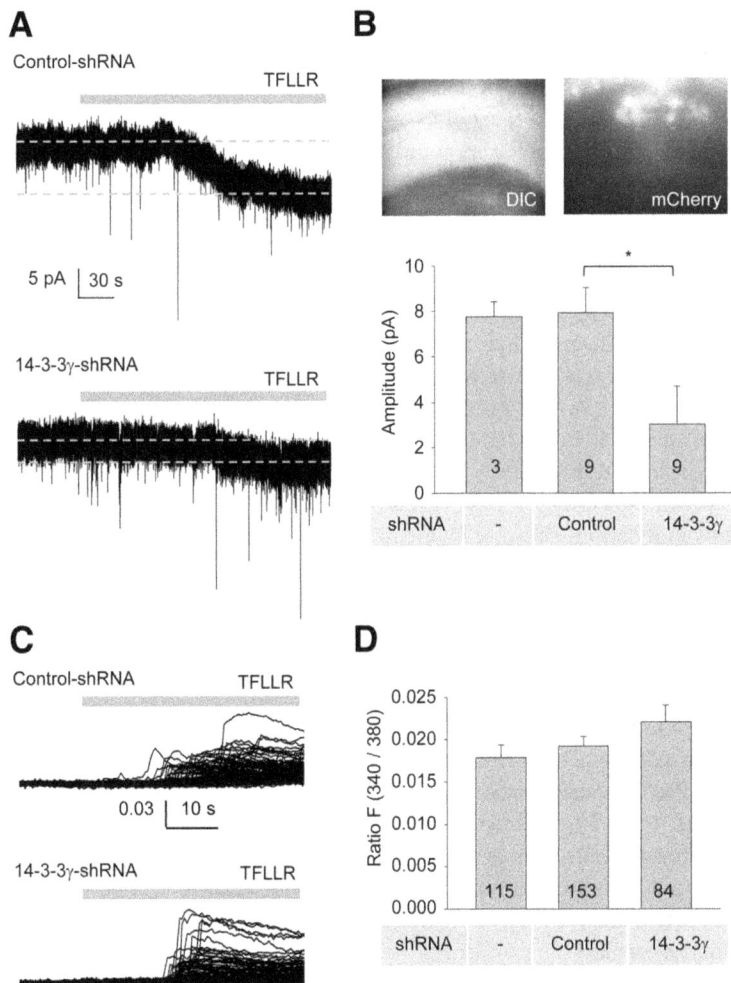

Fig. 5 14–3-3γ-shRNA reduced Best1 mediated glutamate release from hippocampal astrocyte. a Representative measurement of glutamate current in a somatic region of CA1 pyramidal neuron of CaMKIIα-Cre mouse injected with adenovirus expressing control-shRNA or 14–3-3γ-shRNA under voltage clamp held at −60 mV during treatment with TFLLR (30 μM, grey bar). b Upper figures indicate fluorescent protein mCherry images of hippocampal CA1 region injected with adenoviruses transducing either control-shRNA or 14–3-3γ-shRNA. Bar graphs represent the averaged amplitudes (differences between baseline and TFLLR induced current amplitude depicted as dashed lines in (a)). Numbers of tested slices from at least two independent mice are indicated in the bar graph. Asterisk indicates a significant difference determined by one-way ANOVA test (*$p < 0.05$). c Traces from Ca^{2+} imaging recordings performed in naive astrocytes, pSicoR-control-shRNA expressing astrocytes, or pSicoR-14-3-3γ-shRNA expressing astrocytes. Each trace represents a Ca^{2+} response in one cell during treatment with TFLLR (30 μM, grey bar). d Summary bar graph for calcium imaging. Numbers of recorded cells are indicated on the bar graph the surface expression of Best1 in cultured astrocytes, and (iii) PAR-1 induced NMDA current in hippocampal CA1 pyramidal neuron. It raises the possibility that 14–3-3 may be involved in post-translational regulation of channel expression, for example, by participating in channel assembly in the endoplasmic reticulum or by modulating trafficking, retention or retrieval of Best1 channel proteins.

It is possible that through its interaction with Best1, 14–3-3γ modulates gliotransmission not only under physiological condition but also under pathological condition by regulating the surface expression of Best1 in astrocytes. There are numerous reports showing that 14–3-3 proteins have been involved in the pathophysiology of various neurological disorders [19]. 14–3-3γ level is significantly decreased in the cortex of embryos with Down's syndrome and is elevated in several brain regions of patients with AD and in Lewy bodies in Parkinson's disease brains [38]. The elevated level of 14–3-3γ expression in the brain of AD patients could explain the change of Best1 localization from microdomains to the soma and processes in reactive astrocytes [14]. Therefore, the changed expression level of 14–3-3γ in neurological disorders might lead to a possible impairment of synaptic plasticity and signaling pathways which are likely to correlate with transcriptional control or signal transduction, as well as modulation of gliotransmission. Determining the role of 14–3-3 proteins in brain function may lead to advances in understanding how these proteins affect neurological disorders.

Bestrophins including hBest1 and mBest1 have predicted high-stringency phosphorylation sites (scansite.mit.edu) for protein kinase A (PKA), protein kinase C (PKC), and various other kinases. hBest1 interacts physically and functionally with protein phosphatase 2A [39]. Taken together, phosphorylation may play an important role in regulation of surface expression of Bestrophins. Interestingly, putative 14–3-3γ binding motif of Best1 which was tested in this study shares a putative protein kinase C (PKC) phosphorylation site (pSFMGS). It is possible that 14–3-3γ provides a link between Best1 and PKC. Future studies are needed to better understand the potential kinases and phosphatases that are involved in interaction of 14–3-3γ for regulating physiological function of Best1.

Conclusion

In summary, we have provided the first evidence for controlling mechanism for the surface expression of Best1 channels in astrocytes. The regulation of the surface expression of Best1 via 14–3-3γ binding may represent an important determinant of the neuromodulation both in physiological and pathological conditions.

Acknowledgements
Not applicable.

Funding
This work was supported by grants from Creative Research Initiative Program, (2015R1A3A2066619), National Research Foundation (NRF) of Korea (NRF-2014R1A2A1A01007039), and Council of Science & Technology (NST) grant by the Korea government (MSIP) (No. CRC-15-04-KIST).

Authors' contributions
S-JO performed the electrophysiological experiments, Ca^{2+} imaging and immunocytochemistry and was a major contributor in writing the manuscript. JW performed the electrophysiological experiment. MC, EK and YL contributed to the study by performing biochemical experiments (yeast two-hybrid assay, co-ip and BiFC). N-CC and ANP performed molecular modeling and writing the manuscript. J-YP analyzed and reviewed the data from biochemical experiments. C.JL and EMH conceived and supervised the project and wrote the manuscript with all authors' input. All authors read and approved the final manuscript.

Competing interests
The authors declare that they have no competing interests.

Author details
[1]Center for Neuroscience, Korea Institute of Science and Technology, Seoul, Korea. [2]Convergence Research Center for Diagnosis, Treatment and Care System of Dementia, Korea Institute of Science and Technology, Seoul, Korea. [3]Center for Glia-Neuron interaction, Korea Institute of Science and Technology, Seoul, Korea. [4]Center for Functional Connectomics, Korea Institute of Science and Technology, Seoul, Korea. [5]Neuroscience Program, University of Science and Technology (UST), Daejeon, Korea. [6]School of Biosystem and Biomedical Science, College of Health Science, Korea University, Seoul, Korea.

References
1. Wang X, Lou N, Xu Q, Tian GF, Peng WG, Han X, Kang J, Takano T, Nedergaard M. Astrocytic Ca2+ signaling evoked by sensory stimulation in vivo. Nat Neurosci. 2006;9(6):816–23.
2. Haydon PG, Carmignoto G. Astrocyte control of synaptic transmission and neurovascular coupling. Physiol Rev. 2006;86(3):1009–31.
3. Halassa MM, Fellin T, Haydon PG. The tripartite synapse: roles for gliotransmission in health and disease. Trends Mol Med. 2007;13(2):54–63.
4. Lee CJ, Mannaioni G, Yuan H, Woo DH, Gingrich MB, Traynelis SF. Astrocytic control of synaptic NMDA receptors. J Physiol. 2007;581(Pt 3):1057–81.
5. Volterra A, Meldolesi J. Astrocytes, from brain glue to communication elements: the revolution continues. Nat Rev Neurosci. 2005;6(8):626–40.
6. Perea G, Araque A. Astrocytes potentiate transmitter release at single hippocampal synapses. Science. 2007;317(5841):1083–6.
7. Park H, Oh SJ, Han KS, Woo DH, Park H, Mannaioni G, Traynelis SF, Lee CJ. Bestrophin-1 encodes for the Ca2+–activated anion channel in hippocampal astrocytes. J Neurosci. 2009;29(41):13063–73.
8. Park H, Han KS, Oh SJ, Jo S, Woo J, Yoon BE, Lee CJ. High glutamate permeability and distal localization of Best1 channel in CA1 hippocampal astrocyte. Mol Brain. 2013;6:54.
9. Hartzell HC, Qu Z, Yu K, Xiao Q, Chien LT. Molecular physiology of bestrophins: multifunctional membrane proteins linked to best disease and other retinopathies. Physiol Rev. 2008;88(2):639–72.
10. Lee S, Yoon BE, Berglund K, Oh SJ, Park H, Shin HS, Augustine GJ, Lee CJ. Channel-mediated tonic GABA release from glia. Science. 2010; 330(6005):790–6.
11. Han KS, Woo J, Park H, Yoon BJ, Choi S, Lee CJ. Channel-mediated

astrocytic glutamate release via Bestrophin-1 targets synaptic NMDARs. Mol Brain. 2013;6:4.

12. Park H, Han KS, Seo J, Lee J, Dravid SM, Woo J, Chun H, Cho S, Bae JY, An H, et al. Channel-mediated astrocytic glutamate modulates hippocampal synaptic plasticity by activating postsynaptic NMDA receptors. Mol Brain. 2015;8:7.

13. Woo DH, Han KS, Shim JW, Yoon BE, Kim E, Bae JY, Oh SJ, Hwang EM, Marmorstein AD, Bae YC, et al. TREK-1 and Best1 channels mediate fast and slow glutamate release in astrocytes upon GPCR activation. Cell. 2012;151(1):25–40.

14. Jo S, Yarishkin O, Hwang YJ, Chun YE, Park M, Woo DH, Bae JY, Kim T, Lee J, Chun H, et al. GABA from reactive astrocytes impairs memory in mouse models of Alzheimer's disease. Nat Med. 2014;20(8):886–96.

15. Oh SJ, Lee CJ. Distribution and function of the Bestrophin-1 (Best1) channel in the brain. Exp Neurobiol. 2017;26(3):113–21.

16. Dougherty MK, Morrison DK. Unlocking the code of 14-3-3. J Cell Sci. 2004; 117(Pt 10):1875–84.

17. Fu H, Subramanian RR, Masters SC. 14-3-3 proteins: structure, function, and regulation. Annu Rev Pharmacol Toxicol. 2000;40:617–47.

18. Mackintosh C. Dynamic interactions between 14-3-3 proteins and phosphoproteins regulate diverse cellular processes. Biochem J. 2004; 381(Pt 2):329–42.

19. Berg D, Holzmann C, Riess O. 14-3-3 proteins in the nervous system. Nat Rev Neurosci. 2003;4(9):752–62.

20. Jeanclos EM, Lin L, Treuil MW, Rao J, DeCoster MA, Anand R. The chaperone protein 14-3-3eta interacts with the nicotinic acetylcholine receptor alpha 4 subunit. Evidence for a dynamic role in subunit stabilization. J Biol Chem. 2001;276(30):28281–90.

21. Zerangue N, Schwappach B, Jan YN, Jan LY. A new ER trafficking signal regulates the subunit stoichiometry of plasma membrane K(ATP) channels. Neuron. 1999;22(3):537–48.

22. Rajan S, Preisig-Muller R, Wischmeyer E, Nehring R, Hanley PJ, Renigunta V, Musset B, Schlichthorl G, Derst C, Karschin A, et al. Interaction with 14-3-3 proteins promotes functional expression of the potassium channels TASK-1 and TASK-3. J Physiol. 2002;545(Pt 1):13–26.

23. Kilisch M, Lytovchenko O, Arakel EC, Bertinetti D, Schwappach B. A dual phosphorylation switch controls 14-3-3-dependent cell surface expression of TASK-1. J Cell Sci. 2016;129(4):831–42.

24. Liang X, Peters KW, Butterworth MB, Frizzell RA. 14-3-3 isoforms are induced by aldosterone and participate in its regulation of epithelial sodium channels. J Biol Chem. 2006;281(24):16323–32.

25. Liang X, Butterworth MB, Peters KW, Walker WH, Frizzell RA. An obligatory heterodimer of 14-3-3beta and 14-3-3epsilon is required for aldosterone regulation of the epithelial sodium channel. J Biol Chem. 2008;283(41):27418–25.

26. Cho CH, Kim E, Lee YS, Yarishkin O, Yoo JC, Park JY, Hong SG, Hwang EM. Depletion of 14-3-3gamma reduces the surface expression of transient receptor potential Melastatin 4b (TRPM4b) channels and attenuates TRPM4b-mediated glutamate-induced neuronal cell death. Mol Brain. 2014;7:52.

27. Nicole O, Goldshmidt A, Hamill CE, Sorensen SD, Sastre A, Lyuboslavsky P, Hepler JR, McKeon RJ, Traynelis SF. Activation of protease-activated receptor-1 triggers astrogliosis after brain injury. Journal Neurosci. 2005; 25(17):4319–29.

28. Kuruma A, Hartzell HC. Bimodal control of a ca(2+)-activated Cl(−) channel by different ca(2+) signals. J Gen Physiol. 2000;115(1):59–80.

29. Ventura A, Meissner A, Dillon CP, McManus M, Sharp PA, Van Parijs L, Jaenisch R, Jacks T: Cre-lox-regulated conditional RNA interference from transgenes. Proc Natl Acad Sci U S A 2004, 101(28):10380-10385.

30. Kane Dickson V, Pedi L, Long SB. Structure and insights into the function of a ca(2+)-activated Cl(−) channel. Nature. 2014;516(7530):213–8.

31. Yang T, Liu Q, Kloss B, Bruni R, Kalathur RC, Guo Y, Kloppmann E, Rost B, Colecraft HM, Hendrickson WA. Structure and selectivity in bestrophin ion channels. Science. 2014;346(6207):355–9.

32. Yaffe MB, Rittinger K, Volinia S, Caron PR, Aitken A, Leffers H, Gamblin SJ, Smerdon SJ, Cantley LC. The structural basis for 14-3-3:phosphopeptide binding specificity. Cell. 1997;91(7):961–71.

33. Muslin AJ, Tanner JW, Allen PM, Shaw AS. Interaction of 14-3-3 with signaling proteins is mediated by the recognition of phosphoserine. Cell. 1996;84(6):889–97.

34. Hu CD, Chinenov Y, Kerppola TK. Visualization of interactions among bZip and Rel family proteins in living cells using bimolecular fluorescence complementation. Mol Cell. 2002;9(4):789–98.

35. Xu C, Jin J, Bian C, Lam R, Tian R, Weist R, You L, Nie J, Bochkarev A, Tempel W, et al. Sequence-specific recognition of a PxLPxI/L motif by an ankyrin repeat tumbler lock. Sci Signal. 2012;5(226):ra39.

36. Chen XQ, Liu S, Qin LY, Wang CR, Fung YW, Yu AC. Selective regulation of 14-3-3eta in primary culture of cerebral cortical neurons and astrocytes during development. J Neurosci Res. 2005;79(1–2):114–8.

37. Oh SJ, Han KS, Park H, Woo DH, Kim HY, Traynelis SF, Lee CJ. Protease activated receptor 1-induced glutamate release in cultured astrocytes is mediated by Bestrophin-1 channel but not by vesicular exocytosis. Mol brain. 2012;5:38.

38. Shimada T, Fournier AE, Yamagata K. Neuroprotective function of 14-3-3 proteins in neurodegeneration. Biomed Res Int. 2013;2013:564534.

39. Marmorstein LY, McLaughlin PJ, Stanton JB, Yan L, Crabb JW, Marmorstein AD. Bestrophin interacts physically and functionally with protein phosphatase 2A. J Biol Chem. 2002;277(34):30591–7.

7

Reduced synaptic function of Kainate receptors in the insular cortex of Fmr1 Knock-out mice

Shuang Qiu[1,2,3†], Yu Wu[3†], Xinyou Lv[3], Xia Li[4], Min Zhuo[1,2*] and Kohei Koga[1,2,5*]

Abstract

Fragile X syndrome is caused by the loss of fragile X mental retardation protein (FMRP). Kainate receptor (KAR) is a subfamily of ionotropic glutamate receptors (iGluR) that acts mainly as a neuromodulator of synaptic transmission and neuronal excitability. However, little is known about the changes of synaptic KAR in the cortical area of Fmr1 KO mice. In this study, we performed whole-cell patch-clamp recordings from layer II/III pyramidal neurons in the insular cortex of Fmr1 KO mice. We found that KARs mediated currents were reduced in Fmr1 KO mice. KARs were mainly located in the synaptosomal fraction of the insular cortex. The abundance of KAR subunit GluK1 and GluK2/3 in the synaptosome was reduced in Fmr1 KO mice, whereas the total expressions of these KARs subunits were not changed. Finally, lack of FMRP impairs subsequent internalization of surface GluK2 after KAR activation, while having no effect on the surface GluK2 expression. Our studies provide evidence indicating that loss of FMRP leads to the abnormal function and localization of KARs. This finding implies a new molecular mechanism for Fragile X syndrome.

Keywords: FMRP, Fragile X syndrome, Insular cortex, Kainate receptor, Internalization, GluK1, GluK2

Introduction

Fragile X syndrome (FXS) is the most common monogenic cause of autism and inherited mental impairment [1, 2]. The FXS is almost exclusively caused by an expansion of a trinucleotide repeat (CGG) repeat in the 5′ untranslated region of the X-linked fragile X mental retardation 1 (*Fmr1*) gene. Mutation in the Fmr1 gene leads to a failure to express the fragile X mental retardation protein (FMRP), which functions in repressing local translation at the synapse and regulating mRNA trafficking and stability [3–7]. Fmr1 knockout (KO) mice are sufficient to generate a mouse model for FXS and exhibit cognitive deficits and abnormal plasticity in the cortex or hippocampus.

Local protein synthesis is required for long-term synaptic plasticity that stores memories and is orchestrated by the action of glutamate receptors. Activation of metabotropic glutamate receptors (mGluR) produces long-term depression (LTD), which involves local protein synthesis and degradation [8]. In Fmr1 KO mice, mGluR-dependent LTD is strongly increased, mainly due to deregulation of local protein synthesis, and the exaggerated mGluR signaling contributes to many of the synaptic phenotypes in FXS [9, 10].

Besides mGluR, ionotropic glutamate receptors (iGluRs), including N-methyl-D-aspartate receptor (NMDAR) and α-amino-3-hydroxyl-S-methylisoazole-4-propionate receptor (AMPAR), have been identified to be involved in FMRP. FMRP is critical for NMDAR-dependent LTP in the cingulate cortex (ACC) and prefrontal cortex (PFC) [11, 12]. Spike timing-dependent plasticity that requires NMDAR activation is attenuated in neocortical slices from early postnatal Fmr1 KO mice [13]. Moreover, Fmr1 KO mice show impaired performance in an NMDAR-dependent context discrimination task [14]. FMRP is involved in regulating the internalization of AMPARs [15, 16]. Surface expression and phosphorylation of AMPAR subunit GluA1 in response to dopaminergic D_1 receptor stimulation are reduced in PFC neurons from Fmr1 KO mice [17].

Kainate receptor (KAR) is another subtype of iGluRs, which is present at both presynaptic and postsynaptic sites

* Correspondence: min.zhuo@utoronto.ca; kkoga@hotmail.co.jp
†Shuang Qiu and Yu Wu contributed equally to this work.
[1]Center for Neuron and Disease, Frontier Institute of Science and Technology, Xi'an Jiaotong University, Xi'an 710049, China
Full list of author information is available at the end of the article

in the cortex. Both KAR GluK1 and GluK2 subunits involved in KARs mediated transmission in pyramidal neurons from surface layers (layer II/III) of the adult mice ACC and insular cortex [18–20]. Although KAR mediated currents are much smaller in the ACC and insular cortex compared with AMPAR mediated currents, KAR participates in various physiological functions, behaviors and pathological conditions by transgenic mice or pharmacological inhibitors of GluK receptors [18, 21–23]. Recently, it was reported that FMRP plays an important role in GluK1 containing GluKRs dependent pre-LTP in ACC neurons [24]. However, it is still unclear whether the function and expression of KARs is altered in Fmr1 KO mice.

In the present study, we investigate the function and expression of KAR in the insular cortex using Fmr1 KO mice. In vitro whole-cell patch-clamp recordings from layer II/III pyramidal neurons showed that Fmr1 KO mice reduced KARs mediated functions in the insular cortex. KAR was enriched in the synaptosome in Fmr1 WT mice, while the abundance of KAR in the synaptosome was decreased in Fmr1 KO mice. Additionally, Kainate-induced internalization of surface GluK2 was impaired in Fmr1 KO mice. These findings provide evidence that FMRP participates in regulating KAR localization and trafficking in the insular cortex.

Methods
Animals
Adult male Fmr1 wild-type (WT) and Fmr1 knock-out (KO) mice (8 to 12 weeks of age) of the FVB. 129P2-Fmr1tm1Cgr strain used in the experiment were obtained from Dr. WT Greenough (University of Illinois, Champaign, IL). Mice were housed under a 12-h light and dark cycle with food and water provided ad libitum. This study was carried out in accordance with the principles of the Basel Declaration and recommendations followed by the guidelines set from The Canadian Council on Animal Care. In addition, the animal experiments were performed in accordance with the ethical guidelines of the Zhejiang University Animal Experimentation Committee and were in complete compliance with the National Institutes of Health Guide for the Care and Use of Laboratory Animals. All of the protocols were approved by The Animal Care and Use Committee of University of Toronto, Xi'an Jiaotong University and Zhejiang University.

Whole-cell patch-clamp recordings from insular cortex slices
Mice were anesthetized by isoflurane (1–2%). We prepared transverse brain slices of the insular cortex (300 μm) by standard methods [18–20]. Slices were kept in a room temperature submerged recovery chamber with an oxygenated (95% O_2–5% CO_2) solution containing (in mM) 124 NaCl, 25 $NaHCO_3$, 2.5 KCl, 1 KH_2PO_4, 2 $CaCl_2$, 2 $MgSO_4$,

and 10 glucose. After a one hr. recovery period, brain slices were brought into a recording chamber on the stage of an Axioskop 2FS microscope (Carl Zeiss) equipped with infrared differential interference contrast optics for whole-cell patch-clamp recordings. Excitatory postsynaptic currents (EPSCs) were obtained from pyramidal neurons in layer II/III with an Axon 200B amplifier (Axon Instruments) in the insular cortex, and electrical stimulation was given by a bipolar tungsten electrode placed in layer V/VI of the insular cortex [19]. The evoked stimulations were given every 30 s as control test pulses. Repetitive high frequency stimulations were delivered at 200 Hz (5, 10, or 20 shocks) for frequency facilitations. Under the voltage-clamp mode, recording electrodes (2–5 MΩ) with the pipette solution composed of (in mM) 120 Cs-gluconate, 5 NaCl, 1 $MgCl_2$ 0.5 EGTA, 2 Mg-ATP, 0.1 Na_3GTP, 10 HEPES, and 2 lidocanine N-methyl bromide quaternary salt (QX-314), pH 7.2, 280–300 mosmol/l [18, 19]. The initial access resistance was between 15 and 30 MΩ, and was recorded during the experiment. Data were stopped when the access resistance became more that 15% during the experiment. We used the filter at 1 kHz and the data was digitized at 10 kHz. The holding membrane potential was at – 60 mV during the experiments. All experiments were done in the presence of picrotoxin (PTX; 100 μM) and D-2-amino-5-phosphonopentanoic acid (AP-5; 50 μM). We recorded time constants of EPSCs by fitting one exponential function to the falling phase of the currents.

Drugs and antibodies
Kainate (KA) was purchased from Tocris Cookson (Bristol, UK), Picrotoxin (PTX), D-2-amino-5-phosphono-pentanoic acid (AP-5), 1-(4-aminophenyl)-4-methyl-7,8-methylenedioxy- 5H-2,3-benzodiazepine (GYKI53655), 6-cyano-7-nitroquinoxaline-2,3-dione (CNQX), phosphatase inhibitor cocktail 2 and 3 were obtained from Sigma-Aldrich (St. Louis, MO). Antibodies were used: anti-PSD95 (#3450, 1:1000) were from Cell Signaling Technology, anti-synaptophysin (S55768, 1:5000) and anti-β-actin (A2066, 1:1000) were purchased from Sigma, anti-rab5 (sc-46692, 1:500) were from Santa Cruz Biotechnology; anti-GluN2A (AB1555, 1:2000), anti-GluN2B (AB1557, 1:500), anti-GluK1 (07–258, 1:500) and anti-GluK2/3 (04–921, 1:1000) were purchased from Millipore Bioscience Research Reagents.

Primary culture of the cortical neurons
Cortical neuronal cultures from Fmr1 WT or Fmr1 KO mice were prepared by a previously described protocol [25, 26]. Cortical neurons from embryonic day 17 (E17) rats were cultured as described previously [27]. Cultured neurons were incubated in 5% CO_2 humidified incubator at 37 °C and used for experiments at 14 days in vitro (DIV 14).

Brain slices preparations

Brain slices were prepared as previously described [25]. The anatomical terminology was based on the Atlas of Franklin and Paxinos [28]. Fmr1 WT or Fmr1 KO mice were anesthetized with halothane (2%) and 300 μm thickness of brain slices containing the insular cortex were cut with a vibratome in oxygenated artificial cerebrospinal fluid (ACSF) containing 124 mM NaCl, 2 mM KCl, 26 mM NaHCO$_3$, 2 mM CaCl$_2$, 2 mM MgSO$_4$, 1 mM NaH$_2$PO$_4$, and 10 mM D-glucose (pH 7.4) at 4 °C. For performing electrophysiological analysis, the brain slices were put in a submerged recover chamber with oxygenated ACSF at room temperature.

Subcellular fractionation

Subcellular fractionation was conducted by a previous protocol [25, 26]. The insular cortex was dissected in cold ACSF and homogenized in 0.32 M sucrose buffer (10 mM sucrose, 10 mM Hepes, pH 7.4) containing a protease inhibitor cocktail. Samples were centrifuged (1000 g, 10 min, 4 °C) to yield the nuclear enriched pellet and the S1 fraction. The S1 fraction was then centrifuged (12,000 g, 20 min, 4 °C) to obtain the supernant (S2) and pellet (P2; crude synaptosomal membranes) fraction. The P2 pellet was then re-suspended in radioimmunoprecipitation assay (RIPA) buffer [50 mM tris-Cl (pH 7.6), 150 mM NaCl, 1 mM EDTA, 0.1% SDS, 1% NP-40, 0.5% sodium deoxycholate, 1 mM dithiothreitol]. To further digest synaptosomes, we re-suspended the P2 pellet in 4 mM Hepes buffer (4 mM Hepes, 1 mM EDTA, pH 7.4) and then centrifuged (12,000 g, 20 min, 4 °C). Re-suspension and centrifugation were repeated. The resulting pellet was resuspended in buffer A (20 mM Hepes, 0.5% Triton X-100, 100 mM NaCl, pH 7.2) and rotated slowly (15 min, 4 °C), followed by centrifugation (12,000 g, 20 min, 4 °C). The supernatant (Triton X-100 soluble non-PSD fraction) was retained. The pellet was resuspended in buffer B (20 mM Hepes, 0.15 mM NaCl, 1% deoxycholic acid, 1% Triton X-100, 1% SDS, 1 mM dithiothreitol, pH 7.5), followed by gentle rotating (1 h, 4 °C) and centrifugation (10,000 g, 15 min, 4 °C). The supernatant (Triton X-100 insoluble PSD fraction) was retained and the pellet was discarded.

Surface Biotinylation assay of KARs

Surface biotinylation assay was conducted with cultured cortical neurons following a previous protocol [29, 30]. We used primary cultured cortical neurons at DIV 14 treated with or without Kainate for indicated times. The neurons were washed twice with ice-cold PBS containing 1 mM MgCl$_2$ and 0.1 mM CaCl$_2$ (PBS+) and incubated with 1 mg/ml EZ-Link Sulfo-NHS-SS-biotin (Thermo Fisher Scientific) in PBS+ for 30 min at 4 °C with gentle constant shake. Subsequently, the cells were washed with an ice-cold quenching buffer (50 mM glycine in PBS+) and lysed in lysis buffer (1% triton X-100, 0.5% sodium deoxycholate in PBS) at 4 °C for 30 min. Followed by 15 min centrifugation at 4 °C, the supernatant was incubated with streptavidin-Sepharose beads (Thermo Fisher Scientific) overnight at 4 °C. The bound proteins were eluted by a 1.5 × SDS buffer and detected by western blot.

Western blot analysis

Western blot was performed as described previously [25, 31]. Protein concentrations were normalized with the Bradford assay. Equal amounts of protein extract were loaded on SDS-PAGE gels, and separated proteins were transferred onto polyvinylidene membranes at 4 °C. The membranes were blocked with a blocking buffer [5% milk in TBST (tris-buffered saline with Tween 20)] and incubated with primary antibodies (4 °C, overnight). After being washed three times, the membranes were incubated with an appropriate HRP-coupled secondary antibody for another 1 h, and then detected with the Western Lightning Chemiluminescence Reagent Plus. The density of the immunoblots was analyzed with ImageJ.

Data analysis

The data are shown as means ± SEM. Statistical analysis of differences between two groups was conducted by unpaired, two-tailed Student's t-test or Mann-Whitney rank sum test, based on a normality test (Shapiro-Wilk) of the data. We performed a two-way ANOVA and Tukey test for post hoc test when there were 2 independent variables. A probability value of $P < 0.05$ was considered as significant.

Results

Subcellular distribution of KARs in the insular cortex

We examined the subcellular distribution of KARs in the insular cortex of Fmr1 WT mice by synaptosome fractionation. Crude synaptosomal fraction (P2) contains pre- and postsynaptic structures [32]. Further digestion of synaptosome yields a Triton X-100 insoluble PSD fraction and a Triton X-100 soluble non-PSD fraction [25, 33]. As shown in Fig. 1, PSD95 was enriched in the PSD fraction, while Synaptophysin and Rab5 were in the non-PSD fraction (Fig. 1). NMDAR subunits GluN1 and GluN2A were mainly located in the PSD fraction, which is inconsistent with previous findings [25]. GluK1 and GluK2/3 were highly enriched in the P2 fraction (synaptosomal pellet). Unlike NMDARs, both GluK1 and GluK2/3 were mainly distributed in the non-PSD fraction, but not in the PSD fraction (Fig. 1).

Fmr1 KO mice reduced KARs mediated EPSCs in pyramidal neurons from layer II/III of the insular cortex

We tested whether Fmr1 KO mice could alter KARs mediated glutamatergic transmissions in insular cortex

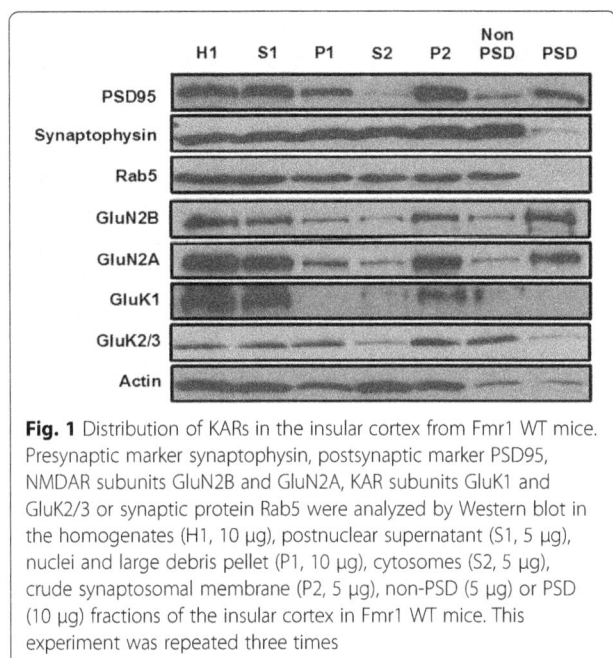

Fig. 1 Distribution of KARs in the insular cortex from Fmr1 WT mice. Presynaptic marker synaptophysin, postsynaptic marker PSD95, NMDAR subunits GluN2B and GluN2A, KAR subunits GluK1 and GluK2/3 or synaptic protein Rab5 were analyzed by Western blot in the homogenates (H1, 10 μg), postnuclear supernatant (S1, 5 μg), nuclei and large debris pellet (P1, 10 μg), cytosomes (S2, 5 μg), crude synaptosomal membrane (P2, 5 μg), non-PSD (5 μg) or PSD (10 μg) fractions of the insular cortex in Fmr1 WT mice. This experiment was repeated three times

neurons. We conducted in vitro whole-cell patch-clamp recordings to visually identify pyramidal cells in layers II/III of the insular cortex slices from adult Fmr1 WT and Fmr1 KO mice [19]. To induce evoked KARs mediated currents, a stimulation electrode was located in layer V/VI of the insular cortex. In the presence of the $GABA_A$ receptor antagonist, PTX (100 μM) and a selective NMDA receptor antagonist, AP-5 (50 μM), single-pulse stimulation evoked EPSCs could be recorded in Fmr1 WT mice (Fig. 2A). After a stable EPSCs baseline of at least 5 min was observed, we applied the potent AMPA receptor antagonist, GYKI53655 (100 μM) in the bath solution. A small residual EPSCs lasted in the presence of GYKI 53655 10 min after the application. The residual EPSCs were considered as KAR mediated currents. Lastly, the AMPAR/KAR antagonist, CNQX (20 μM) was applied, and the bath application of CNQX completely abolished the small GYKI 53655-resistant current. These results suggest that the currents were mediated by KARs (Fig. 2A).

Next, we recorded KAR mediated currents in Fmr1 KO mice. The insular cortex neurons in Fmr1 KO mice showed small KAR mediated currents (Fig. 2B). The avaraged data of KA mediated EPSCs are shown in Fig. 2C. The averaged amplitudes of KARs EPSCs in Fmr1 WT mice were $7.8 \pm 1.2\%$ of the AMPARs/KARs EPSCs as a baseline (averaged AMPA/KA EPSCs: 131.0 ± 5.7 pA; averaged KA EPSCs: 9.8 ± 1.4 pA, $n = 15$ neurons in 11 Fmr1 WT mice). These KAR mediated currents in Fmr1 WT mice are similar to the KA currents in C57BL/6 J mice [18, 19]. KAR EPSCs in Fmr1 KO mice were decreased compared with Fmr1 WT mice (AMPA/KA EPSCs: 125.2 ± 16.7 pA; KA EPSCs: 6.1 ± 1.0 pA, n

$= 13$ neurons in 9 Fmr1 KO mice, $*P < 0.05$ vs Fmr1 WT mice). These results suggest that FMRP is critical for KAR mediated synaptic transmission in the insular cortex.

Fmr1 KO mice show altered kinetics in KAR EPSCs in insular cortex

As shown in Fig. 1D-E, GYKI53655-sensitive and -resistant currents were normalized in Fmr1 WT and Fmr1 KO mice (Fig. 2D). The property of GYKI53655-sensitive currents did not change between the two groups (Fig. 2E). KAR EPSCs (GYKI53655-resistant) displayed slower decay time than AMPA EPSCs (GYKI53655-sensitive) in both groups (82.2 ± 28.0 ms in 13 Fmr1 WT mice, 87.6 ± 10.1 ms in 12 Fmr1 KO mice). However, the rise time (10–90%) of KA EPSCs in Fmr1 KO mice was significantly faster than the time of KAR EPSCs in Fmr1 WT mice (7.1 ± 1.3 ms in Fmr1 WT mice, 3.0 ± 0.4 ms in Fmr1 KO mice, $*P < 0.05$) (Fig. 2E). Since the slow kinetics in insular cortex neurons of Fmr1 WT mice are similar to those in C57BL/6 J mice [19], a lack of FMRP may alter the functions and kinetics of KARs mediated synaptic transmission in the insular cortex.

Fmr1 KO mice reduced summation properties of KAR-EPSCs during repetitive high frequency stimulations

In most synapses in the brain, repetitive stimulations increase KARs mediated EPSCs [18, 19, 34–36]. Thus, we determined that Fmr1 KO mice could alter the summational properties of KARs mediated synaptic transmissions in the insular cortex (Fig. 3A-C). The repetitive high frequency stimulations at 200 Hz were applied by single, 5, 10 and 20 shocks in Fmr1 WT mice and Fmr1 KO mice (Fig. 3A-B). Figure 3A shows that in the presence of GYKI 53655,small residual KAR EPSCs in Fmr1 WT mice significantly increased in amplitude after repetitive stimulation (8.0 ± 1.5 pA by single stimulation, 14.6 ± 2.4 pA by 5 shocks, 18.4 ± 3.1 pA by 10 shocks and 18.9 ± 3.4 pA by 20 shocks, $n = 12$ in 7 Fmr1 WT mice, Fig. 3C). However, in Fmr1 KO mice, KARs mediated currents induced by 5, 10 and 20 shocks at a 200 Hz train were significantly reduced compared with those in Fmr1 WT mice (4.5 ± 1.4 pA by single stimulation, 6.7 ± 1.4 pA by 5 shocks, 8.2 ± 1.1 pA by 10 shocks and 5.0 ± 0.8 pA by 20 shocks n = 12 in 8 Fmr1 KO mice, $*P < 0.05$, Fig. 3C).

In order to further verify these results, we recorded the input (stimulation intensity)-output (KA-EPSC amplitude) relationship of KA EPSCs in Fmr1 WT and Fmr1 KO mice (Fig. 3D, E). Fig. 3D showed that Fmr1 WT mice increased the amplitudes of KARs EPSCs by giving stronger stimulation intensity from 4 to 12 V ($n = 9$ neurons in 7 Fmr1 WT, Fig. 3 Da). However, Fmr1 KO mice did not show the increased KAR EPSCs ($n = 7$ neurons in 5 Fmr1 KO, Fig. 3Db). Compared with Fmr1 WT mice, Fmr1 KO mice reduced

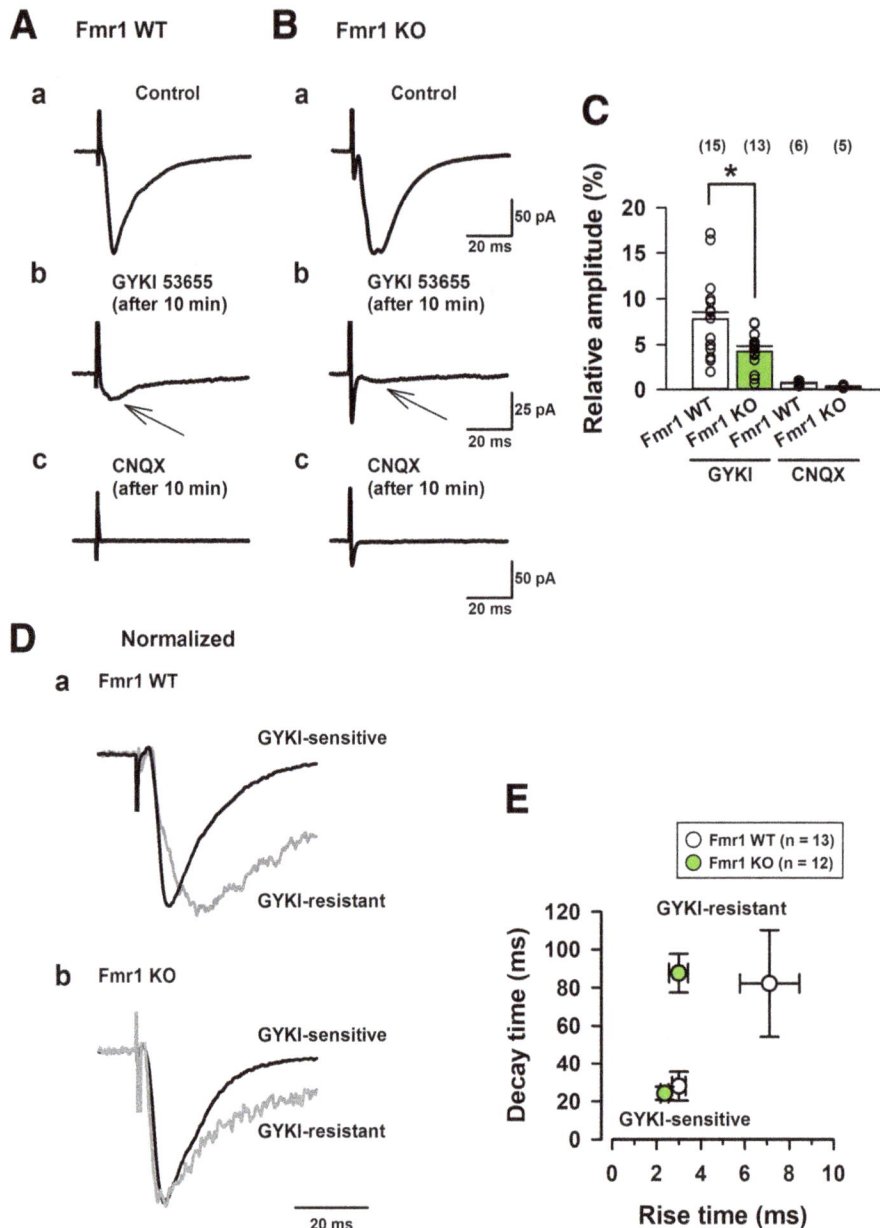

Fig. 2 Fmr1 KO mice reduced KARs-mediated EPSCs in pyramidal neurons of layer II/III insular cortex. **a, b,** To detect KARs-mediated EPSCs, AMPAR/KAR mediated EPSCs were obtained in the presence of GABA$_A$ receptor antagonist, PTX (100 μM) and a NMDARs angatonist, AP-5 (50 μM) for 5 min in Fmr1 WT (Aa) and KO mice (Ba). 10 min after the perfusion of an AMPAR antagonist, GYKI 53655 (100 μM), a residual current remained (A-Bb). The small currents could be totally blocked by a AMPAR/KARs antagonist, CNQX (20 μM) in Fmr1 WT (Ac) and Fmr1 KO mice (Bc). **c,** Statistical results of the percentage of EPSCs in the presence of GYKI 53655 ($n = 15$ in 11 Fmr1 WT mice, $n = 13$ in 9 Fmr1 KO mice), and CNQX ($n = 6$ in 6 Fmr1 WT mice, $n = 5$ in 4 Fmr1 KO mice). Compared with KARs mediated currents in Fmr1 WT mice, KAR-mediated currents in Fmr1 KO mice were significantly decreased (*$P < 0.05$). **d,** KA receptor-mediated EPSCs show slower kinetics in Fmr1 WT and Fmr1 KO mice. Normalized traces of GYKI53655-sensitive and GYKI53655-resistant EPSCs were recorded. **e,** The data of averaged rise time and decay time in GYKI-sensitive and GYKI-resistant traces. The rise time in GYKI53655-resistant EPSCs between Fmr1 WT and Fmr1 KO mice were significantly different (n = 13 in 10 Fmr1 WT mice, $n = 12$ in 10 Fmr1 KO mice) (*$P < 0.05$)

stimulation intensity-dependent amplitudes of KAR EPSCs (*P < 0.05, Fig. 3E). Taken together, these results indicate that FMRP may play important roles in KAR mediated synaptic transmission within the insular cortex.

KARs in the synaptosome is reduced in Fmr1 KO mice
To further investigate whether the expression level of total KAR subunits or the distribution of KAR subunits in the synaptosome is changed in the insular cortex from Fmr1

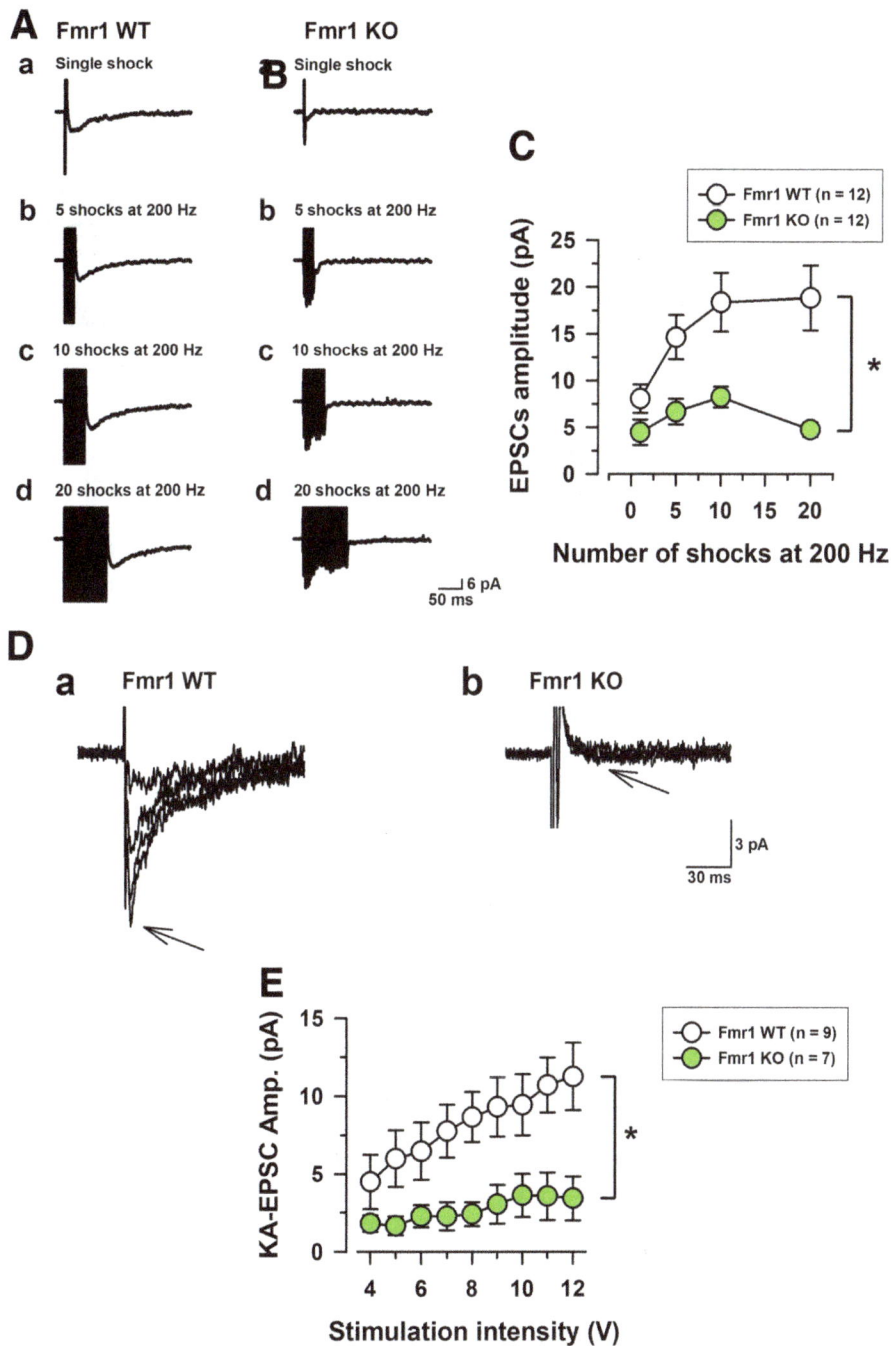

Fig. 3 Fmr1 KO mice decreased high-frequency stimulation-dependent summations of KAR mediated EPSCs in insular cortex neurons. **a, b,** Representative traces of KA EPSCs recorded by different numbers of stimulations (1, 5, 10, and 20 shocks; a-d, respectively) at the frequency of 200 Hz in Fmr1 WT (A) and Fmr1 KO mice (B). **c,** Insular cortex neurons in Fmr1 KO mice show strong reductions by these repetitive stimulations (n = 12 in 7 Fmr1 WT mice, n = 12 in 8 Fmr1 WT mice, *P < 0.05). **d,** KARs mediated input-output relationships for single shock-induced KAR-EPSCs showing intensity dependent summation in Fmr1 WT (A) and Fmr1 KO mice (B). **e,** Neurons in Fmr1 WT mice showed increased amplitudes of KAR-EPSCs that were intensity dependent (n = 9 in 7 Fmr1 WT mice), but neurons in Fmr1 KO mice showed no such significant increase (n = 7 in 5 Fmr1 KO mice, *P < 0.05)

WT and Fmr1 KO mice, we performed a biochemical assay to analyze the amount of GluK1 and GluK2/3 in the homogenate or in the synaptosomal fraction of the insular cortex. As shown in Fig. 4A and B, the amount of GluK1 and GluK2/3 was unaltered in the insular homogenate of Fmr1 KO mice compared to Fmr1 WT mice. However,

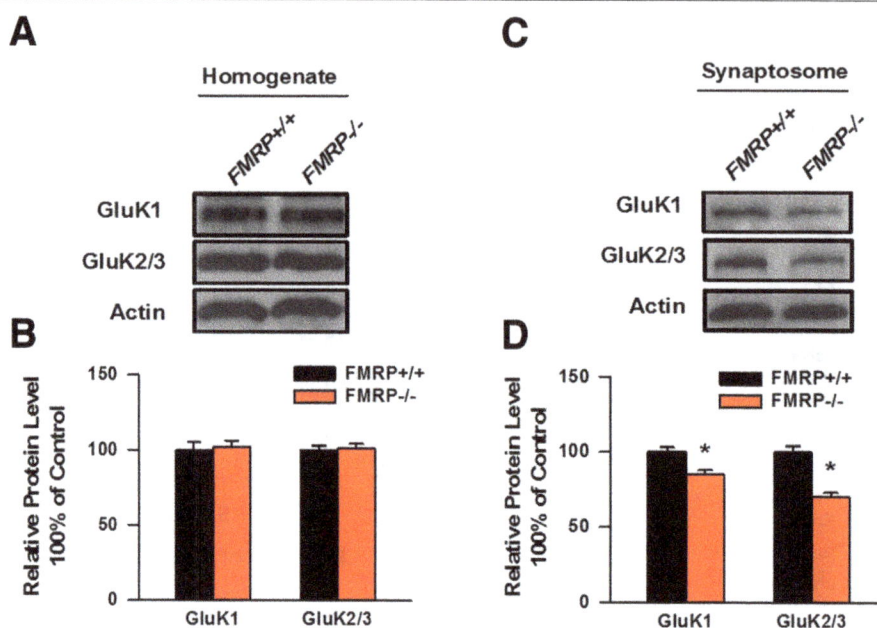

Fig. 4 The abundance of KARs in the synaptosome is decreased in Fmr1 KO mice. **a, b,** Total expression levels of GluK1 and GluK2/3 in the homogenates fraction of the insular cortex conducted from Fmr1 WT and Fmr1 KO mice were detected by Western blot. The expression levels of GluK1 and GluK2/3 in the homogenates were not altered between Fmr1 WT and Fmr1 KO mice ($n = 3$ mice for each group). **c, d,** Expression levels of GluK1 and GluK2/3 in the synaptosome of the insular cortex obtained from Fmr1 WT and Fmr1 KO mice were detected by western blot anaylsis. The expression levels of GluK1 and GluK2/3 in the homogenates was significantly reduced in Fmr1 KO mice compare to Fmr1 WT mice ($n = 5$ mice for each group). *$P < 0.05$

the abundance of GluK1 and GluK2/3 in the synaptosome of the insular cortex was significantly reduced in Fmr1 KO mice compared to Fmr1 WT mice (Fig. 4C and D). These results indicated that deficiency of FMRP results in the reduced synaptic localization of KAR subunits in the insular cortex.

Evoked KAR currents were unchanged in the cultured neurons from Fmr1 KO mice compared with Fmr1 WT mice

To further study the expression and function of KARs, we tested the Kainate-evoked KAR currents in the cultured cortical neurons from Fmr1 WT and Fmr1 KO mice. Kainate (10 μM) was puff-applied (15 psi, 100 ms) in PTX, AP-5 and GYKI 53655 containing ACSF was voltage-clamped under − 60 mV (Fig. 5). The puff application of Kainate produced inward currents in Fmr1 WT and Fmr1 KO mice (Fig. 5A, B). Comparing the KA-mediated currents in cultured neurons from Fmr1 KO mice with those in Fmr1 WT mice, KA-evoked currents were unchanged between Fmr1 KO and Fmr1 WT mice (134.1 ± 32.3 pA, $n = 6$ in 5 Fmr1 WT mice, 119.5 ± 13.6 pA, n = 6 in 6 Fmr1 KO mice, $P > 0.05$, Fig. 5C). These results suggest that the lack of the *Fmr1* gene does not affect the abundance of surface KAR in the cultured cortical neurons.

Total and surface expression of KARs did not change in the cultured cortical neurons from Fmr1 KO mice or Fmr1 WT mice

Next, we cultured cortical neurons from Fmr1 WT and Fmr1 KO mice, and compared the total and surface expression of KARs. As shown in Fig. 6A, the total levels of GluK1 and GluK2/3 showed no significant difference between two groups. We also tested the surface expression level of GluK2/3 in the cultured cortical neurons using surface biotinylation. As shown in Fig. 6B, no difference has been observed between the two groups. These results indicate that FMRP deficiency has no effect on the total expression or surface localization of KARs.

Activity induced endocytosis of KARs was impaired in cultured cortical neurons from Fmr1 KO mice

Previous studies indicate that surface localization of KARs is regulated by neuronal activity. For example, stimulation of neurons with kainate acid induced internalization of GluK2 subunits of KARs in the cultured neurons. To test the role of FMRP in KA receptor trafficking, we first set up a biotinylation assay to test the surface-localized KARs in the cultured cortical neurons obtained from the wild-type rat (Fig. 7A,B). We found that the amount of surface GluK2 was significantly decreased when the neurons were stimulated with Kainate acid. Next, we tested

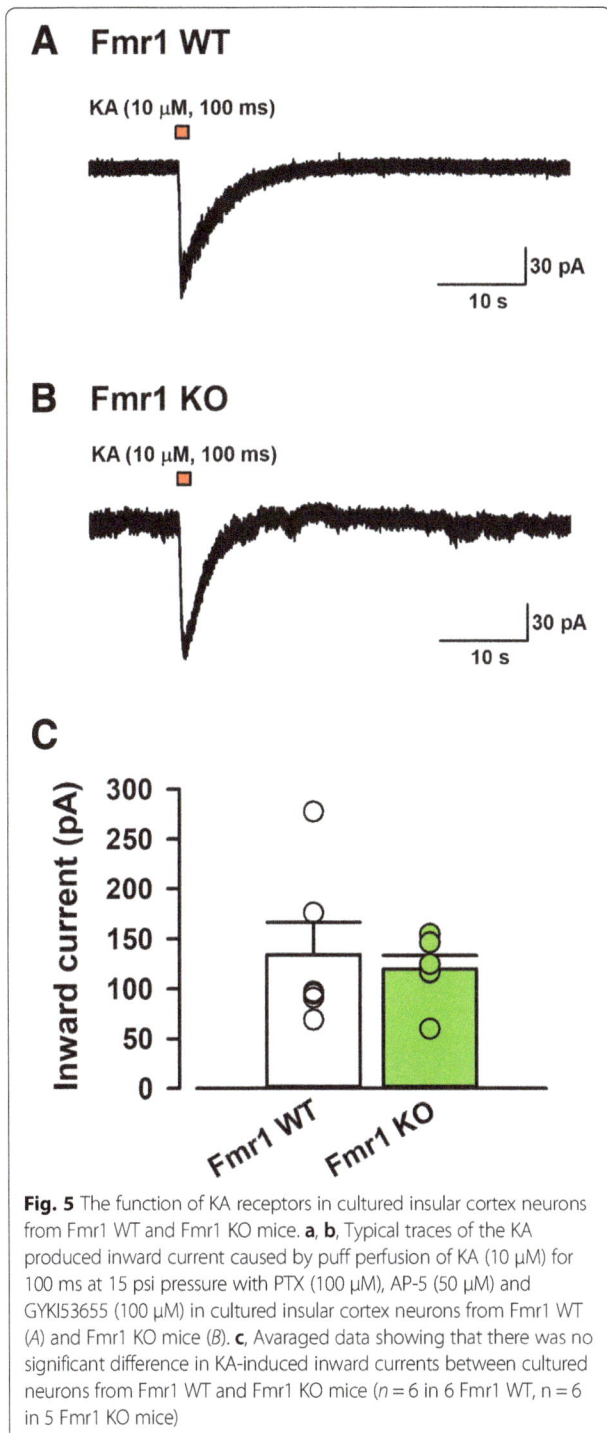

Fig. 5 The function of KA receptors in cultured insular cortex neurons from Fmr1 WT and Fmr1 KO mice. **a**, **b**, Typical traces of the KA produced inward current caused by puff perfusion of KA (10 μM) for 100 ms at 15 psi pressure with PTX (100 μM), AP-5 (50 μM) and GYKI53655 (100 μM) in cultured insular cortex neurons from Fmr1 WT (A) and Fmr1 KO mice (B). **c**, Avaraged data showing that there was no significant difference in KA-induced inward currents between cultured neurons from Fmr1 WT and Fmr1 KO mice (n = 6 in 6 Fmr1 WT, n = 6 in 5 Fmr1 KO mice)

the effects of FMRP deficiency on activity-induced KAR trafficking (Fig. 7C,D). In the cortical neurons cultured from Fmr1 WT mice, stimulation with kainate acid induced the internalization of GluK2/3 subunits. However, KA-induced internalization of GluK2/3 subunits was completely blocked in the neurons cultured from Fmr1 KO mice. These results indicate that lack of FMRP impairs activity-induced trafficking of KARs.

Discussion

The mGluR theory of FXS is well investigated. However, in addition to mGluR, iGluRs are also regulated by FMRP. FMRP is critical for the surface expression and phosphorylation of AMPARs GluA1 subunit in response to dopaminergic D_1 receptor activation [17]. Furthermore, FMRP is important for NMDA receptor-dependent LTP in the ACC and the hippocampal DG region [11, 14]. Here, we demonstrate that synaptic localization and function of KARs are affected in the insular cortex of Fmr1 KO mice, indicating that KARs may also participate in the pathology of the FXS.

In spite of their slow and small currents, KARs play important roles in cortical neurons. Facilitations of GluK1-containing KARs in the ACC and the insular cortex can regulate glutamatergic and GABAergic transmission [19, 37]. The cortical pre-LTP requires activations of KAR [38]. FMRP signaling also involves the KARs dependent cortical pre-LTP [24]. Importantly, Fmr1 KO mice inhibit the expression of the cingulate pre-LTP. One possible reason for the inhibition of pre-LTP is that Fmr1 KO mice alter catalytic and regulatory parts of PKA in the ACC [39]. Therefore, we speculate that FMRP may alter the function of KAR, either directly or indirectly.

KARs may also play important roles in the insular cortex, similar to NMDAR or AMPAR. Indeed, KARs mediated currents are recorded in layer II/II pyramidal neurons of the adult mice insular cortex [19]. The KARs mediated currents require GluK1 and GluK2 receptor subunits because pharmacological blocking and/or gene deletions of both GluK1 and GluK2 receptors reduce the KARs mediated currents [19]. In the present study, we found that Fmr1 KO mice reduced KARs mediated currents induced by single and repetitive electric stimulations, suggesting that FMRP may be important in synaptic KARs mediated transmission in the insular cortex. Although Fmr1 KO mice did not alter total expressions of GluK1 and GluK2 receptors, lacking the *Fmr1* gene reduced these receptors in synaptosomes of the insular cortex. Combined with our biochemical finding, these results indicate that FMRP is crital for regulating the subsynaptic functions of GluK1 and GluK2 receptors in the insular cortex.

We further analyzed the possible molecular mechanism related to the abnormal KAR functions in Fmr1 KO mice using cultured cortical neurons. Both our electrophysiological and biochemical data indicate that knocking-out FMRP has no effect on the surface expression of GluKRs. Interestingly, we found that the kainate activity-induced endocytosis of GluK2 was blocked in the neurons with FMRP knock-out, indicating that the trafficking of KAR is affected. We are still unclear whether FMRP is involved in the regulation of KAR trafficking. Previous work in other labs has shown that the C-terminus of GluK2 may be modulated by protein kinase A (PKA) and/or protein kinase C (PKC)-mediated phosphorylation [40, 41]. The phosphorylation of GluK2 at Ser846

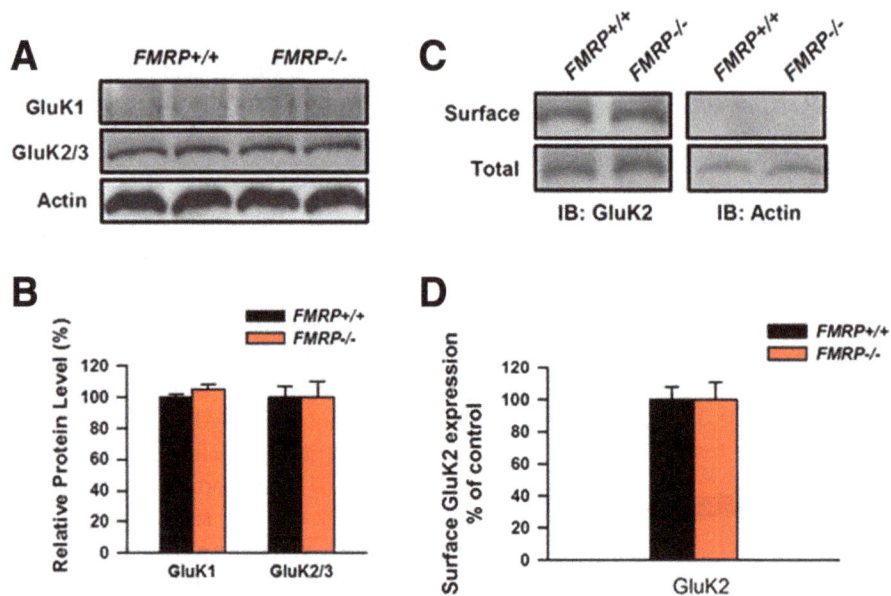

Fig. 6 The expression of KARs in the cultured cortical neurons from Fmr1 WT and Fmr1 KO mice. **a**, **b**, The abundance of GluK1 or GluK2/3 in the homogenate of the cultured cortical neurons from Fmr1 WT mice and Fmr1 KO mice showed no change. **c**, **d**, Surface expression levels of GluK2/3 in insular cortex neurons obtained from Fmr1 WT and Fmr1 KO mice were detected by western blot analysis. The surface expression levels of GluK2/3 were not altered between Fmr1 WT and Fmr1 KO mice (n = 3 independent experiments). Actin was used as negative control for surface biotinylation

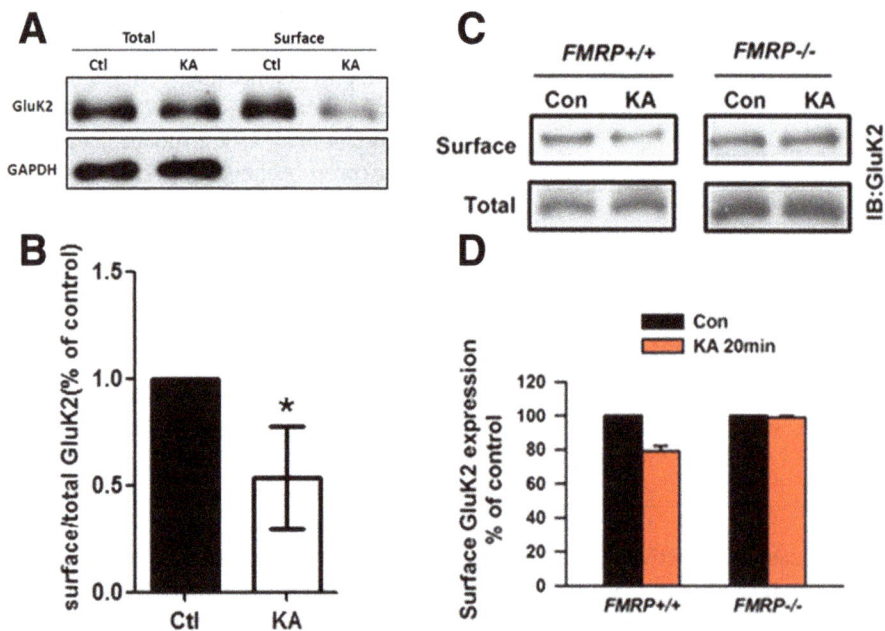

Fig. 7 Activity-induced internalization of GluK2 subunit was impaired in cultured cortical neurons from Fmr1 KO mice. **a**, **b**, GluK2/3 subunit undergoes activity induced internalization in the cultured rat cortical neurons (n = 5 independent experiments). *$P < 0.05$. **c**, **d**, The cultured cortical neurons obtained from Fmr1 WT or Fmr1 KO mice were activated by KA (10 μM) for 20 min and the surface expression of GluK2 was detected by Western blot. The abundance of surface GluK2 in Fmr1 WT mice was significantly decreased upon KA stimulation, whereas that of GluK2 in Fmr1 KO mice did not change (n = 4 independent experiments). *$P < 0.05$

and Ser868 inhibits GluK2 from exiting the ER and trafficking to the cell surface [42]. Moreover, the phosphorylation of GluK2 at Ser846 accelerates KAR endocytosis from the plasma membrane and trafficking to the lateendosome. Importantly, Fmr1 KO mice showed enhanced activity of PKC [43–45]. Therefore, it is possible that the enhanced PKC activity in Fmr1 KO mice impairs the regulation of KAR trafficking. Further research is required to unveil the related signaling pathways.

Abbreviations

ACC: anterior cingulate cortex; AMPAR: α-amino-3-hydroxyl-S-methylisoazole-4-propionate receptor; EPSCs: excitatory postsynaptic currents; FMRP: fragile X mental retardation protein; FXS: Fragile X syndrome; iGluRs: ionotropic glutamate receptors; KA: kainate; KAR: Kainate receptor; KO: knock-out; LTD: long-term depression; LTP: long-term potentiation; mGluR: metabotropic glutamate receptors; NMDAR: N-methyl-D-aspartate receptor; PFC: prefrontal cortex; PKA: protein kinase A; PKC: protein kinase C; WT: wild-type

Acknowledgments
We thank the members of the Laboratory for discussions.

Funding
This work was supported by grants from the EJLB-CIHR Michael Smith Chair in Neurosciences and Mental Health, Canada Research Chair, Canadian Institute for Health Research operating Grants (MOP-124807) and the Azrieli Neurodevelopmental Research Program and Brain Canada. S.Q. and K.K. were supported by the postdoctoral fellowship from Fragile X research foundation of Canada. This work was also supported by Grants National Natural Science Foundation of China (No. 81471125, 81671049 and 91732102 to S.Q., No. 81500904 to X.L.), Zhejiang Science Fund for Distinguished Young Scholars (LR16C090001), National Basic Research Program of China (2013CB910204), the Fundamental Research Funds for the Central Universities of China, and Chinese Ministry of Education Project 111 Program B13026 (S.Q.). In part, K.K. was supported by Takeda Science Foundation.

Authors' contributions
SQ, MZ and KK designed research; SQ, YW, XYL and XL performed the biochemical experiments and KK studied electrophysiological recordings; SQ and KK analyzed data; SQ, MZ and KK wrote the paper. All authors read and approved the final manuscript.

Competing interests
The authors declare that they have no competing interests.

Author details
[1]Center for Neuron and Disease, Frontier Institute of Science and Technology, Xi'an Jiaotong University, Xi'an 710049, China. [2]Department of Physiology, Faculty of Medicine, University of Toronto, Medical Science Building, 1 King's College Circle, Toronto, ON M5S 1A8, Canada. [3]Department of Neurobiology, Key Laboratory of Medical Neurobiology of the Ministry of Health of China, Zhejiang University School of Medicine, Zhejiang 310058, Hangzhou, China. [4]Department of Neurology, The First Affiliated Hospital, Zhejiang University School of Medicine, Zhejiang 310003, Hangzhou, China. [5]Department of Neurophysiology, Hyogo College of Medicine, Nishinomiya, Hyogo 663-8501, Japan.

References
1. Bhakar AL, Dolen G, Bear MF. The pathophysiology of fragile X (and what it teaches us about synapses). Annu Rev Neurosci. 2012;35:417–43.
2. Santoro MR, Bray SM, Warren ST. Molecular mechanisms of fragile X syndrome: a twenty-year perspective. Annu Rev Pathol. 2012;7:219–45.
3. Eichler EE, et al. Length of uninterrupted CGG repeats determines instability in the FMR1 gene. Nat Genet. 1994;8(1):88–94.
4. Pieretti M, et al. Absence of expression of the FMR-1 gene in fragile X syndrome. Cell. 1991;66(4):817–22.
5. Bagni C, Greenough WT. From mRNP trafficking to spine dysmorphogenesis: the roots of fragile X syndrome. Nat Rev Neurosci. 2005;6(5):376–87.
6. Feng Y, et al. Translational suppression by trinucleotide repeat expansion at FMR1. Science. 1995;268(5211):731–4.
7. Darnell JC, Klann E. The translation of translational control by FMRP: therapeutic targets for FXS. Nat Neurosci. 2013;16(11):1530–6.
8. Gladding CM, et al. Tyrosine dephosphorylation regulates AMPAR internalisation in mGluR-LTD. Mol Cell Neurosci. 2009;40(2):267–79.
9. Bear MF, Huber KM, Warren ST. The mGluR theory of fragile X mental retardation. Trends Neurosci. 2004;27(7):370–7.
10. Huber KM, et al. Altered synaptic plasticity in a mouse model of fragile X mental retardation. Proc Natl Acad Sci U S A. 2002;99(11):7746–50.
11. Zhao MG, et al. Deficits in trace fear memory and long-term potentiation in a mouse model for fragile X syndrome. J Neurosci. 2005;25(32):7385–92.
12. Chen T, et al. Pharmacological rescue of cortical synaptic and network potentiation in a mouse model for fragile X syndrome. Neuropsychopharmacology. 2014;39(8):1955–67.
13. Desai NS, et al. Early postnatal plasticity in neocortex of Fmr1 knockout mice. J Neurophysiol. 2006;96(4):1734–45.
14. Eadie BD, et al. NMDA receptor hypofunction in the dentate gyrus and impaired context discrimination in adult Fmr1 knockout mice. Hippocampus. 2012;22(2):241–54.
15. Park S, et al. Elongation factor 2 and fragile X mental retardation protein control the dynamic translation of arc/Arg3.1 essential for mGluR-LTD. Neuron. 2008;59(1):70–83.
16. Waung MW, et al. Rapid translation of arc/Arg3.1 selectively mediates mGluR-dependent LTD through persistent increases in AMPAR endocytosis rate. Neuron. 2008;59(1):84–97.
17. Wang H, et al. FMRP acts as a key messenger for dopamine modulation in the forebrain. Neuron. 2008;59(4):634–47.
18. Wu LJ, et al. Kainate receptor-mediated synaptic transmission in the adult anterior cingulate cortex. J Neurophysiol. 2005;94(3):1805–13.
19. Koga K, et al. Kainate receptor-mediated synaptic transmissions in the adult rodent insular cortex. J Neurophysiol. 2012;108(7):1988–98.
20. Koga K, et al. Coexistence of two forms of LTP in ACC provides a synaptic mechanism for the interactions between anxiety and chronic pain. Neuron. 2015;86(4):1109.
21. Jane DE, Lodge D, Collingridge GL. Kainate receptors: pharmacology, function and therapeutic potential. Neuropharmacology. 2009;56(1):90–113.
22. Wu LJ, Ko SW, Zhuo M. Kainate receptors and pain: from dorsal root ganglion to the anterior cingulate cortex. Curr Pharm Des. 2007;13(15):1597–605.
23. Ko S, et al. Altered behavioral responses to noxious stimuli and fear in glutamate receptor 5 (GluR5)- or GluR6-deficient mice. J Neurosci. 2005; 25(4):977–84.
24. Koga K, et al. Impaired presynaptic long-term potentiation in the anterior cingulate cortex of Fmr1 knock-out mice. J Neurosci. 2015;35(5):2033–43.
25. Qiu S, et al. An increase in synaptic NMDA receptors in the insular cortex contributes to neuropathic pain. Sci Signal. 2013;6(275):ra34.
26. Qiu S, et al. GluA1 phosphorylation contributes to postsynaptic amplification of neuropathic pain in the insular cortex. J Neurosci. 2014; 34(40):13505–15.
27. Wang YB, et al. Adaptor protein APPL1 couples synaptic NMDA receptor with neuronal prosurvival phosphatidylinositol 3-kinase/Akt pathway. J Neurosci. 2012;32(35):11919–29.
28. Franklin KBJ, Paxinos G. The mouse brain in stereotaxic coordinates. 3rd ed. San Deigo: Academic Press; 1997.
29. Lu W, et al. A novel phosphorylation site of N-methyl-D-aspartate receptor GluN2B at S1284 is regulated by Cdk5 in neuronal ischemia. Exp Neurol. 2015;271:251–8.
30. Lu W, et al. Phosphorylation of tyrosine 1070 at the GluN2B subunit is regulated by synaptic activity and critical for surface expression of N-methyl-D-aspartate (NMDA) receptors. J Biol Chem. 2015;290(38):22945–54.

31. Qiu S, et al. An endoplasmic reticulum retention signal located in the extracellular amino-terminal domain of the NR2A subunit of N-methyl-D-aspartate receptors. J Biol Chem. 2009;284(30):20285–98.

32. Milnerwood AJ, et al. Early increase in extrasynaptic NMDA receptor signaling and expression contributes to phenotype onset in Huntington's disease mice. Neuron. 2010;65(2):178–90.

33. Pacchioni AM, Kalivas PW. The role of AMPAR trafficking mediated by neuronal Pentraxins in cocaine-induced neuroadaptations. Mol Cell Pharmacol. 2009;1(2):183–92.

34. Castillo PE, Malenka RC, Nicoll RA. Kainate receptors mediate a slow postsynaptic current in hippocampal CA3 neurons. Nature. 1997;388(6638):182–6.

35. Mulle C, et al. Altered synaptic physiology and reduced susceptibility to kainate-induced seizures in GluR6-deficient mice. Nature. 1998;392(6676):601–5.

36. Vignes M, et al. The synaptic activation of the GluR5 subtype of kainate receptor in area CA3 of the rat hippocampus. Neuropharmacology. 1997; 36(11–12):1477–81.

37. Wu LJ, et al. Genetic and pharmacological studies of GluR5 modulation of inhibitory synaptic transmission in the anterior cingulate cortex of adult mice. Dev Neurobiol. 2007;67(2):146–57.

38. Koga K, et al. Co-existence of two forms of LTP in ACC provides a synaptic mechanism for the interactions between anxiety and chronic pain. Neuron. 2015;85(2):377–89.

39. Koga K, et al. Impaired presynaptic long-term potentiation in the anterior cingulate cortex of Fmr1 knockout mice. J Neurosci. 2015;35(5):2033–43.

40. Kornreich BG, et al. Identification of C-terminal domain residues involved in protein kinase A-mediated potentiation of kainate receptor subtype 6. Neuroscience. 2007;146(3):1158–68.

41. Cho K, et al. Regulation of kainate receptors by protein kinase C and metabotropic glutamate receptors. J Physiol. 2003;548(Pt 3):723–30.

42. Nasu-Nishimura Y, et al. Differential regulation of kainate receptor trafficking by phosphorylation of distinct sites on GluR6. J Biol Chem. 2010;285(4):2847–56.

43. Rackham O, Brown CM. Visualization of RNA-protein interactions in living cells: FMRP and IMP1 interact on mRNAs. EMBO J. 2004;23(16):3346–55.

44. Rivera R, Rozas JL, Lerma J. PKC-dependent autoregulation of membrane kainate receptors. EMBO J. 2007;26(20):4359–67.

45. de Diego-Otero Y, et al. Alpha-tocopherol protects against oxidative stress in the fragile X knockout mouse: an experimental therapeutic approach for the Fmr1 deficiency. Neuropsychopharmacology. 2009;34(4):1011–26.

8

Identification of lncRNA expression profiles and ceRNA analysis in the spinal cord of morphine-tolerant rats

Jiali Shao, Jian Wang, Jiangju Huang, Chang Liu, Yundan Pan, Qulian Guo and Wangyuan Zou[*] ⓘ

Abstract

Morphine tolerance is a challenging clinical problem that limits the use of morphine in pain treatment, but the mechanisms of morphine tolerance remain unclear. Recent research indicates that long noncoding RNAs (lncRNAs) might be a novel and promising target in the pathogeneses of diseases. Therefore, we hypothesized that lncRNAs might play a role in the development of morphine tolerance. Male Sprague-Dawley rats were intrathecally injected with 10 μg morphine twice daily for 7 consecutive days. The animals were then sacrificed for lncRNA microarray tests, and the results were validated by RT-qPCR. Next, functional predictions for the differentially expressed mRNAs (DEmRNAs) were made with the Gene Ontology/Kyoto Encyclopedia of Genes and Genomes (GO/KEGG), and predictions for the differentially expressed lncRNAs (DElncRNAs) were made based on competitive endogenous RNA (ceRNA) analyses. The rats successfully developed morphine tolerance. LncRNA microarray analysis revealed that, according to the criteria of a log2 (fold change) > 1.5 and a P-value < 0.05, 136 lncRNAs and 278 mRNAs were differentially expressed in the morphine tolerance group (MT) compared with the normal saline group (NS). The functions of the DEmRNAs likely involve in the processes of the ion channel transport, pain transmission and immune response. The ceRNA analysis indicated that several possible interacting networks existed, including (MRAK150340, MRAK161211)/miR-219b/Tollip.Further annotations of the potential target mRNAs of the miRNAs according to the gene database suggested that the possible functions of these mRNAs primarily involved the regulation of ubiquitylation, G protein-linked receptors, and Toll-like receptors, which play roles in the development of morphine tolerance. Our findings revealed the profiles of differentially expressed lncRNAs in morphine tolerance conditions, and among these lncRNAs, some DElncRNAs might be new therapeutic targets for morphine tolerance.

Keywords: LncRNA, ceRNA, Morphine tolerance, Spinal cord

Introduction

Morphine tolerance is defined as the diminished analgesic effect and the need for a higher dose to achieve the desired analgesic effect after chronic exposure to morphine [1–4]. Over the past decades, people have attempted to elaborate the mechanisms of morphine tolerance with minimal success. The recent focus of this area is the role of non-coding RNAs (ncRNAs) [5, 6]. Among ncRNAs, some studies have reported that miRNAs are involved in the development of morphine tolerance [7, 8], including the let-7 family, miR-23b [9], miR-133b, miR-339 [10], miR-365 [11] and miR-219-5p

[12]. However, the research regarding long non-coding RNAs (lncRNAs) is still in its infancy.

The sequences of lncRNAs range in size from approximately 200 nt to over 100 kb, and lncRNAs can function in novel mechanisms of the modulation of the expression of genes [13, 14]. Over the past decades, lncRNAs have been the highlight of some studies of cancer, osteoarthritis, nervous system function and development [15–17]. In pain research, recent studies have claimed that Knav2 AS [18], uc.48+ [19] and some other lncRNAs [20] might play roles in the process of the development of neuropathic pain [21, 22]. The function of lncRNAs has been illustrated as follows: lncRNAs can interact with mRNAs, bind to transcription factors, modulate chromatin remodeling, and even directly

---
* Correspondence: wangyuanzou@csu.edu.cn
Department of Anesthesiology, Xiangya Hospital, Central South University, 87 Xiangya Road, Changsha 410008, Hunan, China

regulate the functions of target proteins. Among lncRNAs, some may act as competitive endogenous RNAs (ceRNAs) that target miRNAs [14].

The ceRNA hypothesis was proposed in 2011 with the aim of further elaborating the relationships among RNAs. Salmena et al. [23] highlighted that some RNAs act as ceRNAs that participate in mutual competition for common binding sites of target miRNAs and thus modify the functions of the target miRNAs. Recent research has indicated that ceRNA analysis might shed a light on functional predictions of the effects of lncRNAs [24].

Therefore, in the present study, we hypothesized that lncRNAs might be differentially expressed and act in direct or indirect manners during the development of morphine tolerance. To address this hypothesis, we attempted to identify the lncRNA expression profiles in the spinal cords of rats under normal and morphine tolerance conditions and to predict the possible functions of differentially expressed lncRNAs (DElncRNAs).

Methods

Intrathecal injection of morphine induces a chronic morphine tolerance model in rats

Adult male Sprague-Dawley rats (weight 240–260 g) were obtained from the Hunan SJA Laboratory Animal Company (Hunan, China). The rats were housed in groups and maintained on a 12/12 light-dark cycle at a room temperature of 22 ± 1 °C with food and water freely available. The experimental procedures were approved by the Animal Care and Use Committee of Central South University and conducted in strict accordance with the guidelines of the International Association for the Study of Pain [25]. To establish the rat model of morphine tolerance, rats in the morphine tolerance group (MT, $n = 8$) were intrathecally injected (i.t.) with 10 μg (1 μg/1 μl) of morphine twice daily at 08:00–09:00 am and 16:00–17:00 pm for 7 consecutive days [3, 26]. The normal saline group (NS, n = 8) was injected with equal volumes of normal saline at the same time points.

Tail flick test

The tail flick test was used to measure thermal sensitivity. Before conducting this test, the rats were placed on the plantar surface for 15 min to adapt to the testing environment. Then, we tested one fixed point of the tail 2–3 cm from the tip using the Hargreaves apparatus (Italy, UGO Basile) [26, 27]. The results are expressed as the tail withdrawal latency (TWL), which was ultimately converted to the percent of the maximum possible effect (%MPE). The radiant index was set at 90, and the cut-off was 20 s to avoid tissue damage. The tests were conducted 30 min before and after the morning injection of morphine on days 1, 3, 5, and 7.

Tissue collection and RNA isolation

On day 8, after the morning injection with morphine or saline, the rats were deeply anesthetized with pentobarbital sodium (1%) one hour later. Then, we decapitated the rats, collected the lumbar enlargements and placed the collected tissues into liquid nitrogen as quickly as possible for preservation. Next, we extracted the total RNA from the spinal tissues and tested the RNA quantity and quality with a NanoDrop ND-1000 Spectrophotometer (Thermo,USA) and tested the RNA integrity with agarose gel electrophoresis (2%). Subsequently, we stored the remnant RNA at − 80 °C for later use. The RNA isolation was performed by Kangcheng Bio-tech (Shanghai, China).

Microarray assay

We employed a rat lncRNA microarray 4 × 44 k,V1.0 (Arraystar) containing approximately 9000 lncRNAs to screen the differentially expressed lncRNAs and mRNAs. The total RNAs of the MT and NS groups ($n = 5$) were hybridized with the gene chips. The RNA samples were transcribed into fluorescent cRNAs along the entire lengths of the transcripts without a 3′ bias utilizing random primers. The labeled cRNAs were hybridized to the rat lncRNA microarray. Next, the arrays were scanned with an Agilent DNA Microarray Scanner (part number G2505C). The array images were analyzed with Agilent Feature Extraction software (version 11.0.1.1). Quantile normalization and subsequent data processing were performed using the GeneSpring GX v12.1 software package (Agilent Technologies,USA). The microarray hybridization was performed by Kangcheng Bio-tech (Shanghai, China).

Bioinformatics analysis

We used the criteria of a log2 (fold-change) > 1.5 and a P-value < 0.05 to screen for the deregulated RNAs. Hierarchical clustering was performed with Cluster 3.0, and the heat maps were generated in Java Treeview. The DEmRNAs were analyzed according to the pathway annotations of the Kyoto Encyclopedia of Genes and Genomes (KEGG) and Gene Ontology (GO) functional enrichment using CapitalBion. The -$\log_{10}$ (P-values) of the GO and pathway results are displayed in the histogram. The DElncRNAs were analyzed by ceRNA analyses, which were conducted with Arraystar's homemade miRNA target prediction software, which is based on TargetScan and miRanda [28]. A lncRNA/miRNA/mRNA interaction network was generated to visualize the interactions using Cytoscape. The NCBI Database was used to annotate the functions of the potential target genes.

Real-time quantitative polymerase chain reaction (RT-qPCR)

The microarray results were confirmed by RT-qPCR. The total RNAs of the MT and NS groups ($n = 5$ in each group) were reverse transcribed using random hexamer primers (Arraystar Flash RNA Labeling Kit, Arraystar) according to the manufacturer's description. The expression levels of 18 lncRNAs (MRAK080737, MRAK159688, MRAK046606, DQ266361, XR_005988, uc.48+, uc.310-, XR_009527, XR_008662, S66184, MRAK161211, MRAK 150340, XR_006440, AF196267, MRAK077287, MRAK01 4088, MRAK141001 and MRAK038897), as well as 12 DEmRNAs (S100a8, Batf, Ccl7, RT1-Bb, RatNP-3b, Grm2 and Mmp9, Prrx2, Asb2, Fam111a, Kcnv2 and Tmem119) were examined. GAPDH was used as the house-keeping gene. The sequences of all primers are presented in Table 1. We conducted the RT-qPCR tests with a 10 µL reaction system in a ViiA 7 Real-time qPCR System according to the manufacturer's protocol. Melting-curve analysis was performed to monitor the specificity of the production. All experiments were replicated three times. The gene expression levels in the MT and NS groups were analyzed with the $2^{-\Delta\Delta CT}$ method.

Statistical analysis

All data were presented as mean ± s.e.m. The statistical significance of differences between groups was analyzed with two-way repeated-measures of ANOVA followed by Bonferroni test or with Student's t-test. P values less than 0.05 were considered statistically significant.

Results

Construction of the rat morphine tolerance model

The tail flick test data revealed that there were no significant changes in the thermal sensitivities of NS group ($n = 8$ in each group). However, comparisons between the two groups revealed that, on day 1 post-injection, the %MPE of the MT group (n = 8 in each group) was significantly higher than that of the NS group ($P<0.05$). On day 3 post-injection, the % MPE of the MT group began to decline but remained higher than that of the NS group ($P<0.05$). On day 5 post-injection, the %MPEs did not significantly differ between the two groups ($P>0.05$), and this state continued to day 7 (Fig. 1a), which suggested that a stable morphine tolerance model had been established.

Overview of the lncRNA and mRNA expression profiles

First, we created an overview of the lncRNA and mRNA expression profiles using a using scatter plot, which revealed that large numbers of lncRNAs and mRNAs were differentially expressed between the MT and NS groups ($n = 5$; Fig. 1d). Next, hierarchical cluster analyses of all of the lncRNAs and mRNAs was applied and revealed

that the 5 NS and 5 MT samples clustered independently, and the results also indicated high degrees of consistency in both the NS and MT groups (Fig. 1b, c). All of the microarray results have been uploaded to the GEO database (GSE110115).

Differentially expressed lncRNAs and mRNAs in morphine tolerance

According to the criteria of a log2 (fold change) > 1.5 and a P-value< 0.05, the microarray data identified 136 lncRNAs, including 84 up-regulated and 52 down-regulated lncRNAs, which were significantly altered in the MT group compared with the NS group. The lncRNAs that exhibited the greatest up-regulations were XR_005988, DQ266361, and MRAK046606 with XR_005988 exhibiting the largest up-regulation [log2 (fold change) =12.4243]. The lncRNAs that exhibited the greatest down-regulations were AF196267, XR_009493, and MRAK150340 with AF196267 exhibiting the largest down-regulation [log2 (fold change) =2.2025]. Detailed information, including the top 40 up-regulated and top 40 down-regulated lncRNAs, is provided in Table 2.

Regarding the DEmRNAs, there were 278 genes (176 up-regulated and 102 down-regulated) whose changes met the criteria. These DEmRNAs contained many genes that are known to be involved in pain processing, including Ccl7, Batf, S100a8, Kcnv2, Rgs1, Prrx2, Mmp9, etc. Detailed information about the top 30 up-regulated and top 30 down-regulated mRNAs is listed in Table 3.

Validation of the lncRNA and mRNA expressions

To validate the reliability of the microarray results, 18 DElncRNAs and 12 DEmRNAs were selected and validated by RT-qPCR. The data shown that 11 of 18 selected DElncRNAs (XR_005988, DQ266361, MRAK159688, XR_008662, XR_009527, S66184, MRAK150340, MRAK16 1211, MRAK038897, AF196267 and MRAK141001) and 7 of 12 selected DEmRNAs (Batf, Ccl7, RatNP-3b, Mmp9, Kcnv2, Tmem119 and Asb2) exhibited the same trends in altered expressions and the same significant differences in the microarray and RT-qPCR analyses. On the other hand, the other altered mRNAs and lncRNAs exhibited the trends in changes, but the differences between the two groups were not significant, possibly due to the small sample size (Fig. 2a, b).

Class distributions of the DElncRNAs

The examined lncRNAs were categorized into five groups according to their associations with coding genes: intergenic lncRNAs, antisense overlap lncRNAs, sense overlap lncRNAs, bidirectional lncRNAs, and other. One of the mechanisms by which lncRNAs act is through the interplay with adjacent coding genes [20, 29]; therefore, it was important to classify the locations of the lncRNAs.

Table 1 The detailed information of primer sequence

Sequence name	Primer sequence	Amplicon size (bp)
GAPDH(RAT)	F:5' GCTCTCTGCTCCTCCCTGTTCTA3' R:5' TGGTAACCAGGCGTCCGATA3'	124
MRAK161211	F:5'CTGACCCCAAAGTTTCACATCT3' R:5'CCAGGAGAGGTGTTCCAAGTAA3'	63
MRAK038897	F:5'TGGCAAGAATACCAAAGAGC3' R:5'CACAGCAAGATGTAATGCACAG3'	132
MRAK014088	F:5'GTGTCTATTTCTGGGAGTCTGTGC3' R:5'GCCATTGGTAAGAGAATTAAGCAG3'	102
MRAK080737	F:5'GTGCCAGACCCCAAGGTAAA3' R:5'GAGACAATAATGGAGCCGCC3'	105
MRAK159688	F:5'GTACTGTAGCTCTTCAGCGTCC3' R:5'GTCAGAACATTCAGACCACCTC3'	78
MRAK046606	F:5'GCCAGCATCTCCTACTCACA3' R:5'TGGACTACGGACTACAGTTTACC3'	80
MRAK150340	F:5'ACAGAGTAGGGCAGTCGCAG3' R:5'GGTTGTGGACCATAGAAGAGTTG3'	205
DQ266361	F:5'TGTGGTTAAATCCCCATGC3' R:5'CTTCTCCAAGTCACATCTGCTC3'	63
XR_006440	F:5'GGAGCATCAAATCGAAAGC3' R:5'ACTCGGATCGTCTCAAGGAC3'	162
XR_005988	F:5'TGTGACACCACTGAGACCCTT3' R:5'TGGCCCTCCACACTTTACGA3'	101
uc.48+	F:5' AAATGCAAACTGGATGAGGA 3' R:5' GTTAACACTGTATGTAATTAGGG 3'	279
uc.310-	F:5' CTAATCAAAAACTGACAGCAAGA 3' R:5' GATCTTTCTTAAGCAGAATTTGG 3'	128
XR_009527	F:5' CCAAGGCCCGTATTGAGATTA 3' R:5' AGGGTCCAATGTGCCACGA 3'	116
XR_008662	F:5' TAATGAGGAAGATGAGAATGGC 3' R:5' CCAGATAGGCTTCGTCTTATTC 3'	103
S66184	F:5' TCTTCACATTACCATTACGAGGA 3' R:5' CATCGGAATGATTTTGCTGTGT 3'	51
AF196267	F:5' GCCATCAATTTTCTCTTGACTG 3' R:5' TGAAGGGTCAGTTTGAAGCA 3'	135
MRAK077287	F:5' GCTAATAATTCCTACCAGCAAA 3' R:5' ACCTCACACCCAGTCTCTACAT 3'	151
MRAK141001	F:5' CTTCCCTACCAGTCTATTGAGTG 3' R:5' ACGCTCCACTACAAAATCAGTT 3'	87
S100a8	F:5'GGGAATCACCATGCCCTCTA3' R:5'GCCCACCCTTATCACCAACA3'	168
Batf	F:5'GAGGACCTGGAGAAACAGAATG3' R:5'GCTCAGCACCGATGTGAAGTA3'	87
Ccl7	F:5'GCTGCTATGTCAAGAAACAAAAGA3' R:5'TGATGGGCTTCAGCACAGACT3'	136
RT1-Bb	F:5'GCCCTCAACCACCACAACTT3' R:5'GGTCCAGTCCCCGTTCCTAAT3'	141
Prrx2	F:5'AAGAAGAAGCAGCGTCGGA3' R:5'CAAAGGCGTCAGGGTAGTGT3'	97
Asb2	F:5'TGCTTTTCCTGCCTGTATGG3' R:5'CGACAGGAACTCACAGAACTGC3'	120
RatNP-3b	F:5' CATACGCCAAAGTCTGAAACC 3' R:5' AGCAGTGCCTTTATCCCCTC 3'	168
Grm2	F:5' CCCGGAGAACTTCAACGAA 3'	207

Table 1 The detailed information of primer sequence (Continued)

Sequence name	Primer sequence	Amplicon size (bp)
	R:5' GGCTGGAAAAGGATGATGTG 3'	
Mmp9	F:5' CCCACTTACTTTGGAAACG 3' R:5' GAAGATGAATGGAAATACGC 3'	228
Fam111a	F:5' GACTATTTCTCTCAGGTTCCCA 3' R:5' GTGCTGCATACAAGCTACTTGT 3'	256
Kcnv2	F:5' GGGCTGCGGTAAGCATCTCT 3' R:5' TTGAGAATAATCCCAAAAGCGA 3'	106
Tmem119	F:5' AGACAGTCGAACGGTCTAACAG 3' R:5' TCACAAGTAGCAGCAGAGACAG 3'	127

Our data revealed that, among these DElncRNAs, intergenic lncRNAs and sense overlap lncRNAs accounted for the majority, and only five lncRNAs belonged to the bidirectional category. The concrete data are presented in Fig. 2c.

Functional predictions for the DEmRNAs in the morphine-tolerant rats

To explore the molecular functions of the DEmRNAs in morphine tolerance conditions, we further performed GO and pathway analyses genes that differentially regulated in the MT and NS groups. The pathway analyses indicated that the most significantly enriched pathways of the up-regulated genes included the TNF metabolic pathway and phagocytic processes, and the down-regulated genes were involved in synaptic vesicle activity, the arachidonic acid metabolic pathway, etc. (Fig. 3a, b). The GO results revealed that the most significantly enriched molecular functions of the up-regulated genes in the MT group were peptidase activity, G-protein-coupled receptor activity, and biological processes concentrated on the cytokine response, defense and the immune response. The cell components primarily belonged to extracellular domains and intercellular domains. The most significantly enriched molecular functions of the down-regulated genes in the MT group were voltage-gated channel activity, ion transmembrane activity, and biological processes concentrated on potassium ion transport. The cell components were associated with the sarcolemma, cytoplasmic membrane, and ion channel complexes (Fig. 3c-h).

Functional predictions of the DElncRNAs lncRNA/miRNA/mRNA interactions

We performed coding-noncoding gene co-expression (CNC) analysis, but we found no DEmRNA-associated DElncRNAs, which meant that we were unable to make forecasts about the functions of the DElncRNAs according to the related DEmRNAs. However, ceRNA analysis allowed us to predict the possible functions of the

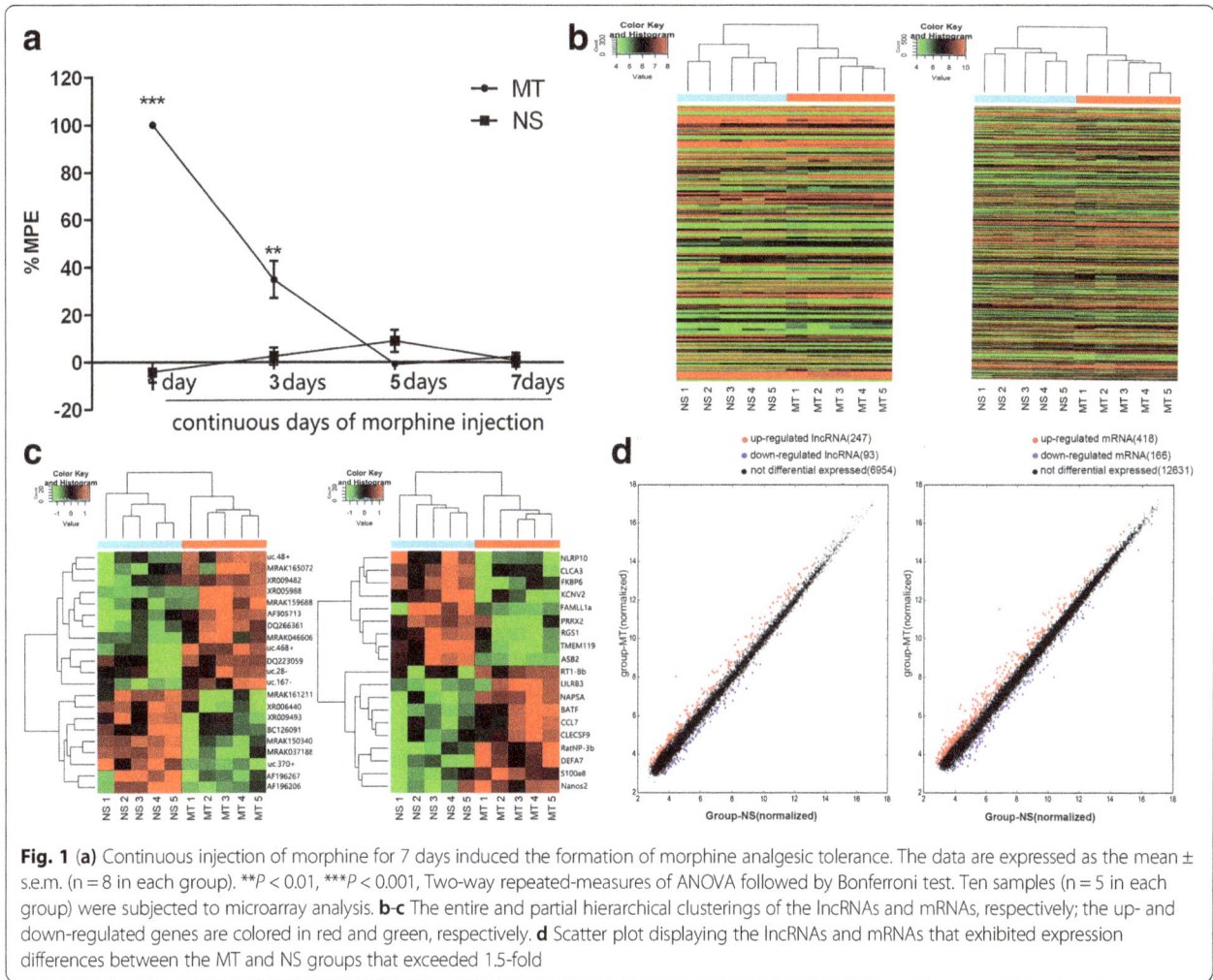

Fig. 1 (a) Continuous injection of morphine for 7 days induced the formation of morphine analgesic tolerance. The data are expressed as the mean ± s.e.m. (n = 8 in each group). **$P < 0.01$, ***$P < 0.001$, Two-way repeated-measures of ANOVA followed by Bonferroni test. Ten samples (n = 5 in each group) were subjected to microarray analysis. b-c The entire and partial hierarchical clusterings of the lncRNAs and mRNAs, respectively; the up- and down-regulated genes are colored in red and green, respectively. d Scatter plot displaying the lncRNAs and mRNAs that exhibited expression differences between the MT and NS groups that exceeded 1.5-fold

DElncRNAs regardless of their adjacent coding genes. According to the ceRNA analysis, we obtained an overview of the potential lncRNA/miRNA/mRNA interactions (Fig. 4a), and we then further identified several promising networks of lncRNA/miRNA/mRNA interactions (Fig. 4b), which included (MRAK161211, MRAK150340)/miR-219b/Tollip and XR_006440/(miR-365, let7)/(Usp31, Usp42, Clcn4−2) networks, and we used these networks to create functional annotations of the predicted target mRNAs by searching the Gene database. The results indicated that the predicted target mRNAs mainly functioned in the process of ubiquitinylation, the GRCP and TLR signaling pathways, and the modulations of transcription, translation and post-translational modification, and these functions might constitute the foundation of morphine tolerance.

Discussion

In the present study, we detected 136 DElncRNAs and 278 DEmRNAs overall and we found that compared with normal rats, DElncRNAs and DEmRNAs were present in the spinal cords of morphine-tolerant rats; GO and KEGG pathway analyses revealed that the potential functions of the DEmRNAs may be concentrated on the processes that are thought be involved in the formation of morphine tolerance; and the ceRNA analysis identified several potential lncRNA/miRNA/mRNA interaction networks that might modulate the development of morphine tolerance.

To identify as many DElncRNAs and DEmRNAs candidates as possible, we set the criteria at a log2 (fold change) > 1.5 and a P-value < 0.05 [30]. Next, we considered several criteria to select lncRNAs and mRNAs from our microarray data for validation. Firstly, we attempted to select the relevant candidates that might be related to our previous studies of morphine tolerance and miRNAs [11, 12]. Secondly, for validation, we chose the lncRNA candidates that exhibited higher fold changes and greater raw expression intensities and had adjacent mRNA that was related to morphine tolerance.

Among the DElncRNAs that we detected, XR_005988 exhibited the most significant up-regulation and was

Table 2 The detailed information of top 40 up-regulated and 40 down-regulated lncRNAs

Up-regulated lncRNAs	Fold change(MT/NS)	P-value	Down-regulated lncRNAs	Fold change(MT/NS)	P-value
XR_005988	12.34156	0.003685	AF196267	2.202529	0.012181
DQ266361	2.486278	0.000882	XR_009493	2.115125	0.019025
MRAK046606	2.367485	0.020344	MRAK150340	2.060765	0.000308
uc.167-	2.199281	0.002987	MRAK037188	1.956905	0.000066
uc.468+	2.137996	0.000249	XR_006440	1.952104	0.003301
XR_009482	2.065426	0.022224	AF196206	1.938910	0.015500
AF305713	2.052460	0.001121	BC126091	1.906750	0.020304
MRAK165072	2.020835	0.015095	uc.370+	1.900405	0.000477
MRAK159688	2.009110	0.008496	MRAK156916	1.879795	0.013478
uc.28-	1.957873	0.033513	XR_008800	1.872603	0.022847
DQ223059	1.911577	0.043779	MRAK077287	1.816863	0.000017
uc.48+	1.897821	0.005311	MRAK014088	1.773360	0.000324
XR_006726	1.887222	0.008923	MRAK161211	1.765669	0.014718
XR_009483	1.883845	0.020077	BC158785	1.742858	0.005583
MRAK013672	1.849562	0.027735	MRuc009dux	1.721422	0.014515
MRAK018927	1.848401	0.025469	MRAK135122	1.718807	0.009117
uc.482-	1.827252	0.000618	MRAK141001	1.690469	0.000352
MRAK138235	1.824250	0.005928	MRuc007nwi	1.688666	0.043028
uc.156-	1.810205	0.037932	uc.264-	1.687839	0.023742
XR_008353	1.802395	0.008201	EF088428	1.673345	0.001656
uc.462+	1.791152	0.001958	uc.363+	1.672870	0.011181
MRAK134839	1.770980	0.033987	BC169026	1.665411	0.007442
MRAK054291	1.760502	0.037076	MRAK008891	1.659204	0.018204
BC093392	1.758918	0.030404	MRAK135686	1.656007	0.005067
MRuc007cgx	1.756746	0.023148	MRAK051195	1.625373	0.000267
MRAK050995	1.742487	0.032134	BC097960	1.619298	0.003837
XR_009527	1.742256	0.022408	MRAK169397	1.617138	0.030259
uc.395-	1.733383	0.035051	MRAK046121	1.614043	0.005023
XR_005532	1.732123	0.042440	MRAK080238	1.594013	0.000840
uc.158-	1.723747	0.010144	BC061963	1.592978	0.002208
MRuc007jeg	1.722591	0.006501	MRAK013677	1.592863	0.000261
XR_008662	1.716865	0.020951	XR_009137	1.575140	0.014863
XR_008674	1.695926	0.047672	BC086373	1.561696	0.008523
S66184	1.680145	0.026505	MRAK083715	1.557152	0.004611
M81783	1.670161	0.011349	MRAK038897	1.555085	0.007252
MRAK083472	1.662885	0.008172	MRAK041309	1.554516	0.000067
XR_009489	1.660491	0.002298	MRAK147844	1.551990	0.000730
XR_008266	1.654757	0.012200	MRAK051810	1.549681	0.022164
uc.310-	1.653784	0.013204	uc.185+	1.545991	0.024361
uc.463-	1.651362	0.021613	BC079474	1.544677	0.000147

classified as a long intergenic non-coding RNA (lincRNA). Although we obtained no information about XR_005988 or its associated genes through searches of all types of gene databases, it is well known that lncRNAs account for the main portion of lncRNAs and exhibit the most substantial biological functions [31], which indicates that XR_005988 is still a promising lncRNA molecule for further study. Additionally, XR_

Table 3 The detailed information of top 30 up-regulated and 30 down-regulated mRNAs

Gene symbol	Description	Fold change(MT/NS)	P-value
Up-regulated genes			
RT1-Bb	RT1 class II, locus Bb	26.0600137	0.03123893
RatNP-3b	defensin RatNP-3 precursor	4.6945682	0.00237615
Lilrb3	leukocyte immunoglobulin-like receptor, subfamily B (with TM and ITIM domains), member 3	4.3359795	0.00815228
Defa7	alpha-defensin 7	4.2552547	0.00156229
Clecsf9	macrophage-inducible C-type lectin	3.4622832	0.01864872
Ccl7	chemokine (C-C motif) ligand 7	3.3728046	0.01483951
Sele	selectin, endothelial cell	3.3632425	0.03028204
Slpi	secretory leukocyte peptidase inhibitor	3.2118152	0.00024306
Lilrc2	leukocyte immunoglobulin-like receptor	3.1471364	0.01375120
V1rj4	vomeronasal 1 receptor, J4	2.9047312	0.03220865
Gja5	gap junction membrane channel protein alpha 5	2.8707048	0.02230140
Mmp9	matrix metallopeptidase 9	2.832538	0.02991875
Batf	basic leucine zipper transcription factor	2.7432184	0.00125327
S100a8	S100 calcium binding protein A8 (calgranulin A)	2.7009035	0.00561932
Birc3	baculoviral IAP repeat-containing 3	2.6968995	0.01058921
Bcl3	B-cell CLL/lymphoma 3	2.6847827	0.00419171
Ccr1	chemokine (C-C motif) receptor 1	2.5775393	0.00007731
Olr463	olfactory receptor 463 (predicted)	2.5772986	0.01425058
Np4	defensin NP-4 precursor	2.4883044	0.00271115
Grm2	glutamate receptor, metabotropic 2	2.4429944	0.00113554
Slpil2	antileukoproteinase-like 2	2.4380328	0.00066484
Cnn1	calponin 1	2.4269788	0.02918954
Olr139	olfactory receptor Olr139	2.4268332	0.01332394
Obp3	alpha-2u globulin PGCL4	2.3723118	0.03995990
Crisp4	cysteine-rich secretory protein 4	2.3633549	0.00810051
Olr1454_predicted	olfactory receptor 1454 (predicted)	2.3350625	0.00247670
Napsa	napsin A aspartic peptidase	2.2770041	0.00035275
Olr1374_predicted	olfactory receptor 1374 (predicted)	2.2313479	0.00040213
LOC497796	Ly49 inhibitory receptor-like	2.2302475	0.00022859
Slpil3	antileukoproteinase-like 3	2.2153032	0.00045886
Down-regulated genes			
Fam111a	hypothetical protein LOC499322	5.1287218	0.02433528
Kcnv2	"potassium channel, subfamily V, member 2"	2.8837136	0.00586212
Fkbp6	FK506 binding protein 6	2.8648794	0.00576975
Nlrp10	"NLR family, pyrin domain containing 10"	2.6101210	0.00386452
Rgs1	regulator of G-protein signaling 1	2.4933037	0.00327101
Ly49i8	Ly49 inhibitory receptor 8	2.3732515	0.01051908
Tmem119	transmembrane protein 119	2.3374630	0.00064129
Cldn14	"*Rattus norvegicus* claudin 14"	2.3184480	0.00751794
Dyrk1a	dual-specificity tyrosine-(Y)-phosphorylation regulated kinase 1A	2.2472669	0.00077705
Ckmt2	sarcomeric mitochondrial creatine kinase	2.2142101	0.00051314
Asb2	ankyrin repeat and SOCS box-containing protein 2	2.1709796	0.00039719
Art2b	ADP-ribosyltransferase 2b	2.1680042	0.00124959
LOC498335	similar to Small inducible cytokine B13 precursor (CXCL13)	2.1501415	0.00012158

Table 3 The detailed information of top 30 up-regulated and 30 down-regulated mRNAs *(Continued)*

Gene symbol	Description	Fold change(MT/NS)	P-value
Prrx2	paired related homeobox 2	2.1294428	0.01452534
LOC364773	aldo-keto reductase family 1, member C12	2.1023343	0.00302323
Cdkn2b	cyclin-dependent kinase inhibitor 2B (p15, inhibits CDK4)	2.0882944	0.00336651
Cd22	CD22 molecule	2.0855279	0.01215534
Nhlrc2	NHL repeat containing 2	2.0426710	0.00054605
Fcrls	Fc receptor-like S, scavenger receptor	2.0407116	0.00627688
Clca3	chloride channel calcium activated 3	2.0188429	0.01580260
Dntt	deoxynucleotidyltransferase, terminal	2.0019106	0.00547055
Grap2	GRB2-related adaptor protein 2	1.9900082	0.00968363
Thrsp	thyroid hormone responsive protein	1.9814822	0.02740488
Plek2	pleckstrin 2	1.9662998	0.00879852
Alox12	arachidonate 12-lipoxygenase	1.9121487	0.00631083
Tnfsf4	tumor necrosis factor (ligand) superfamily, member 4	1.8804698	0.00229007
Mpzl2	myelin protein zero-like 2	1.8783013	0.00003750
Prkag3	protein kinase, AMP-activated, gamma 3	1.8643095	0.00970172
Nr0b2	nuclear receptor subfamily 0, group B, member 2	1.8348501	0.00251892
Traf3ip3	TRAF3 interacting protein 3	1.8326037	0.02787730

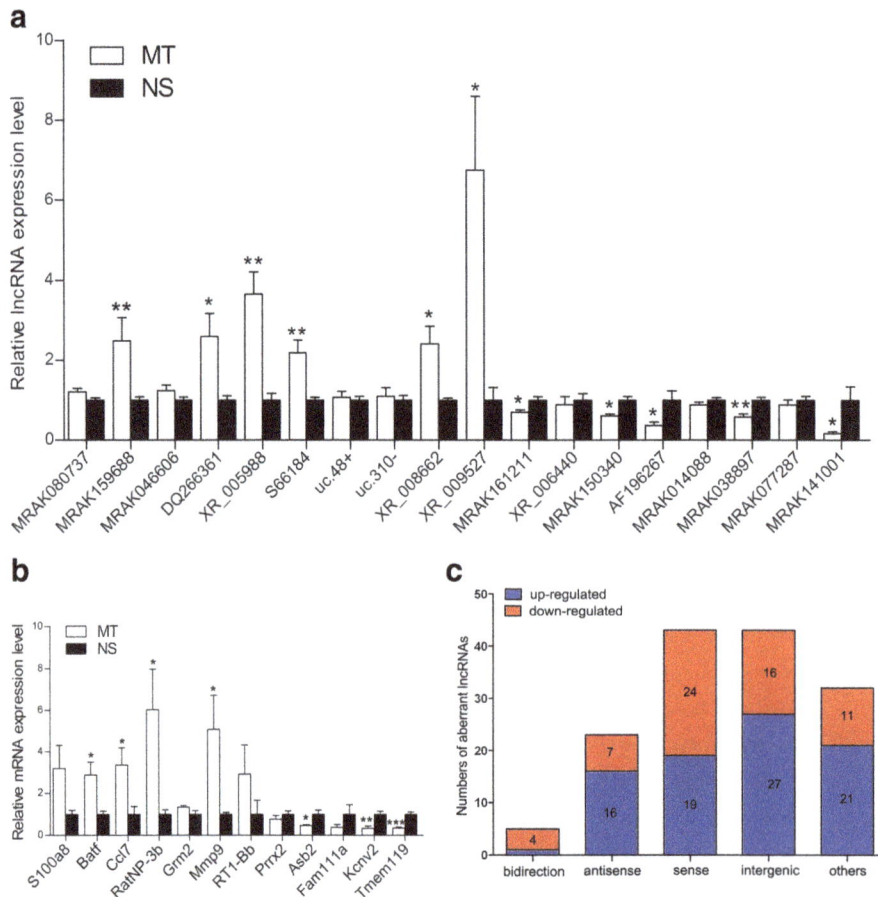

Fig. 2 RT-qPCR validation of eighteen deregulated lncRNAs (**a**) and twelve deregulated mRNAs (**b**) in the lumbar enlargements of both groups. Student's *t*-test. *$P < 0.05$, **$P < 0.01$, ***$P < 0.001$. Distribution of the various types of DElncRNAs. **c** Five classes (bidirectional lncRNAs, antisense lncRNAs, sense lncRNAs, intergenic lncRNAs and the other lncRNAs) were analyzed

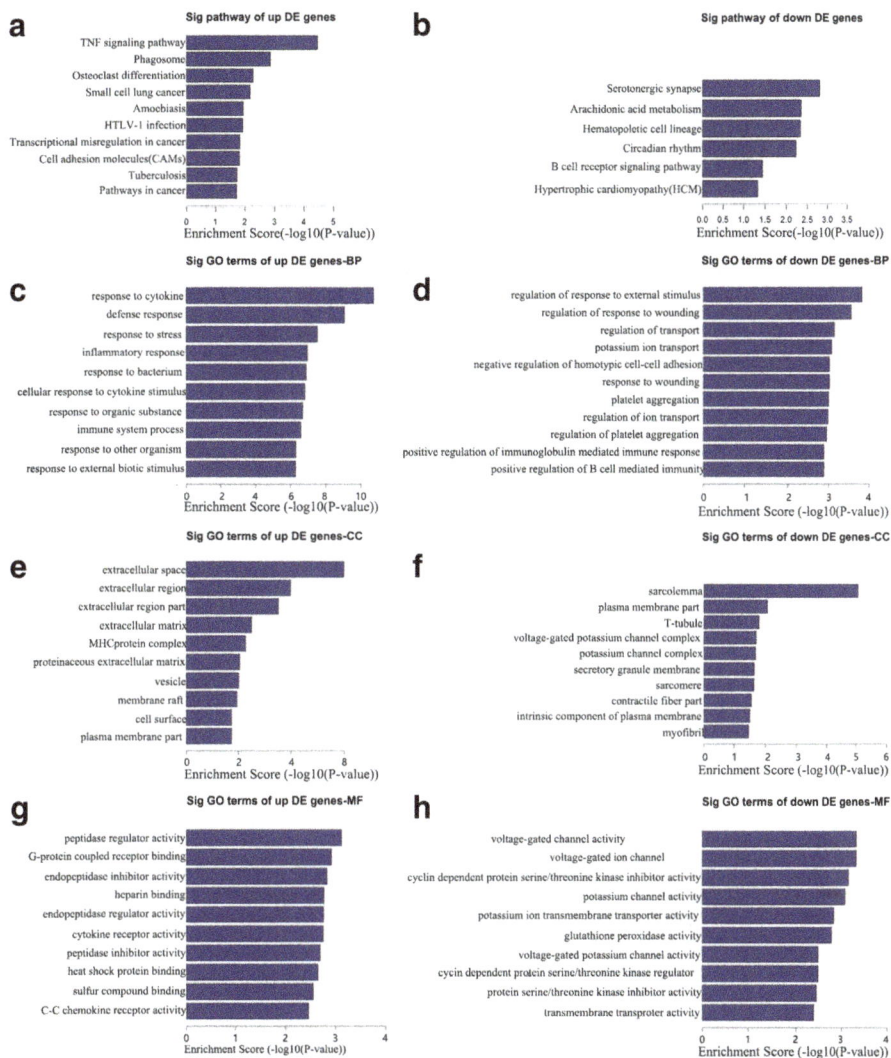

Fig. 3 Pathway analyses of the 176 up-regulated and 102 down-regulated mRNAs with fold changes > 1.5. **a** The significant pathways of the up-regulated genes in the MT group. **b** The significant pathways of the down-regulated genes in the MT group. The biological functions of the differentially expressed mRNAs with fold changes > 1.5 are listed. The significant biological processes (**c**) cellular components (**e**) and molecular functions (**g**) of the up-regulated mRNAs. The significant biological processes (**d**), cellular components (**f**) and molecular functions (**h**) of the down-regulated mRNAs

005988 might bind to some miRNAs according to the ceRNA analysis, which indicates its potential action as a ceRNA. Of course, additional in vivo and in vitro functional research is needed.

MRAK-159688, which was another up-regulated lncRNA identified in our study, is associated with the Fos gene and was named the Fos downstream transcript (FosDT) in a report from Mehta et al. [32] Mehta et al. reported that, in an ischemia/reperfusion model, FosDT interacts with the chromatin-modifying proteins Sin3a and co-repressor of the transcription factor REST (coR-EST) and subsequently represses REST-downstream genes. Moreover, other researchers have indicated that MOR is one of the downstream targets of REST and is negatively modulated by REST in specific neuronal cells [33, 34]. Therefore, the dysregulated MRAK-159688 might be involved in the development of morphine tolerance through interactions with REST.

Since the ceRNA hypothesis was proposed, it has been verified in some tumor diseases. For example, the FER1L4/miRNA106a-5p/PTEN pathway constitutes a novel regulatory pathway that is involved in the occurrence and progression of gastric cancer [35]. Currently, ceRNA analysis is a novel method for predicting the functions of lncRNAs. In our study, we found that several possible interacting pathways among ceRNAs exist, including the following: MRAK161211, MRAK150340/miR-219b/mRNAs (e.g., Tollip, and Ubqln4); XR_

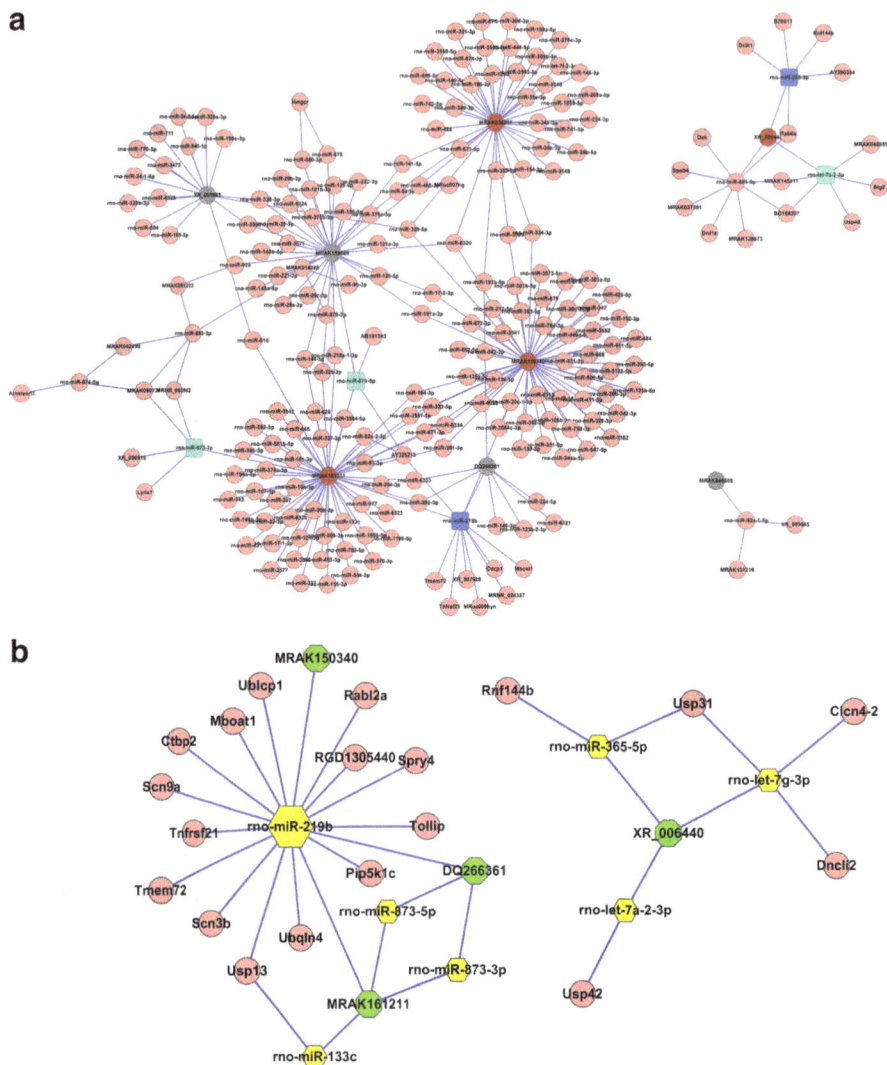

Fig. 4 ceRNA analyses indicated the potential lncRNA/miRNA/mRNA interactions. **a** The potential binding target miRNAs of the verified lncRNAs. The red nodes mean down-regulated lncRNAs, the gray nodes mean up-regulated lncRNAs, the blue squares mean down-regulated miRNAs we are interested in, the green squares mean up-regulated miRNA we are interested in, and the pink nodes mean the other miRNAs and mRNAs. **b** The lncRNA/miRNA/mRNA networks that we are interested in are displayed. The green nodes represent lncRNAs, the yellow pentagons represent miRNAs and the pink nodes represent mRNAs we forecasted

006440/miR-365, let7/mRNAs (e.g., Usp31, Usp42, Clcn4–2); and MRAK161211/miR-133/Usp13.

In our previous study, We have confirmed that miR-219-5p can attenuate morphine tolerance by targeting CaMKIIγ [12]. Furthermore, other researchers have also reported that miR-219 is down-regulated following the continuous application of morphine and can regulate NMDA receptor signaling [36]. Whereas in the present study, we predicted that miR-219b, rather than miR-219-5p, would exert this function. Recent research about miR-219 has mainly concentrated on the functions of miR-219-5p, and the other isoform, i.e., miR-219b, has not been studied in detail. However, on the one hand, we identified miR-219-5p and miR-219b, which have

both previously been reported to function in the suppression of the proliferation, migration and invasion of cells [37, 38]. On the other hand, when we forecasted the downstream targets of miR-219b, we found that their functions were mainly related to the ubiquitination process, G-protein-coupled receptors, alterations in ion channels, and Toll-like receptor signaling pathway regulation, and these function are all involved in the mechanisms of morphine tolerance. Therefore, given its possible target mRNAs, miR-219b is likely to be a new target related to morphine tolerance.

Toll-interacting protein (Tollip) is a potential downstream target of miR-219b and can modulate the expression of the Toll-like receptor (TLR) via its action as an endogenous inhibitor and regulate the IL-1β-induced activation of NF-κB; thus, miR-219b plays an inhibitory role in inflammatory signaling [39, 40]. Previous studies have demonstrated that the TLR-mediated activation of glial cells and TLR4-mediated NF-κB activation might influence the development of morphine tolerance [41, 42]. Therefore, further study is required and we presumed that the MRAK150340, MRAK161211 (i.e., down-regulated lncRNAs)/miRNA-219b/Tollip interaction network potentially functions in morphine tolerance.

On the one hand, previous studies have suggested that let-7 can suppress the expression of MOR [43], and our previous results suggest miR-365 can modulate morphine tolerance by targeting the beta-arrestin 2 protein [11]. On the other hand, Law et al [44] reported that opioid receptor agonists (such as morphine) promote the ubiquitylation of scaffold proteins and thereby change the expression pattern of the receptor signaling pathway. In the present study, the potential downstream genes that we predicted, i.e., Usp31 and Usp42, are both ubiquitylation-related genes. Therefore, the XR_006440/ (let7, miR-365)/(Usp31, Usp42) pathway is likely to be responsible for the formation of morphine tolerance. Moreover, there are other interested candidates other than the validated lncRNAs and mRNAs, and further studies will be needed.

In summary, although our study is preliminary and lacks additional functional experiments, our research has revealed that hundreds of lncRNAs, especially XR_005988 and MRAK159688, are differentially expressed in the spinal cords of morphine-tolerant rats. Further ceRNA analysis revealed that several possible lncRNA/ miRNA/mRNA interaction networks exist, and among these networks, the (MRAK150340, MRAK161211)/ miR-219b/Tollip network holds the most potential for further studies.

Abbreviations

ceRNA: competitive endogenous; DElncRNA: Differentially expressed lncRNA; DEmRNA: Differentially expressed mRNA; GO: Gene Ontology; KEGG: Kyoto Encyclopedia of Genes and Genomes; lncRNA: Long noncoding RNA; MOR: μ-opioid receptor; MT: Morphine tolerance; NCBI: National Center for Biotechnology Information; ncRNA: Noncoding RNA; NS: Normal saline; Tollip: Toll-interacting protein

Funding

This work was supported by grants from the National Natural Science Foundation of China (81471135 and 81771206) and the Natural Science Funds for Distinguished Young Scholars of Hunan Province (2017JJ1036).

Authors' contributions

WZ designed the experiments. JS, JW, JH, CL, YP and WZ performed experiments and analyzed data; JS, QG and WZ drafted the manuscript and finished the final vision of the manuscript. All authors read and approved the final manuscript.

Competing interests

The authors declare that they have no competing interests.

References

1. Ko SW, Wu LJ, Shum F, Quan J, Zhuo M. Cingulate NMDA NR2B receptors contribute to morphine-induced analgesic tolerance. Molecular brain. 2008; 1:2. https://doi.org/10.1186/1756-6606-1-2.
2. Smith SMSMT. Analgesic tolerance to opioids. Pain. 2001;9
3. Song Z, Guo Q, Zhang J, Li M, Liu C, Zou W. Proteomic analysis of PKCgamma-related proteins in the spinal cord of morphine-tolerant rats. PLoS One. 2012;7:e42068. https://doi.org/10.1371/journal.pone.0042068.
4. Song Z, Zou W, Liu C, Guo Q. Gene knockdown with lentiviral vector-mediated intrathecal RNA interference of protein kinase C gamma reverses chronic morphine tolerance in rats. The journal of gene medicine. 2010;12: 873–80. https://doi.org/10.1002/jgm.1514.
5. Bali KK, Kuner R. Noncoding RNAs: key molecules in understanding and treating pain. Trends Mol Med. 2014;20:437–48. https://doi.org/10.1016/j.molmed.2014.05.006.
6. Brianna Marie Lutz AB, Tao Y-X. Noncoding RNAs:new players in chronic pain. Anesthesiology. 2014;121:409–17.
7. Hwang CK, Wagley Y, Law PY, Wei LN, Loh HH. MicroRNAs in opioid pharmacology. Journal of neuroimmune pharmacology : the official journal of the Society on Neuroimmune Pharmacology. 2012;7:808–19. https://doi.org/10.1007/s11481-011-9323-2.
8. Massmo Barbierato MZ, Skaper SD, Giusti P. MicroRNAs: emerging role in the endogenous μ opioid system. CNS Neurol Disord Drug Targets. 2015;14: 239–50.
9. Wu Q, Zhang L, Law PY. Long-term morphine treatment decreases the association of mu-opioid receptor (MOR1) mRNA with polysomes through miRNA23b. Mol Pharmacol. 2009;75:744–50. https://doi.org/10.1124/mol.108.053462.
10. Wu Q, Hwang CK, Zheng H, et al. MicroRNA 339 down-regulates mu-opioid receptor at the post-transcriptional level in response to opioid treatment. FASEB journal : official publication of the Federation of American Societies for Experimental Biology. 2013;27:522–35. https://doi.org/10.1096/fj.12-213439.
11. Wang J, Xu W, Zhong T, Song Z, Zou Y, Ding Z, Guo Q, Dong X, Zou W. miR-365 targets beta-arrestin 2 to reverse morphine tolerance in rats. Sci Rep. 2016;6:38285. https://doi.org/10.1038/srep38285.
12. Wang J, Xu W, Shao J, He Z, Ding Z, Huang J, Guo Q, Zou W. miR-219-5p targets CaMKIIgamma to attenuate morphine tolerance in rats. Oncotarget. 2017;8:28203–14. https://doi.org/10.18632/oncotarget.15997.
13. Brosnan CA, Voinnet O. The long and the short of noncoding RNAs. Curr Opin Cell Biol. 2009;21:416–25. https://doi.org/10.1016/j.ceb.2009.04.001.
14. Wilusz JE, Sunwoo H, Spector DL. Long noncoding RNAs: functional surprises from the RNA world. Genes Dev. 2009;23:1494–504. https://doi.org/10.1101/gad.1800909.
15. Yarmishyn AA, Kurochkin IV. Long noncoding RNAs: a potential novel class of cancer biomarkers. Front Genet. 2015;6:1–10. https://doi.org/10.3389/fgene.2015.00145.
16. Briggs JA, Wolvetang EJ, Mattick JS, et al. Mechanisms of long non-coding RNAs in mammalian nervous system development, plasticity, disease, and evolution. Neuron. 2015;88:861–77. https://doi.org/10.1016/j.neuron.2015.09.045.
17. Jiang SD, Lu J, Deng ZH, Li YS, Lei GH. Long noncoding RNAs in osteoarthritis. Joint, bone, spine : revue du rhumatisme. 2017;84:553–6. https://doi.org/10.1016/j.jbspin.2016.09.006.
18. Zhao X, Tang Z, Zhang H, et al. A long noncoding RNA contributes to neuropathic pain by silencing Kcna2 in primary afferent neurons. Nat Neurosci. 2013;16:1024–31. https://doi.org/10.1038/nn.3438.

19. Wang S, Xu H, Zou L, Xie J, Wu H, Wu B, Yi Z, Lv Q, Zhang X, Ying M, Liu S, Li G, Gao Y, Xu C, Zhang C, Xue Y, Liang S. LncRNA uc.48+ is involved in diabetic neuropathic pain mediated by the P2X3 receptor in the dorsal root ganglia. Purinergic signalling. 2016;12:139–48. https://doi.org/10.1007/s11302-015-9488-x.

20. Jiang BC, Sun WX, He LN, Cao DL, Zhang ZJ, Gao YJ. Identification of lncRNA expression profile in the spinal cord of mice following spinal nerve ligation-induced neuropathic pain. Mol Pain. 2015;11:43. https://doi.org/10.1186/s12990-015-0047-9.

21. Li G, Jiang H, Zheng C, Zhu G, Xu Y, Sheng X, Wu B, Guo J, Zhu S, Zhan Y, Lin W, Ding R, Zhang C, Liu S, Zou L, Yi Z, Liang S. Long noncoding RNA MRAK009713 is a novel regulator of neuropathic pain in rats. Pain. 2017;158:2042–52. https://doi.org/10.1097/j.pain.0000000000001013.

22. Peng H, Zou L, Xie J, Wu H, Wu B, Zhu G, Lv Q, Zhang X, Liu S, Li G, Xu H, Gao Y, Xu C, Zhang C, Wang S, Xue Y, Liang S. lncRNA NONRATT021972 siRNA decreases diabetic neuropathic pain mediated by the P2X3 receptor in dorsal root ganglia. Mol Neurobiol. 2017;54:511–23. https://doi.org/10.1007/s12035-015-9632-1.

23. Salmena L, Poliseno L, Tay Y, et al. A ceRNA hypothesis: the Rosetta stone of a hidden RNA language? Cell. 2011;146:353–8. https://doi.org/10.1016/j.cell.2011.07.014.

24. Tay Y, Rinn J, Pandolfi PP. The multilayered complexity of ceRNA crosstalk and competition. Nature. 2014;505:344–52. https://doi.org/10.1038/nature12986.

25. Zimmermann M. Ethical guidelines for investigations of experimental pain in conscious animals. Pain. 1983;16:109–10.

26. Wei Yu J-XH, Xiao-Jun X, et al. The development of morphine tolerance and dependence in rats with chronic pain. Brain Res. 1997;756:141–6.

27. Zou W, Song Z, Guo Q, Liu C, Zhang Z, Zhang Y. Intrathecal lentiviral-mediated RNA interference targeting PKCgamma attenuates chronic constriction injury-induced neuropathic pain in rats. Hum Gene Ther. 2011;22:465–75. https://doi.org/10.1089/hum.2010.207.

28. Lin SP, Ye S, Long Y, et al. Circular RNA expression alterations are involved in OGD/R-induced neuron injury. *Biochemical and biophysical research communications*. 2016;471:52–6. https://doi.org/10.1016/j.bbrc.2016.01.183.

29. Jia H, Osak M, Bogu GK, Stanton LW, Johnson R, Lipovich L. Genome-wide computational identification and manual annotation of human long noncoding RNA genes. RNA. 2010;16:1478–87. https://doi.org/10.1261/rna.1951310.

30. Huang JF, Guo YJ, Zhao CX, Yuan SX, Wang Y, Tang GN, Zhou WP, Sun SH. Hepatitis B virus X protein (HBx)-related long noncoding RNA (lncRNA) down-regulated expression by HBx (Dreh) inhibits hepatocellular carcinoma metastasis by targeting the intermediate filament protein vimentin. Hepatology. 2013;57:1882–92. https://doi.org/10.1002/hep.26195.

31. Derrien T, Johnson R, Bussotti G, et al. The GENCODE v7 catalog of human long noncoding RNAs: analysis of their gene structure, evolution, and expression. Genome Res. 2012;22:1775–89. https://doi.org/10.1101/gr.132159.111.

32. Mehta SL, Kim T, Vemuganti R. Long Noncoding RNA FosDT promotes ischemic brain injury by interacting with REST-associated chromatin-modifying proteins. The Journal of neuroscience : the official journal of the Society for Neuroscience. 2015;35:16443–9. https://doi.org/10.1523/JNEUROSCI.2943-15.2015.

33. Kim CS, Hwang CK, Choi HS, et al. Neuron-restrictive silencer factor (NRSF) functions as a repressor in neuronal cells to regulate the opioid receptor gene. J Biol Chem. 2004;279:46464–73. https://doi.org/10.1074/jbc.M403633200.

34. Kim CS, Choi HS, Hwang CK, et al. Evidence of the neuron-restrictive silencer factor (NRSF) interaction with Sp3 and its synergic repression to the mu opioid receptor (MOR) gene. Nucleic Acids Res. 2006;34:6392–403. https://doi.org/10.1093/nar/gkl724.

35. Xia T, Chen S, Jiang Z, et al. Long noncoding RNA FER1L4 suppresses cancer cell growth by acting as a competing endogenous RNA and regulating PTEN expression. Sci Rep. 2015;5 https://doi.org/10.1038/srep13445.

36. Kocerha J, Faghihi MA, Lopez-Toledano MA, et al. MicroRNA-219 modulates NMDA receptor-mediated neurobehavioral dysfunction. Proc Natl Acad Sci U S A. 2009;106:3507–12. https://doi.org/10.1073/pnas.0805854106.

37. Long JMQ, Wuren Q, et al. MiR-219-5p inhibits the growth and metastasis of malignant melanoma by targeting BCL-2. Biomed Res Int. 2017;2017:9032502. https://doi.org/10.1155/2017/9032502.

38. Zhao CLX, Han B, et al. Gga-miR-219b targeting BCL11B suppresses proliferation, migration and invasion of Marek's disease tumor cell MSB1. Sci Rep. 2017;7:4247. https://doi.org/10.1038/s41598-017-04434-w.

39. Didierlaurent A, Brissoni B, Velin D, et al. Tollip regulates proinflammatory responses to interleukin-1 and lipopolysaccharide. Mol Cell Biol. 2006;26:735–42. https://doi.org/10.1128/MCB.26.3.735-742.2006.

40. Capelluto DG. Tollip: a multitasking protein in innate immunity and protein trafficking. Microbes Infect. 2012;14:140–7. https://doi.org/10.1016/j.micinf.2011.08.018.

41. Hutchinson MR, Bland ST, Johnson KW, et al. Opioid-induced glial activation: mechanisms of activation and implications for opioid analgesia, dependence, and reward. TheScientificWorldJOURNAL. 2007;7:98–111. https://doi.org/10.1100/tsw.2007.230.

42. Bai L, Zhai C, Han K, et al. Toll-like receptor 4-mediated nuclear factor-kappaB activation in spinal cord contributes to chronic morphine-induced analgesic tolerance and hyperalgesia in rats. Neuroscience bulletin. 2014;30:936–48. https://doi.org/10.1007/s12264-014-1483-7.

43. He Y, Wang ZJ. Let-7 microRNAs and opioid tolerance. Front Genet. 2012;3:1–7. https://doi.org/10.3389/fgene.2012.00110.

44. Law PY, Loh HH, Wei LN. Insights into the receptor transcription and signaling: implications in opioid tolerance and dependence. Neuropharmacology. 2004;(47):300–11. https://doi.org/10.1016/j.neuropharm.2004.07.013.

9

Plasticity changes in forebrain activity and functional connectivity during neuropathic pain development in rats with sciatic spared nerve injury

Tzu-Hao Harry Chao[1], Jyh-Horng Chen[2] and Chen-Tung Yen[1]* ⓘ

Abstract

Neuropathic pain is a major worldwide health problem. Although central sensitization has been reported in well-established neuropathic conditions, information on the acute brain activation patterns in response to peripheral nerve injury is lacking. This study first mapped the brain activity in rats immediately following spared nerve injury (SNI) of the sciatic nerve. Using blood-oxygenation-level-dependent functional magnetic resonance imaging (BOLD-fMRI), we observed sustained activation in the bilateral insular cortices (ICs), primary somatosensory cortex (S1), and cingulate cortex. Second, this study sought to link this sustained activation pattern with brain sensitization. Using manganese-enhanced magnetic resonance imaging (MEMRI), we observed enhanced activity in the ipsilateral anterior IC (AIC) in free-moving SNI rats on Days 1 and 8 post-SNI. Furthermore, enhanced functional connectivity between the ipsilateral AIC, bilateral rostral AIC, and S1 was observed on Day 8 post-SNI. Chronic electrophysiological recording experiments were conducted to confirm the tonic neuronal activation in selected brain regions. Our data provide evidence of tonic activation-dependent brain sensitization during neuropathic pain development and offer evidence that the plasticity changes in the IC and S1 may contribute to neuropathic pain development.

Keywords: Neuropathic pain, Chronic pain, Plasticity, fMRI, MEMRI, Unit recording, Insular cortex

Introduction

Chronic pain is a major health problem affecting up to 20% of the global population. Although acute pain can be properly managed, most people with chronic pain do not have access to adequate pain relief [1]. Among the most difficult cases are those with neuropathic pain initiated by primary lesions or dysfunction in the somatosensory nervous system.

Many studies have investigated brain sensitization in well-established chronic neuropathic conditions. Higher tonic activity or sensitization to peripheral and central stimuli have been detected in many brain regions of humans with such conditions [2–4] and in animal models [5, 6]. Central sensitization at the spinal level was reported as activation-dependent and possibly induced by repeated stimulation [7–10]. In addition, some brain areas have been reported as having similar activation-dependent sensitization properties [11, 12]. By investigating the responses to nerve injury in the peripheral and central brain areas, previous studies have detected the early onset of ectopic discharge in injured nerve fibers [13–15]. One study of trigeminal neuropathic pain in rats showed that nerve injury induced the long-term enhancement of activity in trigeminal ganglion neurons and thalamic neurons [15]. Although strong and continuous brain activation is a possible cause of brain sensitization during neuropathic pain development, experimental data are lacking.

Practically, the study of brain reactions to severe peripheral nerve injury in human subjects is difficult. Therefore, human subjects for such studies are usually selected from people who have received a diagnosis of chronic pain [2, 16, 17]. By contrast, using animal

* Correspondence: ctyen@ntu.edu.tw
[1]Department of Life Science, National Taiwan University, No. 1, Sec. 4, Roosevelt Rd, Taipei 10617, Taiwan
Full list of author information is available at the end of the article

models enables researchers to study brain reactions immediately following peripheral nerve injury [18, 19].

To observe the dynamic changes of brain activity during nerve injury and the possible sustained activation, we designed a nerve cutting device for inducing spared nerve injury (SNI) in the functional magnetic resonance imaging (fMRI) chamber. We used a recoverable anesthesia protocol during blood-oxygenation-level-dependent (BOLD)-fMRI [20–23], and thus could observe neuropathic pain development in the same rat after the BOLD-fMRI experiment.

To correlate the sustained activation with long-term plasticity changes in the brain, we used manganese-enhanced magnetic resonance imaging (MEMRI) to detect plasticity changes in brain activity on Days 1 and 8 after SNI. Recent studies have used MEMRI to assess brain activity in free-moving animals [24–26]. Mn^{2+} can accumulate in excitable cells via voltage-gated Ca^{2+} channels and ionotropic glutamate receptors [27–29], thereby enhancing the signal in T1 contrast images and providing high spatial resolution mapping of brain activations.

Finally, we confirmed the tonic neuronal activations observed in the MR with direct neuronal recording in the insula cortices (ICs) and primary somatosensory cortex (S1). Sustained brain activations induced by SNI were observed by resting fMRI and electrophysiological recording, and these changes correlated with long-term brain plasticity in rats with neuropathic pain.

Methods

Animal subjects
This study used 55 male and 15 female Sprague Dawley rats (National Laboratory Animal Center, Taipei, Taiwan) aged 8–10 weeks and weighing 250–350 g. Vendor health reports indicated that the rats were free of known viruses, bacteria, and parasites. All the rats were housed pairwise in type 3H cages under a 12-h dark/light cycle with an environmental temperature of 22 °C. The cages were filled with C-grade Sani-Chips and food and water were available ad libitum. All experimental procedures were approved by the Institutional Animal Care and Use Committee of National Taiwan University. This study adhered to the guidelines established by the Council of Agriculture of Taiwan for the experimental use of animals.

Seven rats (four males and three females) were used in the BOLD-fMRI study of dynamic brain activity changes during nerve injury. In the MEMRI study of long-lasting changes of brain activity in free-moving rats, the sham ($n = 10$) and SNI ($n = 10$) groups were observed on Day 1 and additional independent sham (n = 10) and SNI ($n = 8$) groups were observed on Day 8 after SNI surgery. At both time points, the naïve ($n = 10$) group was observed. Three additional rats were used to validate the adverse behavioral effects of Mn^{2+}

injection. All the rats in the MEMRI study were male. The electrophysiological study observed the following four groups of rats: ipsilateral rostral anterior insular cortex (RAIC), contralateral RAIC, contralateral anterior cingulate cortex (ACC), and contralateral S1. Each group consisted of three rats. Because skull growth in male rats is relatively rapid, which likely affects electrophysiological recording quality, we used female rats in our electrophysiological study. The BOLD-fMRI data (mixed-gender) revealed similar result when comparing with the electrophysiological data (female only) in acute response to the nerve injury. The basic design of this study is diagrammatically shown in the Fig. 1.

SNI neuropathic pain model
The SNI neuropathic pain model used followed the one established by Decosterd and Woolf [30]. Briefly, rats were anesthetized using ketamine hydrochloride (75 mg/kg, i.p.) and xylazine (15 mg/kg i.p.). An incision was made on the left lateral thigh to expose the sciatic nerve at the level of its trifurcation into the sural, tibial, and common peroneal nerves. The left tibial and common peroneal nerves were tightly ligated using 6.0 silk. Two to 4 mm of the distal nerve was removed and the sural nerve was left intact. After nerve transection, we sutured the muscle by using 6.0 silk and closed the incision with 4.0 silk. Subsequently, the rats were recovered from anesthesia and their allodynia behavior was observed 8 days later. The rats received lincomycin (Lita Pharmacy Co. Ltd., Taiwan; 30 mg/kg/day, i.m. for 3 days) after the surgery to prevent infection.

Behavioral testing
To determine whether the rats had developed neuropathic pain after SNI surgery, we assessed the mechanical allodynia through von Frey filament (North Coast Medical, Inc., Morgan Hill, USA) testing. All behavioral tests were conducted between12:00 and 18:00. Each rat was tested in a $21 \times 12 \times 14$-cm transparent cage after 5 min of habituation. For the mechanical sensitivity test, each rat was placed in a cage with an open wire mesh base and given 15 min for habituation. A set of eight von Frey filaments (0.4, 0.6, 1, 2, 4, 6, 8, and 15 g of bending force) were used to apply increasing amounts of bending force to the lateral plantar surface (the lateral plantar surface was innervated by the sural nerve). If the rat briskly withdrew or one or both of its hind paws flinched, the final lightest von Frey hair force was applied in the subsequent test. Six stimulations were applied in each session and the withdrawal patterns were recorded to determine the 50% withdrawal threshold according to the formula established by Chaplan [31].

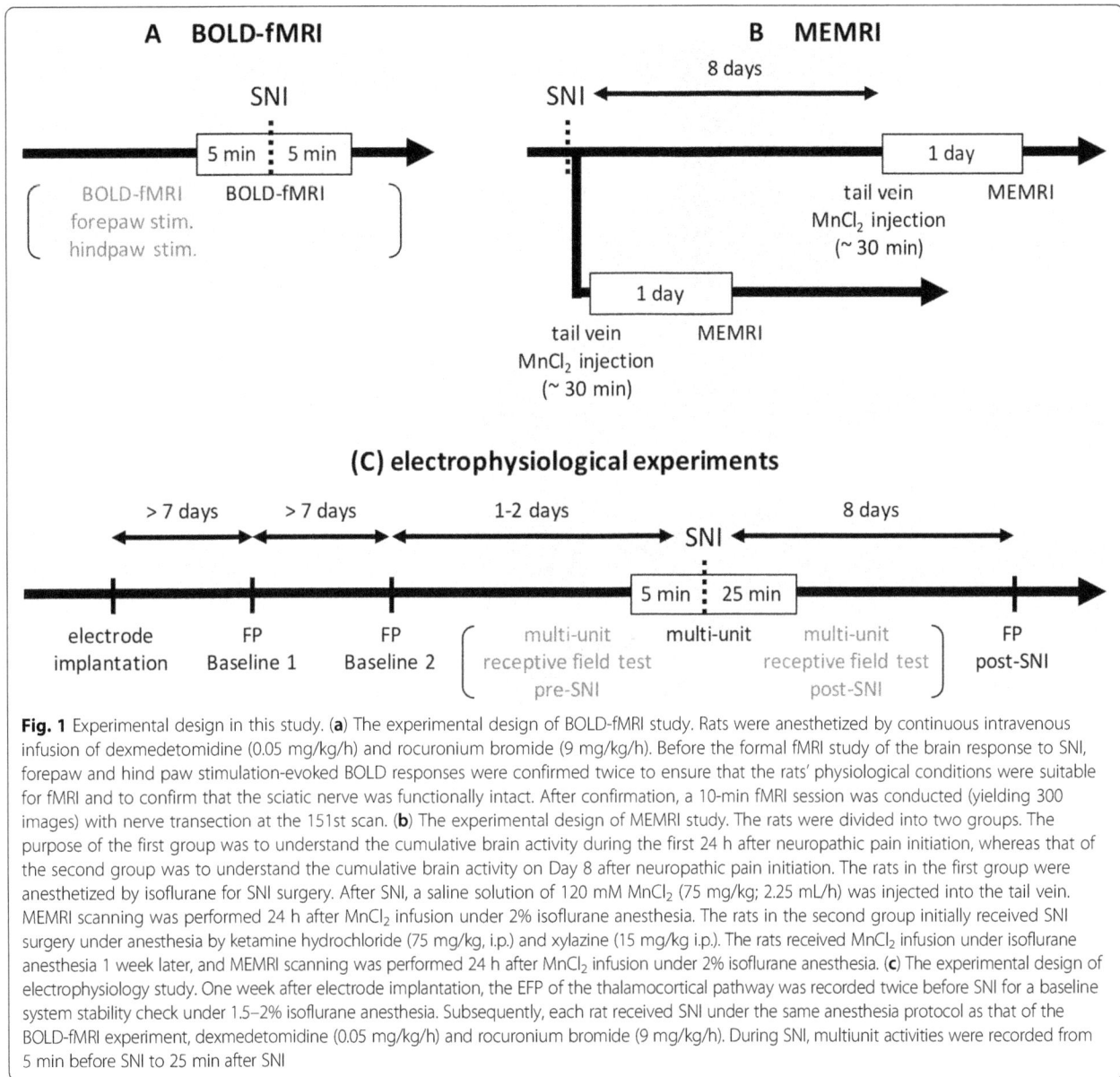

Fig. 1 Experimental design in this study. (**a**) The experimental design of BOLD-fMRI study. Rats were anesthetized by continuous intravenous infusion of dexmedetomidine (0.05 mg/kg/h) and rocuronium bromide (9 mg/kg/h). Before the formal fMRI study of the brain response to SNI, forepaw and hind paw stimulation-evoked BOLD responses were confirmed twice to ensure that the rats' physiological conditions were suitable for fMRI and to confirm that the sciatic nerve was functionally intact. After confirmation, a 10-min fMRI session was conducted (yielding 300 images) with nerve transection at the 151st scan. (**b**) The experimental design of MEMRI study. The rats were divided into two groups. The purpose of the first group was to understand the cumulative brain activity during the first 24 h after neuropathic pain initiation, whereas that of the second group was to understand the cumulative brain activity on Day 8 after neuropathic pain initiation. The rats in the first group were anesthetized by isoflurane for SNI surgery. After SNI, a saline solution of 120 mM $MnCl_2$ (75 mg/kg; 2.25 mL/h) was injected into the tail vein. MEMRI scanning was performed 24 h after $MnCl_2$ infusion under 2% isoflurane anesthesia. The rats in the second group initially received SNI surgery under anesthesia by ketamine hydrochloride (75 mg/kg, i.p.) and xylazine (15 mg/kg i.p.). The rats received $MnCl_2$ infusion under isoflurane anesthesia 1 week later, and MEMRI scanning was performed 24 h after $MnCl_2$ infusion under 2% isoflurane anesthesia. (**c**) The experimental design of electrophysiology study. One week after electrode implantation, the EFP of the thalamocortical pathway was recorded twice before SNI for a baseline system stability check under 1.5–2% isoflurane anesthesia. Subsequently, each rat received SNI under the same anesthesia protocol as that of the BOLD-fMRI experiment, dexmedetomidine (0.05 mg/kg/h) and rocuronium bromide (9 mg/kg/h). During SNI, multiunit activities were recorded from 5 min before SNI to 25 min after SNI

Rat preparation for BOLD-fMRI study

All fMRI experiments were conducted between 12:00 and 18:00. To identify the tonic brain activation after nerve injury, SNI surgery was performed inside the MRI bore during fMRI acquisition. A specially designed nerve transection device consisting of a guidance head and needle with fork tips was implanted before MRI scanning (Fig. 2). Each rat was initially anesthetized using 5% isoflurane and orotracheally intubated for mechanical ventilation. Under isoflurane anesthesia (3.5% mixed with a 30% oxygen and 70% nitrogen mixture), a 1-cm-long incision was made on the lateral surface of the left thigh and the biceps femoris muscle was dissected to expose the sural, common peroneal, and tibial sciatic nerve branches. The nerve transection device was

inserted at the caudal surface of the left thigh, through the muscle layers to the sciatic nerve branches. After the guidance head had been removed, the fork tips were exposed. A stainless steel wire was threaded through the needle and the common peroneal and tibial nerves were fixed to the notches of the fork tips by using a slack noose (Fig. 2). Finally, lidocaine hydrochloride jelly USP 2% (Akorn, Inc., Lake Forest, IL, USA) was applied on the wound carefully without contacting sciatic nerve branches, and then the incision was temporally sutured. This setup enabled the cutting of the common peroneal and tibial nerves during fMRI scanning by pulling on the stainless steel wire. In addition, a set of bipolar stainless steel electrodes each was inserted between the second and third digits of both the left forepaw and left

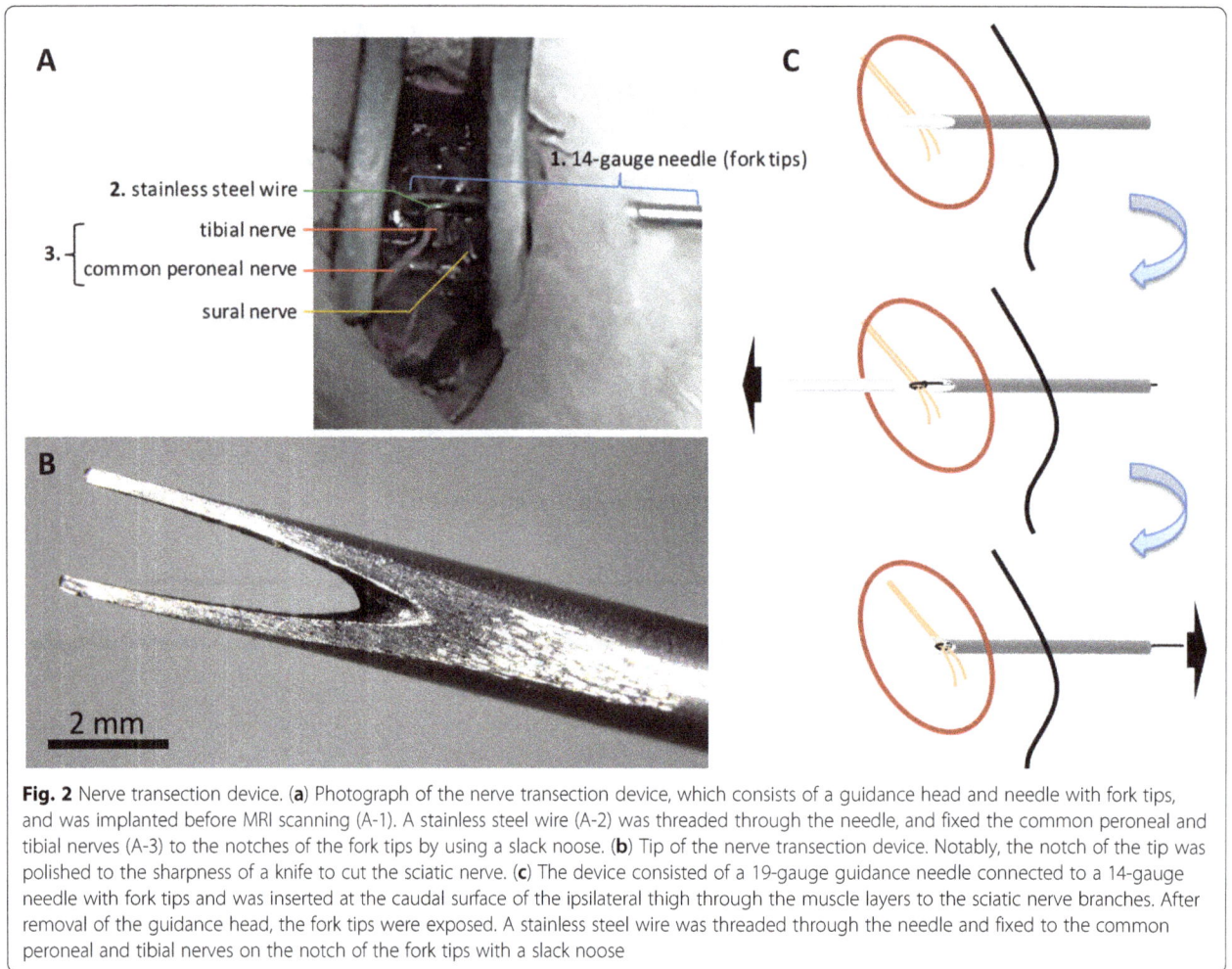

Fig. 2 Nerve transection device. (**a**) Photograph of the nerve transection device, which consists of a guidance head and needle with fork tips, and was implanted before MRI scanning (A-1). A stainless steel wire (A-2) was threaded through the needle, and fixed the common peroneal and tibial nerves (A-3) to the notches of the fork tips by using a slack noose. (**b**) Tip of the nerve transection device. Notably, the notch of the tip was polished to the sharpness of a knife to cut the sciatic nerve. (**c**) The device consisted of a 19-gauge guidance needle connected to a 14-gauge needle with fork tips and was inserted at the caudal surface of the ipsilateral thigh through the muscle layers to the sciatic nerve branches. After removal of the guidance head, the fork tips were exposed. A stainless steel wire was threaded through the needle and fixed to the common peroneal and tibial nerves on the notch of the fork tips with a slack noose

hind paw, respectively. We used forepaw stimulation to induce S1 BOLD responses to confirm the suitability of the conditions for fMRI testing and hind paw stimulation to induce S1 BOLD responses in order to confirm that our settings did not damage the sciatic nerve before nerve transection.

BOLD-fMRI acquisition

Imaging data were acquired using a 7-Tesla scanner with a 30-cm diameter bore (Bruker Biospec 7030 USR, Ettlingen, Germany). The system was equipped with a 670-mT/m (175-μs rise time) actively shielded gradient system (Bruker, BGA12-S) with an inner diameter of 116 mm. A receive-only four-element phased array coil was used to receive radio frequency signals and a linear volume coil was used to transmit radio frequency pulses.

After the rats were secured on the MRI holder, a bolus of dexmedetomidine (0.5 mL; 0.025 mg/kg; Dexdormitor, Orion, Espoo, Finland) was injected into the tail vein. Fifteen minutes after the bolus injection, continuous intravenous infusion of dexmedetomidine (1 mL/h; 0.05 mg/kg/h) and rocuronium bromide (9 mg/kg/h;

Sigma–Aldrich, St. Louis, USA) was initiated and the isoflurane concentration was adjusted to 0.5–1% for the entire scanning period [20]. During the MRI scan, rectal temperature was measured using a thermocouple (Model 1025, SA Instruments, Inc., New York, USA) and maintained at 36.5–37.5 °C by using a circulated hot water bed. The end-tidal CO_2 level was continuously monitored and adjusted to between 2.5–3.0%, a range previously calibrated for invasive blood gas sampling under identical conditions to ensure normal physiological conditions in the rat.

The anatomical images were acquired using a rapid acquisition with relaxation enhancement (RARE) sequence (10 coronal slices, thickness = 1 mm, repetition time (TR) = 2500 ms, echo time (TE) = 33 ms, matrix size = 160 × 160, field-of-view (FOV) = 25 × 25 mm, average = 2). To improve the magnetic field homogeneity of the acquisition site, local shimming of the brain area was performed before BOLD-fMRI data acquisition (Mapshim; Bruker BioSpin). BOLD-fMRI data were acquired using single-shot gradient-echo echo planar imaging (EPI) (10 coronal slices, thickness = 1 mm, TR = 2000 ms, TE =

22 ms, matrix size = 80 × 80, FOV = 25 × 25 mm, bandwidth = 200 kHz).

For standard forepaw and hind paw stimulation fMRI, an isolated stimulator (S48 Square Pulse Stimulator with Stimulus Isolation Unit, Grass Technologies, West Warwick, USA) was used to deliver constant current pulses to the stainless steel electrodes for forepaw and hind paw stimulation. These constant current pulses consisted of monophasic square wave electrical stimulation (0.5 ms, 2 mA, 9 Hz) divided into five blocks of 20-s on/off cycles. Ten dummy scans and ten additional baseline images were acquired, yielding 120 images in total. After the nerve was confirmed to be healthy, a 10-min fMRI session was conducted (yielding 300 images) with nerve transection at the 151st scan. After fMRI, we sutured the muscle using 6.0 silk and closed the incision with 4.0 silk. Subsequently, the rat was recovered from anesthesia and paralysis by receiving atipamezole hydrochloride (3 mg/kg, i.v.; ANTISEDAN, Orion, Espoo, Finland), for the reversal of the sedative and analgesic effects of dexmedetomidine, and sugammadex sodium (4–8 mg/kg, i.v.; Merck Sharp & Dohme Corp., Kenilworth, NJ, USA), for the reversal of the paralytic effect of rocuronium, and its allodynia behavior was tested 8 days later. The rat was administered lincomycin (Lita Pharmacy Co. Ltd., Taichung, Taiwan; 30 mg/kg/day, i.m. for 3 days) after scanning to prevent infection.

Electrode implantation and recordings

Each rat was anesthetized with sodium pentobarbital (50 mg/kg, i.p.), of which supplemental doses (16 mg/kg, i.p.) were administered when necessary. Craniotomies were performed to expose the brain surface vertical to the recording sites. The coordinates for implantation were as follows: (1) mediodorsal thalamic nucleus, medial part (MDM): right or left: 0.4 mm, posterior: 3 mm, depth: 4.5–5.5 mm; (2) rostral anterior insular cortex (RAIC): right or left: 3–5 mm, anterior: 1–4 mm, depth: 5–6 mm; (3) mediodorsal thalamic nucleus, lateral part (MDL): right: 1.2 mm, posterior: 2.5 mm, depth: 4.5–5.5 mm; (4) anterior cingulate cortex (ACC): right: 1.2 mm, anterior: 1–4 mm, depth: 2.5–3 mm; (5) ventral posterolateral thalamic nucleus (VP): right: 2.8–3.3 mm, posterior: 2.8 mm, depth: 5.5–6.5 mm; (6) S1: right: 1–3 mm, posterior: 1 mm, depth: 600–800 μm. For thalamus recording, we used a bundled microarray electrode consisting of seven tungsten microwires with diameters of 35 μm bare and 50 μm insulated (#100211; California Fine Wire) in a 29-G guide tube [32]. The electrode set for the cortex recording consisted of eight stainless steel microwires arranged in a 2–3-mm-wide array. Each rat was implanted with a matching thalamic and cortical target set (MDM-RAIC, MDL-ACC and VP-SI) of electrodes. Only those rats with good evoked cortical responses under low intensity (below 10 μA) thalamic stimulation were used to ensure the accuracy of the cortical implantations. Four stainless steel screws were set in each rat's skull to serve as anchors for the electrode sets. To ground the array electrodes, a copper wire was fixed around the anchoring screw positioned at the occipital bone. When all the electrodes were in place, the surface of the skull was covered with dental cement and the wound was sutured. Lincomycin hydrochloride (30 mg/kg, i.m.) was administered to prevent infection.

After recovering for 1 week, single unit activities were recorded while SNI surgery was conducted. Multiple-channel cortical unit activities were transmitted to a multichannel acquisition processor system (MAP, Plexon, Dallas, USA) through a connecting cable. To record single unit activities while performing SNI surgery, the anesthesia procedure and surgery preparation were identical to those of the fMRI experiment. Single unit recording was initiated 5 min before sciatic nerve transection and continued for 25 min after transection, resulting in 30 min of continuous recording. Spike signals were amplified 7000–32,000-fold, bandpass-filtered at 250 Hz–13 kHz, and digitized at 40 kHz. Well isolated single unit activities in one area were linearly added for a quantitative estimation of the activity change in that cortical area.

Animal preparation for MEMRI study

Two groups of rats underwent MEMRI testing. The first group was tested to determine the cumulative brain activity during the first 24 h of neuropathic pain initiation, whereas the second group was tested to determine the brain activity on Day 8 following neuropathic pain initiation.

Each rat in the first group was initially anesthetized using 5% isoflurane and maintained in a state of anesthesia by using 3.5% isoflurane. SNI surgery was performed as previously described. Following SNI or sham surgery, a solution of 120 mM $MnCl_2$ in saline (75 mg/kg; 2.25 mL/h; $MnCl_2$-$4H_2O$, Sigma–Aldrich, St. Louis, USA) was injected into the tail vein. The $MnCl_2$ injection protocol followed that of a previous study [33]. During surgery, each rat's body temperature was maintained at 36.5–37.5 °C by using a feedback-controlled heating pad. After surgery, each rat was administered lincomycin (30 mg/kg/day, i.m. for 3 days) to prevent infection. MEMRI scanning was performed 24 h after $MnCl_2$ infusion and each rat's allodynia behavior was observed on Days 3 and 8 after scanning.

Following our previous study, each rat in the second group underwent initial SNI or sham surgery under ketamine hydrochloride anesthesia (75 mg/kg, i.p.) and xylazine (15 mg/kg i.p.) [34]. Lincomycin (30 mg/kg/day, i.m. for 3 days) was administered after surgery and all rats were tested for allodynia behavior 1 week later. As previously described, rats in which neuropathic pain was observed were administered MnCl$_2$ infusion under isoflurane anesthesia and MEMRI scanning was performed 24 h later.

MEMRI acquisition

Imaging data were acquired using the 7-Tesla scanner. The receive-only four-element-phased array coil and linear volume coil were used to receive radio frequency signals and transmit radio frequency pulses, respectively. Each rat was initially anesthetized by 5% isoflurane mixed with oxygen and maintained in a state of anesthesia under 2% isoflurane during scanning. The T1-weighted images were acquired using a RARE sequence (30 coronal slices, thickness = 0.7 mm, TR = 870 ms, TE = 8.4 ms, matrix size = 160 × 160, FOV = 25 × 25 mm, average = 16). During scanning, each rat's respiration rate was monitored using a pressure sensor placed below the abdomen. A reading within the range of 40–60 breath/min signified stability. Rectal temperature was measured using a thermocouple and maintained at 36.5–37.5 °C by using a circulated hot water bed.

Image processing and analysis

Statistical parametric maps were generated using the SPM version 8 (www.fil.ion.ucl.ac.uk/spm). All raw images were enlarged by a factor of ten to correlate the image dimensions to human data, thereby facilitating the use of SPM, which was developed for use on humans. For the fMRI data, EPI images obtained from a single session were realigned and resliced to their averaged image to minimize movement artifacts. The realigned images were further coregistered to the average image between subjects. Subsequently, these images were smoothed using a Gaussian kernel with a full width at half maximum (FWHM) of 8 mm (in the space of the enlarged images) to reduce white noise and blur the images. Individual statistical maps were plotted using a general linear model with a hemodynamic response function. A 0.0078-Hz high-pass filter was applied to remove slow signal drift. Group analysis of individual statistical maps was conducted using a single sample t test. The significant BOLD response was determined by an individual voxel threshold of $P < .02$ with a cluster size threshold of 23 continuous voxels (volume = 2.25 mm^3). According to the AlphaSim procedure [35], this threshold combination provides a probability of false-positive clusters within the brain area of $P < .05$.

In the MEMRI data, the images of each subject were coregistered together and the average image from the coregistered images served as the template image. Subsequently, all MEMRI images were coregistered to the template image again and these fine-aligned images were smoothed using a Gaussian kernel with a FWHM of

3 mm (in the space of the enlarged images). The extra brain area was then removed. Statistical parametric maps were generated and one-way analysis of variance (ANOVA) was performed to compare the groups for differences. Grand mean scaling and global normalization scaling were used and an absolute threshold masking of 0 was applied to exclude the extra brain area from the analysis. Significance was determined by an individual voxel threshold of $P < .05$ with a cluster size threshold of 60 continuous voxels (volume = 1.025 mm^3). According to the AlphaSim procedure [35], this threshold combination provides a probability of false positive clusters within the brain area of $P < .03$. The colors of significant areas in statistical maps were encoded from statistical t values. Warm and cold colors indicate increases and decreases in BOLD (or MEMRI) signals, respectively.

Resting-State fMRI Data Analysis Toolkit V1.6 (http://restfmri.net/forum/index.php) was used to conduct functional connectivity analysis of the fMRI data. For fMRI data acquired before and after SNI, EPI images acquired within the first 4 min (first 120 images) and final 4 min (final 120 images) of the 10-min fMRI session were used to generate correlation maps of the pre- and post-SNI groups, respectively. All preprocessed image series were detrended and bandpass-filtered (0.01–0.08 Hz) before the functional connectivity analysis. The correlation maps were transformed into z-statistical parametric maps using REST, and the pre- and post-SNI groups were compared by conducting a paired t test with SPM. The multiple regression analysis function in SPM was used for functional connectivity analysis of the MEMRI images. To determine the brain areas with functional connections to specific regions of interest (ROIs), the inter-subject variability of neural activities in selected ROIs were used as the regressor. These activities were quantified and normalized based on the following equation: average signal intensity within an ROI/average signal intensity of the entire brain.

Statistical analysis

All data are expressed as the mean ± standard error. A P value of <.05 was considered statistically significant. Brain activity in the sham and SNI groups was compared by conducting an independent two-sample t test. The results of the hind paw withdrawal threshold for both groups were compared through one-way repeated measures ANOVA and Tukey's post hoc multiple comparison.

Results

Immediate functional brain changes after spared nerve injury surgery

To analyze the acute brain responses to nerve transection and determine the sustained activated brain areas possibly related to neuropathic pain development, we developed a nerve transection device for conducting SNI inside the MRI machine (Fig. 2). Before the formal fMRI experiment of the brain responses to SNI, forepaw and hind paw stimulation–evoked BOLD responses were obtained to confirm the rat's physiological condition and the healthiness of the sciatic nerve, with the nerve transection devise implanted, respectively. The robust and identical S1 BOLD responses to forepaw stimulation indicated that the rats' physiological conditions were suitable for the fMRI experiment. The S1 BOLD responses to hind paw stimulation indicated that each rat's sciatic nerve was functionally intact before SNI (Fig. 3).

Transection of the left tibial and common peroneal nerves produced significant positive BOLD responses in the medial thalamus, hypothalamus, and S1 hind limb area (S1HL) contralateral to the injured nerve, and cingulate cortex (CC) and RAICs bilaterally. Significant negative BOLD responses were also found in the bilateral caudate putamen (CPu) (Fig. 4A). Moreover, examining each ROI, the increases in the BOLD signal in the bilateral ICs and contralateral S1HL area were continuously enhanced throughout the acquisition period after nerve transection (more than 5 min); the CC exhibited a sustained low level of activation; whereas the CPu showed a robust transient negative BOLD response. The auditory cortex (Aud), selected as a negative control, didn't show significant response during the nerve transection (Fig. 5).

Multi-channel, multiple single unit recording experiments were performed in a separate series of experiment outside the MR chamber to independently examine the neuronal responses in selected forebrain regions to nerve transection. These brain regions included the bilateral RAIC, S1HL and ACC. The locations of the recording sites are shown in Fig. 6. The multiunit recording of the responses to nerve transection in the bilateral RAIC and S1HL area confirmed the sustained enhancement of neural activity (more than 20 min after transection) in both brain regions (Fig. 7).

After fMRI, the rats recovered from anesthesia. The 50% withdrawal threshold of the ipsilateral hind paw was tested on day 3 and day 8 after the fMRI experiment. The thresholds were significantly lower on day 3 and day 8 when comparing with pre-experiment baseline (Fig. 8). This indicated our newly designed

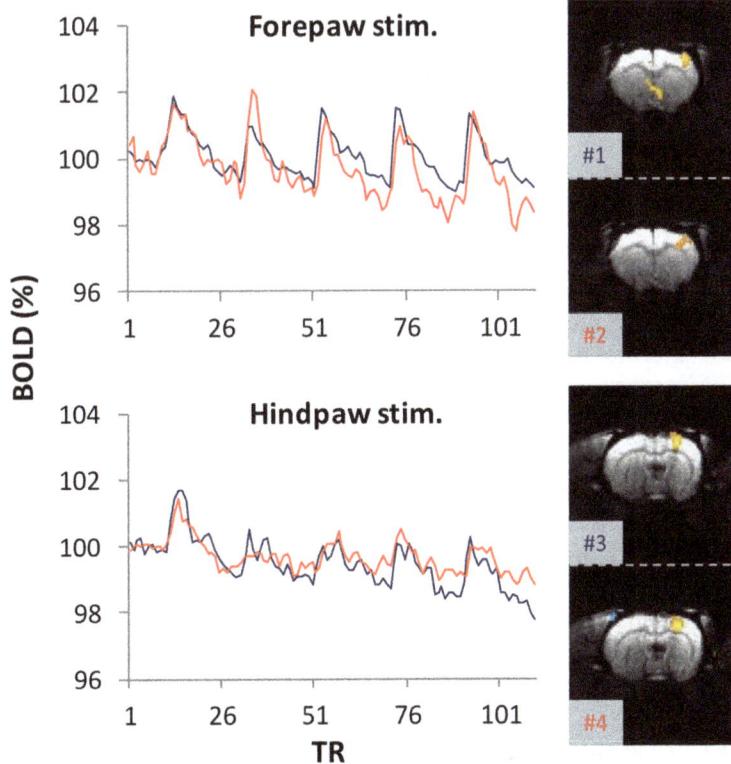

Fig. 3 Represented results of fMRI checkpoints before the formal study. Before the fMRI investigation of the brain responses to SNI nerve transection, we used the S1 BOLD response to forepaw stimulation to confirm whether the experimental conditions were suitable for fMRI scanning (upper panel). Subsequently, we used the S1 BOLD response to hind paw stimulation to verify whether the sciatic nerve was intact after implantation of the nerve transection device (lower panel). In the represented data, the S1 forepaw and hind paw areas exhibited consistent spatial and temporal responses to forepaw and hind paw stimulation, respectively, among the successive scans. #1–4 indicate the scan order. TR stands for the repetition time for each acquisition, which was 2 s in the current study

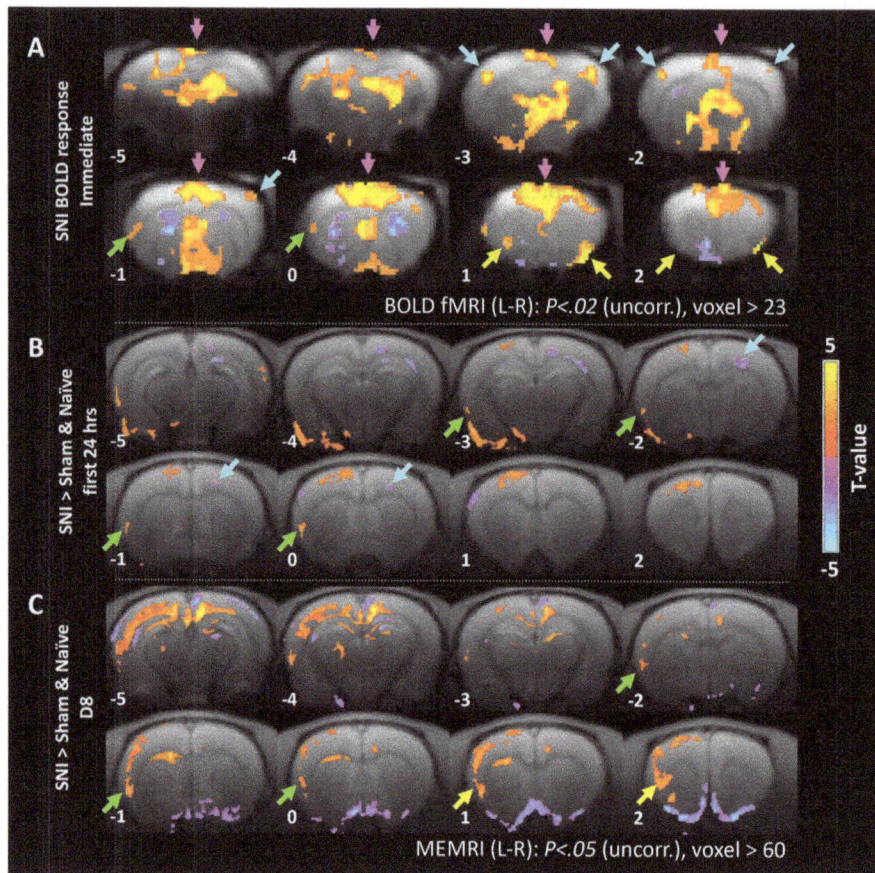

Fig. 4 Functional brain images at various time points after SNI. In each sub-figure, statistical t-maps are shown in 8 consecutive coronal slices of the rat brain, 1 mm each, from the most caudal level (5 mm caudal to the bregma, upper-left corner) to the most rostral (2 mm rostral to the bregma, lower-right). (**a**) Brain responses to SNI surgery during fMRI scanning. Positive BOLD responses are shown in the S1HL area (blue arrows), CC (purple arrows), and RAIC (yellow arrows) ($n = 7$, four males and three females). (**b**) MEMRI voxel-wise comparison of brain activity between the SNI ($n = 10$), sham ($n = 10$), and naïve ($n = 10$) rats on Day 1 after SNI surgery. The SNI group exhibited reduced activity in the S1 contralateral to the injured hind limb (blue arrows) and increased activity in the ipsilateral AIC (green arrows). (**c**) MEMRI voxel-wise comparison of brain activity between the SNI ($n = 10$), sham ($n = 8$), and naïve ($n = 10$) rats on Day 8 after SNI surgery. The SNI group exhibited increased activity in the RAIC and AIC (yellow and green arrows, respectively). The SNI and sham groups respectively shown in (**b**) and (**c**) were independent. Note Robust RAIC activation induced immediately after SNI (yellow arrow in **a**). The enhanced RAIC activity was maintained over 8 days (green arrows in **c**)

nerve cutting device did successfully produced SNI rats.

The significantly enhanced activity immediately after SNI in the RAIC raised the question whether a change in the RAIC functional connectivity network occurred. The EPI images acquired within the first 4 min and the final 4 min of the fMRI experiments were used to generate correlation maps of the pre- and post-SNI groups, respectively. The correlation maps seeded in the contralateral RAIC (the RAIC ROI is shown in Fig. 9a) were transformed into z-statistical parametric maps for comparison between the pre- and post-SNI groups. We found that the functional connections between the contralateral RAIC, contralateral S1, and ipsilateral AIC were enhanced immediately after SNI (Fig. 9b). Upon using the ipsilateral AIC cluster as the ROI to observe the signal time course during the fMRI experiment, we

found that the ipsilateral AIC exhibited sustained activation immediately after SNI (Fig. 9c). These data imply that the sustained activities in the ipsilateral AIC observed during the MEMRI experiment may have started at the time point immediately after SNI.

Subacute changes of functional brain activities and connectivity probed with MEMRI 1 day and 8 day after SNI

In addition to using BOLD-fMRI to study the acute brain responses to nerve transection, we used MEMRI to study the 24-h cumulative brain activity on Day 1 after SNI surgery (Fig. 1b). We found reduced activity in the contralateral S1HL area and enhanced activity in the ipsilateral AIC in the SNI surgery group compared to the naïve and the sham surgery groups (Fig. 4b). To determine whether these brain activity changes would be long-term, we conducted MEMRI to study the brain

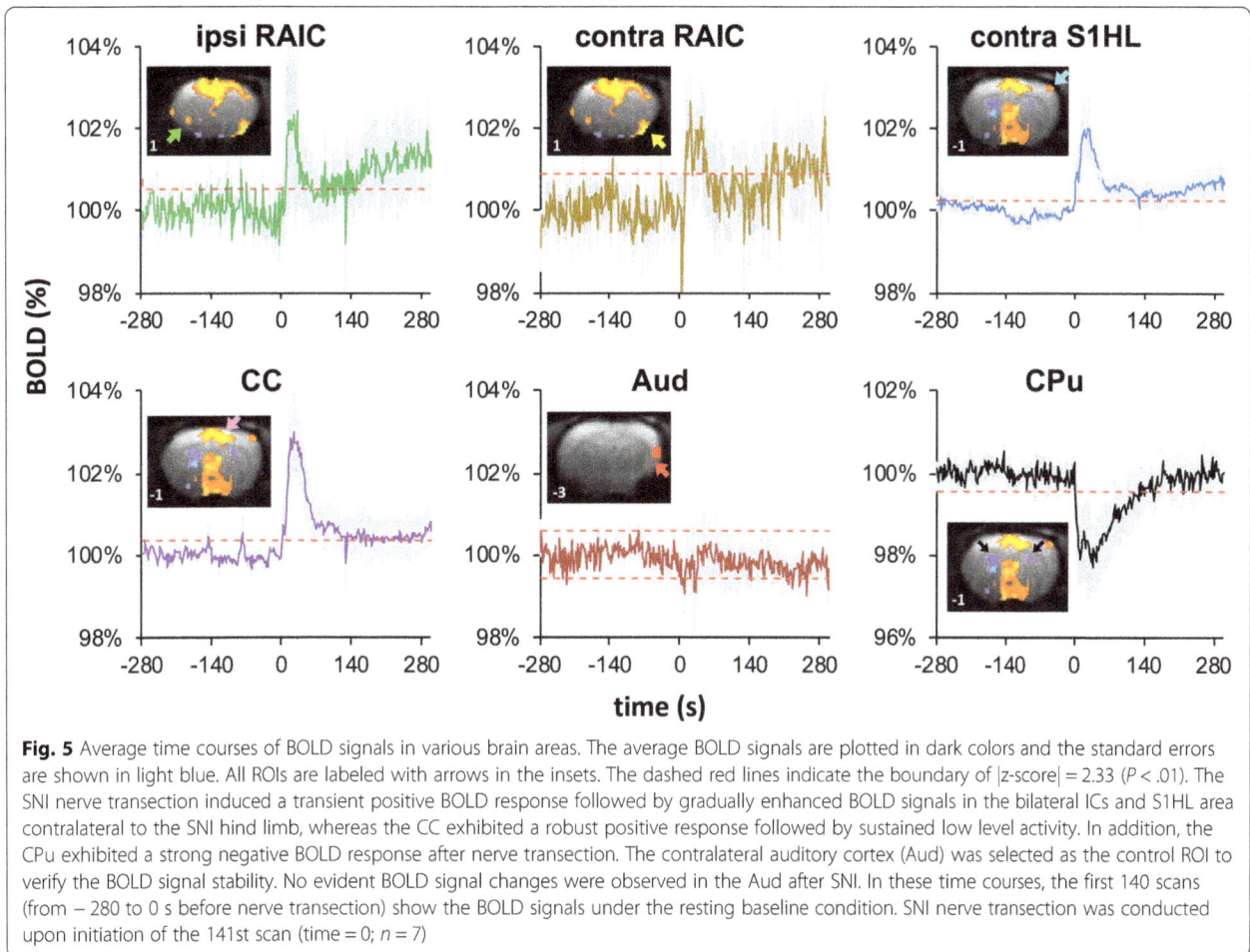

Fig. 5 Average time courses of BOLD signals in various brain areas. The average BOLD signals are plotted in dark colors and the standard errors are shown in light blue. All ROIs are labeled with arrows in the insets. The dashed red lines indicate the boundary of |z-score| = 2.33 (*P* < .01). The SNI nerve transection induced a transient positive BOLD response followed by gradually enhanced BOLD signals in the bilateral ICs and S1HL area contralateral to the SNI hind limb, whereas the CC exhibited a robust positive response followed by sustained low level activity. In addition, the CPu exhibited a strong negative BOLD response after nerve transection. The contralateral auditory cortex (Aud) was selected as the control ROI to verify the BOLD signal stability. No evident BOLD signal changes were observed in the Aud after SNI. In these time courses, the first 140 scans (from − 280 to 0 s before nerve transection) show the BOLD signals under the resting baseline condition. SNI nerve transection was conducted upon initiation of the 141st scan (time = 0; *n* = 7)

activity on Day 8 after SNI surgery. We found ipsilateral AIC and RAIC activities in the SNI group were higher than their counter parts of the sham group (Fig. 4c) on the Day 8. The MEMRI results showed that only in ipsilateral AIC and RAIC, there were long-term changes. Activities in the S1HL area and CC were not significantly changed on day 1 and day 8 after SNI surgery (Fig. 4b and c); in contrast with the fMRI results (Fig. 4a) and unit recording results (Fig. 7) immediately after SNI surgery. These data showed that SNI surgery induced sustained activation in the IC, and the enhanced activity lasted for at least 8 days.

The observation of a continuous increase in ipsilateral AIC activity after SNI surgery implies that long-term plasticity changes may be triggered within the ipsilateral AIC-related networks. To determine how the ipsilateral AIC interacted with the other brain areas in the SNI neuropathic pain rats, we used the MEMRI images acquired on Day 8 after surgery to extract the ipsilateral AIC activity of various subjects and used these quantified activities as regressors to search for other brain areas with synchronized activity fluctuations. The ROI of the ipsilateral AIC was defined as the area of significant

activation in the statistical map in Fig. 4C (SNI > sham and naïve, Day 8) that overlapped within the anatomical AIC region. The green area in Fig. 10A represents the seeding ROI. We found significant cooperation between the ipsilateral AIC versus bilateral RAIC and S1HL area contralateral to the side with nerve injury in the SNI rats (Fig. 10b and c), consistent with our fMRI data (Fig. 9b). This functional correlation was not observed among the sham rats (Fig. 10c); however, although the ipsilateral AIC activity was significantly higher in the SNI rats than the sham rats (*P* = .0038), the contralateral S1HL activity was similar in both groups (Fig. 10d), indicating that under similar somatosensory input conditions, the ipsilateral AIC exhibited an increase in sensory-related activity only in the SNI rats.

We performed a regression analysis using the signal fluctuations extracted from significant clusters in the ipsilateral RAIC area in Fig. 4c (SNI > sham and naïve, D8). The yellow area in Fig. 11a denotes the seeding ROI. We observed a positive correlation between the ipsilateral RAIC and superficial layer of the ACC and prelimbic areas (Fig. 11b). Notably, the ipsilateral RAIC correlated strongly with the bilateral locus coeruleus

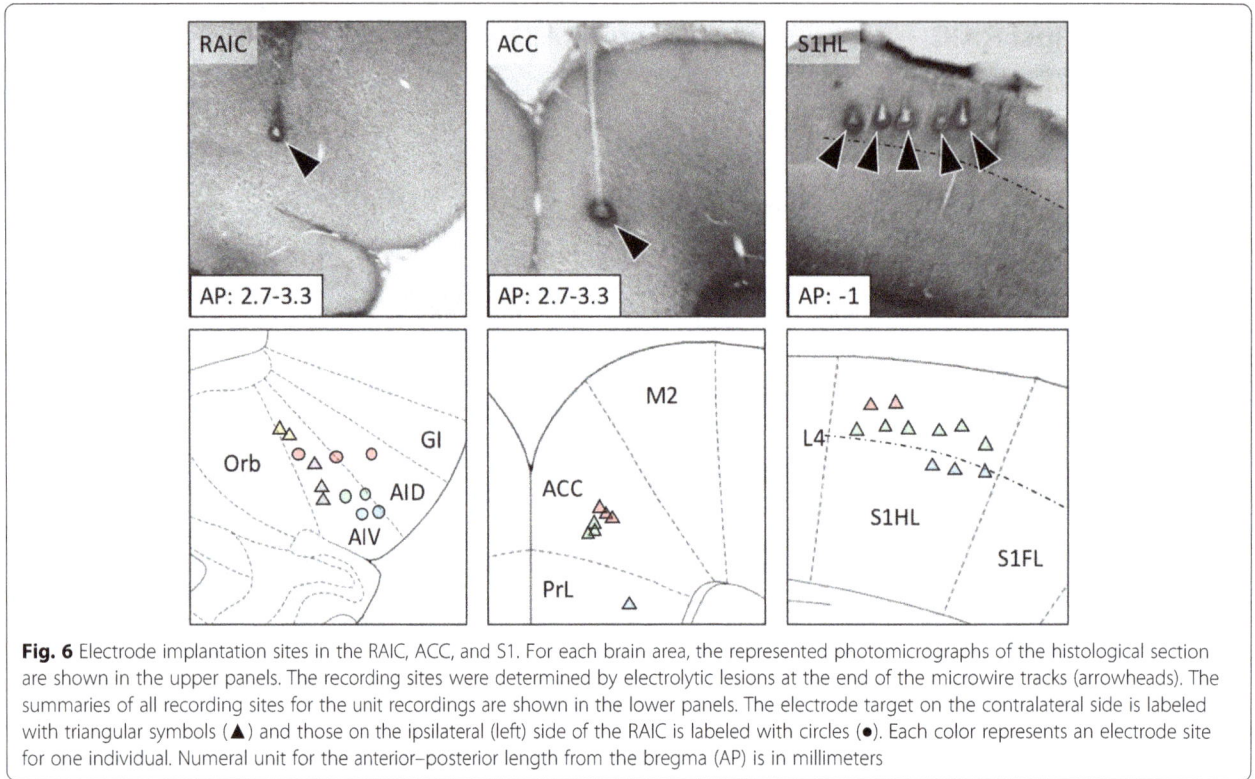

Fig. 6 Electrode implantation sites in the RAIC, ACC, and S1. For each brain area, the represented photomicrographs of the histological section are shown in the upper panels. The recording sites were determined by electrolytic lesions at the end of the microwire tracks (arrowheads). The summaries of all recording sites for the unit recordings are shown in the lower panels. The electrode target on the contralateral side is labeled with triangular symbols (▲) and those on the ipsilateral (left) side of the RAIC is labeled with circles (●). Each color represents an electrode site for one individual. Numeral unit for the anterior–posterior length from the bregma (AP) is in millimeters

(LC) (Fig. 11b) and enhanced activity in the peri-coeruleus regions such as the parabrachial nucleus and nucleus raphe magnus (Fig. 11c). To identify the relative location between the negatively correlated LC and activated peri-coeruleus regions, we overlapped Fig. 11b and c (Fig. 11d). The strong negatively correlated areas are denoted in green ($P < .003$) and the positively correlated areas are shown in magenta (Fig. 11d). Because the LC contributes to descending pain modulations, these results imply that the descending pain modulation pathway may

be involved in the development of neuropathic pain in the SNI model.

Discussion

This study combined functional brain imaging and electrophysiological recording methods to map sustained brain activation regions during early SNI neuropathic pain development in rats. We found nerve injury induced immediate and sustained activity increase in the bilateral ICs and contralateral S1. The elevated activity in the ipsilateral

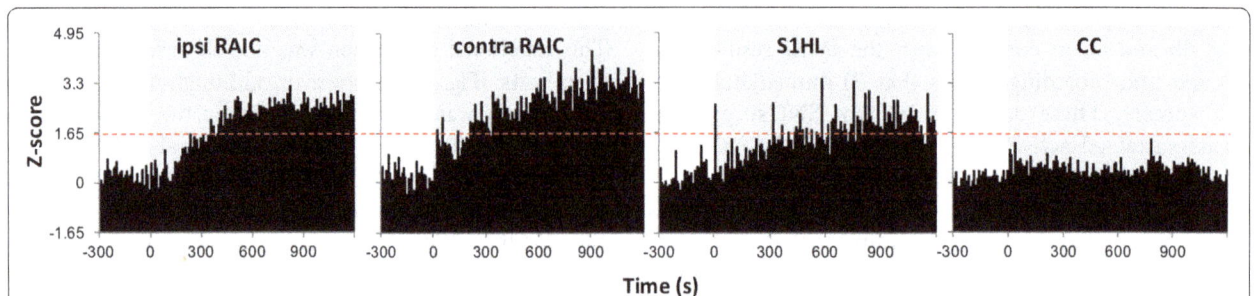

Fig. 7 Unit responses during SNI surgery. SNI nerve transection induced a sustained increase in spike activity in the bilateral RAIC and contralateral S1HL are of the injured hind limb, whereas the CC exhibited no significant changes. The spike rates of each unit were converted to z-scores by using the following equation: (FRi – FRb)/SDb, where FRi is the firing rate in the ith bin of the recording period (5 s for each bin) and FRb and SDb represent the mean firing rate and standard deviation of firing rates before SNI nerve transection, respectively. The group z-scores were averaged from the mean z-scores of individuals. The spike activities under the resting baseline condition from − 300 to 0 s are shown. SNI nerve transection was performed at time = 0 and followed by 1200 s of post-SNI recording (gray area). The dashed red line shows the threshold of $P < .05$ (total unit number/number of rats in each group: 25/3 in the ipsilateral RAIC, 23/3 in the contralateral RAIC, 22/3 in the S1HL area, and 30/3 in the CC)

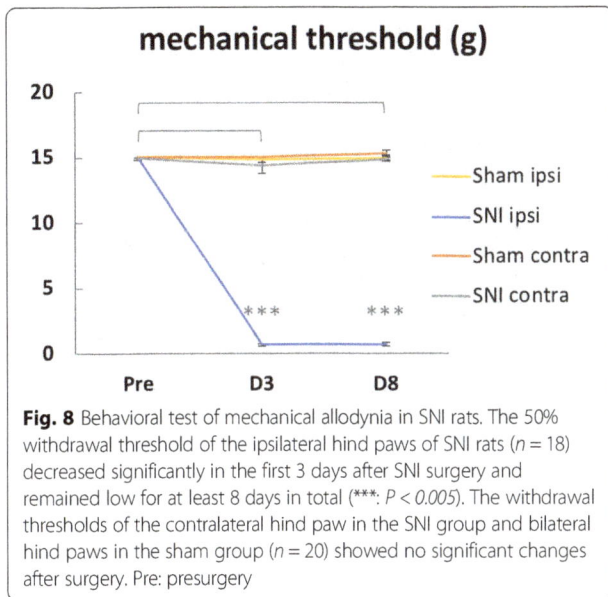

Fig. 8 Behavioral test of mechanical allodynia in SNI rats. The 50% withdrawal threshold of the ipsilateral hind paws of SNI rats (*n* = 18) decreased significantly in the first 3 days after SNI surgery and remained low for at least 8 days in total (***: *P* < 0.005). The withdrawal thresholds of the contralateral hind paw in the SNI group and bilateral hind paws in the sham group (*n* = 20) showed no significant changes after surgery. Pre: presurgery

IC was long-lasting and could be observed on Days 1 and 8 after SNI. Plasticity changes in functional connectivity among the ipsilateral AIC, contralateral S1HL, and bilateral RAIC were observed during the first few days of nerve injury. In addition, the enhanced functional connectivity between the RAIC and LC that spread to the brainstem implied that the descending pain modulation system may be involved in the development of neuropathic pain.

Many functional brain imaging studies of neuropathic pain have been conducted, most of which involved humans with well-established chronic pain. Such studies have focused on the brain responses to various stimulations [36–40] and various brain network patterns [41–43]. However, how nerve injury causes neuropathic pain chronification remains unresolved. Although central sensitization at the spinal level caused by peripheral nerve injury has been reported as activation-dependent [44–47], how nerve injury initially affects brain activity has not been mapped using functional brain imaging methods. Because nerve transection directly activated the peripheral nerve, our findings of brain activation pattern through SNI are similar to those reported in previous studies that use direct peripheral nerve stimulation on rats [48]. The novelty of the current study is the finding that activity in the bilateral ICs, CC, and S1 increased tonically after nerve transection. Such sustained activity may provide a condition for brain sensitization [11, 12].

Some researchers postulate that chronic pain is the result of nociceptive memory in the brain [2, 49, 50]. The center part of this hypothesis is that, similar to memory consolidation, neuropathic pain chronifies inside the brain through a period of sustained high frequency inputs. We tested this hypothesis using resting fMRI, MEMRI and electrophysiological recording experiments. BOLD-fMRI enables the detection of evoked

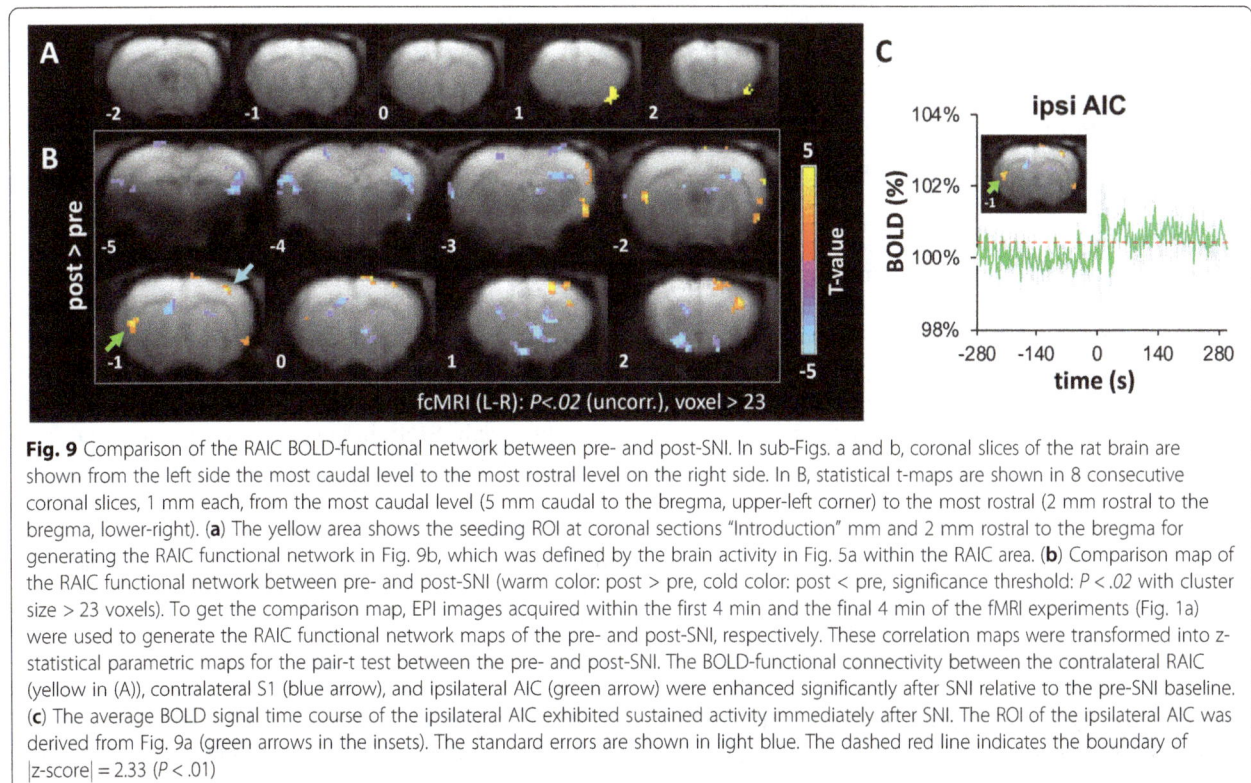

Fig. 9 Comparison of the RAIC BOLD-functional network between pre- and post-SNI. In sub-Figs. a and b, coronal slices of the rat brain are shown from the left side the most caudal level to the most rostral level on the right side. In B, statistical t-maps are shown in 8 consecutive coronal slices, 1 mm each, from the most caudal level (5 mm caudal to the bregma, upper-left corner) to the most rostral (2 mm rostral to the bregma, lower-right). (**a**) The yellow area shows the seeding ROI at coronal sections "Introduction" mm and 2 mm rostral to the bregma for generating the RAIC functional network in Fig. 9b, which was defined by the brain activity in Fig. 5a within the RAIC area. (**b**) Comparison map of the RAIC functional network between pre- and post-SNI (warm color: post > pre, cold color: post < pre, significance threshold: *P* < .02 with cluster size > 23 voxels). To get the comparison map, EPI images acquired within the first 4 min and the final 4 min of the fMRI experiments (Fig. 1a) were used to generate the RAIC functional network maps of the pre- and post-SNI, respectively. These correlation maps were transformed into z-statistical parametric maps for the pair-t test between the pre- and post-SNI. The BOLD-functional connectivity between the contralateral RAIC (yellow in (A)), contralateral S1 (blue arrow), and ipsilateral AIC (green arrow) were enhanced significantly after SNI relative to the pre-SNI baseline. (**c**) The average BOLD signal time course of the ipsilateral AIC exhibited sustained activity immediately after SNI. The ROI of the ipsilateral AIC was derived from Fig. 9a (green arrows in the insets). The standard errors are shown in light blue. The dashed red line indicates the boundary of |z-score| = 2.33 (*P* < .01)

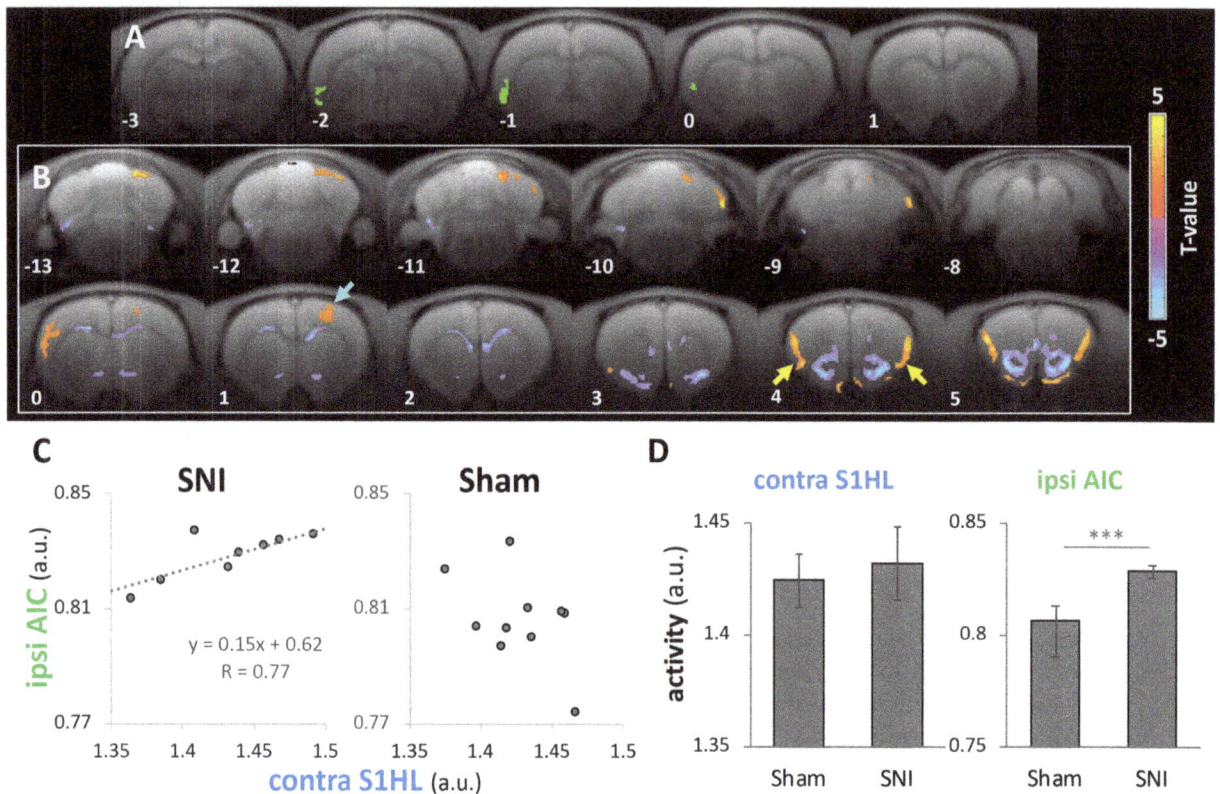

Fig. 10 MEMRI-functional connectivity seeded from ipsilateral AIC of neuropathic pain rats on Day 8 after SNI. In sub-Figs. a and b, coronal slices of the rat brain are shown from the left side the most caudal level to the most rostral level on the right side. In B, statistical t-maps are shown in 12 representative coronal slices, from the most caudal level (13 mm caudal to the bregma, upper-left corner) to the most rostral (5 mm rostral to the bregma, lower-right). (**a**) The green area shows the seeding ROI at coronal sections "Methods" mm, 1 mm and 0 mm caudal to the bregma for the connectivity analysis in Fig. 10b, which was defined by the brain activity in the AIC area shown in Fig. 4c. (**b**) MEMRI-functional connectivity map generated through multiple regression analysis with the inter-subject variability of AIC activations as the regressor. The contralateral S1HL area (blue arrows) and bilateral RAIC (yellow arrows) exhibited significant functional connections with the AIC. (**c**) Activity within the significant area of the contralateral S1HL area (blue arrows) was extracted. Activity in the ipsilateral AIC and contralateral S1HL area are plotted together (sham: $n = 10$; SNI: $n = 8$). The SNI group alone exhibited a significant activity correlation between the ipsilateral AIC and contralateral S1 ($P < .05$). (**d**) Quantitative neural activity in the contralateral S1HL area and ipsilateral AIC. Activity in the ipsilateral AIC was significantly higher in the SNI group than in the sham group ($P < .005$), whereas no difference in contralateral S1HL activity was observed between these two groups

neural activity on the basis of the neurovascular coupling [51–54], however, it is difficult using BOLD-fMRI to quantify the basal neural activity. Although a resting-state fMRI design can be employed to observe large-scale networks inside the brain [55], determining whether activity in a specific brain area is high or low over long periods is difficult. By contrast, MEMRI enables the mapping of cumulative brain activity in free-moving animals over relatively long periods of 3–24 h [24–26, 33, 56, 57]. Furthermore, a recent study used inter-subject variability of brain activity to analyze functional networks during memory consolidation [26]. In the present study, a similar strategy was employed to investigate neuropathic pain chronification. Rather than using the average signals within the atlas-defined ROIs, we used the average signals within the activation cluster as regressors to assess voxel-wise functional connections.

This is because we assumed that only parts of the anatomically defined brain regions exhibited abnormal functional connections; for example, we observed that only part of the contralateral S1HL exhibited plasticity change in functional connectivity with the AIC, possibly because a portion of the right S1HL has been deprived of its input from the tibial and common peroneal nerves.

In many studies, the IC has been consistently activated in various pain paradigms. Some studies have suggested that plasticity in the IC is crucial to the maintenance of neuropathic pain [58–60]. However, the IC is involved in various sensory modalities, as well as motor and emotional functions with complex connections with various brain areas [61]. Craig suggested that the IC is a multimodal homeostatic or interoceptive integration area [62]. Its multimodal input property enables it to serve as a multimodal magnitude estimator or salience detector [61,

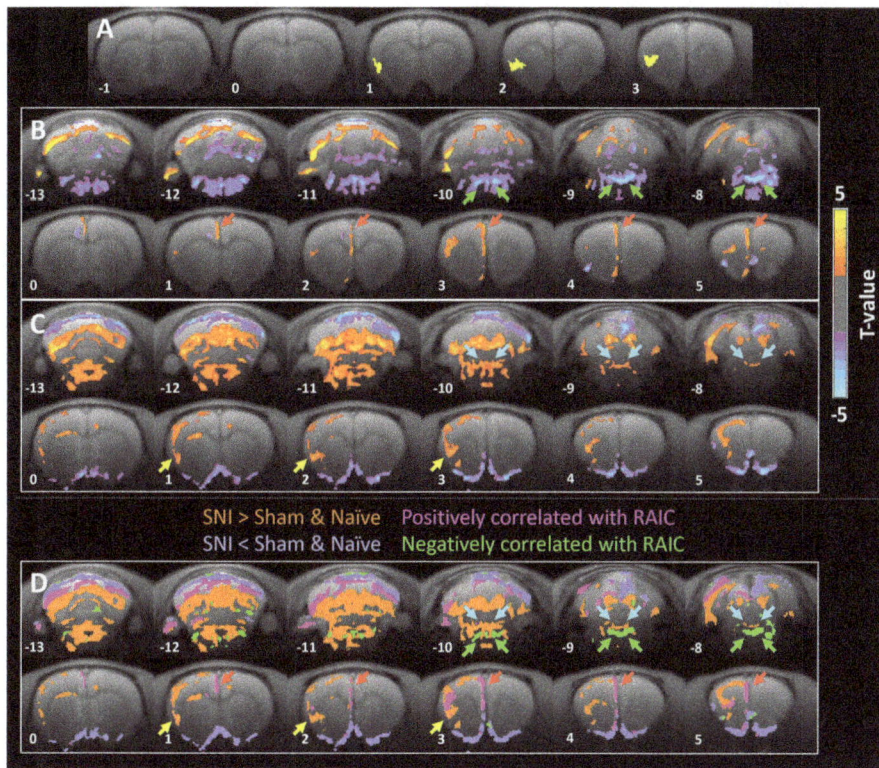

Fig. 11 MEMRI-functional connectivity seeded from ipsilateral RAIC of neuropathic pain rats on Day 8 after SNI. In sub-figures, coronal slices of the rat brain are shown from the left side the most caudal level to the most rostral level on the right side. In **b**, **c** and **d**, statistical t-maps are shown in 12 representative coronal slices, from the most caudal level (13 mm caudal to the bregma, upper-left corner) to the most rostral (5 mm rostral to the bregma, lower-right). (**a**) The yellow area shows the seeding ROI at coronal sections "Introduction" mm, 2 mm and 3 mm rostral to the bregma for the connectivity analysis in Fig. 11b, which was defined by the brain activation in the RAIC area shown in Fig. 4c. (**b**) MEMRI-functional connectivity map generated through multiple regression analysis with the intersubject variability of RAIC activations as the regressor. The contralateral ACC (red arrows) and dorsal brainstem (green arrows) areas exhibited significant functional connections with the RAIC ($P < .05$). (**c**) Voxel-wise comparison of brain activity between SNI and sham group rats on Day 8 day after SNI surgery. The SNI group exhibited increased activity in the RAIC (yellow arrows) and dorsal brainstem (blue arrows) areas ($P < .05$). (**d**) Merged image of (**b**) and (**c**). The strong negatively correlated brainstem areas ($P < .003$) derived from (**b**) are denoted in green and mostly located in the LC. The positively correlated brain areas in (**b**) are denoted in magenta and located around the LC without having a colocalized area

63]. Some studies have found that the IC encodes pain intensity [64, 65]. However, parcellation of the IC into a pain magnitude estimator or salience detector remains controversial [66, 67]. The IC is currently considered a multidimensional integration site for pain [68]. Recent studies have shown that people with IC lesions can rate the magnitude of evoked acute pain. Because the S1 has been reported to encode pain intensity [69, 70], it may serve as a redundancy system for magnitude estimation [66]. In the present study, we found the ipsilateral AIC exhibited consistently enhanced activity after SNI surgery; and the functional connection between the AIC with the contralateral S1HLalso enhanced under the neuropathic pain condition. These data thereby imply that a plasticity change of the pain magnitude estimation standard may have occurred in the SNI neuropathic pain rats.

Peripheral nerve injury induces S1 reorganization and causes the input-deprived cortex to be occupied by neighborhood expansion [71]. Our data showed that activity within the S1HL decreased on Day 1 after SNI surgery but recovered to a similar level as that of the sham group by Day 8. This recovery may be the result of cortical reorganization and the expanded representation of the neighboring nerves. The association between S1 reorganization and neuropathic pain development is not yet understood. Furthermore, we found the S1HL area began to cooperate with the AIC under the neuropathic pain condition; however, the overall S1HL activity did not differ between the SNI and sham groups. In our previous study, we observed no variations in S1HL responses to von Frey hair stimulation between SNI and naïve rats [34]. Whether and how the S1 is involved in allodynia is the subject of debate. Some studies on people with neuropathic pain have reported increase activity in the S1 with allodynic stimulations [40, 72, 73], whereas others with similar experimental designs have not observed any variations in S1 response [37, 74]. Nevertheless, our data shows the enhanced functional connection between the reorganized S1HL area and AIC in SNI neuropathic pain rats, thereby shedding new light on the association between the S1 and neuropathic pain development.

In this study, the RAIC exhibited sustained activity in response to SNI and strongly enhanced activity on Day 8 after SNI. A previous anatomical study revealed that the RAIC received considerable input from the centrolateral thalamus (CL) and mediodorsal thalamus (MD) [75], which showed strong activity in response to SNI in the fMRI result. The CL and MD are major sites of termination for the spinothalamic tract [76–79] and are implicated in the sensorimotor integration of nociceptive processing [80]. Our data showed that after SNI, RAIC activity was strongly and negatively correlated with the LC and several brainstem areas, whereas the peri-coeruleus region exhibited enhanced neural activity. According to a previous anatomical study, the RAIC projects to the peri-coeruleus region, rostroventral medulla, lateral hypothalamus, parabrachial area, dorsal raphe, and periaqueductal gray [75], all of which have been directly linked to brainstem-mediated descending modulation in spinal nociceptive neurons [81–87]. However, a previous study demonstrated that the activation of RAIC projection neurons can cause hyperalgesia in a top-down manner [88]. Two groups of RAIC projection neurons respectively act upon two independent subcortical nuclei to modulate the nociceptive threshold. The first group projects to the gamma-aminobutyric acid (GABA) interneurons in the peri-coerulear zone, and these GABAergic interneurons inhibit the LC neurons and affect the noradrenergic bulbospinal projections. The second group projects to the amygdala and causes hyperalgesia when activated [88]. Therefore, our data may imply a plasticity change in the pain threshold through a top-down modulation from the RAIC after SNI.

The limitation of the present study is the relatively small number of rats used in the BOLD fMRI and its supplementary electrophysiological studies. The classical spared nerve injury model transected the 2 larger branch of the sciatic nerve and leaves only the minor sural nerve intact. This is a major trauma to the rat. SNI is a very robust neuropathic pain model with minimal variations. This has been described by Decosterd & Woolf in the abstract of their original paper: *"The spared nerve injury model results in early (<24 h), prolonged (>6 months), robust (all animals are responders) behavioral modifications."* [30]. The robustness of the SNI model has been repeated in our lab in several previously published papers [34, 89] and can be clearly observed in the Fig. 8 of the present study. Nevertheless, the small number of animal used prevents a meaningful analysis of possible difference between male and female rats.

In summary, this study constitutes the first experimental observation of the forebrain regions with tonically enhanced activity induced by peripheral nerve injury and the first study to correlate this tonic brain activity with long-term brain plasticity. The SNI-induced plasticity changes in the ipsilateral AIC, bilateral RAICs, and S1 may contributed to the neuropathic pain development through changes in the sensorimotor integration of nociceptive information. Moreover, the negative functional correlation between the RAIC and LC suggested a change in the descending pain modulation system under the condition of neuropathic pain development.

Abbreviations
ACC: anterior cingulate cortex; AIC: anterior insular cortex; BOLD-fMRI: blood-oxygenation-level-dependent functional magnetic resonance imaging; CC: cingulate cortex; CL: centrolateral thalamus; CPu: caudate putamen; EPI: echo planar imaging; FWHM: full width at half maximum; GABA: gamma-aminobutyric acid; IC: insular cortex; MD: mediodorsal thalamus; MDL: mediodorsal thalamic nucleus, lateral part; MDM: mediodorsal thalamic nucleus, medial part; MEMRI: manganese-enhanced magnetic resonance imaging; RAIC: rostral anterior insular cortex; ROIs: regions of interest; S1: primary somatosensory cortex; S1HL: S1 hind limb; SNI: spared nerve injury; VP: ventral posterolateral thalamic nucleus

Acknowledgements
The authors thank 7 T animal MRI Core Lab of the Neurobiology and Cognitive Science Center, National Taiwan University for technical and facility supports.

Funding
This study was supported by a grant from Ministry of Science and Technology, Taiwan, MOST105–2311-B-002 -029.

Authors' contributions
THHC conceived and designed the experiment under the supervision of CTY. THHC performed the experiment, analyzed the data and prepare the first draft of the manuscript. JHC gave technical supports and suggestions. CTY finalized the manuscript.

Competing interests
The authors declare that they have no competing interests.

Author details
[1]Department of Life Science, National Taiwan University, No. 1, Sec. 4, Roosevelt Rd, Taipei 10617, Taiwan. [2]Interdisciplinary MRI/MRS Lab, Department of Electrical Engineering, National Taiwan University, No. 1, Sec. 4, Roosevelt Rd, Taipei 10617, Taiwan.

References

1. Goldberg DS, McGee SJ. Pain as a global public health priority. BMC Public Health 2011;11(1):1.
2. Apkarian AV, Baliki MN, Geha PY. Towards a theory of chronic pain. Prog Neurobiol. 2009;87(2):81–97.
3. Li X-Y, Ko H-G, Chen T, Descalzi G, Koga K, Wang H, et al. Alleviating neuropathic pain hypersensitivity by inhibiting PKMzeta in the anterior cingulate cortex. Science. 2010;330:1400–4.
4. Tan W, Yao W-L, Hu R, Lv Y-Y, Wan L, Zhang C-H, et al. Alleviating neuropathic pain mechanical allodynia by increasing Cdh1 in the anterior cingulate cortex. Mol Pain. 2015;11:56.
5. Han J, Kwon M, Cha M, Tanioka M, Hong S-K, Bai SJ, et al. Plasticity-related PKMζ signaling in the insular cortex is involved in the modulation of neuropathic pain after nerve injury. Neural Plast. 2015:2015.
6. Li X-Y, Ko H-G, Chen T, Descalzi G, Koga K, Wang H, et al. Alleviating neuropathic pain hypersensitivity by inhibiting PKMζ in the anterior cingulate cortex. Science. 2010;330(6009):1400–4.
7. Woolf CJ. Evidence for a central component of post-injury pain hypersensitivity. Nature. 1983.
8. Woolf CJ, Wall PD. Relative effectiveness of C primary afferent fibers of different origins in evoking a prolonged facilitation of the flexor reflex in the rat. J Neurosci. 1986;6(5):1433–42.
9. Cook AJ, Woolf CJ, Wall PD, McMahon SB. Dynamic receptive field plasticity in rat spinal cord dorsal horn following C-primary afferent input. Nature. 1987;325(6100):151–3.
10. Ji R-R, Kohno T, Moore KA, Woolf CJ. Central sensitization and LTP: do pain and memory share similar mechanisms? Trends Neurosci. 2003; 26(12):696–705.
11. Collingridge GL, Isaac JT, Wang YT. Receptor trafficking and synaptic plasticity. Nat Rev Neurosci. 2004;5(12):952–62.
12. Morimoto K, Fahnestock M, Racine RJ. Kindling and status epilepticus models of epilepsy: rewiring the brain. Prog Neurobiol. 2004;73(1):1–60.
13. Ali Z, Ringkamp M, Hartke TV, Chien HF. Flavahan Na, Campbell JN, et al. uninjured C-fiber nociceptors develop spontaneous activity and alpha-adrenergic sensitivity following L6 spinal nerve ligation in monkey. J Neurophysiol. 1999;81:81.
14. Liu C-N, Wall PD, Ben-Dor E, Michaelis M, Amir R, Devor M. Tactile allodynia in the absence of C-fiber activation: altered firing properties of DRG neurons following spinal nerve injury. Pain. 2000;85(3):503–21.
15. Tseng W-T, Tsai M-L, Iwata K, Yen C-T. Long-term changes in trigeminal ganglionic and thalamic neuronal activities following inferior alveolar nerve transection in behaving rats. J Neurosci. 2012;32:16051–63.
16. Baliki MN, Petre B, Torbey S, Herrmann KM, Huang L, Schnitzer TJ, et al. Corticostriatal functional connectivity predicts transition to chronic back pain. Nat Neurosci. 2012;15:1117–9.
17. Burgmer M, Pfleiderer B, Maihöfner C, Gaubitz M, Wessolleck E, Heuft G, et al. Cerebral mechanisms of experimental hyperalgesia in fibromyalgia. Eur J Pain. 2012;16(5):636–47.
18. Kim S, Nabekura J. Rapid synaptic remodeling in the adult somatosensory cortex following peripheral nerve injury and its association with neuropathic pain. J Neurosci. 2011;31:5477–82.
19. Li R, Hettinger PC, Machol JA, Liu X, Stephenson J, Pawela CP, et al. Cortical plasticity induced by different degrees of peripheral nerve injuries: a rat functional magnetic resonance imaging study under 9.4 tesla. Journal of brachial plexus and peripheral nerve injury. 2013;8(1):4.
20. Chao THH, Chen JH, Yen CT. Repeated BOLD-fMRI imaging of deep brain stimulation responses in rats. PLoS One. 2014;9.
21. Weber R, Ramos-Cabrer P, Wiedermann D, Van Camp N, Hoehn M. A fully noninvasive and robust experimental protocol for longitudinal fMRI studies in the rat. NeuroImage 2006;29:1303–1310.
22. Niskanen J-P, Airaksinen AM, Sierra A, Huttunen JK, Nissinen J, Karjalainen PA, et al. Monitoring Functional Impairment and Recovery After Traumatic Brain Injury in Rats by fMRI. J Neurotrauma. 2012(ja).
23. Weber R, Ramos-Cabrer P, Justicia C, Wiedermann D, Strecker C, Sprenger C, et al. Early prediction of functional recovery after experimental stroke: functional magnetic resonance imaging, electrophysiology, and behavioral testing in rats. J Neurosci. 2008;28(5):1022–9.
24. Eschenko O, Canals S, Simanova I, Beyerlein M, Murayama Y, Logothetis NK. Mapping of functional brain activity in freely behaving rats during voluntary running using manganese-enhanced MRI: implication for longitudinal studies. NeuroImage. 2010;49:2544–55.
25. Hattori S, Hagihara H, Ohira K, Aoki I, Saga T, Suhara T, et al. In vivo evaluation of cellular activity in αCaMKII heterozygous knockout mice using manganese-enhanced magnetic resonance imaging (MEMRI). Front Integr Neurosci. 2013;7:76.
26. Chen KH, Chen DY, Liang KC. Functional connectivity changes during consolidation of inhibitory avoidance memory in rats: a manganese-enhanced MRI study. The Chinese journal of physiology. 2013;56:269–81.
27. Itoh K, Sakata M, Watanabe M, Aikawa Y, Fujii H. The entry of manganese ions into the brain is accelerated by the activation of N-methyl-d-aspartate receptors. Neuroscience. 2008;154:732–40.
28. Hankir MK, Parkinson JR, Bloom SR, Bell JD. The effects of glutamate receptor agonists and antagonists on mouse hypothalamic and hippocampal neuronal activity shown through manganese enhanced MRI. NeuroImage. 2012;59:968–78.
29. Silva AC, Bock NA. Manganese-enhanced MRI: An exceptional tool in translational neuroimaging. Schizophr Bull 2008;34:595–604.
30. Decosterd I, Woolf CJ. Spared nerve injury: an animal model of persistent peripheral neuropathic pain. Pain. 2000;87(2):149–58.
31. Chaplan SR, Bach FW, Pogrel JW, Chung JM, Yaksh TL. Quantitative assessment of tactile allodynia in the rat paw. J Neurosci Methods. 1994;53:55–63.
32. Tseng W-T, Yen C-T, Tsai M-L. A bundled microwire array for long-term chronic single-unit recording in deep brain regions of behaving rats. J Neurosci Methods. 2011;201(2):368–76.
33. Chuang KH, Koretsky AP, Sotak CH. Temporal changes in the T1 and T2 relaxation rates (??R1 and ??R2) in the rat brain are consistent with the tissue-clearance rates of elemental manganese. Magn Reson Med. 2009; 61:1528–32.
34. Lin H-C, Huang Y-H, Chao T-HH, Lin W-Y, Sun W-Z, Yen C-T. Gabapentin reverses central hypersensitivity and suppresses medial prefrontal cortical glucose metabolism in rats with neuropathic pain. Mol Pain. 2014;10:63.
35. Ward BD. Simultaneous Inference for fMRI Data. 2000:1–16.
36. Apkarian AV, Hashmi JA, Baliki MN. Pain and the brain: specificity and plasticity of the brain in clinical chronic pain. Pain. 2011;152:S49–64.
37. Witting N, Kupers RC, Svensson P, Jensen TS. A PET activation study of brush-evoked allodynia in patients with nerve injury pain. Pain. 2006; 120:145–54.
38. Schweinhardt P, Glynn C, Brooks J, McQuay H, Jack T, Chessell I, et al. An fMRI study of cerebral processing of brush-evoked allodynia in neuropathic pain patients. NeuroImage. 2006;32:256–65.
39. Samuelsson M, Leffler AS, Hansson P. Dynamic mechanical allodynia: on the relationship between temporo-spatial stimulus parameters and evoked pain in patients with peripheral neuropathy. Pain. 2005;115:264–72.
40. Peyron R, Schneider F, Faillenot I, Convers P, Barral F-G, Garcia-Larrea L, et al. An fMRI study of cortical representation of mechanical allodynia in patients with neuropathic pain. Neurology. 2004;63:1838–46.
41. Baliki MN, Geha PY, Apkarian AV, Chialvo DR. Beyond feeling: chronic pain hurts the brain, disrupting the default-mode network dynamics. J Neurosci. 2008;28:1398–403.
42. Welsh RC, Chen AC, Taylor SF. Low-frequency BOLD fluctuations demonstrate altered thalamocortical connectivity in schizophrenia. Schizophr Bull. 2010;36: 713–22.
43. Cardoso-Cruz H, Lima D, Galhardo V. Impaired spatial memory performance in a rat model of neuropathic pain is associated with reduced hippocampus-prefrontal cortex connectivity. J Neurosci. 2013;33:2465–80.
44. Sandkühler J, Liu X. Induction of long-term potentiation at spinal synapses by noxious stimulation or nerve injury. Eur J Neurosci. 1998;10:2476–80.
45. Gruber-Schoffnegger D, Drdla-Schutting R, Hönigsperger C, Wunderbaldinger G, Gassner M, Sandkühler J. Induction of thermal hyperalgesia and synaptic long-term potentiation in the spinal cord lamina I by TNF-α and IL-1β is mediated by glial cells. J Neurosci. 2013;33:6540–51.
46. Zhang H-M, Zhou L-J, Hu X-D, Hu N-W, Zhang T, Liu X-G. Acute nerve injury induces long-term potentiation of C-fiber evoked field potentials in spinal dorsal horn of intact rat. Sheng li xue bao : [Acta physiologica Sinica]. 2004;56:591–6.
47. Liu X-G, Zhou L-J. Long-term potentiation at spinal C-fiber synapses: a target for pathological pain. Curr Pharm Des. 2015;21:895–905.

48. Cho YR, Jones SR, Pawela CP, Li R, Kao DS, Schulte ML, et al. Cortical brain mapping of peripheral nerves using functional magnetic resonance imaging in a rodent model. J Reconstr Microsurg. 2008;24:551–7.

49. Yi M, Zhang H. Nociceptive memory in the brain: cortical mechanisms of chronic pain. J Neurosci. 2011;31:13343–5.

50. Mansour AR, Farmer MA, Baliki MN, Apkarian AV. Chronic pain: the role of learning and brain plasticity. Restor Neurol Neurosci. 2014;32:129–39.

51. Pasley B, Freeman R. Neurovascular coupling. Scholarpedia. 2008;3:5340.

52. Harder DR, Alkayed NJ. Lange aR, Gebremedhin D, Roman RJ. Functional hyperemia in the brain: hypothesis for astrocyte-derived vasodilator metabolites. Stroke. 1998;29:229–34.

53. Attwell D, Iadecola C. The neural basis of functional brain imaging signals. Trends Neurosci. 2002;25(12):621–5.

54. Logothetis NK. The neural basis of the blood-oxygen-level-dependent functional magnetic resonance imaging signal. Philos Trans R Soc Lond Ser B Biol Sci. 2002;357:1003–37.

55. Biswal B, Yetkin FZ, Haughton VM, Hyde JS. Functional connectivity in the motor cortex of resting human brain using echo-planar MRI. Magnetic resonance in medicine : official journal of the Society of Magnetic Resonance in Medicine / Society of Magnetic Resonance in Medicine. 1995;34:537–41.

56. Silva AC, Lee JH, Aoki I, Koretsky AP. Manganese-enhanced magnetic resonance imaging (MEMRI): methodological and practical considerations. NMR Biomed. 2004;17:532–43.

57. Jeong K-Y, Lee C, Cho J-H, Kang J-H, Na H-S. New method of manganese-enhanced magnetic resonance imaging (MEMRI) for rat brain research. Experimental animals / Japanese Association for Laboratory Animal Science. 2012;61:157–64.

58. Ferrier J, Bayet-Robert M, Dalmann R. El Guerrab a, Aissouni Y, Graveron-Demilly D, et al. cholinergic neurotransmission in the posterior insular cortex is altered in preclinical models of neuropathic pain: key role of muscarinic M2 receptors in donepezil-induced Antinociception. J Neurosci. 2015;35:16418–30.

59. Qiu S, Zhang M, Liu Y, Guo Y, Zhao H, Song Q, et al. GluA1 phosphorylation contributes to postsynaptic amplification of neuropathic pain in the insular cortex. J Neurosci. 2014;34:13505–15.

60. Han J, Kwon M, Cha M, Tanioka M. Hong S-k, Bai SJ, et al. Plasticity-Related PKM ζ Signaling in the Insular Cortex Is Involved in the Modulation of Neuropathic Pain after Nerve Injury Neural Plasticity. 2015;2015:1–10.

61. Circuitry and functional aspects of the insular lobe in primates including humans, (1996).

62. Craig AD. Interoception: the sense of the physiological condition of the body. Curr Opin Neurobiol. 2003;13:500–5.

63. Downar J, Crawley AP, Mikulis DJ, Davis KD. A cortical network for the detection of novel events across multiple sensory modalities. NeuroImage. 2001;13:S310-S.

64. Coghill RC, Sang CN, Maisog JM, Iadarola MJ. Pain intensity processing within the human brain: a bilateral, distributed mechanism. J Neurophysiol. 1999;82:1934–43.

65. Baliki MN, Geha PY. Apkarian aV. parsing pain perception between nociceptive representation and magnitude estimation. J Neurophysiol. 2009;101:875–87.

66. Moayedi M, Weissman-Fogel I. Is the insula the "how much" intensity coder? J Neurophysiol. 2009;102:1345–7.

67. Downar J, Mikulis DJ, Davis KD. Neural correlates of the prolonged salience of painful stimulation. NeuroImage. 2003;20:1540–51.

68. Brooks JCW, Tracey I. The insula: A multidimensional integration site for pain. Pain2007. p. 1–2.

69. Ea M, Keaser ML, Gullapalli RP, Greenspan JD. Regional intensive and temporal patterns of functional MRI activation distinguishing noxious and innocuous contact heat. J Neurophysiol. 2005;93:2183–93.

70. Rainville P, Carrier B, Hofbauer RK, Bushnell MC, Duncan GH. Dissociation of sensory and affective dimensions of pain using hypnotic modulation. Pain. 1999;82:159–71.

71. Kaas JH, Merzenich MM, Killackey HP. The reorganization of somatosensory cortex following peripheral nerve damage in adult and developing mammals. Annu Rev Neurosci. 1983;6:325–56.

72. Petrovic P, Ingvar M, Stone-Elander S, Petersson KM, Hansson P. A PET activation study of dynamic mechanical allodynia in patients with mononeuropathy. Pain. 1999;83:459–70.

73. Peyron R, Faillenot I, Pomares FB, Le Bars D, Garcia-Larrea L, Laurent B. Mechanical allodynia in neuropathic pain. Where are the brain representations located? A positron emission tomography (PET) study. Eur J Pain 2013;17:1327–1337.

74. Kim CE, Kim YK, Chung G, Im HJ, Lee DS, Kim J, et al. Identifying neuropathic pain using 18F-FDG micro-PET: a multivariate pattern analysis. NeuroImage. 2014;86:311–6.

75. Jasmin L, Granato A, Ohara PT. Rostral agranular insular cortex and pain areas of the central nervous system: a tract-tracing study in the rat. J Comp Neurol. 2004;468(3):425–40.

76. Cliffer K, Burstein R, Giesler G. Distributions of spinothalamic, spinohypothalamic, and spinotelencephalic fibers revealed by anterograde transport of PHA-L in rats. J Neurosci. 1991;11(3):852–68.

77. Ma W, Peschanski M, Ralston HJ. Fine structure of the spinothalamic projections to the central lateral nucleus of the rat thalamus. Brain Res. 1987;414(1):187–91.

78. Ganchrow D. Intratrigeminal and thalamic projections of nucleus caudalis in the squirrel monkey (Saimiri sciureus): a degeneration and autoradiographic study. J Comp Neurol. 1978;178(2):281–311.

79. Craig A. Distribution of trigeminothalamic and spinothalamic lamina I terminations in the macaque monkey. J Comp Neurol. 2004;477(2):119–48.

80. Itoh K, Mizuno N. Topographical arrangement of thalamocortical neurons in the centrolateral nucleus (CL) of the cat, with special reference to a spino-thalamo-motor cortical path through the CL. Exp Brain Res. 1977;30(4):471–80.

81. Aimone L, Bauer C, Gebhart G. Brain-stem relays mediating stimulation-produced antinociception from the lateral hypothalamus in the rat. J Neurosci. 1988;8(7):2652–63.

82. Basbaum AI, Fields HL. Endogenous pain control systems: brainstem spinal pathways and endorphin circuitry. Annu Rev Neurosci. 1984;7(1):309–38.

83. Carstens E, Fraunhoffer M, Suberg S. Inhibition of spinal dorsal horn neuronal responses to noxious skin heating by lateral hypothalamic stimulation in the cat. J Neurophysiol. 1983;50(1):192–204.

84. Chiang C, Hu JW, Sessle BJ. Parabrachial area and nucleus raphe magnus-induced modulation of nociceptive and nonnociceptive trigeminal subnucleus caudalis neurons activated by cutaneous or deep inputs. J Neurophysiol. 1994;71(6):2430–45.

85. Chiang CY, Sessle BJ, Hu JW. Parabrachial area and nucleus raphe magnus-induced modulation of electrically evoked trigeminal subnucleus caudalis neuronal responses to cutaneous or deep A-fiber and C-fiber inputs in rats. Pain. 1995;62(1):61–8.

86. Millan MJ. Descending control of pain. Prog Neurobiol. 2002;66(6):355–474.

87. Prado WA, Faganello FA. The anterior pretectal nucleus participates as a relay station in the glutamate-, but not morphine-induced antinociception from the dorsal raphe nucleus in rats. Pain. 2000;88(2):169–76.

88. Jasmin L, Rabkin SD, Granato A, Boudah A, Ohara PT. Analgesia and hyperalgesia from GABA-mediated modulation of the cerebral cortex. Nature. 2003;424(6946):316–20.

89. Lee K-S, Huang Y-H, Yen C-T. Periaqueductal gray stimulation suppresses spontaneous pain behavior in rats. Neurosci Lett. 2012;514(1):42–5.

10

The Rap activator Gef26 regulates synaptic growth and neuronal survival via inhibition of BMP signaling

Keunjung Heo[1,2], Minyeop Nahm[3], Min-Jung Lee[1,2], Young-Eun Kim[4], Chang-Seok Ki[4], Seung Hyun Kim[3] and Seungbok Lee[1*] (iD)

Abstract

In *Drosophila*, precise regulation of BMP signaling is essential for normal synaptic growth at the larval neuromuscular junction (NMJ) and neuronal survival in the adult brain. However, the molecular mechanisms underlying fine-tuning of BMP signaling in neurons remain poorly understood. We show that loss of the *Drosophila* PDZ guanine nucleotide exchange factor Gef26 significantly increases synaptic growth at the NMJ and enhances BMP signaling in motor neurons. We further show that Gef26 functions upstream of Rap1 in motor neurons to restrain synaptic growth. Synaptic overgrowth in *gef26* or *rap1* mutants requires BMP signaling, indicating that Gef26 and Rap1 regulate synaptic growth via inhibition of BMP signaling. We also show that Gef26 is involved in the endocytic downregulation of surface expression of the BMP receptors thickveins (Tkv) and wishful thinking (Wit). Finally, we demonstrate that loss of Gef26 also induces progressive brain neurodegeneration through Rap1- and BMP signaling-dependent mechanisms. Taken together, these results suggest that the Gef26-Rap1 signaling pathway regulates both synaptic growth and neuronal survival by controlling BMP signaling.

Keywords: *Drosophila*, Gef26, Synaptic growth, Neurodegeneration, Endocytic regulation of BMP signaling

Introduction

Transsynaptic retrograde signaling from postsynaptic cells controls the development and survival of presynaptic neurons [1–3]. At the *Drosophila* larval neuromuscular junction (NMJ), the bone morphogenetic protein (BMP) ligand glass bottom boat (Gbb) is secreted from the postsynaptic muscle and acts as a key retrograde signal that promotes the expansion of synaptic arbors [4–7]. In motoneurons, the Gbb signal is processed by a tetrameric presynaptic complex containing the type II BMP receptor wishful thinking (Wit) and either of two type II BMP receptors, thickveins (Tkv) and saxophone (Sax). Upon Gbb binding, this receptor complex phosphorylates the R-Smad mothers against decapentaplegic (Mad). Phosphorylated Mad (P-Mad) translocates into the nucleus through its interaction with the co-Smad Medea to regulate transcription of target genes [8]. Mutations disrupting this canonical BMP signaling pathway,

including *gbb*, *wit*, *tkv*, *sax*, and *mad*, all display NMJ undergrowth and defective basal transmission [4–7]. In sharp contrast, genetic conditions to elevate presynaptic BMP signaling cause NMJ overgrowth with excessive formation of small "satellite" boutons [9–12], which bud off the main axis of the motor axon terminal. Based on these findings, it has been proposed that the level of BMP signaling is instructive for the regulation of NMJ synapse growth [10]. Subsequent work on the *Drosophila* brain has begun to reveal the importance of precise regulation of BMP signaling in the maintenance of adult neurons. It has been demonstrated that, in addition to synaptic overgrowth, elevation of BMP signaling induces abnormal brain neurodegeneration in the adult fly [9].

Drosophila NMJ studies have identified various endocytic proteins as negative regulators of BMP-dependent synaptic growth. For example, loss of two endocytosis regulators, Dap160/intersectin and endophilin, leads to an increase in synaptic P-Mad levels and NMJ overgrowth with excessive satellite bouton formation [10, 13]. In addition, a similar phenotype is also induced by loss of spichthyin (Spict),

---

* Correspondence: seunglee@snu.ac.kr
[1]Department of Brain and Cognitive Sciences, College of Natural Sciences, Seoul National University, Seoul 08826, South Korea
Full list of author information is available at the end of the article

Spartin, and endosomal maturation defective (Ema), all of which are involved in endolysosomal trafficking of BMP receptors [9, 11, 14]. Importantly, these endocytic genes are shown to functionally interact with BMP signaling pathway components at the NMJ [9–11, 14]. These findings imply that endocytosis and subsequent lysosomal degradation of BMP receptors are important mechanisms involved in attenuating Gbb-induced signaling at the NMJ.

In a genetic screen for mutations that affect synaptic morphology at the *Drosophila* NMJ, we identified the *gef26* gene, which encodes a PDZ guanine nucleotide exchange factor (PDZ-GEF) for the small GTPase Rap1. Gef26 was originally known to control the development of various organs primarily by regulating cadherin-mediated cell-cell adhesion and integrin-dependent cell-matrix interactions [15–19]. Here, we report a novel role for the Gef26-Rap1 pathway in the regulation of BMP-dependent synaptic growth and neuronal survival. Null mutations in the *gef26* or *rap1* gene cause NMJ overgrowth characterized by excessive satellite bouton formation, recapitulating the phenotype induced by elevated BMP signaling. Genetic interactions between *gef26*, *rap1*, and components of the BMP pathway suggest that Gef26 acts through Rap1 to restrain BMP-dependent synaptic growth at the NMJ. Importantly, Gef26 promotes endocytic downregulation of surface expression of the BMP receptors Tkv and Wit. Finally, our genetic data indicate that regulation of BMP signaling by the Gef26-Rap1 pathway is critical for neuronal survival in the adult brain.

Results

Drosophila gef26 is required presynaptically for normal synaptic growth

To identify genes involved in the regulation of synaptic development, we performed an anatomical screen on 1500 independent EP insertion lines [20, 21]. We inspected third instar larval NMJs using the axonal membrane marker anti-HRP. In this screen, we isolated an insertion (G3533) localized in the first intron of the *Drosophila gef26* gene (CG9491). These mutants displayed NMJ overgrowth with an excessive formation of small "satellite" boutons (data not shown), which protrude from parental boutons located at primary axon terminal arbors.

To determine the null phenotype of *gef26* at the NMJ, we utilized the transheterozygous combination of *gef26^6*, a previously reported null allele [19, 22], and the *Df(2 L)BSC5* deficiency (henceforth referred to as *Df*) to delete the *gef26* locus. A significant synaptic overgrowth phenotype was observed at every glutamatergic type-I NMJ in *gef26^6/Df* third instar larvae. To quantify the *gef26* phenotype, we measured overall bouton number and satellite bouton number at NMJ 6/7 and NMJ 4 from abdominal segment 2 (Fig. 1a, b; Additional file 1:

Table S1). Compared with wild-type controls (w^{1118}), bouton number normalized to muscle surface area in *gef26^6/Df* larvae was increased by 24% at NMJ 6/7 and by 51% at NMJ 4. At the same time, satellite bouton number in *gef26^6/Df* was increased by 39% at NMJ 6/7 and by 219% at NMJ 4. Comparable synaptic growth defects were observed in larvae homozygous for *gef26^6* (Fig. 1a, b).

To determine whether *gef26* function is required pre- or postsynaptically for normal synaptic growth regulation, we expressed a *gef26* cDNA transgene (*UAS-gef26*) in *gef26^6/Df* mutants under the control of tissue-specific GAL4 drivers. Expression of *UAS-gef26* using a neuronal driver (*C155-GAL4*) fully rescued the NMJ growth defect of *gef26* mutants (Fig. 1b). In contrast, expression of *UAS-gef26* in all somatic muscles using the *BG57-GAL4* driver failed to rescue the NMJ growth defect (Fig. 1b), suggesting that Gef26 functions presynaptically to restrain synaptic growth at the NMJ.

Additional evidence for a presynaptic requirement for Gef26 was provided by assessment of the effect of RNA interference (RNAi)-mediated knockdown of Gef26 expression. Neuronal expression of a dsRNA-fragment of *gef26* (*UAS-gef26^RNAi*) using *C155-GAL4* increased both bouton number and satellite bouton number and mimicked the *gef26* loss-of-function mutation, whereas muscular expression of the same dsRNA using *BG57-GAL4* had no effect (Additional file 2: Figure S1a, b; Additional file 3: Table S2). This result supports the notion that Gef26 acts in presynaptic neurons to restrain synaptic growth at the NMJ.

We further characterized satellite boutons at *gef26* mutant NMJs using several synaptic markers. Satellite boutons contained the active zone antigen NC82 and the synaptic vesicle marker cysteine-string protein (CSP) (Additional file 2: Figure S1c, d). In addition, satellite boutons were found to recruit the subsynaptic reticulum (SSR) marker discs-large (Dlg). Finally, NC82 in satellite boutons was nicely juxtaposed to the essential glutamate receptor subunit GluRIIC (Additional file 2: Figure S1e, f). Thus, satellite boutons in *gef26* mutants display the anatomical hallmarks of functional synapses.

Gef26 acts through Rap1 to regulate synaptic growth

Since Gef26 acts via Rap1 to mediate various developmental processes [15–17, 19, 22], we decided to investigate whether Rap1 is the major target for Gef26 in the regulation of synaptic growth. We began by investigating whether loss of *rap1* produces NMJ phenotypes similar to those caused by *gef26* loss-of-function mutations. For this purpose, we analyzed NMJ morphology in third instar larvae homozygous for the *rap1^MI11950* allele (hereafter referred to as *rap1^M*) harboring a Minos element within the *rap1* gene. Compared with wild-type controls,

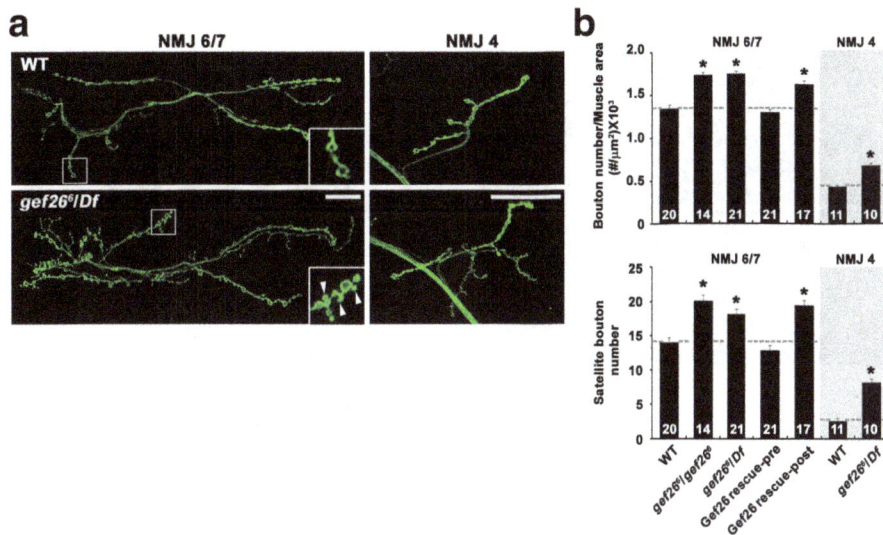

Fig. 1 Loss of presynaptic *gef26* function leads to synaptic overgrowth at the NMJ. **a** Confocal images of anti-HRP-labeled NMJs 6/7 (left) and NMJs 4 (right) in wild-type (w^{1118}) and *gef26^6/Df* third-instar larvae. *gef26* mutant NMJs have increased numbers of total and satellite boutons compared with wild type. Arrowheads mark satellite boutons. Scale bars, 20 μm. **b** Quantification of total bouton number normalized to muscle surface area and satellite bouton number at NMJ 6/7 and NMJ 4 in wild-type, *gef26^6/gef26^6*, *gef26^6/Df*, *C155-GAL4/+*; *gef26^6/Df*, *UAS-gef26/+* (Gef26 rescue-pre), and *gef26^6/Df*; *BG57-GAL4/UAS-gef26* (Gef26 rescue-post) third-instar larvae. The number of NMJs analyzed is indicated in each bar. Data are expressed as mean ± SEM. All comparisons are made with wild-type (*$P < 0.001$)

both overall bouton number and satellite bouton number in *rap1^M* mutants were significantly increased (Fig. 2a, b; Additional file 4: Table S3). To confirm the requirement for *rap1* in the proper regulation of synaptic growth, we also examined NMJ morphology in third instar larvae expressing *rap1* dsRNA (*UAS-rap1^RNAi*) under the control of *C155-GAL4*. This genetic manipulation significantly increased overall bouton number and satellite bouton number (Additional file 5: Figure S2a, b; Additional file 6: Table S4). In contrast, muscular expression of *UAS-rap1^RNAi* did not noticeably alter NMJ morphology (Additional file 5: Figure S2a, b; Additional file 6: Table S4). Thus, loss of presynaptic *rap1* produces *gef26*-like phenotypes at the NMJ.

Next, we assayed the transheterozygous interaction between *gef26* and *rap1* during synaptic growth. Heterozygous *gef26^6/+* or *rap1^M/+* larvae displayed normal NMJ morphology. However, overall bouton number and satellite bouton number were both significantly increased in transheterozygous *gef26^6/+*; *rap1^M/+* larvae compared with single *gef26^6/+* or *rap1^M/+* heterozygotes (Fig. 2b). This type of genetic interaction suggests that Gef26 and Rap1 function in the same pathway.

Finally, we explored the epistatic relationship between *gef26* and *rap1*. Neuronal overexpression of dominant-active Rap1-Q63E (*UAS-rap1^CA*) using *C155-GAL4* produced an NMJ undergrowth phenotype with fewer synaptic boutons (Fig. 2b). Importantly, neuronal overexpression of *UAS-rap1^CA* was able to induce a similar phenotype even in the *gef26^6/Df* background (Fig. 2b), indicating that the overactivity of Rap1 completely suppresses the synaptic

overgrowth in *gef26* mutants. These results suggest that Gef26 acts upstream of Rap1 to restrain synaptic growth at the NMJ.

Gef26 and Rap1 regulate synaptic growth via inhibition of BMP signaling

Previous studies have identified Gbb as a key retrograde signal that stimulates synaptic growth at the NMJ [4–7, 23]. Consistently, elevation of BMP signaling, which can be achieved by either presynaptic overexpression of a dominantly active Tkv receptor or loss of the inhibitory Smad Daughters against decapentaplegic (Dad), causes synaptic overgrowth with excessive satellite bouton formation [9, 10], recapitulating phenotypes exhibited by *gef26* or *rap1* mutants. Therefore, we wondered whether Gef26 and Rap1 might regulate synaptic growth by inhibiting BMP signaling. To test this possibility, we first examined the transheterozygous interaction between *gef26* or *rap1* and *dad* at the NMJ. Like *gef26^6/+* and *rap1^M/+* larvae, heterozygous *dad^J1E4/+* larvae displayed normal NMJ morphology (Fig. 3a, b; Additional file 7: Table S5). In contrast, both overall bouton number and satellite bouton number were significantly increased in transheterozygous *gef26^6/+*; *dad^J1E4/+* and *rap1^M,+/+,dad^J1E4* larvae compared with wild-type controls (Fig. 3a, b), suggesting a functional link between Gef26/Rap1 and the BMP signaling pathway during synaptic growth.

We next examined whether synaptic overgrowth in *gef26* or *rap1* mutants depends on BMP signaling. Heterozygosity for the BMP receptor gene *tkv* (*tkv^7/+*), which had no effect on NMJ morphology in a wild-type

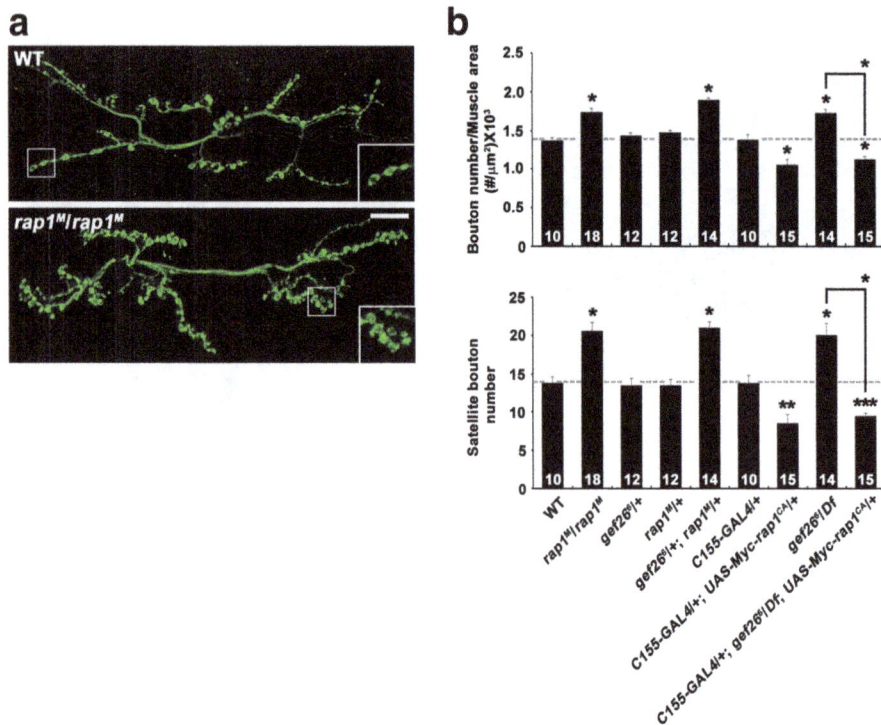

Fig. 2 *gef26* interacts genetically with *rap1* at the NMJ. **a** Confocal images of anti-HRP-labeled NMJ 6/7 in wild-type and *rap1^M^/rap1^M^* third-instar larvae. Scale bar, 20 μm. **b** Quantification of total bouton number normalized to muscle surface area and satellite bouton number at NMJ 6/7 in wild-type, *rap1^M^/rap1^M^*, *gef26^6^/+*, *rap1^M^/+*, *gef26^6^/+; rap1^M^/+*, *C155-GAL4/+*, *C155-GAL4/+; UAS-Myc-rap1^CA^/+*, *gef26^6^/Df*, and *C155-GAL4/+; gef26^6^/Df, UAS-Myc-rap1^CA^/+* backgrounds. The number of NMJs analyzed is indicated in each bar. Data are expressed as mean ± SEM. All comparisons are made with wild-type (*$P < 0.001$; **$P < 0.01$; ***$P < 0.05$)

background, suppressed synaptic overgrowth in *gef26^6^/Df* or *rap1^M^/rap1^M^* mutants (Fig. 3c, d; Additional file 7: Table S5). Moreover, removal of both copies of *tkv* (*tkv^1^/tkv^7^*) in the *gef26^6^/Df* background caused a synaptic undergrowth phenotype, which was similar to that of *tkv^1^/tkv^7^* mutants (Fig. 3c, d). Thus, BMP signaling is necessary for synaptic overgrowth in *gef26* or *rap1* mutants.

Finally, we directly tested the role of Gef26/Rap1 in inhibiting BMP signaling by assaying P-Mad levels in *gef26* and *rap1* mutants. P-Mad accumulation at NMJ synapses and in the nuclei of ventral nerve cord (VNC) motoneurons was significantly increased in *gef26^6^/Df* or *rap1^M^/rap1^M^* larvae compared with wild-type controls (Fig. 3e, f). Neuronal expression of *UAS-gef26* in *gef26^6^/Df* mutants was capable of reversing the increase of P-Mad in motoneurons (Fig. 3f), establishing the roles of Gef26 and Rap1 as negative regulators of BMP signaling. These results support a model in which Gef26 and Rap1 restrain synaptic growth by inhibiting BMP signaling.

Gef26 and Rap1 control BMP-dependent synaptic growth by regulating *Drosophila fragile X mental retardation 1* (*dfmr1*) expression and microtubule stability

At the *Drosophila* NMJ, BMP signaling has been shown to repress the expression of the *dfmr1* gene [9]. The *dfmr1*

product (dFMRP) in turn negatively regulates the expression of the microtubule-associated protein 1B (MAP1B) Futsch [24], which promotes synaptic growth by stabilizing synaptic microtubules [25]. Therefore, we hypothesized that Gef26/Rap1 might control synaptic growth by regulating microtubule stability via the dFMRP-Futsch pathway. To test the involvement of dFMRP in Gef26/Rap1-dependent regulation of synaptic growth, we first examined the transheterozygous interaction between *gef26* or *rap1* and *dfmr1* at the NMJ. Total bouton number and satellite bouton number were significantly higher in transheterozygous *gef26^6^/+; dfmr1^Δ50M^/+* and *rap1^M^, +/+,dfmr1^Δ50M^* larvae than in wild-type controls, although the single heterozygotes displayed normal synaptic growth (Fig. 4a, b; Additional file 8: Table S6). In a subsequent experiment, we directly tested whether loss of Gef26 or Rap1 alters *dfmr1* expression. Levels of *dfmr1* mRNA were significantly lower in *gef26* and *rap1* mutants than in wild-type controls, as demonstrated by quantitative real-time PCR (Fig. 4c). Given the roles of Gef26 and Rap1 in inhibiting BMP signaling, these results imply that Gef26/Rap1 restrains synaptic growth by relieving BMP-dependent repression of *dfmr1* transcription.

Next, we investigated whether *gef26* and *rap1* mutants affect synaptic Futsch levels. In wild-type NMJs, Futsch was detected as a filamentous bundle occupying the

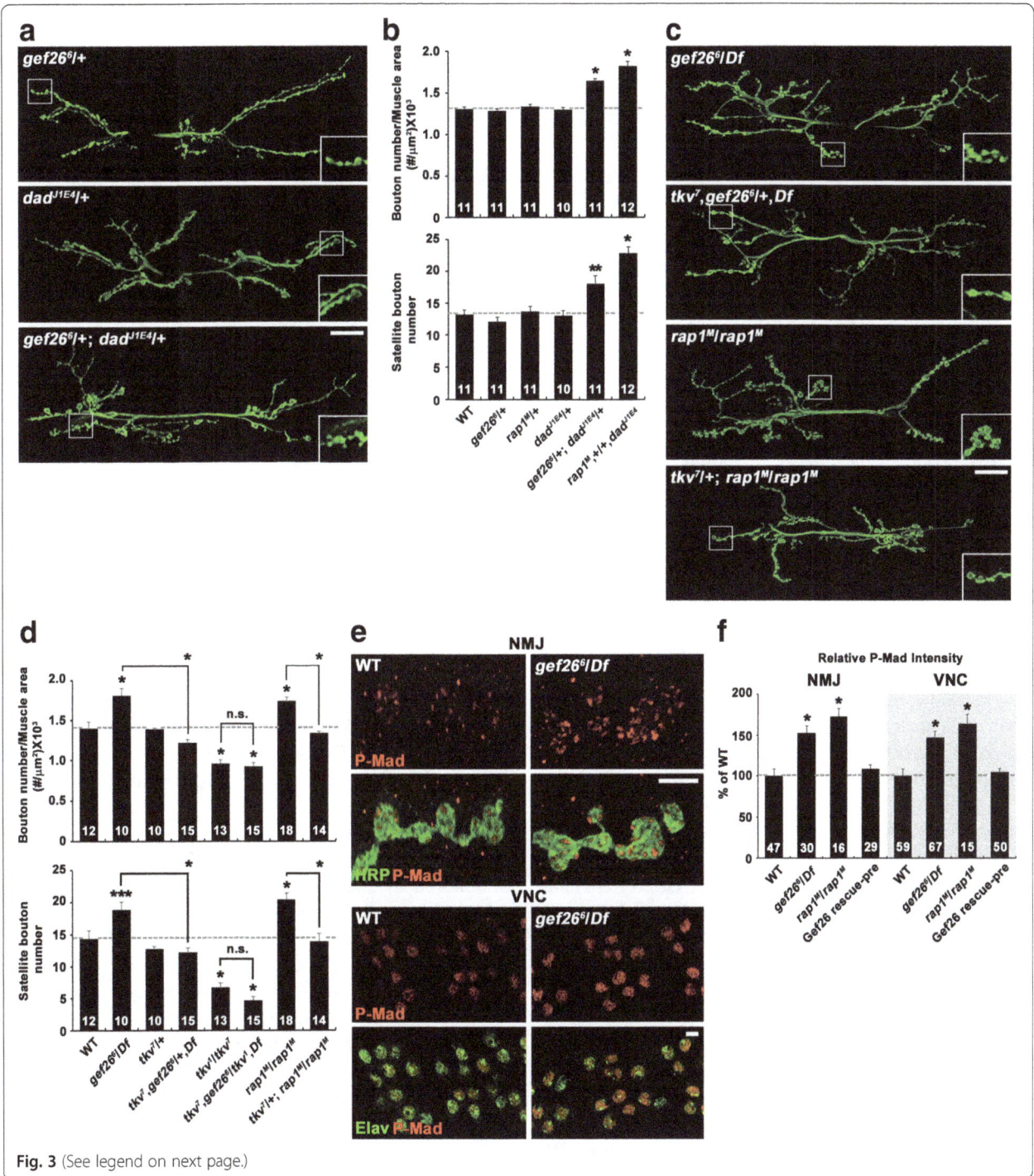

Fig. 3 (See legend on next page.)

Fig. 3 Gef26 and Rap1 inhibit BMP signaling to restrain synaptic growth. **a–d** *gef26/rap1* interacts with BMP signaling pathway components. **a** and **b** Transheterozygous interactions between *gef26* or *rap1* and *dad*. **a** Confocal images of anti-HRP-labeled NMJ 6/7 in *gef26⁶/+*, *dad^{J1E4}/+*, and *gef26⁶/+; dad^{J1E4}/+* third-instar larvae. Scale bar, 20 μm. **b** Quantification of total bouton number and satellite bouton number at NMJ 6/7 in the following genotypes: wild-type, *gef26⁶/+*, *rap1^M/+*, *dad^{J1E4}/+*, *gef26⁶/+; dad^{J1E4}/+*, and *rap1^M, +/+,dad^{J1E4}*. **c** and **d** Synaptic overgrowth in *gef26* and *rap1* depends on BMP signaling. **c** Confocal images of anti-HRP-labeled NMJ 6/7 in *gef26⁶/Df*, *tkv⁷,gef26⁶/+,Df*, *rap1^M/rap1^M*, and *tkv⁷/+; rap1^M/rap1^M* third-instar larvae. Scale bar, 20 μm. **d** Quantification of total bouton number and satellite bouton number at NMJ 6/7 in the following genotypes: wild-type, *gef26⁶/Df*, *tkv⁷/+*, *tkv⁷,gef26⁶/+,Df*, *tkv¹/tkv⁷*, *tkv⁷,gef26⁶/tkv¹,Df*, *rap1^M/rap1^M*, and *tkv⁷/+; rap1^M/rap1^M*. Note that synaptic overgrowth in *gef26* and *rap1* mutants is significantly suppressed by loss of one copy of *tkv*. **e** and **f** Levels of pMad are increased in *gef26* and *rap1* mutants. **e** Confocal images of NMJ 6/7 and ventral nerve cord (VNC) labeled with anti-P-Mad and anti-HRP or anti-Elav in wild-type and *gef26⁶/Df* third-instar larvae. Scale bars, 5 μm. **f** Quantification of the ratio of the average levels of P-Mad to HRP or Elav. Genotypes include wild-type, *gef26⁶/Df*, *rap1^M/rap1^M*, and *C155-GAL4/+; gef26⁶/Df; UAS-gef26/+* (Gef26 rescue-pre). The number of NMJs or VNCs analyzed is indicated in each bar. Data are expressed as mean ± SEM. All comparisons are made with wild-type unless otherwise indicated (*$P < 0.001$; **$P < 0.01$; ***$P < 0.05$; n.s., not significant)

center of the presynaptic terminals. However, Futsch staining was fainter or not detectable in newly formed or terminal boutons. Futsch immunoreactivity was significantly increased in *gef26* and *rap1* mutant axons compared with wild-type controls (Fig. 4d, e). In addition, the number of terminal boutons with Futsch immunoreactivity (visualized as a looped or punctate structure) was significantly higher in *gef26⁶/Df* or *rap1^M/rap1^M* mutants (Fig. 4d, arrowheads). These results indicate that Gef26 and Rap1 function to limit presynaptic Futsch level.

Futsch reliably labels microtubules in presynaptic motor terminals [25]. Therefore, the above results suggest the involvement of microtubule stability in Gef26/Rap1-mediated regulation of synaptic growth. To directly test this possibility, we assayed the extent of synaptic growth in *gef26* and *rap1* mutants fed vinblastine, a microtubule-severing drug [26]. When vinblastine was fed at a low concentration (1 μM) that did not affect synaptic growth, it completely suppressed the synaptic overgrowth phenotype of *gef26⁶/Df* or *rap1^M/rap1^M* larvae (Fig. 4f, g; Additional file 8: Table S6). These results support the idea that Gef26/Rap1 controls synaptic growth by regulating microtubule stability via the Futsch pathway.

Gef26 regulates the endocytic internalization of the BMP receptors Tkv and Wit

We next attempted to determine how Gef26 attenuates BMP signaling. Mutations disrupting endocytosis, including *endophilin* (*endo*) and *dap160*, increase presynaptic P-Mad levels at the NMJ along with simultaneous synaptic overgrowth and the formation of excessive satellite boutons [10, 13, 27], suggesting that endocytosis of surface BMP receptors is an important mechanism to inhibit BMP-dependent synaptic growth. Since a similar phenotype was observed in *gef26* mutants, we wondered if Gef26 regulates BMP signaling through endocytosis. To test this possibility, we first investigated genetic interactions between *gef26* and mutations in endocytic genes. In heterozygous *gef26⁶/+*, *endoA^{Δ4}/+*, and *dap160^{Δ1}/+* larvae, total bouton number and satellite bouton number were at wild-type levels (Fig. 5a, b; Additional file 9: Table S7). In sharp contrast,

both parameters were significantly increased in transheterozygous *gef26⁶/+; endoA^{Δ4}/+*, or *gef26⁶/dap160^{Δ1}* larvae (Fig. 5a, b), raising the possibility that Gef26 regulates BMP-dependent synaptic growth through an endocytic mechanism. It has been proposed that Dap160 interacts with the endosomal protein Nervous wreck (Nwk) to negatively regulate synaptic growth [10, 28]. However, total bouton number and satellite bouton number were normal in transheterozygous *gef26⁶/+; nwk²/+* larvae (Fig. 5b), suggesting that Gef26 and Nwk regulate BMP signaling through distinct pathways.

We then examined the impact of *gef26* knockdown on the endocytic internalization of BMP receptors in neuronal BG2-c2 cells. We transiently transfected a Myc-Tkv-Flag or Myc-Wit-Flag construct into control or *gef26*-knockdown cells (Fig. 5c) and prelabeled the cells with an anti-Myc antibody at 4 °C. We then initiated endocytosis by incubating the cells at 25 °C for 10 min and visualized the internalization of the labeled surface receptors by Myc staining. Total Myc-Tkv-Flag or Myc-Wit-Flag was also monitored by staining for the intracellular Flag-tag after cellular permeabilization. In controls cells, we observed several Myc-Tkv-Flag- or Myc-Wit-Flag-positive intracellular puncta (Fig. 5d; data not shown). Importantly, when examined in only cells with similar fluorescence intensities of Flag staining, the number of intracellular Myc-Tkv-Flag- or Myc-Wit-Flag-positive puncta per cell was dramatically reduced in *gef26*-knockdown cells (Fig. 5d, e), suggesting that Gef26 is required for the endocytic internalization of BMP receptors.

Next, we determined the impact of *gef26* loss-of-function on the levels of surface Tkv at the NMJ. To do this, we expressed *UAS-Myc-tkv* in wild-type and *gef26* mutants using *C155-GAL4*. Surface Myc-Tkv and total HRP were measured by sequential staining with anti-Myc and anti-HRP antibodies under nonpermeant and permeant conditions, respectively. The ratio of Myc-Tkv signal to HRP signal intensity was significantly increased in *gef26* compared with wild-type NMJs (Fig. 5f, g). Levels of Myc-Tkv expression were not significantly different between wild-type and *gef26⁶/Df* animals (Fig. 5h, i). These

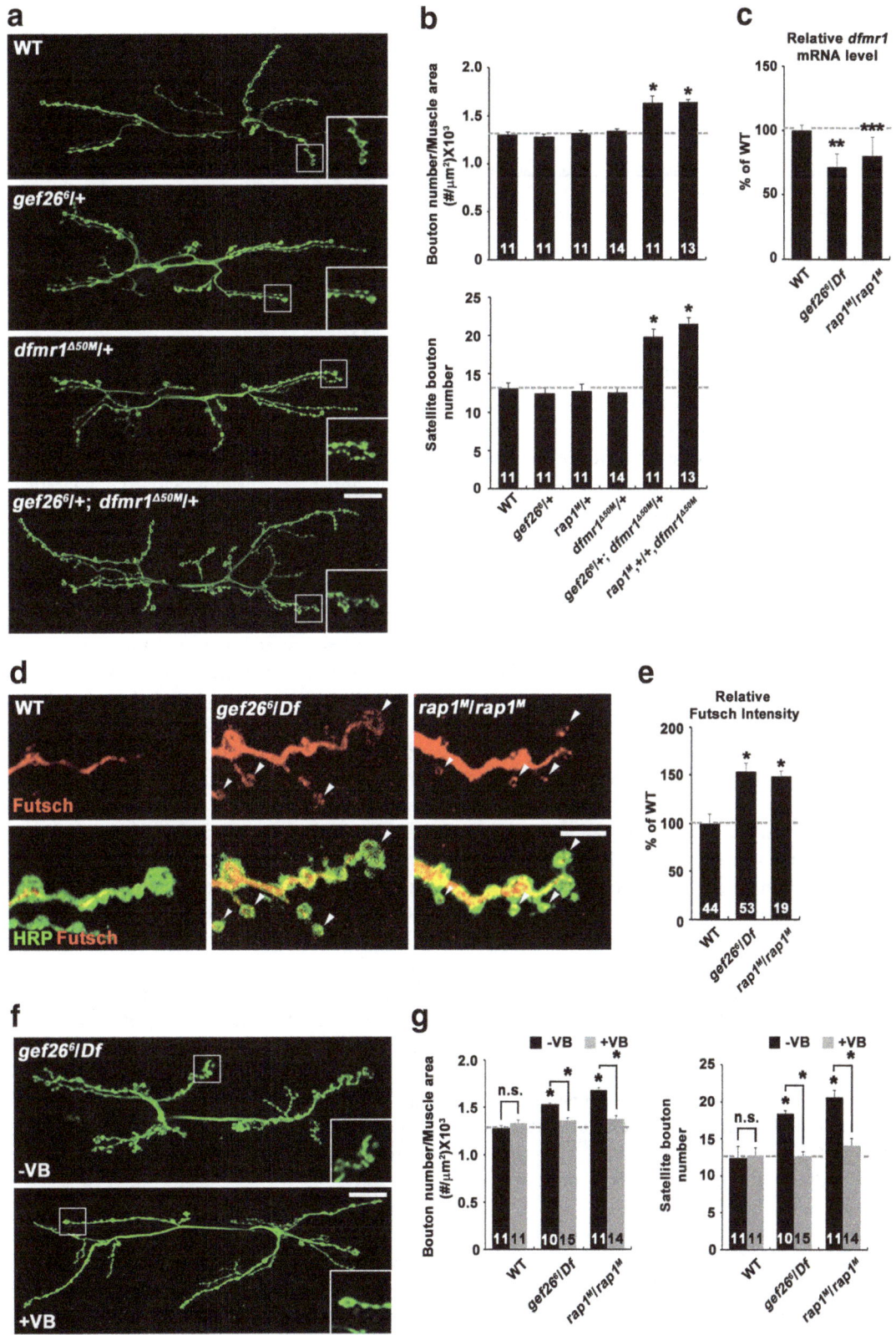

Fig. 4 (See legend on next page.)

(See figure on previous page.)

Fig. 4 Altered *dfmr1* expression and microtubule stability cause synaptic overgrowth in *gef26* and *rap1* mutants. **a** and **b** Transheterozygous interactions between *gef26* or *rap1* and *dfmr1*. **a** Confocal images of anti-HRP-labeled NMJ 6/7 in wild-type, *gef26^6/+*, *dfmr1^{Δ50M}/+*, and *gef26^6/+; dfmr1^{Δ50M}/+* third-instar larvae. Scale bar, 20 μm. **b** Quantification of total bouton number and satellite bouton number at NMJ 6/7 in the following genotypes: wild-type, *gef26^6/+*, *rap1^M/+*, *dfmr1^{Δ50M}/+*, *gef26^6/+; dfmr1^{Δ50M}/+*, and *rap1^M,+/+,dfmr1^{Δ50M}*. **c** Quantification of *dfmr1* RNA levels using quantitative real-time PCR in the CNS of wild-type, *gef26^6/Df*, and *rap1^M/rap1^M* third-instar larvae. *rp49* was used as an internal control. **d** and **e** Levels of synaptic Futsch are increased in *gef26* and *rap1* mutants. **d** Confocal images of anti-Futsch and anti-HRP staining from NMJ 6/7 of wild-type, *gef26^6/Df*, and *rap1^M/rap1^M* third-instar larvae. Arrowheads indicate Futsch-positive terminal loops. Scale bar, 5 μm. **e** Quantification of the ratio of the average anti-Futsch to anti-HRP staining intensities. **f** and **g** Synaptic overgrowth in *gef26* and *rap1* mutants is suppressed by vinblastine administration. **f** Confocal images of NMJ 6/7 immunostained with anti-HRP are shown for *gef26^6/Df* mutants raised in the absence (-VB) or presence (+VB) of 1 μM vinblastine. Scale bar, 20 μm. **g** Quantification of total bouton number and satellite bouton number at NMJ 6/7 in the indicated genotypes. The number of NMJs analyzed is indicated in each bar. Data are expressed as mean ± SEM. All comparisons are made with wild-type unless otherwise indicated (*$P < 0.001$; **$P < 0.01$; ***$P < 0.05$; n.s., not significant)

data support a role for Gef26 in endocytic internalization of the Tkv receptor.

Given the role of Gef26 in BMP receptor internalization, we examined whether synaptic vesicle endocytosis is affected in *gef26* mutant NMJs. We stimulated third instar fillets with 90 mM K^+ in the presence of the styryl dye FM1–43FX. During a 1-min labeling period, dye uptake into synaptic boutons was not significantly different between wild-type and *gef26^6/Df* mutant animals (Additional file 10: Figure S3a, b). This result indicates that loss of Gef26 does not grossly affect endocytosis at the presynaptic terminal of the NMJ.

Gef26/Rap1 regulation of BMP signaling is essential for neuronal survival in the adult brain

Overactivation of BMP signaling in the adult *Drosophila* brain induces age-dependent progressive motor dysfunction and neurodegeneration [9]. Since we established the role of Gef26 in downregulating BMP signaling at the NMJ, we investigated whether *gef26* knockdown induces adult phenotypes similar to elevated BMP signaling. We first assayed the locomotor performance of *C155-GAL4/ +; UAS-gef26^{RNAi}/+* flies in a geotactic climbing assay. Compared with age-matched *C155-GAL4/+* controls, 20-day-old *C155-GAL4/+; UAS-gef26^{RNAi}/+* flies displayed a significantly reduced climbing response within 30 s (*C155-GAL4/+*: 16.56 ± 0.57 cm, *C155-GAL4/+; UAS-gef26^{RNAi}/+*: 9.33 ± 0.11 cm, $P < 0.001$; Fig. 6a, b).

We then investigated whether knockdown of *gef26* expression is associated with neurodegeneration by examining histological sections of adult brains. At 2 days after eclosion, *C155-GAL4/+; UAS-gef26^{RNAi}/+* brains had normal anatomical and histological organization (Fig. 6c). However, aged *C155-GAL4/+; UAS-gef26^{RNAi}/+* brains exhibited progressive vacuolization (Fig. 6c, arrowheads), which is a hallmark of neurodegeneration in the *Drosophila* brain [29]. Vacuolization progressed at a much slower rate in *C155-GAL4/+* control brains (Fig. 6d). To further characterize neurodegeneration, we performed caspase-3 and TUNEL staining on 20-day-old brains. Caspase-3- or TUNEL-positive cells were detected in *C155-GAL4/+; UAS-gef26^{RNAi}/+* brains, but

not in *C155-GAL4/+* control brains (Fig. 6e; Additional file 11: Figure S4a, b). In addition, TUNEL staining revealed that neuronal knockdown of *gef26* induces cell death in an age-dependent, progressive manner (Additional file 11: Figure S4b). Importantly, anti-caspase-3 signals overlapped with the neuronal marker anti-Elav, but not with the glial marker anti-Repo (Fig. 6e, arrowheads). Together, these results indicate that Gef26 activity is essential for neuronal survival in the adult brain.

Finally, we investigated whether Gef26 collaborates with Rap1 and the BMP pathway to maintain normal locomotor ability and neuronal survival. To this end, we first examined transheterozygous combinations of *gef26* and *rap1* or *dad* with respect to locomotor dysfunction. At 20 days of age, transheterozygous *gef26^6/+; rap1^M/+* and *gef26^6/+; dad^{J1E4}/+* flies displayed mildly reduced climbing response compared with age-matched *gef26^6/+*, *rap1^M/+*, or *dad^{J1E4}/+* flies (data not shown). However, these transheterozygous flies at 30 days of age exhibited severely reduced climbing ability (Additional file 11: Figure S4c, d). We also examined transheterozygous interactions between *gef26* and *rap1* or *dad* with respect to brain neurodegeneration. At 20 days of age, heterozygous *gef26^6/+*, *rap1^M/+*, or *dad^{J1E4}/+* flies were not distinguishable from wild-type controls with respect to the total number of vacuoles (Fig. 6f). In sharp contrast, there was a significant vacuolization in the brains of transheterozygous *gef26^6/+; rap1^M/+* or *gef26^6/+; dad^{J1E4}/+* flies (Fig. 6f), supporting a functional link between Gef26, Rap1, and the BMP signaling pathway in the regulation of neuronal survival in the adult brain.

Discussion

In the mammalian nervous system, PDZ-GEF1 (also called RAPGEF2) and its downstream GTPase Rap1 play an important role in homeostatic synaptic plasticity by decreasing the density of dendritic spines [30], the primary postsynaptic compartment for excitatory synapses. However, the presynaptic function of these molecules has not been addressed. In this study, we identified the *Drosophila* homologs (Gef26 and Rap1, respectively) as

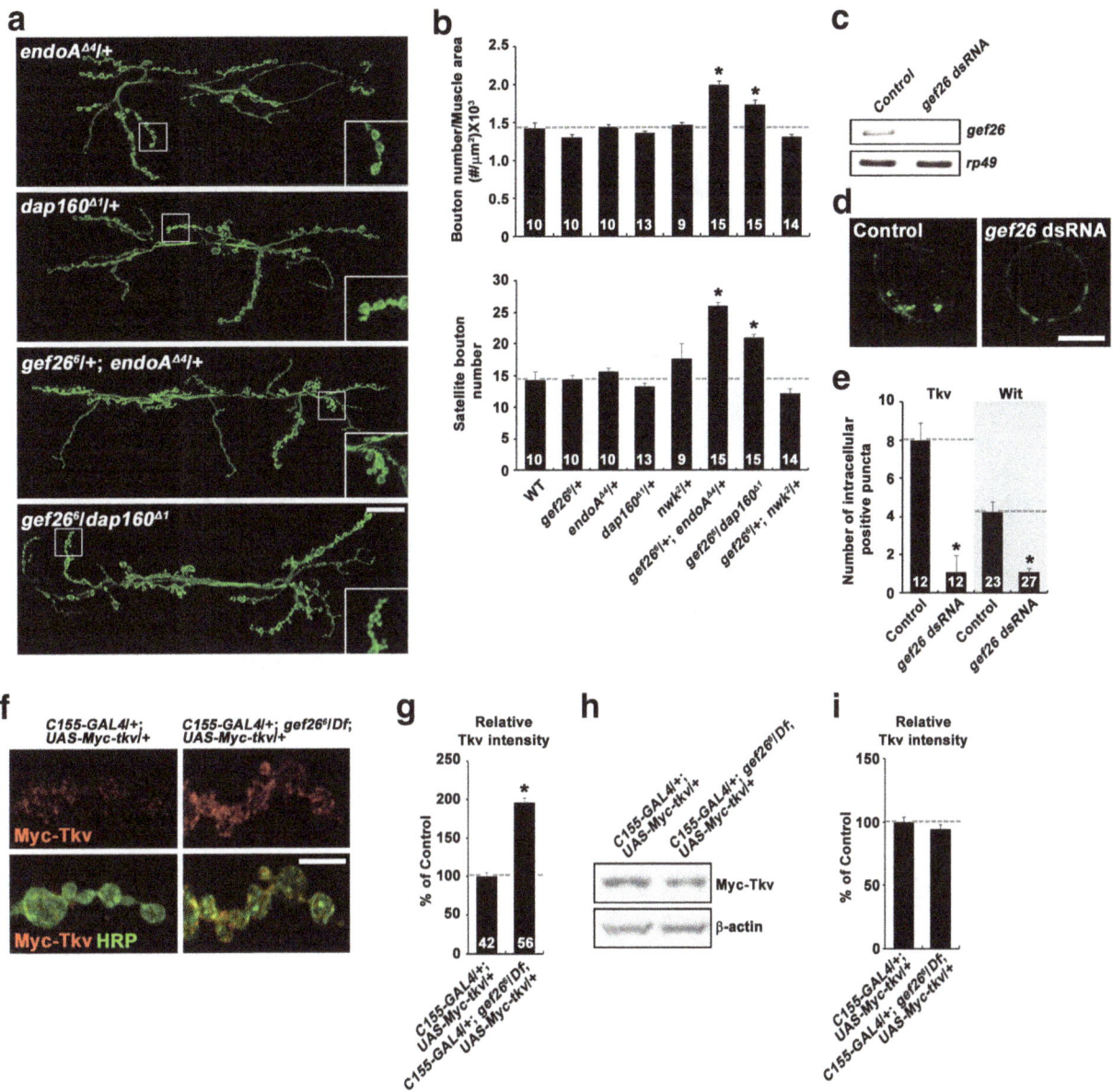

Fig. 5 Gef26 regulates endocytic internalization and surface expression of BMP receptors. **a** and **b** *gef26* interacts with endocytic mutations during synaptic growth. **a** Confocal images of anti-HRP-labeled NMJ 6/7 in *endoA*$^{\Delta4}$/+, *dap160*$^{\Delta1}$/+, *gef26*^{6}/+; *endoA*$^{\Delta4}$/+, and *gef26*^{6}/*dap160*$^{\Delta1}$ third-instar larvae. Scale bar, 20 μm. **b** Quantification of total bouton number and satellite bouton number at NMJ 6/7 in the following genotypes: wild-type, *gef26*^{6}/+, *endoA*$^{\Delta4}$/+, *dap160*$^{\Delta1}$/+, *nwk*^{2}/+, *gef26*^{6}/+; *endoA*$^{\Delta4}$/+, *gef26*^{6}/*dap160*$^{\Delta1}$, and *gef26*^{6}/+; *nwk*^{2}/+. **c-e** Gef26 is required for endocytic internalization of surface BMP receptors. BG2-c2 cells were transfected with *pAc-Myc-tkv-Flag* or *pAc-Myc-wit-Flag* in the absence (control) and presence of *gef26* dsRNA. Live control and Gef26-depleted cells were prelabeled with anti-Myc (green) at 4 °C, followed by incubation at 25 °C for 10 min to allow internalization of the labeled surface receptors. After fixation and permeabilization, cells were sequentially stained with anti-Flag (red) and fluorescently-labeled secondary antibodies. **c** Reverse transcription (RT)-PCR analysis to confirm knockdown efficiency of Gef26. **d** Single confocal sections through the middle of control and *gef26*-knockdown cells are shown for the green channel only. Scale bar, 5 μm. **e** Quantification of the number of intracellular Myc-positive puncta per cell. Only cells with similar Flag signal (red) intensities were analyzed. **f** and **g** Steady-state levels of surface Tkv are increased at the NMJ of *gef26* mutants. **f** Representative confocal images of NMJ 6/7 in *C155-GAL4*/+; *UAS-Myc-tkv*/+ and *C155-GAL4*/+; *gef26*^{6}/*Df*; *UAS-Myc-tkv*/+ larvae. NMJ preparations were sequentially stained with anti-Myc (red) and anti-HRP (green) under nonpermeant and permeant conditions. Scale bar, 5 μm. **g** Quantification of the ratio of surface Myc-Tkv to HRP fluorescence intensities. **h** and **i** Transgenic expression of Myc-Tkv in neurons is not altered by loss of Gef26. **h** Western blot of central nervous system (CNS) extracts from *C155-GAL4*/+; *UAS-Myc-tkv*/+ and *C155-GAL4*/+; *gef26*^{6}/*Df*; *UAS-Myc-tkv*/+ larvae. The blot was probed with anti-Myc and anti-β-actin. **i** Quantitative analysis of three independent blots by densitometric measurements. For each sample, the band intensity of Myc-Tkv was normalized to that of β-actin. The number of NMJs (**b**), cells (**e**), or synaptic boutons (**g**) analyzed is indicated in each bar. Data are expressed as mean ± SEM. *$P < 0.001$

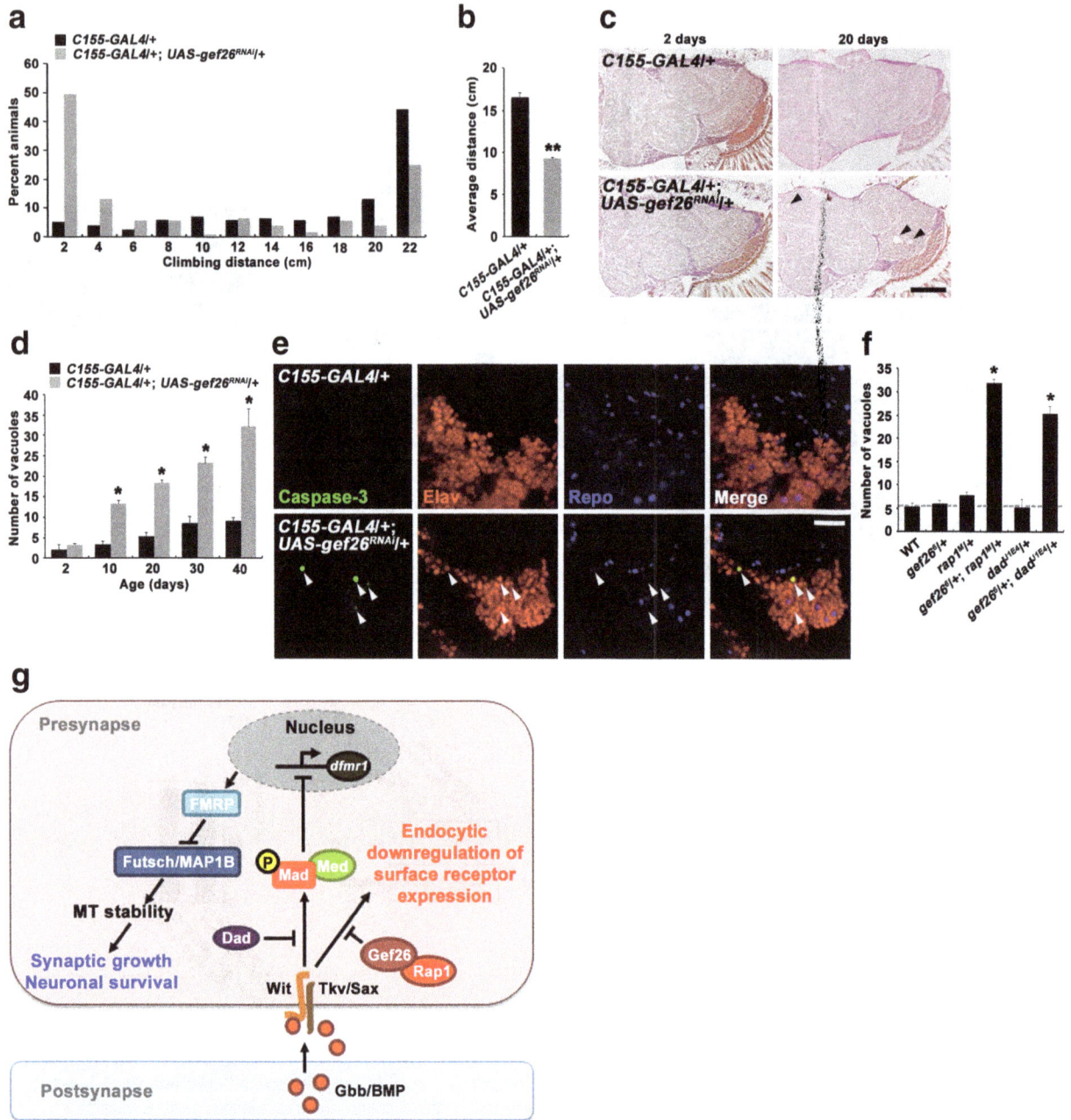

Fig. 6 Loss of Gef26 induces motor dysfunction and progressive brain neurodegeneration in the adult fly. **a** and **b** Adult locomotor activity is impaired by neuron-specific Gef26 knockdown. **a** Distribution of the distance climbed by 20-day-old *C155-GAL4/+* and *C155-GAL4/+; UAS-gef26^RNAi/+* flies over a 30 s period. **b** Quantification of average climbing distance. **c** and **d** Neuron-specific Gef26 knockdown causes brain neurodegeneration in an age-dependent manner. **c** Frontal brain sections (5 μm) stained with H&E are shown for *C155-GAL4/+* and *C155-GAL4/+; UAS-gef26^RNAi/+* flies at 2 or 20 days of age. Note the presence of numerous vacuoles (arrowheads) in the brain of 20-day-old *C155-GAL4/+; UAS-gef26^RNAi/+* flies. Scale bar, 20 μm. **d** Quantification of vacuoles with a diameter greater than 5 μm in *C155-GAL4/+* and *C155-GAL4/+; UAS-gef26^RNAi/+* brains at different ages. $n > 10$. **e** Confocal sections of 20-day-old *C155-GAL4/+* and *C155-GAL4/+; UAS-gef26^RNAi/+* brains stained with anti-caspase-3 (green), anti-Elav (red), and anti-Repo (blue). Anti-caspase-3 signals overlaps with the neuronal cell marker anti-Elav (arrowheads) but not with the glial cell marker anti-Repo. Scale bar, 20 μm. **f** Quantification of brain vacuolization in 20-day-old wild-type ($n = 5$), *gef26^6/+* ($n = 5$), *rap1^M/+* ($n = 6$), *gef26^6/+; rap1^M/+* ($n = 5$), *dad^J1E4/+* ($n = 5$), and *gef26^6/+; dad^J1E4/+* ($n = 6$) flies. **g** Model for Gef26/Rap1 regulation of BMP-dependent synaptic growth and neuronal survival

new presynaptic regulators of BMP-dependent synaptic growth. First, *gef26* and *rap1* mutant NMJs display a distinctive phenotype of excessive satellite bouton formation, recapitulating synaptic defects induced by elevated BMP signaling [9, 10, 12]. Second, genetic epistasis analysis and several independent genetic experiments demonstrate that Gef26 acts upstream of Rap1 at presynaptic NMJ terminals. Third, synaptic overgrowth in *gef26* and *rap1* mutants depends on the level of BMP signaling. Fourth, *gef26* and *rap1* mutants show a significant increase in the level of P-Mad, the readout of BMP signaling. Fifth, Gef26 and Rap1 negatively regulate the stability of presynaptic microtubules via dFMRP, which is known to be a major target for BMP signaling in the regulation of synaptic growth [9]. Based on these data, we propose that the presynaptic GEF26-Rap1 pathway regulates synaptic growth by modulating microtubule stability via the BMP-dFMRP pathway.

How might Gef26 regulate BMP signaling? Increasing evidence suggests that endocytosis of surface BMP receptors is a key mechanism of signal attenuation at presynaptic NMJ terminals. In support of this notion, our data imply that Gef26 inhibits BMP signaling by regulating the endocytic internalization of its receptor(s). *gef26* displays transheterozygous interactions with mutations disrupting endocytosis (i.e., *dap160* and *endoA*) during synaptic growth. In addition, *gef26* mutant NMJs show an increase in the level of surface Tkv, supporting the role of Gef26 in receptor endocytosis. Most directly, we show that Gef26 facilitates the endocytic internalization of the BMP receptors Tkv and Wit in cultured cells. These findings imply a model in which Gef26 attenuate BMP signaling through facilitating endocytosis of BMP receptors (Fig. 6g).

Elevated BMP signaling has been implicated in the pathogenesis of hereditary spastic paraplegia (HSP), a group of neurodegenerative motor disorders. In mammalian cells, several HSP proteins, including NIPA1, Spastin, and Spartin, have been shown to inhibit BMP signaling [31]. At the *Drosophila* NMJ, the NIPA1 homologue Spichthyin (Spict) and Spartin also inhibit BMP signaling to restrain synaptic growth [9, 11]. Importantly, it has now been demonstrated that elevation of BMP signaling in adult *spartin* flies causes progressive neurodegeneration and locomotor dysfunction [9]. Consistent with these studies and the proposed role of Gef26 as an inhibitor of BMP signaling, depletion of *gef26* in the adult fly induces neurodegeneration and locomotor function. Thus, the current study solidifies the notion that precise regulation of BMP signaling is critical for the maintenance of adult neurons. A future challenge will be to investigate whether PDZ-GEF1 and other human Gef26 homologues contribute to the maintenance of the human motor system and, if so, whether this neuroprotective role involves the regulation of retrograde BMP transsynaptic signaling.

A final point of interest is the mechanism of how the Gef26-Rap1 pathway facilitates BMP receptor endocytosis. In various experimental systems, Rap1 has been identified to regulate actin-driven cellular processes. For example, mammalian Rap1 promotes cell spreading by localizing the RacGEFs Vav2 and Tiam1 to sites of lamellipodia extension [32], which is driven by Rac-dependent actin polymerization. In addition, *Dictyostelium* Rap1 is also involved in chemotaxis by activating the Rac signaling pathway through RacGEF1 [33]. Since actin polymerization is known to provide mechanical forces required for multiple stages of endocytosis [34], it is tempting to speculate that Rap1 facilitates endocytosis by regulating actin polymerization through the RacGEF-Rac signaling pathway. Interestingly, the Rac signaling pathway has been implicated in the regulation of BMP-dependent synaptic growth at the *Drosophila* NMJ [35]. In future studies, it will be interesting to investigate the role of the Rac signaling pathway in Rap1-dependent endocytosis.

Methods

Drosophila stocks

Flies were maintained on standard medium at 25 °C. w^{1118} was used as the wild-type control. $gef26^6$ was generously provided by S. Hou (National Institutes of Health National Cancer Institute, Frederick, MD, USA) [19], and nwk^2 was obtained from K. O'Connor-Giles (University of Wisconsin, Madison, WI, USA) [10]. *Df(2 L)BSC5* (a deficiency of the *gef26* locus), $rap1^{MI1950}$, tkv^1, tkv^7, dad^{J1E4}, $endoA^{\Delta4}$, and $dap160^{\Delta1}$ were obtained from the Bloomington Stock Center (Bloomington, IN, USA). Transgenic lines carrying *UAS-gef26*, *UAS-Myc-rap1^{CA}*, and *UAS-Myc-tkv* were generated in the w^{1118} background using standard protocols. RNA interference (RNAi) lines PDZ-GEF^{KK102612} (referred to here as *UAS-gef26^{RNAi}*) and Rap1^{KK107785} (*UAS-rap1^{R-NAi1}*) were obtained from the Vienna Drosophila Resources Center (Vienna, Austria). Another RNAi line Rap1^{HMJ21898} (*UAS-rap1^{RNAi2}*) was obtained from the Bloomington Stock Center. Neural and muscle-specific expression of UAS transgenes was achieved using *C155-GAL4* [36] and *BG57-GAL4* [37], respectively.

Cell culture and transient transfection

Drosophila neuronal BG2-c2 cells were maintained at 25 °C in M3 medium (Sigma-Aldrich, St. Louis, MO, USA) supplemented with 10% heat-inactivated fetal bovine serum (Gibco, Carlsbad, CA, USA), 10 μg/ml insulin (Sigma-Aldrich), and penicillin/streptomycin. Cells were transfected in 12-well plates with 1 μg plasmid DNA in the presence or absence of 5 μg double-stranded RNA (dsRNA) using Cellfectin II (Invitrogen, Carlsbad, CA, USA).

Molecular biology

Full-length cDNAs for *gef26* and *rap1* were obtained by reverse transcription PCR of total RNA extracted from *Drosophila* S2R+ cells and introduced into the pUAST or pUAST-Myc vector to generate *UAS-gef26* and *UAS-Myc-rap1*. For *UAS-Myc-rap1^CA^*, glutamine 63 was mutated to glutamate by overlapping PCR using *UAS-Myc-rap1* (the template DNA) and the primers 5'-ATGGCCGT-GAACTCCTCCGTACCC-3' and 5'-TACGGAGGAGTT-CACGGCCATGCG-3' in combination with the BglII-Myc-linked primer 5'-GGGAGATCTGCCACCATG-GAACAAAAACTCATCTCAGAAGAG-GATCT-GATGCGTGAGTACAAAATC-3' and the XbaI-linked primer 5'-GGGTCTAGATAGCAGAACACATAGGGAC-3', respectively, and the assembled product was introduced into pUAST. For *pAc-Myc-tkv-Flag*, a full-length cDNA (clone ID: LD45557) for *tkv* (*CG14026*) was obtained from the Drosophila Genomics Resource Center (Bloomington, IN, USA). The cDNA insert was PCR-amplified and then introduced into the pTOP Blunt V2 vector (Enzynomics, Daejeon, Republic of Korea). Myc and Flag epitope-tag sequences were introduced immediately downstream of the signal sequence and at the C-terminus of Tkv, respectively, by PCR-based mutagenesis. The resulting *Myc-tkv-Flag* insert was subcloned into the pAc5.1 vector. For *pAc-Myc-wit-Flag*, Flag epitope-tag sequence was introduced downstream of the *wit* sequence of *pAc-Myc-wit* [9] by PCR-based mutagenesis. The resulting *Myc-wit-Flag* fragment was re-introduced into the pAc5.1 vector.

To measure levels of *dfmr1* expression, total RNA was extracted from the third instar brain and ventral ganglion using the TRIsure kit (Bioline, Taunton, MA, USA) and reverse transcribed using the SuperScript III cDNA synthesis kit (Invitrogen). Quantitative real-time PCR reactions were performed using SYBR Select Master Mix (Applied Biosystems, Foster City, CA, USA) on an Applied Biosystems 7500 Real-Time PCR System. The mean Ct of triplicate reactions was used to determine relative expression of *dfmr1* using the $2^{-\Delta\Delta CT}$ method. Expression of *rp49* was used as the internal control. The primers used were: *dfmr1*, 5'-GGATCAGAACATAC-CACGTG-3' and 5'-CTGGCAGCTATCGTGGAGGCG-3'; and *rp49*, 5'-CACCAGTCGGATCGATATGC-3' and 5'-CACGTTGTGCACCAGGAACT-3'.

For RNA interference (RNAi) experiments in BG2-c2 cells, *gef26* dsRNA was produced by in vitro transcription of a DNA template containing T7 promoter sequences at both ends, as described previously [38]. The DNA template was produced by PCR from the *UAS-gef26* vector using primers containing a T7 promotor sequence followed by *gef26*-specific sequences: 5'-GTGGCCGGCTCTACCAGT-3' and 5'-TGGTACGC-GAGTCGAACG-3'.

Western blot analysis

Larval CNS (the brain lobes and the ventral nerve cord) preparations were homogenized in ice-cold lysis buffer (25 mM Tris-HCl, pH 7.5, 150 mM NaCl, 0.5% Triton X-100, and protease inhibitors) and subjected to western blotting as described previously [20]. The following primary antibodies were used: anti-Myc (1:1000, Cell Signaling, Danvers, MA, USA) and anti-β-actin (1:1000, Sigma-Aldrich).

BMPR internalization assay

BG2-c2 cells were transfected with *pAc-Myc-tkv-Flag* or *pAc-Myc-wit-Flag* in the presence or absence of *gef26* dsRNA. At 72 h post-transfection, live cells were incubated with an anti-Myc antibody (1:200, Cell Signaling) at 4 °C for 1 h to label Myc-Tkv-Flag or Myc-Wit-Flag proteins expressed on the cell surface, followed by incubation at 25 °C for 10 min to allow internalization of the labeled receptors. Cells were subsequently washed in an ice-cold acidic buffer (0.5 M NaCl, 0.2 M acetic acid, pH 4.0) for 15 min to remove any remaining bound anti-Myc antibody and fixed in PBS containing 4% formaldehyde for 10 min. Fixed cells were permeabilized in PBT-0.2 (PBS, 0.2% Triton X-100) for 10 min, blocked with PBS containing 1% BSA for 1 h, and sequentially incubated with a mouse anti-Flag primary antibody (1:500, Sigma-Aldrich) and a FITC-conjugated anti-mouse secondary antibody (1:200, Jackson ImmunoResearch, West Grove, PA, USA) in PBS containing 1% BSA. Stained cells were mounted with SlowFade antifade medium (Invitrogen) and imaged with a LSM 800 laser-scanning confocal microscope (Carl Zeiss, Jena, Germany) using a Plan Apo 63 × 1.4 NA oil objective. The number of intracellular Myc-positive puncta was measured in cells with similar fluorescence intensities of Flag staining.

Immunostaining of larval NMJs

Wandering third-instar larvae were dissected in Ca^{2+}-free HL3 solution and fixed in PBS containing 4% formaldehyde for 20 min. Fixed larval fillets were washed with PBT-0.1 (PBS, 0.1% Triton X-100) and blocked with PBT-0.1 containing 0.2% BSA for 1 h. Samples were sequentially incubated with primary antibodies overnight at 4 °C and fluorescently-labeled secondary antibodies for 1 h at room temperature. The following monoclonal antibodies from the Developmental Studies Hybridoma Bank (DSHB, Iowa City, IA, USA) were used as primary antibodies: anti-HRP (1:200), anti-Futsch (1:50), anti-CSP (1:300), anti-NC82 (1:50), and anti-Dlg (1:500). Additional primary antibodies used were anti-P-Mad/PS1 (1:500) [39], anti-GluRIIC (1:200) [40], anti-P-Mad (1:100, Cell Signaling), and anti-Myc (1:200, Cell Signaling). FITC- and Cy3-conjugated secondary antibodies (Jackson ImmunoResearch) were used at 1:200. Images were captured with an LSM 800 laser-scanning confocal microscope using a C Apo 40× W or Plan Apo 63 × 1.4 NA objective.

Quantification of bouton number and satellite bouton number was performed at NMJ 6/7 and NMJ 4 in abdominal segment 2, as previously described [20]. Bouton number was normalized to muscle surface area. Statistical analysis was performed using SigmaPlot (Systat Software, San Jose, CA, USA). Comparisons were made by one-way ANOVA analysis with a post-hoc Turkey test. For comparison of only two samples, an unpaired Student's t-test was used. Data are presented as mean ± SEM.

FM1–43FX uptake assay

FM1–43FX dye uptake experiments were performed as described previously [9, 41]. Briefly, wandering third-instar larvae were dissected in Ca^{2+}-free HL3 saline and then incubated in HL3 saline with 90 mM KCl, 5 mM $CaCl_2$, and 4 µM FM1–43FX (Molecular Probes, Eugene, OR, USA) for 1 min. FM1–43FX-loaded samples were vigorously washed with Ca^{2+}-free HL3 saline for 10 min, and fixed in PBS containing 4% formaldehyde, and washed three times in PBS. Images were collected using a Plan Apo 40 × 0.90 NA water-immersion objective on FV300 laser-scanning confocal microscope (Olympus, Tokyo, Japan).

Histology, immunostaining, and TUNEL staining of adult brains

Heads from adult flies at 2, 10, 20, 30, and 40 days post-eclosion were fixed overnight in PBS containing 4% para-formaldehyde at 4 °C, embedded in paraffin, and subjected to serial 5-µm sectioning in a frontal orientation. Serial sections covering the entire brain were placed on a single slide and stained with hematoxylin and eosin (H&E) using a standard protocol. Vacuoles larger than 5 µm were counted throughout the entire brain.

For immunostaining analysis, brains from 20-day-old flies were dissected in ice-cold PBS, and fixed overnight in PBS containing 4% formaldehyde at 4 °C. Fixed brains were subsequently permeabilized in PBT-0.3 (PBS, 0.3% Triton X-100) for 1 h and blocked with PBT-0.3 containing 5% BSA for 1 h. The brains were sequentially incubated with primary antibodies for 48 h at 4 °C and fluorescently-labeled secondary antibodies for 24 h at 4 °C. The following primary antibodies were used in this study: anti-Elav (7E8A10, DSHB) at 1:10, anti-Repo (8D12, DSHB) at 1:10, and anti-cleaved caspase-3 (Cell Signaling) at 1:100. Antibody-stained brains were mounted in SlowFade anti-fade medium (Invitrogen). Fluorescent images were acquired with a LSM 800 laser-scanning confocal microscope using a C Apo 40× W objective.

TUNEL assays on paraffin sections of adult brains were performed using the In Situ Cell Death Detection Kit (Roche, Mannheim, Germany). Briefly, paraffin sections were dewaxed according to standard procedures. After washed with PBS, the sections were permeabilized in PBS containing 0.1% sodium citrate and 0.1% Triton X-100 for 15 min at room temperature. After washing with PBS, the samples were incubated with the TUNEL reaction mixture in a dark humid chamber for 1 h at 37 °C, prior to DAPI staining for 5 min at room temperature. TUNEL- and DAPI-positive cells were counted in three consecutive, middle frontal sections of adult brains.

Adult climbing test

Adult locomotor ability was assayed as described previously [9]. For each genotype tested, approximately 100 flies were collected within 1 day of eclosion; aged for 2, 10, 20, 30, and 40 days; and placed into a glass graduated cylinder. After 5 min of adaptation to their environment, flies were gently vortexed for 5 s. The distance climbed by individual flies in a 30 s period was measured. Climbing assays were repeated 3 times for each genotype, and the results were averaged.

Conclusions

In summary, our findings establish a novel role for the Gef26-Rap1 pathway in regulating BMP-dependent synaptic growth and neuronal survival. Regulation of surface expression of BMP receptors via endocytosis may represent an important underlying mechanism.

Additional files

Additional file 1: Table S1. Quantification of NMJ parameters for the experiments in Fig. 1b.

Additional file 2: Figure S1. Presynaptic requirement for Gef26 in synaptic growth regulation and characterization of satellite boutons. **a** Confocal images of anti-HRP-labeled NMJ 6/7 in *C155-GAL4/+*, *C155-GAL4/+; UAS-gef26^{RNAi}/+*, *BG57-GAL4/+*, and *BG57-GAL4/UAS-gef26^{RNAi}* third-instar larvae. Scale bar, 20 µm. **b** Quantification of total bouton number and satellite bouton number. **c-e** Confocal images of NMJ 6/7 stained with anti-HRP and anti-NC82 (**c**), anti-CSP (**d**), or anti-Dlg (**e**) for wild-type and *gef26^6/Df* third-instar larvae. **f** Confocal images of NMJ 6/7 stained with anti-NC82 and anti-GluRIIC in wild-type and *gef26^6/Df* third-instar larvae. The number of NMJs analyzed is indicated in each bar. Data are expressed as mean ± SEM. *$P < 0.001$.

Additional file 3: Table S2. Quantification of NMJ parameters for the experiments in Additional file 2: Figure S1B.

Additional file 4: Table S3. Quantification of NMJ parameters for the experiments in Fig. 2b.

Additional file 5: Figure S2. *rap1* is required presynaptically for normal synaptic growth. **a** Confocal images of anti-HRP-labeled NMJ 6/7 in *C155-GAL4/+*, *C155-GAL4/+; UAS-rap1^{RNAi1}/+*, *C155-GAL4/+; UAS-rap1^{RNAi2}/+*, *BG57-GAL4/+*, *BG57-GAL4/UAS-rap1^{RNAi1}*, and *BG57-GAL4/UAS-rap1^{RNAi2}* third-instar larvae. Scale bar, 20 µm. **b** Quantification of total bouton number and satellite bouton number. The number of NMJs analyzed is indicated in each bar. Data are expressed as mean ± SEM. *$P < 0.001$.

Additional file 6: Table S4. Quantification of NMJ parameters for the experiments in Additional file 5: Figure S2B.

Additional file 7: Table S5. Quantification of NMJ parameters for the experiments in Fig. 3.

Additional file 8: Table S6. Quantification of NMJ parameters for the experiments in Fig. 4.

Additional file 9: Table S7. Quantification of NMJ parameters for the experiments in Fig. 5b.

Additional file 10: Figure S3. *gef26* mutant NMJs show normal FM1–43FX dye uptake after nerve stimulation. **a** Confocal images of NMJ 6/7 boutons in wild-type and *gef26⁶/Df* third instar larvae. NMJ synapses were stimulated for 1 min with 90 mM K$^+$ and 5 mM Ca^{2+} in the presence of FM1–43FX. Scale bar, 20 μm. **b** Quantification of FM1–43FX fluorescence intensity.

Additional file 11: Figure S4. Progressive apoptotic cell death in *gef26* knockdown brains and reduced locomotor activities of flies transheterozygous for *gef26* and *rap1* or *dad*. **a** and **b** Neuron-specific knockdown of *gef26* expression causes age-dependent apoptotic cell death in the adult brain. **a** Confocal slices of 20-day-old *C155-GAL4/+* and *C155-GAL4/+; UAS-gef26^{RNAi}/+* brains labeled with TUNEL and DAPI. Scale bars, 20 μm. **b** Quantification of TUNEL-positive cells in three consecutive, middle frontal sections (5 μm thick) of *C155-GAL4/+* and *C155-GAL4/+; UAS-gef26^{RNAi}/+* brains. *n* = 4. **c** and **d** Reduced locomotor activities of flies transheterozygous for *gef26* and *rap1* or *dad*. **c** Distribution of the distance climbed by 30-day-old flies of the indicated genotypes over a 30 s period. **d** Quantification of average climbing distance for the genotypes indicated. All comparisons are with the *C155-GAL4/+* control (**b**) or wild type (**d**): *$P < 0.001$.

Abbreviations

BMP: Bone morphogenetic protein; CSP: Cysteine-string protein; *dfmr1*: *Drosophila* fragile X mental retardation 1; Dlg: Discs-large; Gbb: Glass bottom boat; GEF: Guanine nucleotide exchange factor; NMJ: Neuromuscular junction; P-Mad: Phosphorylated Mad; Tkv: Thickveins

Acknowledgements

The authors thank Dr. Steve Hou and the Bloomington Stock Center for providing the fly strains used in this study.

Authors' contribution

CSK, SHK, and SL designed the study. KH, MN, MJL, and YEK performed the experiments and analyzed the data. KH and SL wrote the manuscript. All authors read and approved the final manuscript.

Funding

This work was supported by a grant from the National Research Foundation of Korea (No. 2017M3C7A1025368) and by the BK21+ program of the National Research Foundation of Korea.

Competing interests

The authors declare that they have no competing interests.

Author details

¹Department of Brain and Cognitive Sciences, College of Natural Sciences, Seoul National University, Seoul 08826, South Korea. ²Department of Cell & Developmental Biology, Dental Research Institute, Seoul National University, Seoul 03080, South Korea. ³Department of Neurology, Hanyang University College of Medicine, Seoul 04763, South Korea. ⁴Department of Laboratory Medicine and Genetics, Samsung Medical Center, Sungkyunkwan University School of Medicine, Seoul 06351, South Korea.

References

1. Marques G, Zhang B. Retrograde signaling that regulates synaptic development and function at the drosophila neuromuscular junction. Int Rev Neurobiol. 2006;75:267–85.
2. Poon VY, Choi S, Park M. Growth factors in synaptic function. Front Synaptic Neurosci. 2013;5:6.
3. Zweifel LS, Kuruvilla R, Ginty DD. Functions and mechanisms of retrograde neurotrophin signalling. Nat Rev Neurosci. 2005;6:615–25.
4. Aberle H, Haghighi AP, Fetter RD, McCabe BD, Magalhaes TR, Goodman CS. (2002) wishful thinking encodes a BMP type II receptor that regulates synaptic growth in drosophila. Neuron. 2002;33:545–58.
5. Marques G, Bao H, Haerry TE, Shimell MJ, Duchek P, Zhang B, et al. The drosophila BMP type II receptor wishful thinking regulates neuromuscular synapse morphology and function. Neuron. 2002;33:529–43.
6. McCabe BD, Marques G, Haghighi AP, Fetter RD, Crotty ML, Haerry TE, et al. The BMP homolog Gbb provides a retrograde signal that regulates synaptic growth at the drosophila neuromuscular junction. Neuron. 2003;39:241–54.
7. Rawson JM, Lee M, Kennedy EL, Selleck SB. Drosophila neuromuscular synapse assembly and function require the TGF-beta type I receptor saxophone and the transcription factor mad. J Neurobiol. 2003;55:134–50.
8. Keshishian H, Kim YS. Orchestrating development and function: retrograde BMP signaling in the drosophila nervous system. Trends Neurosci. 2004;27:143–7.
9. Nahm M, Lee MJ, Parkinson W, Lee M, Kim H, Kim YJ, et al. Spartin regulates synaptic growth and neuronal survival by inhibiting BMP-mediated microtubule stabilization. Neuron. 2013;77:680–95.
10. O'Connor-Giles KM, Ho LL, Ganetzky B. Nervous wreck interacts with thickveins and the endocytic machinery to attenuate retrograde BMP signaling during synaptic growth. Neuron. 2008;58:507–18.
11. Wang X, Shaw WR, Tsang HT, Reid E, O'Kane CJ. Drosophila spichthyin inhibits BMP signaling and regulates synaptic growth and axonal microtubules. Nat Neurosci. 2007;10:177–85.
12. Zhao G, Wu Y, Du L, Li W, Xiong Y, Yao A, et al. Drosophila S6 Kinase like inhibits neuromuscular junction growth by downregulating the BMP receptor thickveins. PLoS Genet. 2015;11:e1004984.
13. Dickman DK, Lu Z, Meinertzhagen IA, Schwarz TL. Altered synaptic development and active zone spacing in endocytosis mutants. Curr Biol. 2006;16:591–8.
14. Kim S, Wairkar YP, Daniels RW, DiAntonio A. The novel endosomal membrane protein Ema interacts with the class C Vps-HOPS complex to promote endosomal maturation. J Cell Biol. 2010;188:717–34.
15. Boettner B, Van Aelst L. The rap GTPase activator drosophila PDZ-GEF regulates cell shape in epithelial migration and morphogenesis. Mol Cell Biol. 2007;27:7966–80.
16. Huelsmann S, Hepper C, Marchese D, Knoll C, Reuter R. The PDZ-GEF dizzy regulates cell shape of migrating macrophages via Rap1 and integrins in the drosophila embryo. Development. 2006;133:2915–24.
17. Lee JH, Cho KS, Lee J, Kim D, Lee SB, Yoo J, et al. Drosophila PDZ-GEF, a guanine nucleotide exchange factor for Rap1 GTPase, reveals a novel upstream regulatory mechanism in the mitogen-activated protein kinase signaling pathway. Mol Cell Biol. 2002;22:7658–66.
18. Spahn P, Ott A, Reuter R. The PDZ-GEF protein dizzy regulates the establishment of adherens junctions required for ventral furrow formation in drosophila. J Cell Sci. 2012;125:3801–12.
19. Wang H, Singh SR, Zheng Z, SW O, Chen X, Edwards K, et al. Rap-GEF signaling controls stem cell anchoring to their niche through regulating DE-cadherin-mediated cell adhesion in the drosophila testis. Dev Cell. 2006;10:117–26.
20. Nahm M, Kim S, Paik SK, Lee M, Lee S, Lee ZH, et al. dCIP4 (drosophila Cdc42-interacting protein 4) restrains synaptic growth by inhibiting the secretion of the retrograde glass bottom boat signal. J Neurosci. 2010; 30:8138–50.
21. Nahm M, Long AA, Paik SK, Kim S, Bae YC, Broadie K, et al. The Cdc42-selective GAP rich regulates postsynaptic development and retrograde BMP transsynaptic signaling. J Cell Biol. 2010;191:661–75.

22. Singh SR, SW O, Liu W, Chen X, Zheng Z, Hou SX. Rap-GEF/rap signaling restricts the formation of supernumerary spermathecae in Drosophila Melanogaster. Develop Growth Differ. 2006;48:169–75.

23. Sweeney ST, Davis GW. Unrestricted synaptic growth in spinster-a late endosomal protein implicated in TGF-beta-mediated synaptic growth regulation. Neuron. 2002;36:403–16.

24. Zhang YQ, Bailey AM, Matthies HJ, Renden RB, Smith MA, Speese SD, et al. Drosophila Fragile X-related gene regulates the MAP1B homolog Futsch to control synaptic structure and function. Cell. 2001;107:591–603.

25. Roos J, Hummel T, Ng N, Klambt C, Davis GW. Drosophila Futsch regulates synaptic microtubule organization and is necessary for synaptic growth. Neuron. 2000;26:371–82.

26. Jordan MA, Thrower D, Wilson L. Effects of vinblastine, podophyllotoxin and nocodazole on mitotic spindles. Implications for the role of microtubule dynamics in mitosis. J Cell Sci. 1992;102(Pt 3):401–16.

27. Marie B, Sweeney ST, Poskanzer KE, Roos J, Kelly RB, Davis GW. Dap160/intersectin scaffolds the periactive zone to achieve high-fidelity endocytosis and normal synaptic growth. Neuron. 2004;43:207–19.

28. Rodal AA, Motola-Barnes RN, Littleton JT. Nervous wreck and Cdc42 cooperate to regulate endocytic actin assembly during synaptic growth. J Neurosci. 2008;28:8316–25.

29. Muqit MM, Feany MB. Modelling neurodegenerative diseases in drosophila: a fruitful approach? Nat Rev Neurosci. 2002;3:237–43.

30. Lee KJ, Lee Y, Rozeboom A, Lee JY, Udagawa N, Hoe HS, et al. Requirement for Plk2 in orchestrated ras and rap signaling, homeostatic structural plasticity, and memory. Neuron. 2011;69:957–73.

31. Tsang HT, Edwards TL, Wang X, Connell JW, Davies RJ, Durrington HJ, et al. The hereditary spastic paraplegia proteins NIPA1, spastin and spartin are inhibitors of mammalian BMP signalling. Hum Mol Genet. 2009;18:3805–21.

32. Arthur WT, Quilliam LA, Cooper JA. Rap1 promotes cell spreading by localizing Rac guanine nucleotide exchange factors. J Cell Biol. 2004;167:111–22.

33. Mun H, Jeon TJ. Regulation of actin cytoskeleton by Rap1 binding to RacGEF1. Mol Cells. 2012;34:71–6.

34. Mooren OL, Galletta BJ, Cooper JA. Roles for actin assembly in endocytosis. Annu Rev Biochem. 2012;81:661–86.

35. Ball RW, Warren-Paquin M, Tsurudome K, Liao EH, Elazzouzi F, Cavanagh C, et al. Retrograde BMP signaling controls synaptic growth at the NMJ by regulating trio expression in motor neurons. Neuron. 2010;66:536–49.

36. Lin DM, Goodman CS. Ectopic and increased expression of Fasciclin II alters motoneuron growth cone guidance. Neuron. 1994;13:507–23.

37. Budnik V, Koh YH, Guan B, Hartmann B, Hough C, Woods D, et al. Regulation of synapse structure and function by the drosophila tumor suppressor gene dlg. Neuron. 1996;17:627–40.

38. Lee S, Nahm M, Lee M, Kwon M, Kim E, Zadeh AD, et al. The F-actin-microtubule crosslinker shot is a platform for Krasavietz-mediated translational regulation of midline axon repulsion. Development. 2007;134:1767–77.

39. Persson U, Izumi H, Souchelnytskyi S, Itoh S, Grimsby S, Engstrom U, et al. The L45 loop in type I receptors for TGF-beta family members is a critical determinant in specifying Smad isoform activation. FEBS Lett. 1998;434:83–7.

40. Marrus SB, Portman SL, Allen MJ, Moffat KG, DiAntonio A. Differential localization of glutamate receptor subunits at the drosophila neuromuscular junction. J Neurosci. 2004;24:1406–15.

41. Verstreken P, Ohyama T, Bellen HJ. FM 1-43 labeling of synaptic vesicle pools at the drosophila neuromuscular junction. Methods Mol Biol. 2008; 440:349–69.

11

Suppression of cortical seizures by optic stimulation of the reticular thalamus in PV-mhChR2-YFP BAC transgenic mice

Wei Jen Chang[1], Wei Pang Chang[2] and Bai Chuang Shyu[1]* ⓘ

Abstract

Deep brain stimulation in thalamic regions has been proposed as a treatment for epilepsy. The electrical current excites thalamocortical activity which is controlled by γ-aminobutyric acid (GABA)ergic interneurons in the reticular thalamic nucleus (nRT). Previous studies showed that enhancing GABAergic inhibitory strength in the nRT reduces the duration and power of seizures, indicating that the thalamus plays an important role in modulating cortical seizures. The aim of the present study was to apply optogenetics to study the role of the nRT in modulating cortical seizures. We used PV-ChR2-EYFP transgenic mice from Jackson Laboratories, in which only Channelrhodopsin-2 (ChR2) is expressed in parvalbumin-expressing interneurons. Cortical seizure-like activity was induced by electrical stimulation of the corpus callosum after applying 4-aminopyridine. ChR2 expression was abundant in the nRT and cerebellum in PV-ChR2-EYFP transgenic mice. Light stimulation in the nRT caused burst firing in regions of the thalamus and nRT in vitro. Multi-unit activity increased during high-frequency (100 and 50 Hz) light stimulation in the S1 region and thalamus in vivo. Corpus callosum stimulation-induced seizure-like activity was effectively suppressed by high-frequency (100 Hz) and long-duration (10 s) light stimulation. The suppressive effects were reversed by applying a GABA$_B$ receptor antagonist but not a GABA$_A$ receptor antagonist in the cortex. The results indicated that light stimulation affected thalamocortical relay neurons by activating ChR2-expression neurons in the nRT. High-frequency and long-duration light stimulation was more effective in suppressing cortical seizure-like activity. GABA$_B$ receptors may participate in suppressing seizure-like activity.

Keywords: Channelrhodopsin, Optogenetics, Reticular thalamic nucleus, Primary somatosensory cortex, Thalamus, Seizure, GAGA antagonists

Introduction

Epilepsy is a neurological disorder that is characterized by seizure activity associated with abnormal synchronous neural overexcitation [1]. Epilepsy affects 50 million people worldwide, and nearly 0.1% die from seizure-related disorders every year in the United States. More than 30% of patients suffer from drug-resistant epilepsy [2]. For these patients, several alternative therapeutic approaches have been employed, such as transcranial direct current stimulation, transcranial magnetic stimulation, and deep brain stimulation (DBS). Deep brain stimulation has been adapted for both clinical treatment and animal studies. Different brain regions have been targeted to treat such neuronal disorders as epilepsy, Alzheimer's disease, Parkinson's disease, essential tremor, dystonia, cluster headache, and chronic pain [3]. Deep brain stimulation has been applied to several brain nuclei, including the cerebellum, hippocampus, amygdala, and thalamus, among others. The thalamus plays an important role in seizure development and inhibition [4, 5]. The centromedial and anterior nuclei of the thalamus have been targeted for the treatment of epilepsy. These two nuclei can suppress refractory epilepsy and generalized seizure disorder [3, 6]. Despite the successful application of DBS for the treatment of epileptic disorders, the mechanism by which the DBS acts on the nervous system is still unclear.

The reticular thalamic nucleus (nRT) is an important region that lies between thalamocortical circuits [7]. Most of the nRT contains GABAergic neurons that innervate

* Correspondence: bmbai@gate.sinica.edu.tw
[1]Institute of Biomedical Sciences, Academia Sinica, Taipei 11529, Taiwan, ROC
Full list of author information is available at the end of the article

the thalamus and produce inhibitory postsynaptic potentials (IPSPs) and provide synaptic inhibition of excitatory thalamocortical relay neurons [8]. Previous studies found that nRT stimulation can suppress limbic motor seizures [9]. Enhancing GABAergic inhibitory strength in the nRT reduced the duration and power of absence seizures [10]. Furthermore, several studies have shown that nRT plays a critical role in the modulation of cortical activity during sleep and arousal through their strong impact on thalamocortical neurons [11–14]. The aforementioned studies used electrical stimulation approaches that might lead to unwanted side effects. The nRT also receives inputs from the cortex, and thalamocortical and thalamocortical pathways lie in the vicinity of the nRT. Electrical or pharmacological stimulation of the nRT can excite these passing fibers. Optogenetic methods have recently been developed, in which light-sensitive channels are engineered to be expressed in target cells, which may provide a better method of DBS [15]. Cortical injury that was induced by thalamocortical seizures was interrupted by suppressing the activity of thalamic nuclei using a closed-loop optogenetic strategy [16]. However, the involvement of nRT in cortical seizures requires further investigation. The present study investigated whether optic stimulation of the nRT suppresses cortical seizure activity. We use transgenic mice in which Channelrhodopsin-2 (ChR2) is expressed in parvalbumin (PV)-expressing neurons in the nRT. These neurons can be specifically activated by a blue light laser (473 nm) [17]. This optogenetic approach can selectively activate the nRT and control its activity in real time, while not affecting adjacent neurons or having side effects that typically occur with traditional pharmacological or electrical stimulation methods. The present study may be critically important in laying the groundwork for understanding the role of the nRT in thalamocortical seizures.

Methods

Animals

Prv-mhChR2-YFP BAC transgenic mice were purchased from Jackson Laboratories (stock no. 012355, Bar Harbor, ME, USA). These mice express channelrhodopsin-2/EYFP fusion protein (mhChR2::YFP) that is directed to neuronal populations by the mouse PV promoter on the BAC transgene. Prv-mhChR2-YFP mice were genotyped using the Jackson Laboratories genotyping protocol. Polymerase chain reaction (PCR)-positive mice were mated with C57BL/6 J mice to establish transgenic lines. All of the mouse experiments were performed according to the guidelines established by the Academia Sinica Institutional Animal Care and Utilization Committee. Efforts were made to minimize animal suffering and reduce the number of animals used.

Genotyping

To determine ChR2 gene expression in individual mice, we examined each mouse based on tail DNA. Tail samples were clipped about 0.3 cm per mice for DNA extraction, the tail samples were incubated for approximately 16 h in tail extraction buffer (50 mM Tris [pH 8.0], 100 mM ethylenediaminetetraacetic acid [pH 0.8], and 10% sodium dodecyl sulfate) that contained 20 mg/ml proteinase K (Qiagen, Hilden, Germany). Proteinase K was then inactivated by incubation for 5 min at 95 °C. The samples were then centrifuged at $20,000 \times g$ for 1 min, and the supernatant was collected. Polymerase chain reaction amplification was used to detect the Prv-mhChR2-YFP transgene in somatic DNA. DNA polymerase was purchased from Thermo Scientific (Waltham, USA) and used according to the manufacturer's instructions. The PCR conditions were the following: 95 °C for 2 min, followed by 30 × [95 °C for 30 s, 56.8 °C for 30 s, and 72 °C for 30 s], with final extension at 72 °C for 5 min. The PCR products were run on 2% agarose gels with ethidium bromide, visualized using a gel imaging system.

Functional assessment in brain slices in vitro

Brains from 6 to 8 week old PV-ChR2 mice were sliced into 400 μm coronal sections using a vibratome (Microslicers, DTK-1000). The slices were kept fresh by artificial cerebrospinal fluid (aCSF) that contained the following: 124 mM NaCl, 25 mM $NaHCO_3$, 10 mM D-glucose, 4.4 mM KCl, 1 mM NaH_2PO_4, 2 mM $MgSO_4$, and 2 mM $CaCl_2$ (pH 7.4). The slices were incubated in oxygenated aCSF (95% O_2 and 5% CO_2) for at least 1 h for recovery.

The recording pipettes were constructed from borosilicate glass with a pipette puller (P-97, Sutter Instruments (Novato, USA). The pipettes were filled with aCSF and inserted into the nRT or thalamic regions to record local field potentials. Blue light was generated by a blue light laser (473 nm, Sol-473-050MFL, Shanghai Dreamlaser, Shanghai, China). A 62.5 μm diameter optic fiber (GIF625, Thorlabs, New Jersey, USA) that was connected to the blue light laser was placed in the nRT region for light stimulation. Light power (422.4 mW/mm^2) was measured by LaserCheck (LaserCheck, Coherent, California, USA) to activate expressing ChR2 neurons. Analog signals were amplified by Axon MultiClamp 700B and processed using the Power 1401 Mk II CED data acquisition system (Cambridge Electronic Design, Cambridge, England). Spike2 software (Cambridge Electronic Design, Cambridge, England) was used for offline analysis.

Surgery for in vivo electrophysiological measurements

PV-Chr2 mice were initially anesthetized with 4% isoflurane mixed in oxygenated air and then placed in a stereotaxic apparatus. The animals were maintained under anesthesia with 1.75% isoflurane in oxygen during surgery. Body temperature was maintained at 36.5–37.5 °C with a homeothermic blanket system (Model 50–7079, Harvard Apparatus, Holliston, MA, ISA). Craniotomy was performed over the skull regions on top of the primary somatosensory cortex (S1). Small parts of the dura over S1 were carefully removed using a 23-gauge needle. After surgical preparation, the animals were anesthetized with 1.6% isoflurane during the recording session. The depth of anesthesia was periodically monitored and maintained by pinching the paw or tail so that no overt body movement occurred.

Recording evoked field potentials in the S1 and thalamus in vivo

Extracellular field potentials that were evoked by electrical pulses were first mapped by a silver-sliver chloride (Ag-AgCl) tip electrode in the S1 region (~1.5 mm posterior and 3.5 mm lateral to bregma). To induce a cortical response, a pair of stainless-steel needles was inserted into the mouse whisker region or hind paw and used to deliver bipolar electrical stimulation (5 mA, 0.5 ms duration, model 2100, AM Systems, Washington, USA). The position in S1 that resulted in a maximal local field potential that was evoked by electrical stimulation was identified and designated as the insertion point for the multichannel recording probe (16 contact points, 100 μm interval spacing). The probe was inserted perpendicular to the S1 region. Another multichannel recording probe was used to record extracellular field potentials in the thalamus (~3.5 mm posterior and ~1.8 mm lateral to bregma; probe inserted 40° from vertical). In some of the experiments, an optoelectrode that combined an optic fiber and electrode (OAx16-10 mm-100-177, Neuronexus, Michigan, USA) was inserted into thalamic regions for simultaneous light stimulation and field potential recording. For optic stimulation, the optic fiber was inserted into the nRT for light stimulation (10–1000 ms continuous light or 10–100 Hz stimulation) by a blue light laser. An Ag-AgCl reference electrode was placed in the olfactory bulb. The sampling rate of recorded analog signals was 6 kHz, and data were processed using a multichannel data acquisition system (TDT, Florida USA) and computer.

Cortical seizure induction

Spontaneous cortical seizure activity was induced by local application of the potassium channel blocker 4-aminopyridine (4-AP; 50 mM) on the cortical surface. A tungsten electrode was inserted into contralateral side of the corpus callosum. Electrical stimulation was performed with a 500 μA pulse current intensity, 0.5 ms pulse duration, and 10 Hz in 4 s pulse width using a constant-current pulse generator (Model 2100, A-M Systems, Washington, USA). Cortical seizure activity was induced every 10 s electrical stimulation. The induction

of cortical seizure activity by electrical stimulation occurred simultaneously with optic stimulation of the nRT to evaluate possible suppressive effects.

Chronic electroencephalographic recording and behavioral assessment in freely moving mice

A silver-ball electrode with an omnetic connector (A79014, Omnetics Connectors, Minnesota, USA) was fixed over the S1 region for electroencephalographic (EEG) recording. An optic fiber (BFL37–200, Thorlabs, New Jersey, USA) was inserted into the nRT for optic stimulation. The mice were allowed to recover from the surgical procedures at least for 1 week. EEG signals over the S1 region were recording and calculated by short-time Fourier transform (STFT). EEG signals in the S1 region were divided into shorter segments (1 s) of equal length, and the Fourier transform was computed. Computations were performed using the stft function in Matlab software (MathWorks, Natick, MA, USA). The optic fiber was inserted in the nRT and connected with a LC Ferrule (MM-FER2007C-1270, Precision Fiber Products, California, USA) and ceramic split sleeve (SM-CS, Precision Fiber Products, California, USA) that were fixed on the head by dental cement. Another optic fiber with a fiber optic rotary joint (FRJ_1X1 FC-FC, Doric Lenses, Quebec, Canada) was connected to the ferrule and sleeve to avoid optic fiber interruption when the mice were freely moving.

Verification of electrode placement and immunohistochemistry

At the end of the experiment, a small lesion was made by passing an anodal current (25 μA, 5 s) through the deepest electrode of the electrode probe. Another lesion was made at the same lead after the electrode probe was withdrawn by 500 μm. The brains were fixed by perfusion with normal saline followed by 4% paraformaldehyde in 0.1 M phosphate-buffered saline (PBS; pH 7.4). The brains were removed, postfixed for 72 h, sectioned at 60 μm on a cryostat, and processed for immunohistochemistry. The brain slices were incubated with 1% bovine serum albumin, 0.02% sodium azide, and 0.3% Triton in PBS for 1 h. The sections were incubated with rabbit polyclonal anti-PV (GTX11427, GeneTex, California, USA) and anti-DAPI at dilutions of 1:500 for 24 h at 4 °C. Immunohistochemistry was performed using rabbit secondary IgG (H + L) antibody (pre-adsorbed, DyLight 594) and rabbit IgG (H + L) antibody (pre-adsorbed, DyLight 405, GTX 76756, GeneTex, California, USA).

Drug administration

4-Aminopyridine (100 mM), the $GABA_A$ receptor antagonist bicuculline (100 μM), and the $GABA_B$ antagonist CGP52432 (100 μM) were purchased from Tocris Cookson (Ellisville, MO, USA), dissolved in physiological saline, and administered by local application on the S1 region. For seizure induction in freely moving animals, pentylenetetrazol (PTZ; 50 mg/kg), which causes alterations in excitatory and inhibitory neurotransmitter systems, was dissolved in saline and intraperitoneally injected.

Data analysis

Field potential data were recorded by Spike2 and Signal software (Cambridge Electronic Design, Cambridge, England), and multi-unit activity in the behavioral and electrophysiological experiments was analyzed by Matlab software (MathWorks, Natick, MA, USA). Multi-unit activity was counted when the amplitude of the field response was two-times greater than the background threshold. Average EEG discharges were based on the average field potential after CC stimulation for 1 min. The EEG signals and field potentials were first averaged every 5 s (one bin) for the entire period (12 bins). The average discharges were based on the average of all 12 bins during the 1 min period. Correlations between seizure-like activity in the S1 and thalamus, recorded at different locations, were evaluated by cross-correlation analysis. Computations were performed using the xcorr function in Matlab software. If data follow normal distribution in normality test, significant changes after drug application were determined using one-way analysis of variance (ANOVA) and Systat (SPSS) software. The data were plotted using Microsoft Excel software. One-way ANOVA with repeated test was used to analyze the data of neuronal discharges in multiple groups and FFT power of EEG recordings in freely moving animals. Values

of $p < 0.05$ were considered statistically significant. Tukey's post hoc test was used to detect the sources of group differences in the ANOVA.

Results

Expression of channelrhodopsin

ChR2 expression was found in the nRT in coronal brain sections in PV-ChR2-EYFP transgenic mice (Fig. 1a). Green fluorescence indicates endogenous ChR2 expression. The retrograde dye fluorogold was injected into the S1 region to confirm the thalamocortical pathway (Fig. 1a). Retrogradely labeled fluorogold dye was detected in thalamic neuron fibers (yellow fluorescence) and nRT neuron fibers (green fluorescence), which innervated thalamic neurons (Fig. 1a [square enlarged in Fig. 1b], Fig. 1b [square enlarged in Fig. 1c]). Most neurons in the nRT were PV-type interneurons (Fig. 1d, red fluorescence). Endogenous ChR2 was expressed on PV interneuron membranes in the nRT region (Fig. 1e, g, green fluoresce). Parvalbumin interneurons and ChR2 and DAPI staining are merged in Fig. 1g.

Functional verification of ChR2

Brain slices that contained the nRT and thalamus were prepared to verify the functional activation of ChR2. A blue light laser (473 nm) was used to stimulate the nRT, and multi-unit activity was recorded in the nRT and thalamus (Fig. 2a). Multi-unit activity was induced in the nRT by different light frequencies and durations (Fig. 2b). Burst firing with short and long latencies was optically stimulated in the nRT and recorded in the nRT and

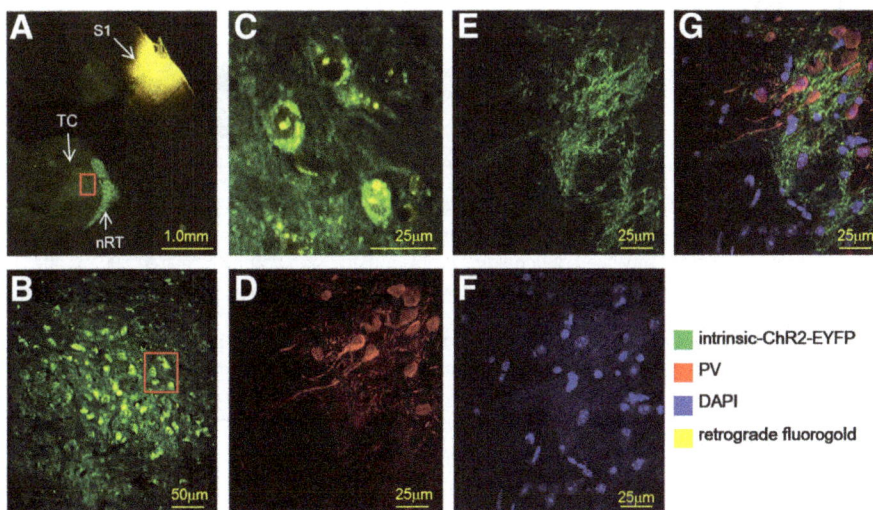

Fig. 1 Expression of endogenous PV-ChR2-EYFP in the nRT and labeling of the retrograde dye fluorogold that was injected in the S1 region. **a** ChR2 (*green* fluorescence) and fluorogold (*yellow* fluorescence). TC denotes thalamocortical relay neurons. **b** Enlarged thalamic region that shows cells that were retrogradely labeled with fluorogold in the thalamic region. **c** Enlarged thalamic region, showing that nRT neuron fibers (*green* fluorescence) surrounded thalamocortical neurons (fluorogold retrogradely labeled neurons). **d** Immunostaining of PV in the nRT. **e** Enlarged nRT region. Endogenous ChR2 was expressed only in the nRT. **f** Chemical fluorescence stain results of DAPI in the nRT. **g** Merged image of DAPI, PV, and ChR2

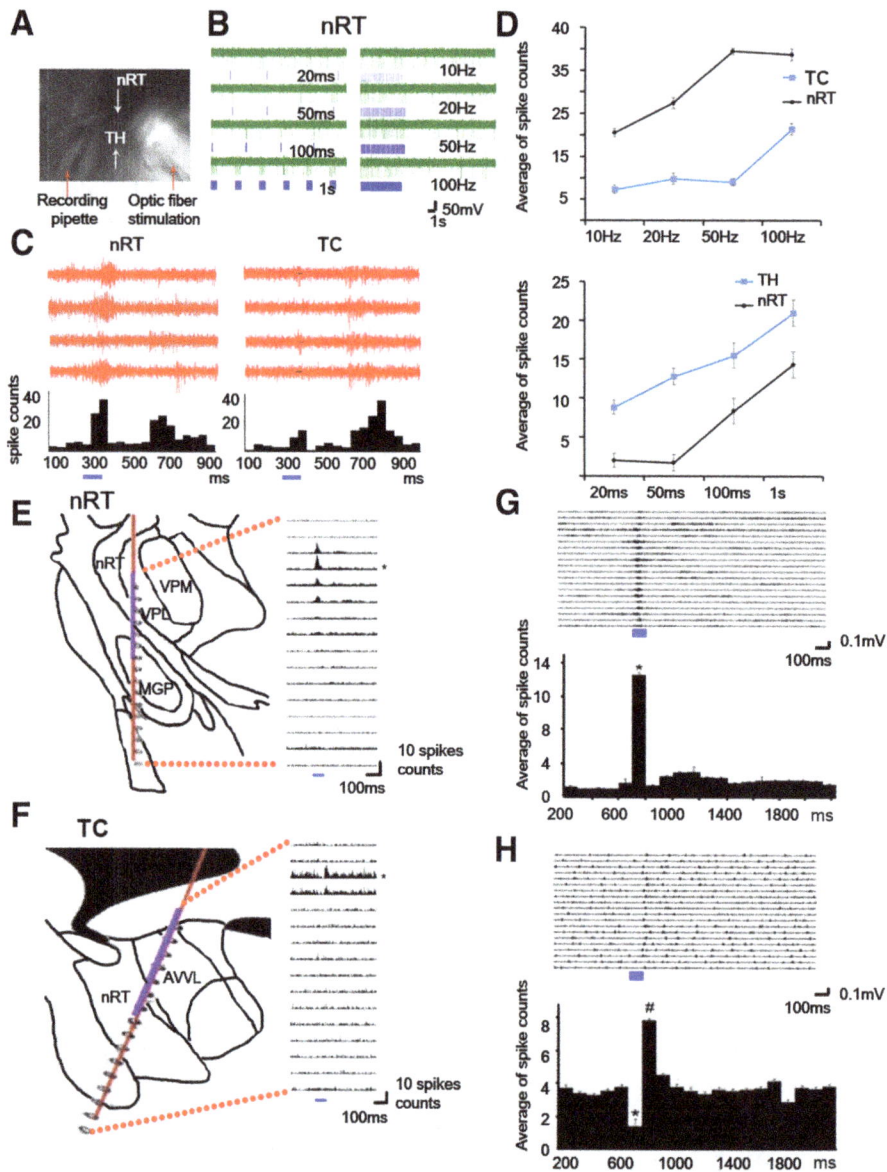

Fig. 2 Functional verification of ChR2 in vitro (**a-d**) and in vivo (E-H). **a** Horizontal brain slice (400 μm) that contained the nRT and thalamus. **b** nRT neurons in response to 10 Hz, 20 Hz, 50 Hz, 100 Hz, 20 ms, 50 ms, 100 ms, and 1 s light stimulation. **c** Spikes from nRT (*left*) and thalamocortical relay neurons (TC) (*right*) neurons in response to light stimulation. Multi-unit activity in the nRT significantly increased during light stimulation. Multi-unit activity in the thalamus was slightly enhanced during light stimulation and significantly increased 500 ms after light stimulation (*blue*). **d** Averaged spike counts from nRT and thalamus neurons in response to different pulse durations of light stimulation. **e** Position of optoelectrode aligned on the histology atlas. Upper channels 3–7 are in the nRT. (Right) Summation of multi-unit activity from 10 sweeps. During laser stimulation (100 ms blue line), spike activity was evoked in channels that were located in the nRT. **f** Position of optoelectrode aligned on the histology atlas. Upper channels 2–9 are in the thalamus. (Right) Summation of multi-unit activity from 10 sweeps. During laser stimulation (*blue* line), spike activity decreased and rebounded in channels that were located in the thalamus. **g** Multi-unit activity from 20 sweeps in channel 4 in the nRT. **h** Multi-unit activity from 20 sweeps in channel 3 in the thalamus. During laser stimulation, multi-unit activity in the thalamus significantly decreased and rebounded after laser stimulation was terminated

thalamus (Fig. 2c). Spike counts that were evoked by different light stimulation conditions are shown in Fig. 2d. To test the functional activation of ChR2-expressing neurons in vivo, an optoelectrode was inserted in the nRT (Fig. 2e) and thalamus (Fig. 2f) to record multi-unit spike responses to light stimulation. Twenty trials of optic stimulation in the nRT (Fig. 2g) and thalamus (Fig. 2h) were averaged. A rebound response was detected after light stimulation in the thalamus (Fig. 2h, bottom). These results indicate that ChR2-EYFP neurons were activated by blue light stimulation and relayed signals to lateral thalamic regions.

Cortical and thalamic responses evoked by different light stimulation durations and frequencies

To test thalamic and cortical responses to light stimulation in the nRT, multichannel recording electrodes were inserted in the S1 and thalamus (Fig. 3a). Optic light stimulation-evoked multi-unit activity was recorded and analyzed in the S1 region and thalamus (Fig. 3b). Firing activity in thalamocortical relay regions (S1 and thalamus) responded to different durations and frequencies of light stimulation in vivo. Multi-unit activity increased during high-frequency (100 and 50 Hz) light stimulation in the S1 region and thalamus (Fig. 3c). These results indicate that optic light stimulation in the nRT induced multi-unit activity through the thalamocortical pathway to the S1 region.

Closed loop of cortical and thalamic seizure activity

Cortical seizures were induced by the local application of 4-AP (100 mM) on the S1 surface and electrical stimulation of the contralateral corpus callosum (Fig. 4a). Seizure-like activity was recorded by simultaneously detecting local field potentials and frequency spectra in the S1 region and thalamus (Fig. 4b). The sweeps of seizure activity were divided into five time bins. Cross correlations of seizure-like activity (Fig. 4c, lower panel) were analyzed and are presented as correlograms (Fig. 4c, upper panel). Correlation coefficients of the relative bins between S1 and the thalamus indicated positive correlations ($r = 0.5904$) in the pre-seizure period (Fig. 4 Da). Correlation coefficients between S1 and the thalamus became negative ($r = -0.4008$ [Fig. 4 Db], $r = -0.3348$ [Fig. 4Dc], $r = -0.4884$ [Fig. 4Dd], $r = 0.4992$ [Fig. 4De]) during the electrically induced seizure-like activity period (Fig. 4Cb-d). During the seizure onset period, the peak time of the cross-correlation coefficient was delayed, with a maximal peak latency of 15 ms (Fig. 4e). These results show that seizures were initiated in the cortex and then propagated to the thalamus, indicating that seizure-like activity in the cortex and thalamus was highly correlated. Seizure-like activity in the cortex preceded thalamic activity and was initiated earlier. Thus, thalamic activity was affected by seizure progression though the thalamocortical pathway.

Suppressive effects of the nRT on electrically evoked cortical seizures

The setup for cortical seizure induction, recording, and optic stimulation is shown in Fig. 5a. Spontaneous cortical and thalamic seizure-like activity was induced by the application of 4-AP and could be induced by electrical stimulation of the contralateral corpus callosum (Fig. 5b, left panel, yellow). This seizure-like activity was significantly suppressed by 10 s light stimulation and recovered after the light stimulation was terminated (Fig. 5b, middle

and right panels). Sweeps of seizure activity were analyzed every 5 s. Corpus callosum activation-induced seizure-like activity was suppressed by 10 s light stimulation after corpus callosum stimulation. Seizure activity recovered when light stimulation of the nRT was terminated (Fig. 5c). The suppressive effect was tested using various frequencies (10 Hz ~100 Hz, 10 s duration) and durations (1 s ~ 10s) of continuous light stimulation. Corpus callosum activation-induced seizure-like activity was effectively suppressed by high-frequency (100 Hz) and long-duration (10 s) light stimulation. The one-way ANOVA with repeated test (electrical stimulation vs. different light stimulation conditions) indicated significant effects of group in the S1 region ($F_{7,564} = 19.61$, $p < 0.05$) and thalamus ($F_{7,385} = 4.9$, $p < 0.05$). The suppressive effects were significant for both high-frequency and long-duration light stimulation (Fig. 6). The distribution of lesion sites indicated that multichannel probe recording sites were located in the thalamus and nRT. These results demonstrate that corpus callosum activation-induced cortical seizures could be effectively suppressed by light stimulation of the nRT.

Effects of GABA antagonism on cortical seizure suppression

The suppressive effect may be caused by feedforward inhibition that is mediated by GABA receptors [18, 19]. The effects of GABA$_A$ and GABA$_B$ antagonism were tested by applying receptor antagonists on the cortical surface. Seizure-like activity in the S1 region and thalamus was induced by applying 4-AP (100 mM) and electrical stimulation of the corpus callosum (Fig. 7a, left). Seizure-like activity was suppressed by 10 s light stimulation (Fig. 7a, middle). Application of the GABA$_B$ antagonist reversed these suppressive effects (Fig. 7a, right). Figure 7b shows the effects of application of the GABA$_A$ and GABA$_B$ antagonists on the suppressive effects, summarized as average cortical evoked discharges. Statistical analysis showed that averaged discharges were significantly different in different treatments. Seizure activity was significantly decreased by light stimulation of the nRT for 10 s. These suppressive effects were abolished by application of the GABA$_B$ receptor antagonist. The GABA$_A$ antagonist bicuculline was less effective than the GABA$_B$ antagonist CGP52432. The one-way ANOVA with repeated test (electrical stimulation vs. different light stimulation conditions) indicated significant effects of group ($F_{5,439} = 51.30$, $p < 0.05$). The suppressive effects of light stimulation could be reversed by applying the GABA$_B$ antagonist but not the GABA$_A$ antagonist (Fig. 7b, left panel). Seizure activity in the thalamic region was also suppressed by 10 s light stimulation, and this suppressive effect was reversed by the GABA$_B$ antagonist and GABA$_A$ antagonist ($F_{5,479} = 165.444$, $p < 0.05$; Fig. 7b, right panel).

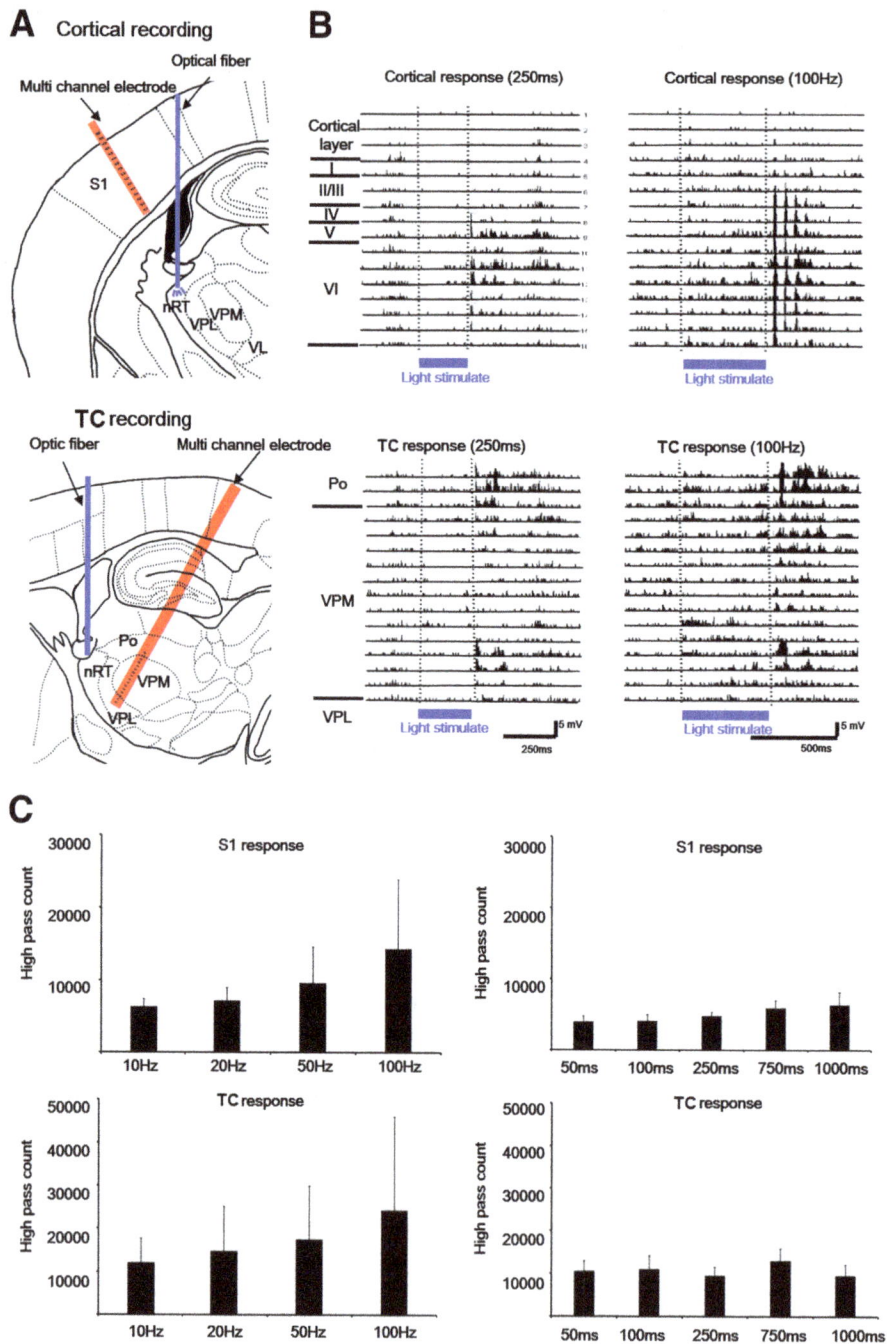

Fig. 3 Cortical and thalamic responses with different durations and frequencies of light stimulation. **a** In the upper panel, the multichannel electrode is positioned in S1. One optic fiber was implanted in the nRT. In the lower panel, another multichannel electrode was located in the VPM. **b** High-pass field potentials of S1 and thalamus after different light stimulation conditions in the nRT. **c** Statistical analysis of spike counts recorded in the cortex and thalamus with different light stimulation conditions in the nRT, the target brain area S1 showed that non-significant differences occurred at different durations of stimulation (F4, 20 = 1.70, $p > 0.05$) and frequency of stimulation (F3, 15 = 0.82, $p > 0.05$) after one-way ANOVA with repeated test. In addition, another target side thalamus showed that non-significant differences occurred at different durations of stimulation (F4, 20 = 0.59, $p > 0.05$) and frequency of stimulation (F3, 15 = 1.37, $p > 0.05$, $n = 6$)

Evaluation of optic stimulation of the nRT in awake freely moving mice

Silver-ball electrodes with an omnetic connector were attached to the cortical surface over S1 to record EEG activity in freely moving animals. Spontaneous local field potentials (Fig. 8a, left panel) and STFT (Fig. 8a, right panel) were recorded in freely moving animals. The theta band frequency was noted in freely moving animals.

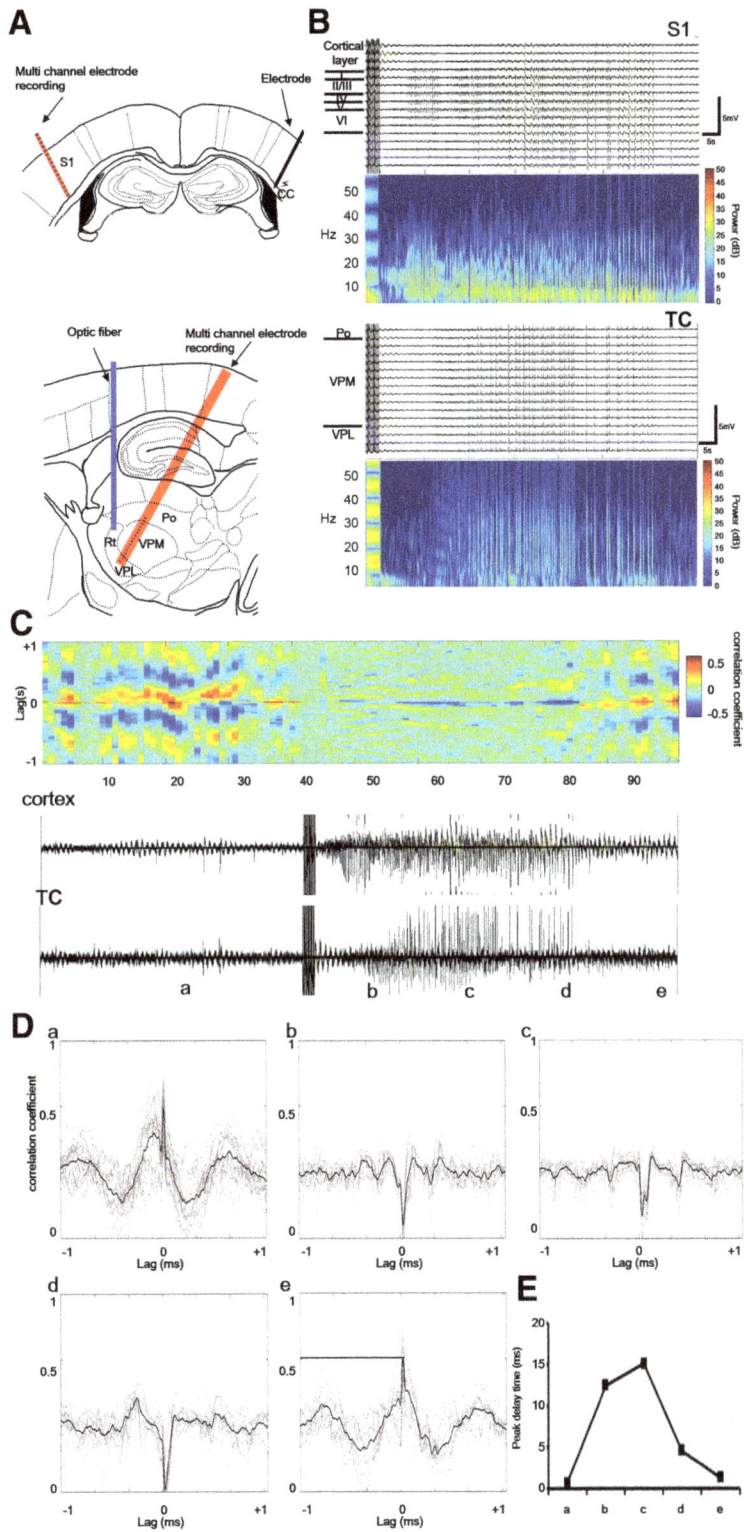

Fig. 4 (See legend on next page.)

(See figure on previous page.)
Fig. 4 Closed-loop cortical and thalamic seizure activity was induced by corpus callosum stimulation after applying 4-AP. **a** The left panel shows the electrical probe location in the corpus callosum (*blue bar*) and a multichannel recording probe in the S1 and thalamus. The optic fiber was inserted above the nRT. **b** The right panel shows field potentials that were recorded by a multichannel electrode in S1 and the fast Fourier transform (FFT). The FFT power significantly increased at the onset of seizure activity. Vertical lines are artifacts from corpus callosum stimulation. Seizure oscillations in the S1 and thalamus were recorded after corpus callosum stimulation. **c** Cross correlation of cortical and thalamic seizure activity. The sweep period was divided into pre-seizure (**a**) and post-seizure (**b-d**) periods. **d** Cross correlograms of activity in periods **a** to **e**. The results showed a positive correlation in the pre-seizure period (**a**) and negative correlations in the post-seizure periods (**b-e**). **e** Plot of peak latency of cross correlation coefficients during the post-seizure periods (**b-e**)

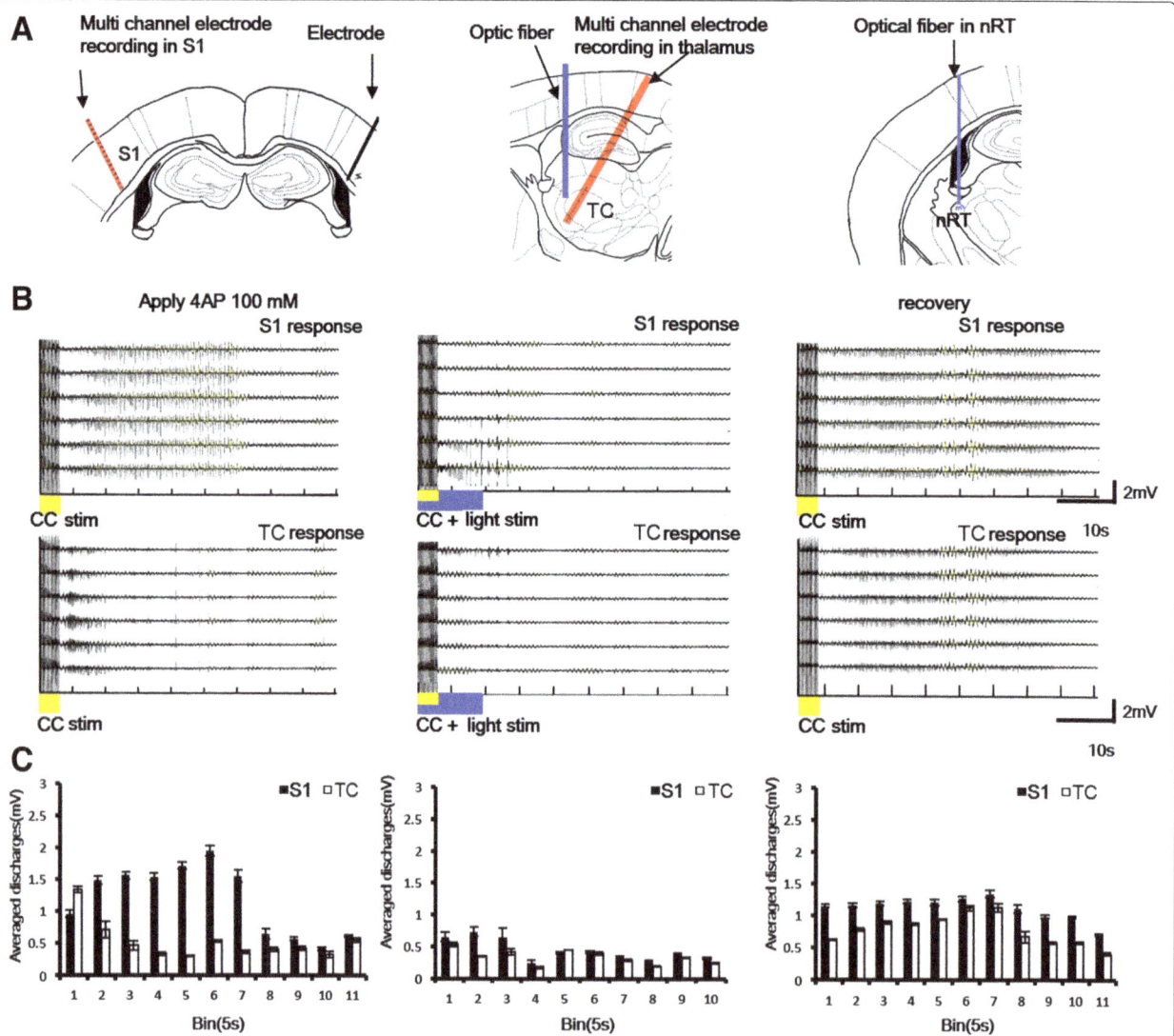

Fig. 5 Example of cortical and thalamic seizure activity that was suppressed by nRT stimulation. **a** Probe and stimulation sites. Optical fiber targeted on the nRT. Multichannel recording electrodes were placed in S1 and VPM&VPL of the thalamus. **b** In the *left* panel, cortical and thalamic seizure-like activity was induced by electrical stimulation of the corpus callosum (4 s, 10 Hz, 500 µA) (*yellow bar*) after applying 4-AP. In the middle panel, light stimulation (*blue bar*) was applied immediately following electrical stimulation. In the right panel, only electrical stimulation was applied without light stimulation. **c** Effect of optic stimulation on seizure activity. In the middle panel, sweeps were analyzed every 5 s. Corpus callosum stimulation-induced seizure-like activity was suppressed by 10 s light stimulation (*blue mark*) after corpus callosum stimulation. In the *right* panel, seizure activity recovered when light stimulation in the nRT was terminated

Suppression of cortical seizures by optic stimulation of the reticular thalamus...

143

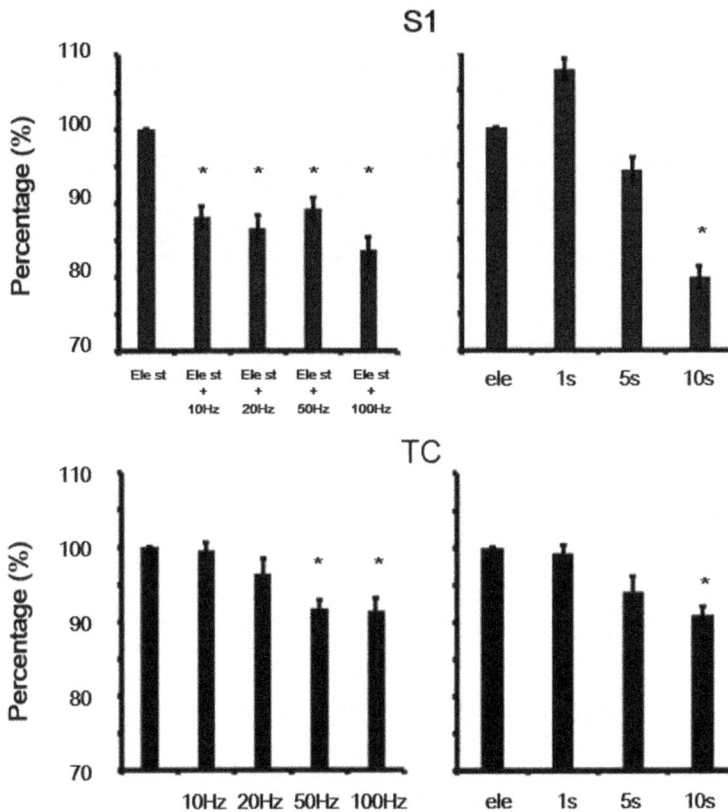

Fig. 6 Statistical analysis of suppressive effect of light stimulation on cortical and thalamic seizures. Various frequencies (10 Hz ~100 Hz, 10 s duration) and durations (1 s ~ 10s) of continuous light stimulation were applied. High-frequency 10s and long-duration continuous light stimulation significantly decreased seizure activity. $*p < 0.05$, compared with electrical stimulation only (one-way ANOVA with repeated test followed by post hoc test). Error bars indicate the SEM

Electroencephalographic recordings showed that seizure activity spikes were induced 5 min after the intraperitoneal injection of PTZ (Fig. 8b). Light stimulation (100 Hz, 5 s) was delivered during the period of seizure induction. Seizure activity spikes were suppressed by light stimulation of the nRT (Fig. 8c, blue). Different light stimulation conditions (control without light stimulation, 10 Hz light stimulation, 100 Hz light stimulation) were applied during the pre-seizure period (black column) and seizure period (white column) in the S1 region. The statistical analysis of different frequency wave bands showed that the power of all of the wave bands was significantly decreased by low-frequency (10 Hz) and high-frequency (100 Hz) light stimulation compared with the seizure period without light stimulation. The one-way ANOVA with repeated test revealed significant effects for each band (theta band, $F_{2,496} = 151.572$; alpha band, $F_{2,2399} = 403.663$; beta band, $F_{2,5999} = 647.974$; all $p < 0.05$). These results indicated that GABAergic neurons in the nRT played an important role in suppressing cortical seizure-like activity in freely moving animals.

Discussion

The present study found that 4-AP-induced seizures in the cortex and thalamus were suppressed by optogenetically activating the nRT. We also found that the suppressive effect of light stimulation on cortical seizures was related to GABA_B receptor transmission. Overall, cortical seizures were effectively suppressed by light stimulation in freely moving mice.

ChR2-EYFP was abundantly expressed in PV-expressing neurons in the nRT in Prv-mhChR2-YFP BAC transgenic mice, and these neurons responded to light stimulation. ChR2 has been shown to have low expression in the thalamus, striatum, cortex, and hippocampus [17, 20]. The low transgene expression in the cortex may be caused by transcription regulatory elements that are inherent to the BAC construct or post-translational processes. Low expression can be rescued by reconstructing PV-expressing neurons with tdTomato, and these neurons were shown to be expressed throughout the nRT and other areas [21]. We further found innervation of thalamocortical projection neurons by these nRT neurons, confirmed by the observation of connections between

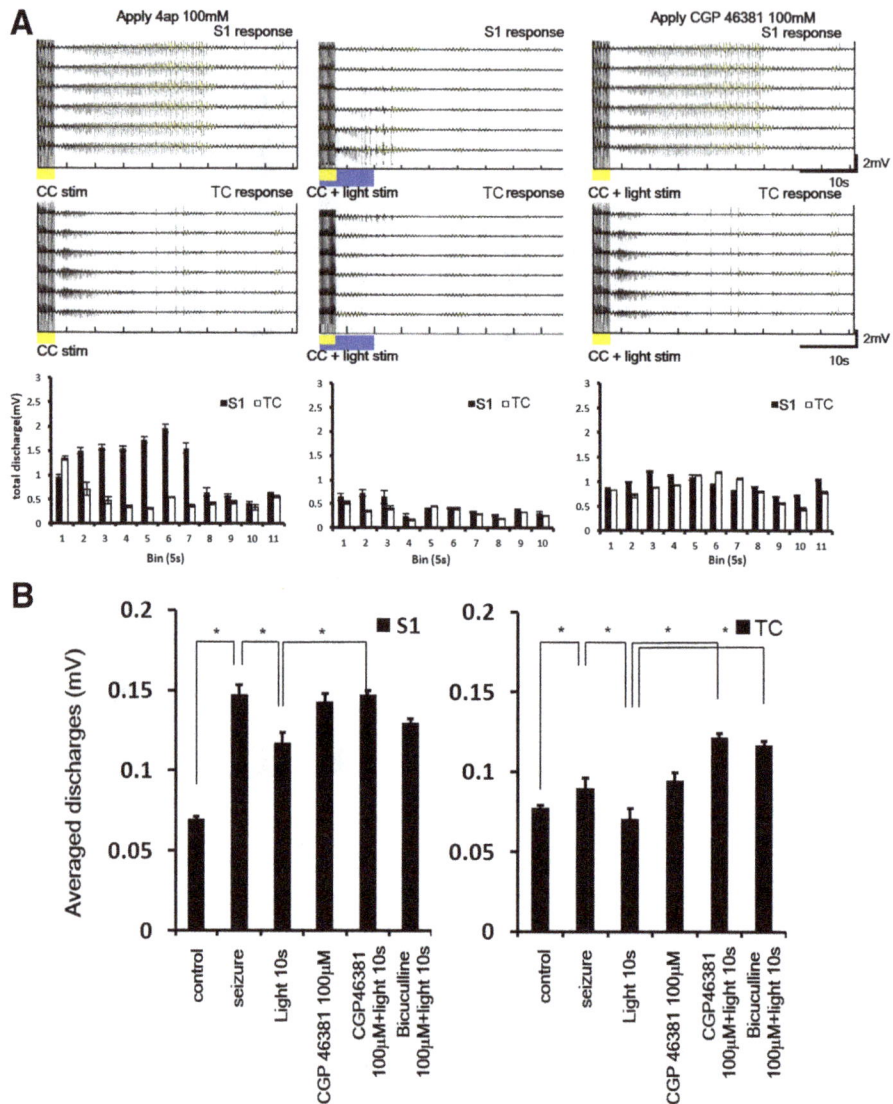

Fig. 7 Seizure-like activity was partially reversed by the GABA$_B$ antagonist CGP46381 (100 µM). **a** In the left panel, cortical and thalamic seizure-like activity was induced by electrical stimulation of the corpus callosum (yellow bar) after applying 4-AP. In the middle panel, corpus callosum stimulation-induced seizure-like activity was suppressed by 10 s light stimulation (*blue mark*) after corpus callosum stimulation. In the right panel, seizure-like activity was partially reversed by the GABA$_B$ antagonist CGP46381 (100 µM). **b** Average discharges induced by different light stimulation conditions and drug applications in the S1 region (*left panel*) and thalamus (*right panel*). The suppressive effects of 10 s light stimulation were reversed by the GABA$_B$ antagonist. $p < 0.05$, one-way ANOVA with repeated test followed by post hoc test. $n = 3$

extended processes of PV-ChR2 neurons and the retrogradely labeled thalamic neurons. The nRT has two types of interneurons: projection neurons that innervate thalamic relay neurons and local interneurons. ChR2 is expressed in both types of neurons, and the optical stimulation likely indiscriminately excited both types of neurons. The effects of excitation would be conveyed by projection neurons and exert effects on thalamic relay neurons. The functional role of GABAergic interneurons in the nRT was demonstrated in a recent study in which deletion of the GABA$_A$ receptor α1 subunit increased inhibition in the nRT and reduced absence seizures, in which abnormal

oscillations are believed to develop in thalamocortical pathways [22–24].

4-Aminopyridine has been widely used to induce focal epileptic discharges in different region in vitro, including the hippocampus [25], cingulate cortex [26–28], neocortex [29], amygdala [30], brain slice of guinea pig [31] and optical imaging study in Ferrets in vivo [32]. The application of 4-AP in the somatosensory cortex induced seizure-like activity and affected the neighboring cortex [33]. Our previous studies showed that the thalamus regulates 4-AP-induced cingulate cortex seizure-like activity by regulating gap junctions [28, 34]. Seizure-like activity that was induced

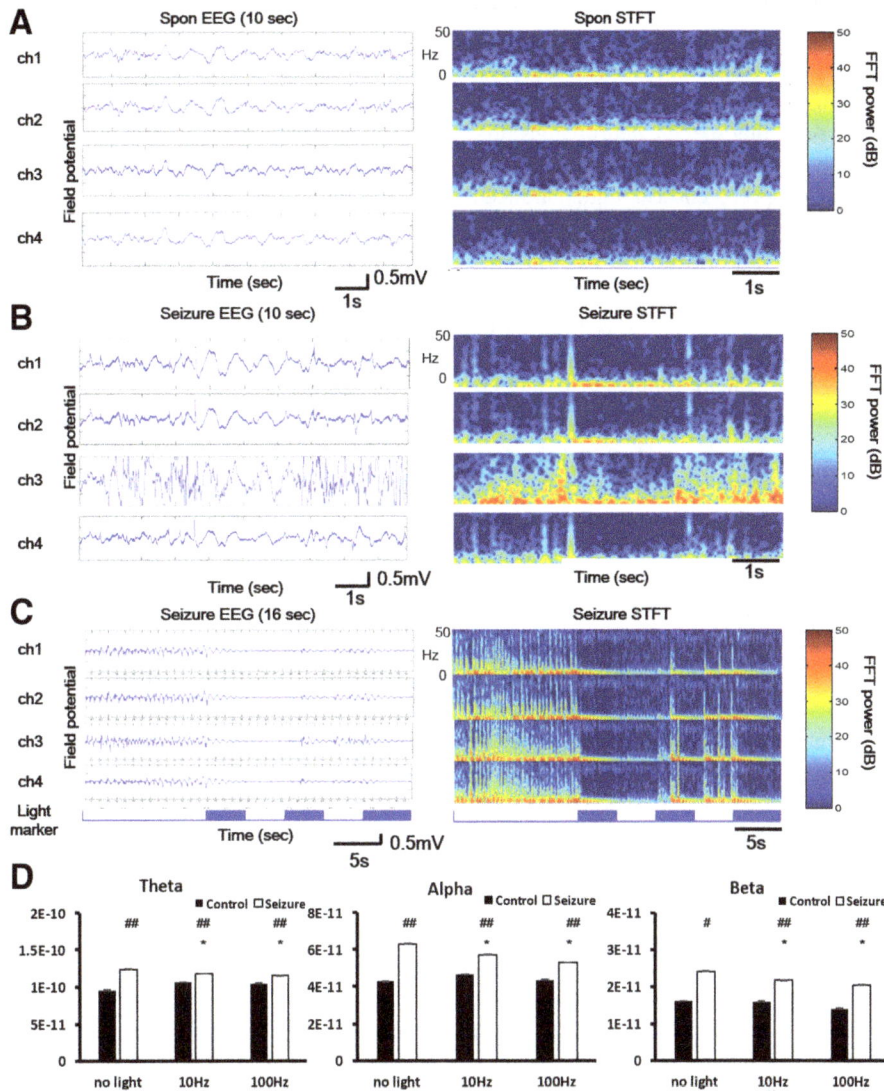

Fig. 8 Seizure-like activity was suppressed by light stimulation in the nRT in freely moving mice. **a** The left column shows spontaneous field potentials in the S1 region based on EEG recordings. The right column shows spontaneous field potentials after STFT. **b** Seizure-like activity was induced by PTZ (50 mg/kg, i.p.). The right column shows the field potentials of seizure-like activity. **c** The left column showed EEG waves in the S1 region in seizure onset period. Blue marks represent the light stimulation periods in the nRT. Seizure like activities were suppressed when light stimulation turned on. Right column presented STFT in seizure-like activities and seizure suppression period. **d** Different light stimulation conditions in the pre- and post-seizure periods. FFT power was analyzed and divided into three frequency bands (theta, 4–7 Hz; alpha, 8–15 Hz; beta, 16–30 Hz). In the post-seizure periods, the frequency power significantly decreased in all three bands when 10 and 100 Hz light stimulation was applied. *$p < 0.05$ compared with different light stimulation, ##$p < 0.05$ compared with control and seizure groups. Error bars indicate SEM. (one-way ANOVA with repeated test followed by post hoc test)

by 4-AP application in the somatosensory cortex may have affected ventrobasal complex (VB) regions through the thalamocortical pathway, revealed by synchronous discharges in the cortex and thalamus (Fig. 4). Cortical stroke-induced seizure-like activity is known to produce long-distance synchronization in the cortex and thalamus [15]. Long-distance synchronization is modulated by ascending cholinergic and serotonergic systems and thalamocortical feedback loops. When seizures occur, extracellular K^+ concentrations increase and extracellular Ca^{2+}

concentrations decrease, leading to changes in synaptic transmission, in which low Ca^{2+} concentrations inhibit the normal release of transmitters [34]. 4-Aminopyridine induced seizure-like activity in the cortex, which may have altered synaptic neurotransmitter release and led to synchronous oscillatory activity through thalamocortical feedback loops.

Electrical stimulation of the nRT has been suggested for the treatment of temporal lobe epilepsy [10]. However, electrical stimulation has side effects. Electrical stimulation can affect neurons that surround the target region, and all types of neurons are activated by such stimulation. Furthermore, damage or lesions can occur in the target region if the stimulation duration is too long. Optogenetics may solve these problems by activating specific neuronal groups. Previous studies used this new optogenetic method to control thalamic activity to suppress cortical injury-induced seizures [16] and to control different types of interneurons for the treatment of epilepsy [35]. In the present study, we used different durations and frequencies of light stimulation of the nRT. Seizure activity and behavior were suppressed by nRT neuron activation (Figs. 5 and 8). These suppressive effects were more robust with high-frequency and long-duration light stimulation, which may have resulted from augmented GABA release when the nRT was activated. Previous studies found that a halorodopsin-expressing adeno-associated virus in the hippocampus suppressed kainic acid-induced temporal lobe epilepsy [36, 37]. Neocortical epilepsy is usually drug-resistant. A halorodopsin-expressing lentivirus also suppressed tetrodotoxin-induced focal cortical seizures [38]. The inhibition of neuronal activity in the CA3 area of the hippocampus suppressed kainic acid-induced seizures [39, 40]. Seizures that were induced by cortical stroke through the thalamocortical pathway were suppressed by the halorodopsin-induced inhibition of VB neuron activity [16]. High-frequency optic stimulation (20 and 50 Hz) of the CA3 area of the hippocampus suppressed 4-AP-induced seizures in Thy1-ChR2 transgenic mice [41]. We also observed suppressive effects of high-frequency optic stimulation. Such high frequencies may thus be better for regulating GABA neurotransmitter release in the nRT to suppress cortical seizures.

The suppression of cortical seizures by the activation of thalamocortical pathways likely occurred through a cortical feedforward inhibitory mechanism. Thalamocortical feedforward inhibition has been related to inhibitory GABAergic interneurons in the cortex [42, 43]. $GABA_A$ receptor-mediated IPSCs were abolished by the $GABA_A$ antagonist picrotoxin in thalamocortical slices [18]. However, whether $GABA_B$ receptors mediate thalamocortical feedforward inhibition is still unclear. GABA receptors play an important role in mediating seizure activity. $GABA_A$ receptors mediate 4-AP-induced synchronous events in the hippocampus and entorhinal cortex. $GABA_A$ receptors also participate in the initiation, maintenance, and termination of ictal discharges [44, 45]. $GABA_B$ receptors mediate 4-AP-induced long-lasting depolarization and asynchronous excitatory and inhibitory potentials in the rat hippocampal region [46]. CGP35348 blocks presynaptic $GABA_B$ receptors and leads to an increase in GABA release and elevation of $[K^+]_o$ [47]. In the present study, GABAergic interneurons in the nRT were activated by blue light, which strongly hyperpolarized VB neurons, results in the generation of Ca^{2+} spikes, and triggers rebound burst firing

in the somatosensory cortex. [48]. We hypothesize that 4-AP-induced seizures in the cortex are suppressed by cortical GABAergic neurons that receive inputs from the VB and release GABA. Ventrobasal inputs affect both cortical excitatory and inhibitory cells. Our results showed that the $GABA_B$ antagonist CGP46381 had no effect on seizure activity when it was applied alone (Fig. 7b), thus excluding the possible confounding effects of cortical disinhibition. The involvement of $GABA_B$ receptors in cortical feedforward inhibition has been reported previously, in which $GABA_B$ but not $GABA_A$ receptors regulate thalamocortical inputs of cortical neurons presynaptically and modulate the thalamocortical excitation of excitatory and inhibitory neurons in layer IV of the barrel cortex [49].

GABAergic interneurons and glutamatergic principal cells are excited by each other. Their interaction is reciprocal, and cortical interneuron excitation can directly suppress local networks through inhibitory feedback. Cortical interneurons can be excited by receiving long-range excitatory inputs from other subcortical nuclei, thus generating feedforward inhibition [50]. Thalamocortical axons were afferents on cortical fast-spiking inhibitory neurons but not afferent in regular-spiking neurons which are pyramidal neurons in rodents [51]. Thalamocortical relay neuron activation corresponds with synchronous discharges of S1 cortical neurons, leading GABAergic interneurons in the S1 region to release GABA and inhibit postsynaptic neurons [42]. Spiny fast-spiking interneurons receive thalamocortical neuron inputs and mediate IPSCs. Thalamocortical relay neurons can precisely and reliably activate spiny fast-spiking interneurons in the S1 region and provide feedforward inhibition of postexcitatory neurons [52]. Feedforward inhibition plays an important role in mature cortical function. $GABA_A$ receptor-mediated transmission regulates thalamocortical circuit function. GABAergic transmission was also shown to be strongly engaged in stellate cells that received strong thalamocortical inputs in mature mice, whereas this engagement was weaker in neonatal mice [53]. These studies suggest that 4-AP-induced seizure activity was suppressed by the excitation of cortical interneurons through thalamocortical inputs and a mechanism of feedforward inhibition.

Our results showed that light stimulation affected thalamocortical relay neurons by activating ChR2-expressing neurons in the nRT. High-frequency and long-duration light stimulation may be more effective in suppressing cortical seizure-like activity. Histological examination verified that the stimulation of areas near the nRT and thalamus were more effective in suppressing cortical seizures, and $GABA_B$ receptors may participate in suppressing seizure-like activity.

Conclusions

The reticular thalamic nucleus (nRT) is a potential target for deep brain stimulation. It can affect ventrobasal thalamic regions, thus regulating the somatosensory cortex through the thalamocortical pathway. The present study found that evoking the activity of specifically nRT neurons by light stimulation of ChR2 protein attenuated cortical seizures. The mechanism of these suppressive effects involved γ-aminobutyric acid-B (GABA$_B$) receptors in cortical regions. The findings suggest that neuronal firing in the nRT mediates cortical GABA neurons, which may be an effective target for deep brain stimulation to suppress cortical seizures.

Acknowledgements
We are thankful for technical support from the Neural Circuit Electrophysiology Core at Academia Sinica. This work was undertaken at the Institute of Biomedical Sciences, which received funding from Academia Sinica.

Funding
The present study was supported by Ministry of Science and Technology grants (NSC 99-2320-B-001-016-MY3 and NSC 100-2311-B-001-003-MY3) and a National Health Research Institutes grant (NHRI-EX106-10439NI).

Authors' contributions
WJC conducted the experiments in vitro and in vivo, analyzed experimental data and wrote the manuscript. WPC participated the initial stage of experiments and help in experimental design. BCS conceived the experiments, and was a major contributor in writing the manuscript. All authors read and approved the final manuscript.

Competing interests
The authors declare that they have no competing interests.

Author details
[1]Institute of Biomedical Sciences, Academia Sinica, Taipei 11529, Taiwan, ROC. [2]Department of Anesthesiology and Perioperative Medicine, School of Medicine, University of Alabama, Birmingham, AL 35211, USA.

References
1. Fisher RS, van Emde Boas W, Blume W, Elger C, Genton P, Lee P, et al. Epileptic seizures and epilepsy: definitions proposed by the international league against epilepsy (ILAE) and the International Bureau for Epilepsy (IBE). Epilepsia [internet]. 2005;46:470–2. Available from: http://www.ncbi.nlm.nih.gov/pubmed/15816939.
2. Kwan P, Brodie MJ. Early identification of refractory epilepsy. N Engl J med [internet]. 2000;342:314–9. Available from: http://www.ncbi.nlm.nih.gov/pubmed/10660394.
3. Lyons MK. Deep brain stimulation: current and future clinical applications. Mayo Clin proc [internet]. 2011;86:662–72. Available from: http://www.ncbi.nlm.nih.gov/pubmed/21646303.
4. Kahane P, Depaulis A. Deep brain stimulation in epilepsy: what is next? Curr Opin Neurol [internet]. 2010;23:177–82. Available from: http://www.ncbi.nlm.nih.gov/pubmed/20125010.
5. Graber KD, Fisher RS. Deep Brain Stimulation for Epilepsy: Animal Models. In: Noebels JL, Avoli M, Rogawski MA, Olsen RW, Delgado-Escueta AV, editors. Jasper's Basic Mech. Epilepsies [Internet]. 4th ed. Bethesda (MD); 2012. Available from: http://www.ncbi.nlm.nih.gov/pubmed/22787652.
6. Lim SN, Lee ST, Tsai YT, Chen IA, Tu PH, Chen JL, et al. Electrical stimulation of the anterior nucleus of the thalamus for intractable epilepsy: a long-term follow-up study. Epilepsia [internet]. 2007;48:342–7. Available from: http://www.ncbi.nlm.nih.gov/pubmed/17295629.
7. Pinault D. The thalamic reticular nucleus: structure, function and concept. Brain res brain res rev [internet]. 2004;46:1–31. Available from: http://www.ncbi.nlm.nih.gov/pubmed/15297152.
8. Kim U, Sanchez-Vives M V, McCormick DA. Functional dynamics of GABAergic inhibition in the thalamus. Science (80-.). [internet]. 1997;278:130–4. Available from: http://www.ncbi.nlm.nih.gov/pubmed/9311919.
9. Nanobashvili Z, Chachua T, Nanobashvili A, Bilanishvili I, Lindvall O, Kokaia Z. Suppression of limbic motor seizures by electrical stimulation in thalamic reticular nucleus. Exp Neurol [internet]. 2003;181:224–30. Available from: http://www.ncbi.nlm.nih.gov/pubmed/12781995.
10. Nanobashvili ZI, Surmava AG, Bilanishvili IG, Barbaqadze MG, Mariamidze MD, Khizanishvili NA. Significance of the thalamic reticular nucleus GABAergic neurons in normal and pathological activity of the brain. J Behav Brain Sci. 2012;2:436–44.
11. Halassa MM, Siegle JH, Ritt JT, Ting JT, Feng G, Moore CI. Selective optical drive of thalamic reticular nucleus generates thalamic bursts and cortical spindles. Nat Neurosci. 2011;14:1118–20.
12. Kim A, Latchoumane C, Lee S, Kim GB, Cheong E, Augustine GJ, Shin HS. Optogenetically induced sleep spindle rhythms alter sleep architectures in mice. Proc Natl Acad Sci U S A. 2012;109:20673–8.
13. Lewis LD, Voigts J, Flores FJ, Schmitt LI, Wilson MA, Halassa MM, Brown EN. Thalamic reticular nucleus induces fast and local modulation of arousal state. elife. 2015;13:e08760.
14. Ni KM, Hou XJ, Yang CH, Dong P, Li Y, Zhang Y, Jiang P, Berg DK, Duan S, Li XM. Selectively driving cholinergic fibers optically in the thalamic reticular nucleus promotes sleep. elife. 2016;5:e10382.
15. Creed M, Pascoli VJ, Luscher C. Addiction therapy. Refining deep brain stimulation to emulate optogenetic treatment of synaptic pathology. Science (80-.). [internet]. 2015;347:659–64. Available from: http://www.ncbi.nlm.nih.gov/pubmed/25657248.
16. Paz JT, Davidson TJ, Frechette ES, Delord B, Parada I, Peng K, et al. Closed-loop optogenetic control of thalamus as a tool for interrupting seizures after cortical injury. Nat Neurosci [internet]. 2013;16:64–70. Available from: http://www.ncbi.nlm.nih.gov/pubmed/23143518.
17. Zhao S, Ting JT, Atallah HE, Qiu L, Tan J, Gloss B, et al. Cell type-specific channelrhodopsin-2 transgenic mice for optogenetic dissection of neural circuitry function. Nat methods [internet]. 2011;8:745–52. Available from: http://www.ncbi.nlm.nih.gov/pubmed/21985008.
18. Sasaki S, Huda K, Inoue T, Miyata M, Imoto K. Impaired feedforward inhibition of the thalamocortical projection in epileptic Ca2+ channel mutant mice, tottering. J Neurosci [internet]. 2006;26:3056–3065. Available from: http://www.ncbi.nlm.nih.gov/pubmed/16540584.
19. Yang JW, Shih HC, Shyu BC. Intracortical circuits in rat anterior cingulate cortex are activated by nociceptive inputs mediated by medial thalamus. J Neurophysiol [internet]. 2006;96:3409–22. Available from: http://www.ncbi.nlm.nih.gov/pubmed/16956990.
20. Asrican B, Augustine GJ, Berglund K, Chen S, Chow N, Deisseroth K, et al. Next-generation transgenic mice for optogenetic analysis of neural circuits. Front neural circuits [internet]. 2013;7:160. Available from: http://www.ncbi.nlm.nih.gov/pubmed/24324405.
21. Kaiser T, Ting JT, Monteiro P, Feng G. Transgenic labeling of parvalbumin-expressing neurons with tdTomato. Neuroscience [Internet]. 2015; Available from: http://www.ncbi.nlm.nih.gov/pubmed/26318335.
22. Arain FM, Boyd KL, Gallagher MJ. Decreased viability and absence-like epilepsy in mice lacking or deficient in the GABAA receptor alpha1 subunit. Epilepsia [internet]. 2012;53:e161–5. Available from: http://www.ncbi.nlm.nih.gov/pubmed/22812724.
23. Avoli M. A brief history on the oscillating roles of thalamus and cortex in absence seizures. Epilepsia [internet]. 2012;53:779–89. Available from: http://www.ncbi.nlm.nih.gov/pubmed/22360294.

24. Zhou C, Ding L, Deel ME, Ferrick EA, Emeson RB, Gallagher MJ. Altered intrathalamic GABAA neurotransmission in a mouse model of a human genetic absence epilepsy syndrome. Neurobiol dis [internet]. 2015;73:407–17. Available from: http://www.ncbi.nlm.nih.gov/pubmed/25447232.

25. Avoli M, Louvel J, Kurcewicz I, Pumain R, Barbarosie M. Extracellular free potassium and calcium during synchronous activity induced by 4-aminopyridine in the juvenile rat hippocampus. J Physiol [Internet]. 1996;493 (Pt 3:707–717). Available from: http://www.ncbi.nlm.nih.gov/pubmed/8799893.

26. Panuccio G, Curia G, Colosimo A, Cruccu G, Avoli M. Epileptiform synchronization in the cingulate cortex. Epilepsia [internet]. 2009;50:521–36. Available from: http://www.ncbi.nlm.nih.gov/pubmed/19178556.

27. Chang WP, Wu JS, Lee CM, Vogt BA, Shyu BC. Spatiotemporal organization and thalamic modulation of seizures in the mouse medial thalamic-anterior cingulate slice. Epilepsia [internet]. 2011;52:2344–55. Available from: http://www.ncbi.nlm.nih.gov/pubmed/22092196.

28. Chang WP, Wu JJ, Shyu BC. Thalamic modulation of cingulate seizure activity via the regulation of gap junctions in mice thalamocingulate slice. PLoS one [internet]. 2013;8:e62952. Available from: http://www.ncbi.nlm.nih.gov/pubmed/23690968.

29. Zhao M, Ma H, Suh M, Schwartz TH. Spatiotemporal dynamics of perfusion and oximetry during ictal discharges in the rat neocortex. J Neurosci [internet]. 2009;29:2814–23. Available from: http://www.ncbi.nlm.nih.gov/pubmed/19261877.

30. Klueva J, Munsch T, Albrecht D, Pape HC. Synaptic and non-synaptic mechanisms of amygdala recruitment into temporolimbic epileptiform activities. Eur J Neurosci [internet]. 2003;18:2779–91. Available from: http://www.ncbi.nlm.nih.gov/pubmed/14656327.

31. Uva L, Trombin F, Carriero G, Avoli M, de Curtis M. Seizure-like discharges induced by 4-aminopyridine in the olfactory system of the in vitro isolated guinea pig brain. Epilepsia [internet]. 2013;54:605–15. Available from: http://www.ncbi.nlm.nih.gov/pubmed/23505998.

32. Schwartz TH, Bonhoeffer T. In vivo optical mapping of epileptic foci and surround inhibition in ferret cerebral cortex. Nat med [internet]. 2001;7:1063–7. Available from: http://www.ncbi.nlm.nih.gov/pubmed/11533712.

33. Harris S, Bruyns-Haylett M, Kennerley A, Boorman L, Overton PG, Ma H, et al. The effects of focal epileptic activity on regional sensory-evoked neurovascular coupling and postictal modulation of bilateral sensory processing. J Cereb blood flow Metab [internet]. 2013;33:1595–604. Available from: http://www.ncbi.nlm.nih.gov/pubmed/23860375.

34. Chang WP, Shyu BC. Anterior cingulate epilepsy: mechanisms and modulation. Front Integr Neurosci [internet]. 2014;7:104. Available from: http://www.ncbi.nlm.nih.gov/pubmed/24427123.

35. Ledri M, Madsen MG, Nikitidou L, Kirik D, Kokaia M. Global optogenetic activation of inhibitory interneurons during epileptiform activity. J Neurosci [internet]. 2014;34:3364–77. Available from: http://www.ncbi.nlm.nih.gov/pubmed/24573293.

36. Krook-Magnuson E, Armstrong C, Oijala M, Soltesz I. On-demand optogenetic control of spontaneous seizures in temporal lobe epilepsy. Nat Commun [internet]. 2013;4:1376. Available from: http://www.ncbi.nlm.nih.gov/pubmed/23340416.

37. Krook-Magnuson E, Szabo GG, Armstrong C, Oijala M, Soltesz I. Cerebellar directed Optogenetic intervention inhibits spontaneous hippocampal seizures in a mouse model of temporal lobe epilepsy. eNeuro [internet]. 2014;1. Available from: http://www.ncbi.nlm.nih.gov/pubmed/25599088.

38. Wykes RC, Heeroma JH, Mantoan L, Zheng K, MacDonald DC, Deisseroth K, et al. Optogenetic and potassium channel gene therapy in a rodent model of focal neocortical epilepsy. Sci Transl Med [internet]. 2012;4:161ra152. Available from: http://www.ncbi.nlm.nih.gov/pubmed/23147003.

39. Sukhotinsky I, Chan AM, Ahmed OJ, Rao VR, Gradinaru V, Ramakrishnan C, et al. Optogenetic delay of status epilepticus onset in an in vivo rodent epilepsy model. PLoS one [internet]. 2013;8:e62013. Available from: http://www.ncbi.nlm.nih.gov/pubmed/23637949.

40. Berglind F, Ledri M, Sorensen AT, Nikitidou L, Melis M, Bielefeld P, et al. Optogenetic inhibition of chemically induced hypersynchronized bursting in mice. Neurobiol dis [internet]. 2014;65:133–41. Available from: http://www.ncbi.nlm.nih.gov/pubmed/24491965.

41. Chiang CC, Ladas TP, Gonzalez-Reyes LE, Durand DM. Seizure suppression by high frequency optogenetic stimulation using in vitro and in vivo animal models of epilepsy. Brain Stimul [internet]. 2014;7:890–9. Available from: http://www.ncbi.nlm.nih.gov/pubmed/25108607.

42. Swadlow HA. Thalamocortical control of feed-forward inhibition in awake somatosensory "barrel" cortex. Philos trans R Soc L. B biol Sci [internet]. 2002;357: 1717–27. Available from: http://www.ncbi.nlm.nih.gov/pubmed/12626006.

43. Gabernet L, Jadhav SP, Feldman DE, Carandini M, Scanziani M. Somatosensory integration controlled by dynamic thalamocortical feed-forward inhibition. Neuron [internet]. 2005;48:315–27. Available from: http://www.ncbi.nlm.nih.gov/pubmed/16242411.

44. Perreault P, Avoli M. 4-aminopyridine-induced epileptiform activity and a GABA-mediated long-lasting depolarization in the rat hippocampus. J Neurosci [internet]. 1992;12:104–15. Available from: http://www.ncbi.nlm.nih.gov/pubmed/1309571.

45. Lopantsev V, Avoli M. Participation of GABAA-mediated inhibition in ictallike discharges in the rat entorhinal cortex. J Neurophysiol [internet]. 1998;79:352–60. Available from: http://www.ncbi.nlm.nih.gov/pubmed/9425204.

46. Motalli R, Louvel J, Tancredi V, Kurcewicz I, Wan-Chow-Wah D, Pumain R, et al. GABA(B) receptor activation promotes seizure activity in the juvenile rat hippocampus. J Neurophysiol [internet]. 1999;82:638–47. Available from: http://www.ncbi.nlm.nih.gov/pubmed/10444662.

47. Motalli R, D'Antuono M, Louvel J, Kurcewicz I, D'Arcangelo G, Tancredi V, et al. Epileptiform synchronization and GABA(B) receptor antagonism in the juvenile rat hippocampus. J Pharmacol Exp Ther [internet]. 2002;303:1102–13. Available from: http://www.ncbi.nlm.nih.gov/pubmed/12438533.

48. Huguenard JR, McCormick DA. Thalamic synchrony and dynamic regulation of global forebrain oscillations. Trends Neurosci [internet]. 2007;30:350–6. Available from: http://www.ncbi.nlm.nih.gov/pubmed/17544519.

49. Porter JT, Nieves D. Presynaptic GABAB receptors modulate thalamic excitation of inhibitory and excitatory neurons in the mouse barrel cortex. J Neurophysiol [internet]. 2004;92:2762–70. Available from: http://www.ncbi.nlm.nih.gov/pubmed/15254073.

50. Isaacson JS, Scanziani M. How inhibition shapes cortical activity. Neuron [internet]. 2011;72:231–43. Available from: http://www.ncbi.nlm.nih.gov/pubmed/22017986.

51. Bruno RM, Simons DJ. Feedforward mechanisms of excitatory and inhibitory cortical receptive fields. J Neurosci [internet]. 2002;22:10966–75. Available from: http://www.ncbi.nlm.nih.gov/pubmed/12486192.

52. Sun QQ, Huguenard JR, Prince DA. Barrel cortex microcircuits: thalamocortical feedforward inhibition in spiny stellate cells is mediated by a small number of fast-spiking interneurons. J Neurosci [internet]. 2006;26:1219–30. Available from: http://www.ncbi.nlm.nih.gov/pubmed/16436609.

53. Daw MI, Ashby MC, Isaac JT. Coordinated developmental recruitment of latent fast spiking interneurons in layer IV barrel cortex. Nat Neurosci [internet]. 2007;10:453–61. Available from: http://www.ncbi.nlm.nih.gov/pubmed/17351636.

12

5-HTR$_{2A}$ and 5-HTR$_{3A}$ but not 5-HTR$_{1A}$ antagonism impairs the cross-modal reactivation of deprived visual cortex in adulthood

Nathalie Lombaert[1], Maroussia Hennes[1], Sara Gilissen[1], Giel Schevenels[1], Laetitia Aerts[1], Ria Vanlaer[1], Lieve Geenen[1], Ann Van Eeckhaut[2], Ilse Smolders[2], Julie Nys[1,3] and Lutgarde Arckens[1*]

Abstract

Visual cortical areas show enhanced tactile responses in blind individuals, resulting in improved behavioral performance. Induction of unilateral vision loss in adult mice, by monocular enucleation (ME), is a validated model for such cross-modal brain plasticity. A delayed whisker-driven take-over of the medial monocular zone of the visual cortex is preceded by so-called unimodal plasticity, involving the potentiation of the spared-eye inputs in the binocular cortical territory. Full reactivation of the sensory-deprived contralateral visual cortex is accomplished by 7 weeks post-injury. Serotonin (5-HT) is known to modulate sensory information processing and integration, but its impact on cortical reorganization after sensory loss, remains largely unexplored. To address this issue, we assessed the involvement of 5-HT in ME-induced cross-modal plasticity and the 5-HT receptor (5-HTR) subtype used. We first focused on establishing the impact of ME on the total 5-HT concentration measured in the visual cortex and in the somatosensory barrel field. Next, the changes in expression as a function of post-ME recovery time of the monoamine transporter 2 (vMAT2), which loads 5-HT into presynaptic vesicles, and of the 5-HTR$_{1A}$ and 5-HTR$_{3A}$ were assessed, in order to link these temporal expression profiles to the different types of cortical plasticity induced by ME. In order to accurately pinpoint which 5-HTR exactly mediates ME-induced cross-modal plasticity, we pharmacologically antagonized the 5-HTR$_{1A}$, 5-HTR$_{2A}$ and 5-HTR$_{3A}$ subtypes. This study reveals brain region-specific alterations in total 5-HT concentration, time-dependent modulations in vMAT2, 5-HTR$_{1A}$ and 5-HTR$_{3A}$ protein expression and 5-HTR antagonist-specific effects on the post-ME plasticity phenomena. Together, our results confirm a role for 5-HTR$_{1A}$ in the early phase of binocular visual cortex plasticity and suggest an involvement of 5-HTR$_{2A}$ and 5-HTR$_{3A}$ but not 5-HTR$_{1A}$ during the late cross-modal recruitment of the medial monocular visual cortex. These insights contribute to the general understanding of 5-HT function in cortical plasticity and may encourage the search for improved rehabilitation strategies to compensate for sensory loss.

Keywords: Brain plasticity, Visual cortex, Adult mice, Monocular enucleation, Neuromodulator, Serotonin

* Correspondence: lut.arckens@kuleuven.be
[1]Laboratory of Neuroplasticity and Neuroproteomics, Katholieke Universiteit Leuven, Naamsestraat 59, Box 2467, B-3000 Leuven, Belgium
Full list of author information is available at the end of the article

Introduction

Even though the mammalian brain is most susceptible to changes in sensory inputs during so-called critical periods early in life [1–4], it retains the intrinsic capacity to recover from sensory deprivation well into adulthood [1, 5–7]. In human patients, for example, late-onset vision loss triggers two types of cross-modal brain plasticity [8]: 'compensatory plasticity' is the result of experience-dependent refinement of the spared senses, whereas 'cross-modal recruitment' involves the take-over of the deprived visual cortical territory for the active processing of non-visual information, leading to enhanced sound localization abilities or improved tactile acuity as with Braille reading [9–13].

In an animal model of one-eyed vision, due to monocular enucleation (ME) in adult (P120) mice, we could previously establish extensive neuronal reactivation of both the binocular zone (Bz) and the medial monocular zone (Mmz) of the deprived contralateral visual cortex

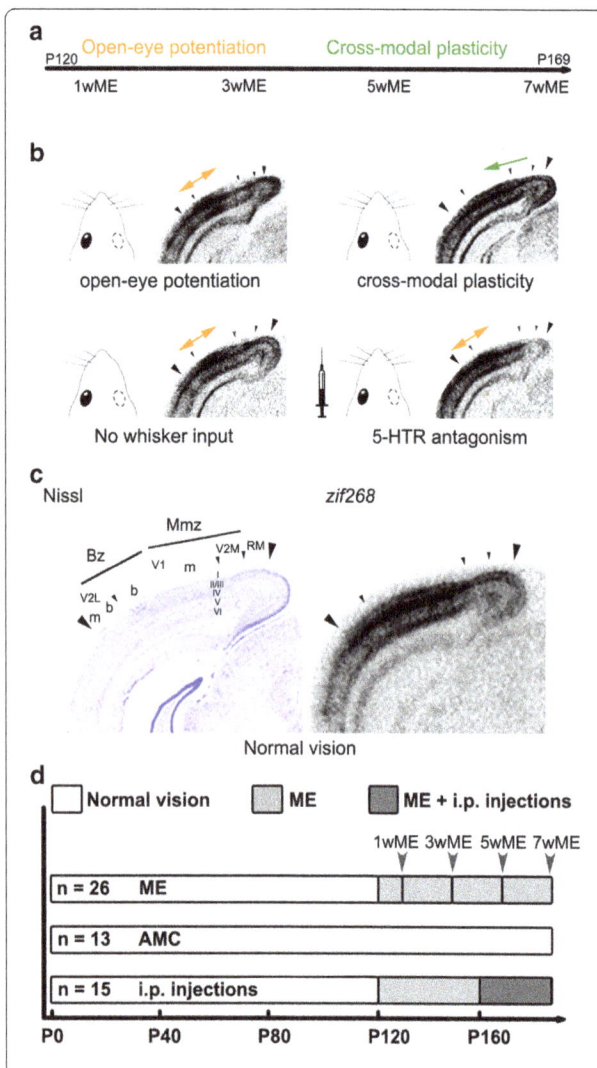

Fig. 1 Schematic overview of the different cortical plasticity phases occurring in the adult ME-mouse model and illustration of the experimental setup. **a** Timeline indicating the early unimodal plasticity phase (week 1–3 post-ME) and the subsequent cross-modal plasticity phase (week 4–7 post-ME). **b** Overview of the ISH *zif268*-based reactivation pattern of the uni-and cross-modal plasticity phase in adult mice upon ME. Whisker deprivation and 5-HTR antagonism specifically suppress reactivation of the Mmz. **c** Illustration of the anatomical delineation of the visual cortex regions on a Nissl-stained coronal section which are then overlaid on the matching ISH *zif268* section. The delineated visual cortical areas are indicated between large arrowheads: V2L, V1, V2M and RM with the distinction between monocular (m) and binocular (b) segments. The binocular zone (Bz) comprises V2Lb-V1b while the medial monocular zone (Mmz) includes V1m-V2M. The different cortical layers are indicated with Roman numbers: I-VI. **d** All animals had normal vision up to the age of P120 or in case of the non-deprived age-matched control mice (AMC), up to P169 (white bars). Mice that underwent monocular enucleation (ME, light gray bars) at P120 recovered under standard housing conditions during 1 week (1wME, *n* = 5; representing ongoing open-eye potentiation), 3 weeks (3wME, *n* = 5, representing the end of the open-eye potentiation phase), 5 weeks (5wME, *n* = 5; representing ongoing cross-modal plasticity phase) or 7 weeks (7wME, *n* = 11; representing the end of the cross-modal plasticity phase). All drug-treated ME mice recovered for 7 weeks and received daily intraperitoneal (i.p.) injections of either saline (*n* = 6), 5-HTR_{1A} antagonist (WAY-100635, *n* = 3), 5-HTR_{2A} antagonist (ketanserin, *n* = 3) or 5-HTR_{3A} antagonist (ondansetron, *n* = 3) during the last 3 weeks of the 7 weeks post-ME period (dark gray bar, representing the time window of whisker-driven cross-modal plasticity). The number of animals (n) is represented in the bars

within a 7 week recovery period (7wME) (Fig. 1a, b). This functional recovery not only relied on the expected unimodal potentiation of spared-eye inputs occurring in the Bz during the first 3 weeks post-ME, but also on an ensuing tactile whisker-related reactivation of especially the Mmz from week four onwards [14–16]. This cross-modal effect was most pronounced in the infragranular layers of the Mmz [15]. The level of neuronal activity reached in the Mmz 7 weeks post-ME could be experimentally manipulated by reducing or intensifying whisker inputs, respectively by means of whisker removal or via natural whisker stimulation during exploration of a new, enriched cage environment in complete darkness. These observations confirmed the manifestation of the cross-modal recruitment of the medial monocular cortical territory by the whiskers [15]. The post-ME recovery period is thus characterized by the recruitment of the deprived visual areas by the spared senses in adult mice just as in human patients.

Despite the current understanding of molecular and cellular aspects of visual cortex plasticity [12, 17–22] and the well-described role of neuromodulators in brain plasticity [19, 23–27], only little is known about sensory deprivation-induced alterations in serotonin (5-HT) signaling across sensory areas or, in concreto, about how 5-HT is involved in the different types of cortical plasticity in the context of acquired blindness. A wide range of axonal projections, originating from the serotonergic

Raphe Nucleus in the brain stem [28], reach the different sensory cortices, where 5-HT and several of the 14 identified mammalian 5-HT receptor subtypes are involved in the integration of neuronal signals and in the processing of sensory information [29–35].

Of particular interest to the field of cortical plasticity are the serotonergic G-protein coupled receptors 5-HTR_{1A} and 5-HTR_{2A}, and ion channel 5-HTR_{3A}. These receptors are most abundantly expressed in the mammalian neocortex, predominantly on excitatory, excitatory and inhibitory, and exclusively on inhibitory neurons respectively. In addition, 5-HTR_{1A} and 5-HTR_{2A} have already been implicated in either unimodal or cross-modal plasticity [18, 27, 32, 36–41]. On the one hand, administration of the selective serotonin reuptake inhibitor (SSRI) fluoxetine during a period of visual deprivation via eyelid suture reinstated juvenile-like unimodal ocular dominance plasticity in adulthood. This extraordinary phenomenon was found to be mediated through, amongst others, changes in 5-HTR_{1A} receptor function leading to an experience-dependent shift in the cortical excitation/inhibition balance (E/I) [26, 27, 36, 42, 43]. On the other hand, 2 days of visual deprivation in young rats mediated a 5-$HTR_{2A/2C}$-dependent delivery of AMPAR1 specifically at layer IV-II/III synapses of the primary somatosensory barrel cortex (S1BF), ultimately leading to compensatory plasticity in the form of a sharpened whisker-barrel map and more fine-tuned barrel neuron responses to primary whisker stimulation [32].

Adult cortical plasticity in response to sensory deprivation was further found to involve the activation of dis-inhibitory cortical circuits including the vasoactive intestinal polypeptide (VIP)-positive interneurons [44–51]. VIP cells are a type of 5-HTR_{3A} expressing interneurons, which account for approximately $1/3^{rd}$ of the entire interneuron population [52]. We discovered before that $GABA_AR_{\alpha 1}$-mediated intracortical inhibition elicits a pivotal role in the different response of the Bz and the Mmz to ME [53]. Since 5-HT and the 5-HT receptors are considered important regulators of the cortical E/I balance [37, 54, 55], they may well exert a major impact on the excitability of the specific brain circuits involved in different types of cortical plasticity.

All these findings indicate that 5-HT may indeed elicit a very important role in the cortical response to sensory loss. We therefore initiated a set of experiments to elucidate if and how exactly 5-HT or one of the three above described 5-HT receptor subtypes, take part in ME-induced plasticity in adult mice. HPLC analysis was performed on whole-tissue homogenates of the visual cortex and S1BF to study the long-term impact of ME on the total 5-HT concentration in these two sensory cortices, known to functionally adapt upon vision loss [15]. Western blotting experiments were conducted to

investigate the longitudinal effect of ME on the vesicular monoamine transporter 2 (vMAT2), 5-HTR_{1A} and 5-HTR_{3A} protein expression levels. Different time-points post-ME were chosen to enable distinction between the earlier effects occurring in the Bz, during the unimodal open-eye potentiation phase, and those occurring in the Mmz, during the subsequent cross-modal phase. We pharmacologically antagonized 5-HTR_{1A}, 5-HTR_{2A} and 5-HTR_{3A} receptor function, to pinpoint via which of these receptors 5-HT mediates ME-induced cross-modal plasticity in the visual cortex and in S1BF. As before, we relied on in situ hybridization for the neuronal activity reporter gene zif268 as a high-throughput read-out to differentiate the distinct post-ME plasticity phases (Fig. 1c, d). We demonstrate brain region-specific and time-dependent alterations in pre- and postsynaptic aspects of 5-HT neurotransmission in the adult brain upon ME. A role for 5-HTR_{1A} in unimodal open-eye potentiation was confirmed and we provide evidence for the involvement of 5-HTR_{2A} and 5-HTR_{3A} but not 5-HTR_{1A} in ME-induced cross-modal plasticity. The potential of a defined pharmacological and spatiotemporal control on cross-modal plasticity holds promise towards future refinements of rehabilitation strategies to treat acquired sensory loss.

Methods
Animals
In total 54 C57Bl/6 J mice (Janvier Elevage, Le Genest-St-Isle, France) of either sex (32 male/22 female) were used in this study. All mice were housed under standard laboratory conditions with constant room temperature and humidity, an 10/14-h dark/light cycle with food and water available ad libitum. All experiments have been approved by the Ethical Research Committee of KU Leuven and were in strict accordance with the European Communities Council Directive of 22 September 2010 (2010/63/EU) and with the Belgian legislation (KB of 29 May 2013). Every effort was made to minimize animal suffering and to reduce the number of animals. Figure 1 illustrates the experimental manipulations and the number of mice used per condition (Fig. 1b, d). The different phases of cortical plasticity under study have been determined previously based on the impact of either visual stimulation via the spared eye, or somatosensory deprivation/stimulation based on whisker clipping/natural whisker use during the exploration of new toys in complete darkness, on neuronal activity in the visual cortex of adult ME mice [15]. Specifically, 1 week post-ME (1wME) mice are in an ongoing unimodal open-eye potentiation phase. Mice with a 3 week post-ME recovery period (3wME) are at the end of the open-eye potentiation phase, which restores normal visually driven activity levels in an extended binocular

zone (Bz). 5 weeks post-ME (5wME) mice are in an on-going cross-modal phase whereas mice with a 7 week post-ME recovery period (7wME) have undergone maximal cross-modal visual cortex reactivation in which normal activity levels are restored in the monocular zone of the visual cortex, especially medial to the Bz (Mmz), only now relying on whisker inputs. Cortical regions of interest therefore are the visual cortex, Bz and Mmz, and the primary somatosensory barrel field (S1BF).

Monocular enucleation paradigm and tissue preparation
The removal of the right eye, or monocular enucleation (ME), was performed as described previously [14]. Briefly, adult (P120) mice were anaesthetized by intraperitoneal injection of a mixture of ketamine hydrochloride (75 mg/kg, Dechra Veterinary Products, Eurovet) and medetomidine hydrochloride (1 mg/kg Orion Corporation, Janssen Animal Health). Eye ointment (Tobrex, Alcon) was administered to the left eye to prevent dehydration. The right eye was carefully removed and the orbit was filled with hemostatic cotton wool (Qualiphar, Bornem, Belgium) in case of bleeding. Analgesics were injected subcutaneously (Metacam, 2 mg/kg, 0.1 mL) and atipamezol hydrochloride was administered to reverse anaesthesia (1 mg/kg i.p., Orion Corporation, Elanco Animal Health). Following ME, the mice were housed in their home cages under standard laboratory conditions for a 1 to 7 week recovery period. Control mice are age-matched (AMC) to the 7 week ME mice, the time point of maximal recovery of neuronal activity [56]. At the end of the ME period, the mice were sacrificed by cervical dislocation. For HPLC-based determination of the total 5-HT concentration in visual and somatosensory tissue samples, the brains were rapidly extracted and immediately frozen in 2-methylbutane (Merck, Overijse, Belgium) at a temperature of − 40 °C. All brains were stored at − 80 °C until sectioning. A tissue blotting device (Model PA 002 Mouse Brain Blocker, 1 mm, David KOPF instruments, California) was used to prepare approximately 1 mm-thick coronal slices to subsequently isolate the whole visual cortex and the primary somatosensory cortex (S1BF) with sterile scalpels. Separate analysis of medial monocular and binocular cortex was technically impossible with this method. For Western blotting experiments, 100 μm-thick coronal cryosections were collected on baked glass slides and stored at − 80 °C. Specifically for radioactive in situ hybridization (ISH) experiments, the mice were placed overnight in their home cages in a dark room to reduce *zif268*-expression to basal levels. The following day, the mice were placed in a high-lit environment to upregulate sensory driven *zif268*-mRNA expression. After 45 min, at peak *zif268*-mRNA expression levels, the mice were sacrificed by cervical dislocation. The brains were rapidly

removed, immersed in 2-methylbutane at a temperature of − 40 °C (Merck, Overijse, Belgium) and stored at − 80 °C until sectioning. Serial sections with a thickness of 25 μm were prepared on a cryostat (HM 500 OM, Microm, Thermo Scientific, Walldorf, Germany), mounted on 0.1% poly-L-Lysine-coated (Sigma-Aldrich) slides, and stored at − 20 °C until further processing.

Quantification of the total serotonin content in mouse brain homogenates
The total serotonin (5-HT) content in the visual and barrel cortex (HPLC total $n = 15$, AMC: $n = 9$; 7wME: $n = 6$) was measured based on previously reported methods [57–59]. In summary, after weighing cortical tissue, 190 μL of an antioxidant solution (0.1 M acetic acid, 3.3 mM L-cysteine, 0.27 mM Na_2EDTA and 0.0125 mM ascorbic acid) and 10 μL of an internal standard solution (3,4-dihydroxybenzylamine solution 1 μg/mL in antioxidant) were added to the tissue. After homogenization, the samples were centrifuged (20 min, 9500 g, 4 °C). The supernatant was diluted 5-fold in 0.5 M acetic acid and 20 μL was injected automatically on a reversed phase liquid chromatography system (autosampler ASI-100 and HPLC pump P680 A HPG/2, Dionex, Amsterdam, The Netherlands) with electrochemical detection (potential = + 700 mV) (Amperometric Detector LC-4C, BAS, Indiana, USA). With this liquid chromatography method, we are able to measure within one run the monoamines noradrenaline, dopamine and 5-HT, some of their major metabolites (such as 3,4-dihydroxyphenylacetic acid; 5-hydroxy-indoleacetic acid; homovanillic acid) as well as the internal standard 3,4-dihydroxybenzylamine (Fig. 2). The separation between the different compounds was achieved using a narrowbore C18 column (Alltech®, Alltima™, 5 μm, 150 × 2.1 mm, Grace, Deerfield, IL, USA). The mobile phase buffer contained 0.1 M sodium acetate, 20 mM citric acid, 1 mM sodium octane sulfonic acid, 1 mM dibutylamine and 0.1 mM Na_2EDTA adjusted to pH 3.7 (mobile phase composition: 97 buffer / 3 methanol (v/v)). For this study, we specifically quantified the 5-HT content of the different samples. Tissue concentration was expressed as ng 5-HT /g wet tissue (ng/g).

Western analysis
Western blotting (WB) was used to investigate the changes in relative expression of pre- and postsynaptic proteins involved in serotonergic neurotransmission. Time-course samples were prepared to separately examine the protein expression in the Mmz, Bz and S1BF over a 7-week period. The experimental conditions included: 1, 3, 5, 7 weeks post-ME. For each of the experimental conditions, as well as for the control mice

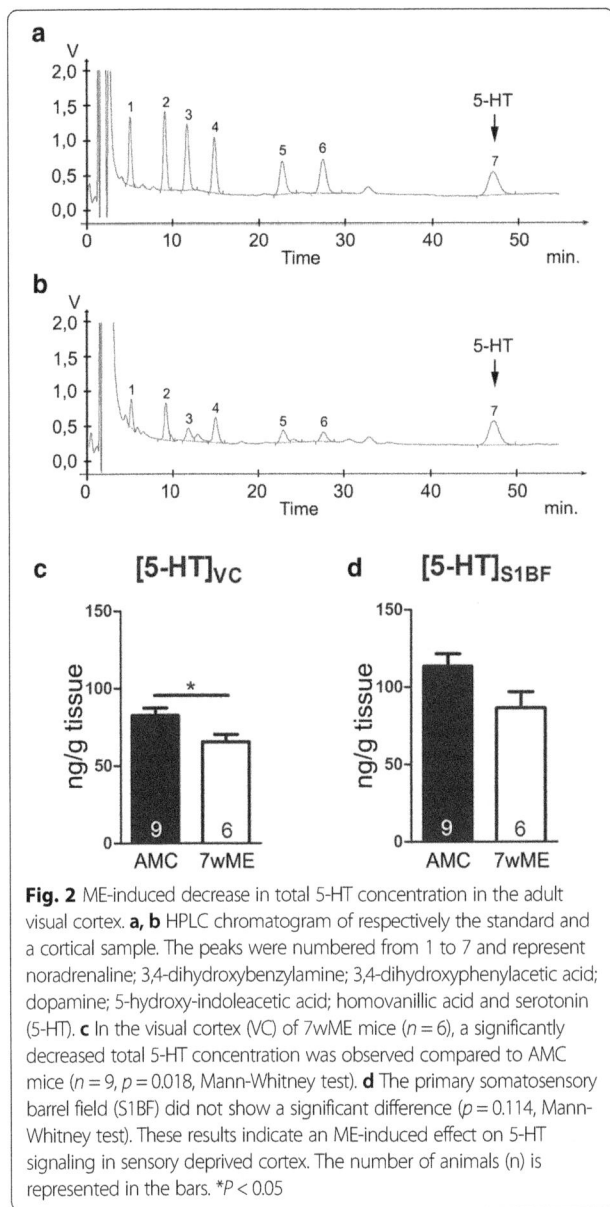

Fig. 2 ME-induced decrease in total 5-HT concentration in the adult visual cortex. **a, b** HPLC chromatogram of respectively the standard and a cortical sample. The peaks were numbered from 1 to 7 and represent noradrenaline; 3,4-dihydroxybenzylamine; 3,4-dihydroxyphenylacetic acid; dopamine; 5-hydroxy-indoleacetic acid; homovanillic acid and serotonin (5-HT). **c** In the visual cortex (VC) of 7wME mice ($n = 6$), a significantly decreased total 5-HT concentration was observed compared to AMC mice ($n = 9$, $p = 0.018$, Mann-Whitney test). **d** The primary somatosensory barrel field (S1BF) did not show a significant difference ($p = 0.114$, Mann-Whitney test). These results indicate an ME-induced effect on 5-HT signaling in sensory deprived cortex. The number of animals (n) is represented in the bars. *$P < 0.05$

Protein extraction from tissue slices

Based on the mouse brain atlas of Paxinos and Franklin (2013) [63], the primary somatosensory barrel field (S1BF: 0.5-(– 2); 3–4.5; 1, relative to Bregma in A-P; M-L; D), the medial monocular zone (Mmz, comprising monocular V1 and V2M: – 2.7-(– 4.7); 1–2.5; 1, relative to Bregma and the binocular zone (Bz, comprising binocular V2L and V1: – 2.7-(– 4.7); 2.5–4; 1, relative to Bregma) were microscopically excised and collected separately from 100 μm-thick coronal cryosections (Fig. 1c). Tissue was collected in a mix of 4 μL of complete protease inhibitor cocktail (Roche Diagnostics, GmbH) and 100 μL ice-cold lysis buffer (2% SDS, 65 mM Tris-HCl in MQ) optimized for the enrichment of membrane (–associated) proteins [64, 65]. Proteins were extracted from the tissue by mechanical homogenization using drill-driven, sterile disposable pestles (Argos Technologies), sonication (5 × 10 s), incubation at 70 °C (5 min) and centrifugation (15 min, 13000 rpm, 4 °C). The supernatant was collected and the total protein concentration was determined using the Qubit fluorometer (Invitrogen). Samples were stored at – 80 °C.

Immunoblotting

To obtain the optimal primary antibody working concentration, a protein dilution series ranging from 5 to 30 μg was analyzed. A concentration within the linear range of the detection system that resulted in a good signal to noise ratio was chosen for monocular, binocular and somatosensory samples separately. For vMAT2, 5-HTR$_{1A}$ and 5-HTR$_{3A}$ analysis, this resulted in 15 μg for samples of all three regions. 5-HTR$_{2A}$ was excluded from the analyses due to the lack of a specific antibody. Reference sample (pool) consisting of a mixture of equal amounts of each prepared tissue sample was run for monocular, binocular and somatosensory cortex, with the same optimal amount of protein on each gel to gauge blot-to-blot variability. After the addition of 5 μl reducing agent (10×, Invitrogen, Paisley, United Kingdom) and 2 μl LDS sample buffer (4×, Invitrogen), the samples were denatured (10 min, 70 °C). The protein samples were separated on 4–12% Bis-Tris Midi-gels in the XCell4 SureLock Midi-Cell (Invitrogen). The Spectra™ Multicolor Broad range protein ladder (Thermo-Scientific) was used as molecular weight standard. Subsequently, the samples were transferred to a polyvinylidene fluoride (PVDF) membrane. After 1–2 h incubation in a 5% ECL blocking agent (GE Healthcare, Buckinghamshire, UK) in Tris-saline (0.01 M Tris, 0.9% NaCl, 0.1% TX-100, pH 7.6), the membrane was incubated overnight with a primary antibody rabbit anti-vMAT2 (1:1000, R&D Systems, Novus Biologicals), with rabbit anti-5-HTR$_{1A}$ (1:200, Alomone Labs), with rabbit anti-5-HTR$_{3A}$ (1:200, Alomone Labs). The next

age-matched to the 7wME mice (AMC), at least 4 mice were included (Figs. 3 and 4, WB total $n = 24$, AMC: $n = 4$; 1wME: $n = 5$; 3wME: $n = 5$; 5wME: $n = 5$; 7wME: $n = 5$). All ME samples were analyzed relative to the AMC samples (absolute OD-values measured in the Mmz, Bz or S1BF of the AMC as mean ± SEM for vMAT2 (Mmz: 2.824 ± 0.483; Bz: 0.691 ± 0.044; S1BF: 0.953 ± 0.130), 5-HTR$_{1A}$ (Mmz: 0.855 ± 0.126; Bz: 0.667 ± 0.076; S1BF: 0.700 ± 0.073) and 5-HTR$_{3A}$ (Mmz: 0.955 ± 0.087; Bz: 0.854 ± 0.138; S1BF: 0.764 ± 0.273)). We chose to analyze vMAT2 protein expression levels since they provide information on the presynaptic loading of vesicles with 5-HT and because vMAT2 expression levels positively correlate with the total 5-HT concentration present in a given brain region of interest [60–62].

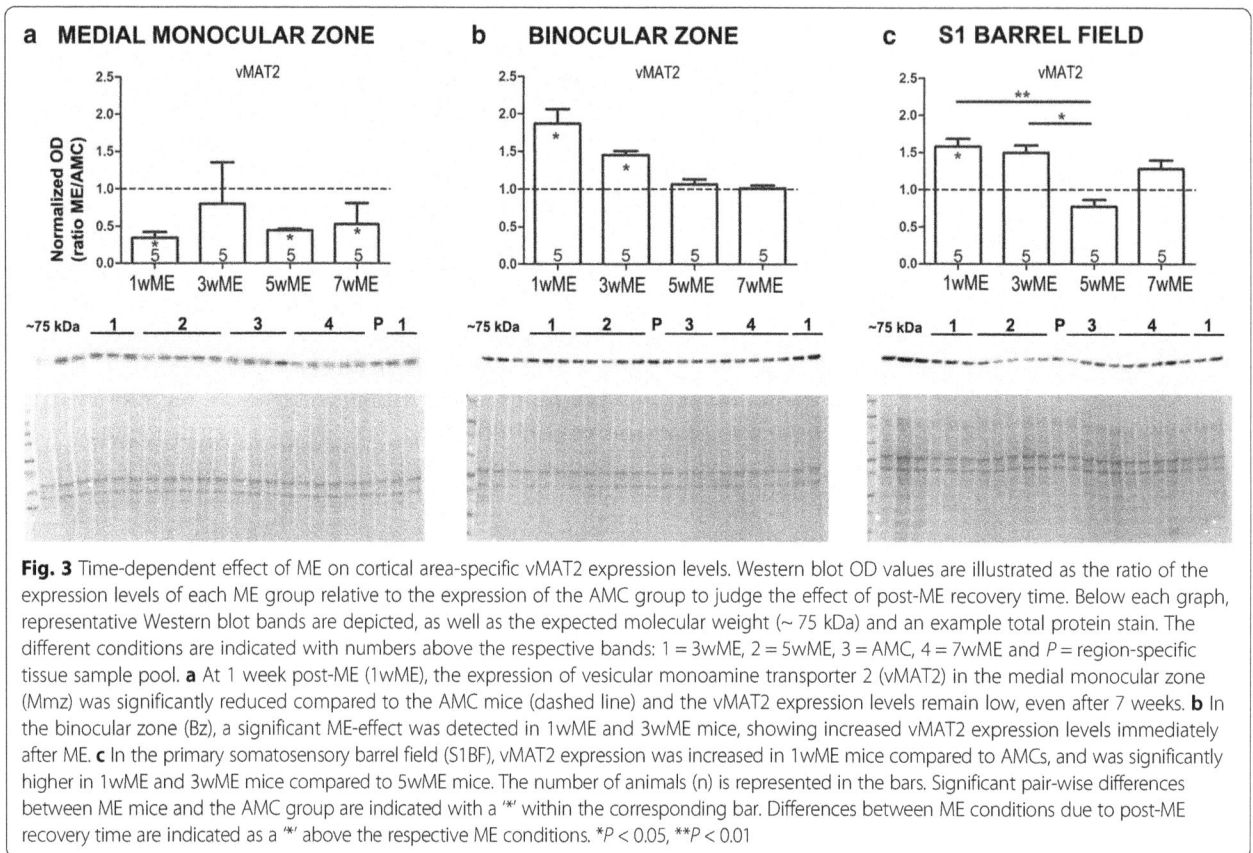

Fig. 3 Time-dependent effect of ME on cortical area-specific vMAT2 expression levels. Western blot OD values are illustrated as the ratio of the expression levels of each ME group relative to the expression of the AMC group to judge the effect of post-ME recovery time. Below each graph, representative Western blot bands are depicted, as well as the expected molecular weight (~ 75 kDa) and an example total protein stain. The different conditions are indicated with numbers above the respective bands: 1 = 3wME, 2 = 5wME, 3 = AMC, 4 = 7wME and P = region-specific tissue sample pool. **a** At 1 week post-ME (1wME), the expression of vesicular monoamine transporter 2 (vMAT2) in the medial monocular zone (Mmz) was significantly reduced compared to the AMC mice (dashed line) and the vMAT2 expression levels remain low, even after 7 weeks. **b** In the binocular zone (Bz), a significant ME-effect was detected in 1wME and 3wME mice, showing increased vMAT2 expression levels immediately after ME. **c** In the primary somatosensory barrel field (S1BF), vMAT2 expression was increased in 1wME mice compared to AMCs, and was significantly higher in 1wME and 3wME mice compared to 5wME mice. The number of animals (n) is represented in the bars. Significant pair-wise differences between ME mice and the AMC group are indicated with a '*' within the corresponding bar. Differences between ME conditions due to post-ME recovery time are indicated as a '*' above the respective ME conditions. $*P < 0.05$, $**P < 0.01$

day, the blots were successively washed in Tris-saline (4×5 min), 30 min incubated with HRP-conjugated secondary antibody (goat anti-rabbit IgG, 1:50.000, Dako, Glostrup, Denmark), rinsed in Tris-saline (5×5 min) and Tris-stock (1×5 min) (0.05 M Tris, pH 7.6). The immunoreactive bands were visualized using a chemiluminescent reaction (1×5 min, Super Signal West Dura, ThermoScientific, Pierce) combined with the BIO-RAD ChemiDoc™ MP Imaging System. In order to correct for intra- and inter-gel variability and to normalize the concentration of the specific detected proteins to the total amount of protein present, we performed a total protein stain (TPS) with Swift Membrane Stain (G-Biosciences) according to manufacturer's instructions. Immediately after the staining, blots were scanned with the BIO-RAD ChemiDoc™ MP Imaging System.

Semi-quantitative Western analysis

The immunostained protein bands were semi-quantitatively evaluated by densitometry (Image Lab™ software) separately for monocular, binocular and somatosensory cortex samples (Figs. 3 and 4). First, to account for intra-gel and inter-gel variability including loading differences or incomplete transfer onto the membrane, a TPS was employed rather than the use of a single reference protein [53, 66, 67]. For each protein of interest, the optical density value per mouse was normalized to its corresponding TPS. Also, to compare samples between different gels, normalized data were expressed relative to the region-specific reference sample (pool).

Pharmacology

ME mice (pharmacology total $n = 15$, saline: $n = 6$; WAY-100635: $n = 3$; ketanserin: $n = 3$; ondansetron: $n = 3$) received daily injections (i.p.), at 2 pm exactly, of a specific 5-HT receptor antagonist at a dose based on prior literature, and specifically during the 3-week period of cross-modal plasticity from week 5 to 7 post-ME (Fig. 1d). Systemic drug delivery was chosen because a long-term treatment with a locally implanted slow release system (e.g. Alzet minipump) would lead to cortical tissue damage and scar formation, potentially influencing the local neuromodulator levels [68]. Drugs used were the 5-HTR$_{1A}$ antagonist WAY-100635 maleate (Abcam Ab120550, 1 mg/kg, 0.2 mL i.p.) [37, 36, 69, 70], the 5-HTR$_{2A}$ antagonist ketanserin tartrate (R&D Systems, Tocris Bioscience, 5 mg/kg, 0.2 mL i.p.) [71–74] and the 5-HTR$_{3A}$ antagonist ondansetron hydrochloride (R&D Systems, Tocris Bioscience, 5 mg/kg, 0.2 mL i.p.) [75]. Control animals were housed under the same standard conditions and received saline injections (0.9%, i.p.) following the same injection regimen. All animals were sacrificed by cervical dislocation. Brains were rapidly removed and stored as described above.

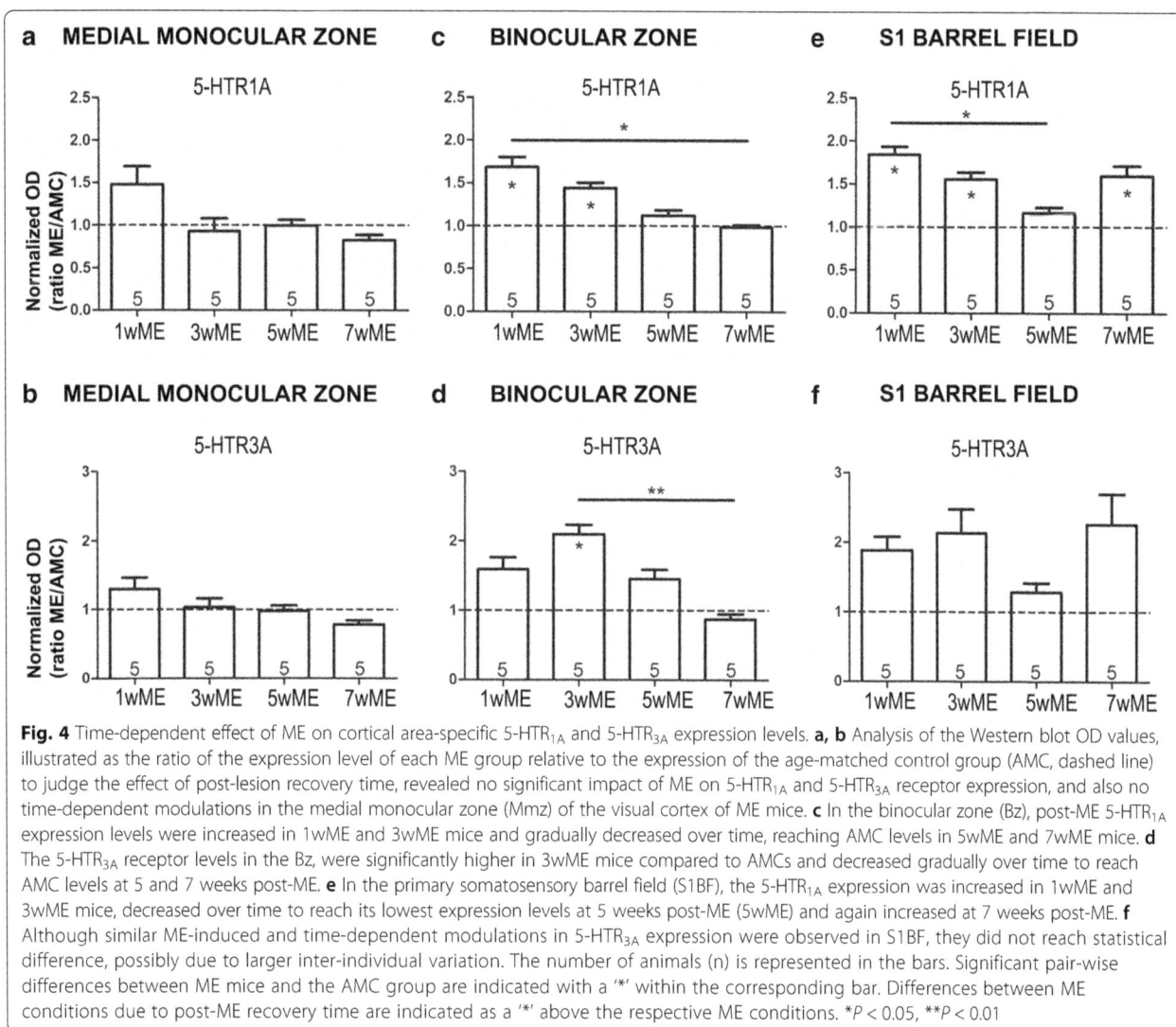

Fig. 4 Time-dependent effect of ME on cortical area-specific 5-HTR$_{1A}$ and 5-HTR$_{3A}$ expression levels. **a, b** Analysis of the Western blot OD values, illustrated as the ratio of the expression level of each ME group relative to the expression of the age-matched control group (AMC, dashed line) to judge the effect of post-lesion recovery time, revealed no significant impact of ME on 5-HTR$_{1A}$ and 5-HTR$_{3A}$ receptor expression, and also no time-dependent modulations in the medial monocular zone (Mmz) of the visual cortex of ME mice. **c** In the binocular zone (Bz), post-ME 5-HTR$_{1A}$ expression levels were increased in 1wME and 3wME mice and gradually decreased over time, reaching AMC levels in 5wME and 7wME mice. **d** The 5-HTR$_{3A}$ receptor levels in the Bz, were significantly higher in 3wME mice compared to AMCs and decreased gradually over time to reach AMC levels at 5 and 7 weeks post-ME. **e** In the primary somatosensory barrel field (S1BF), the 5-HTR$_{1A}$ expression was increased in 1wME and 3wME mice, decreased over time to reach its lowest expression levels at 5 weeks post-ME (5wME) and again increased at 7 weeks post-ME. **f** Although similar ME-induced and time-dependent modulations in 5-HTR$_{3A}$ expression were observed in S1BF, they did not reach statistical difference, possibly due to larger inter-individual variation. The number of animals (n) is represented in the bars. Significant pair-wise differences between ME mice and the AMC group are indicated with a '*' within the corresponding bar. Differences between ME conditions due to post-ME recovery time are indicated as a '*' above the respective ME conditions. *$P < 0.05$, **$P < 0.01$

In situ hybridization for *zif268*-mRNA

High-throughput radioactive ISH experiments were performed on series of coronal brain sections between Bregma levels – 1.5 mm and – 5 mm and changes in the mRNA expression level of the immediate early gene (IEG) *zif268*, a proven excellent activity reporter gene in the mammalian brain, were quantified (mouse: [15, 16, 51, 53, 56, 76–78], cat: [79–82]. As such, the spatial extent and the exact anatomical location of experience-induced, predominantly excitatory [6, 83–87], neuronal activity changes were analyzed and compared throughout all cortical layers of the visual and somatosensory neocortex. This high-throughput approach allows the molecular visualization of cortical reactivation patterns in response to ME. ISH for *zif268*-mRNA was performed with a mouse-specific synthetic oligonucleotide probe (Eurogentec, Seraing, Belgium) with sequence 5′-ccgtt gctcagcagcatcatctcctccagtttggggtagttgtcc-3′. As described previously [51, 53, 77, 88], each probe was 3′-end

labeled with [^{33}P] dATP using terminal deoxynucleotidyl transferase (Invitrogen, Carlsbad, CA). Unincorporated nucleotides were separated from the labeled probe by means of miniQuick Spin Oligo Columns (Roche Diagnostics, Vilvoorde, Belgium). The cryostat sections were fixed, dehydrated and delipidated. The radioactively labeled probes were added to a hybridization cocktail (50% (v/v) formamide, 4× standard SSC buffer, 1× Denhardt's solution, 10% (w/v) dextran sulfate, 100 μg/ml herring sperm DNA, 250 μg/ml tRNA, 60 mM dithiothreitol, 1% (w/v) N-lauroyl sarcosine, and 20 mM NaHPO$_4$, pH 7.4) and applied to the cryostat sections (10^6 cpm/section). After an overnight incubation at 37 °C in a humid chamber, the sections were rinsed in 1× standard SSC buffer at 42 °C, dehydrated, air-dried and exposed to an autoradiographic film (Biomax MR; Kodak, Rochester, NY). After 7 days, the films were developed in EMS replacement for Kodak developer D-19 (Electron Microscopy Sciences, Hatfield) and fixed in Rapid fixer (Ilford

Hypam; Kodak). Autoradiographic images of adjacent sections per examined cortical area per mouse were scanned at 1200 dpi (CanoScan LIDE 600F; Canon, Tokyo, Japan), and all images were similarly adjusted for brightness and contrast in Adobe Photoshop Elements 2018 (version 16.0, × 64, Adobe Systems Incorporated).

Histology and localization of visual and somatosensory areal boundaries with Nissl patterns

Upon ISH, the cryostat sections were Nissl-counterstained (1% cresyl violet; Fluka, Sigma-Aldrich) according to standard procedures to visualize cortical boundaries between different visual and somatosensory areas and to aid the interpretation of the *zif268*-activity patterns (Fig. 1c). Images of the stained coronal sections were obtained at 5× (NA: 0.16) with a light microscope (Zeiss Axio Imager Z1) equipped with an AxioCam MRm camera (1388 × 1040 pixels) using the software program Zen (Zen Pro 2012, Carl Zeiss, Benelux). Comparisons were made with the stereotaxic mouse brain atlas [63] to delineate visual and somatosensory cortical borders as described previously [53, 56]. In all figures illustrating visual or somatosensory cortex, large arrowheads indicate the total extent of the cortex, whereas small arrowheads indicate the inter-areal borders. In the visual cortex, five subregions can be distinguished from lateral to medial (Figs. 1c, 5): the lateral extrastriate cortex (V2L), which is subdivided into a monocular (V2Lm, segments 1–4) and binocular region (V2Lb, segments 4–8), the primary visual cortex (V1) which is subdivided further into a binocular (V1b, segments 8–15) and monocular region (V1 m, segments 15–21), and the medial extrastriate cortex (V2M, segments 21–24) [51, 53, 56, 89]. For the *zif268* analysis, we focused specifically on the Bz (V2Lb-V1b) and the Mmz (V1 m-V2M) as these regions undergo open-eye potentiation and cross-modal plasticity respectively. In the somatosensory cortex, we distinguished the primary somatosensory barrel field (S1BF) from the more lateral secondary somatosensory cortex (S2) and the more medial primary somatosensory cortex (S1), as the primary receiver of whisker inputs (Fig. 6) [63].

Quantitative analysis of ISH results

To quantify the optical density (OD; mean gray value per pixel) of the ISH autoradiograms, a custom-made Matlab (Matlab R2017a; Mathworks) script was used as described previously [51, 53]. We analyzed at least three mice per condition. Per mouse, three ISH sections with an inter-distance of 100 μm were investigated (for visual cortex: − 3.5-(− 3.7); 1–4; 1, relative to Bregma; for somatosensory cortex: − 1.7-(− 1.9); 2.5–4; 1, relative to Bregma). The region of interest in the left hemisphere was demarcated by determining the top edge of the cortex, the boundary between the supra-and granular layers

(II-III and IV) and the infragranular layers (V and VI), and the border between the infragranular layers and the corpus callosum. The region of interest was then divided equally into 24 segments from lateral to medial to create two lattices of 24 quadrangles, corresponding to the upper (II-IV) and lower (V-VI) layers. To compensate for possible variation in brain size and morphology, the lattices were translated on each autoradiogram over the cortical curvature, fixing the border of a specific segment to an areal border (border segment 20/21 is the area border V1 m/V2M). For each segment created this way, the relative OD was calculated as the mean gray value of all pixels contained within a particular quadrangle and was normalized to the mean gray value of a square measured in the corpus callosum (a defined region with no *zif268*-mRNA expression above background) in order to compare autoradiograms across experiments. Relative neuronal activity was expressed in percentages based on the following formula: 1 − (cortical *zif268*/background) × 100. Results are presented as profiles of neuronal activity per brain area and are illustrated in subregion-specific bar graphs. Pseudo-color maps were generated through a second custom-made Matlab script (Matlab R2017a; Mathworks, Natick, MA) and represent a false color coding of the gray values ranging from black (0) to white (225); high gray values are represented in white/yellow on the false color scale bar (0–50), medium high gray values are represented in red (50–100) or blue (100–150) and low gray values are represented in green/black (150–255).

Statistics

All HPLC results, Western blotting data and relative OD-values in ISH-sections were presented as mean ± SEM. Normal distribution and in parallel, equal variance between groups was tested. A non-parametric test (Mann-Whitney) was applied for pairwise comparison. A Kruskal-Wallis test followed by a Dunn's multiple comparisons post-hoc test was used to determine the recovery time-dependent modulations of protein expression levels upon ME. For all tests, a probability level (α level was set to 0.05) of < 0.05 was accepted as statistically significant ($*p < 0.05$, $**p < 0.01$, $***p < 0.001$). Statistical analyses were performed using GraphPad Prism 5.01 (GraphPad Software, Inc).

Results

Reduced visual cortex 5-HT concentration in response to monocular enucleation

To investigate if 5-HT is involved in adult ME-induced cross-modal plasticity and to better understand its role therein, we first examined whether the total 5-HT concentration was affected in the two cortices that functionally adapt upon ME. The total 5-HT concentration was

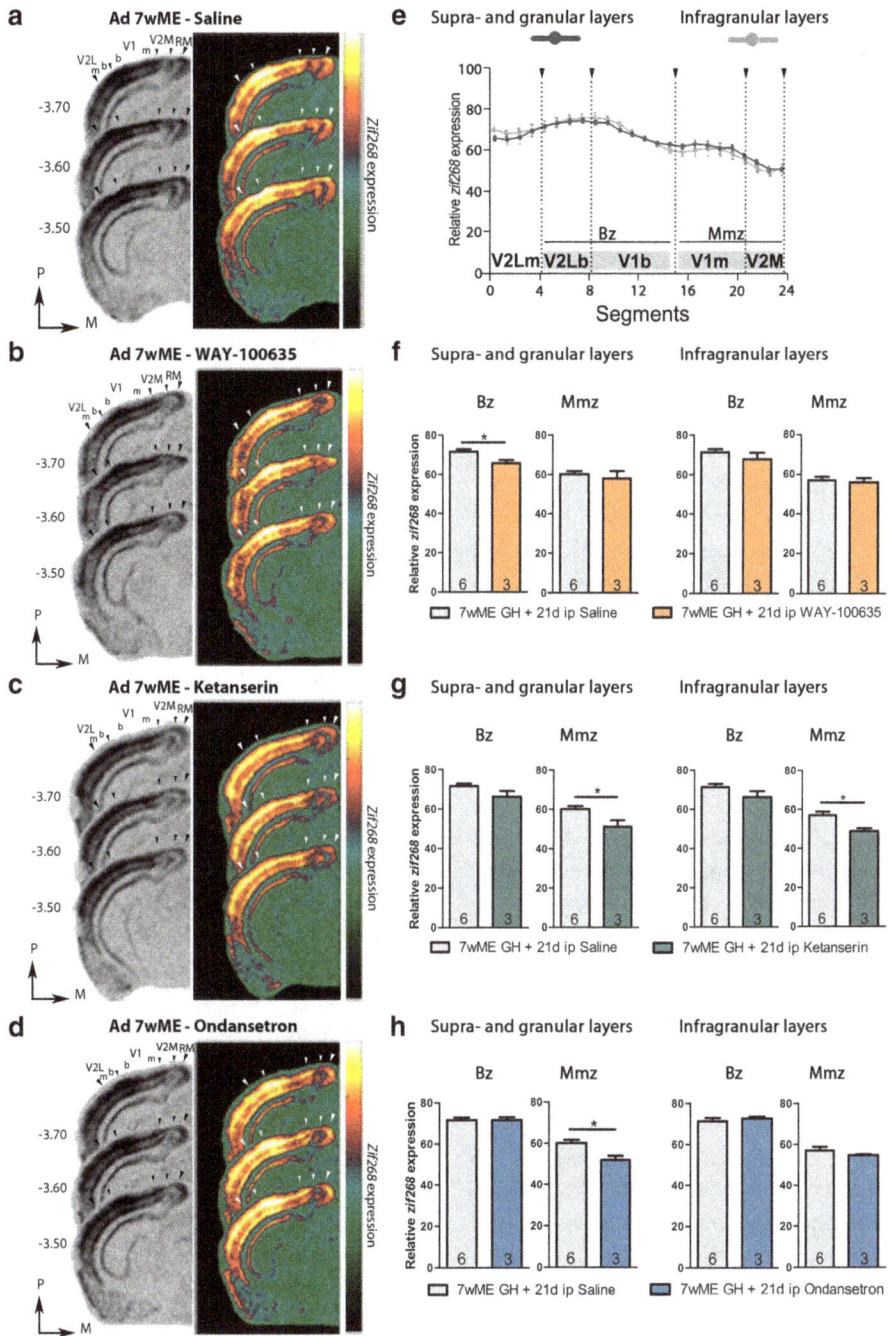

Fig. 5 (See legend on next page.)

(See figure on previous page.)

Fig. 5 5-HTR antagonist treatment from week 5–7 post-ME affects neuronal activity levels in Mmz and Bz. **a-d** Images of 3 adjacent sections (− 3.5-(− 3.7); 1–4; 1, relative to Bregma) from adult 7wME mice, drug or sham-treated during the last 3 weeks of the 7wME recovery period: (**a**) saline, (**b**) 5-HTR$_{1A}$-antagonist WAY-100635, (**c**) 5-HTR$_{2A}$-antagonist ketanserin, (**d**) 5-HTR$_{3A}$-antagonist ondansetron. Corresponding pseudocolor representations are displayed next to their respective ISH sections. **e** Line graphs illustrating relative *zif268*-mRNA expression levels, measured as the average OD-value/segment, for saline-injected 7wME mice. For supra- and granular layers II/III-IV (e, left panel, dark gray line) and for infragranular layers V-VI (e, right panel, light gray line) the expression levels are displayed along the 5 predefined visual subdivisions (black arrowheads are in accordance with the small arrowheads in a-d, including the subdivision between monocular zones m and binocular zones b in V2L and V1). Error bars represent the SEM of the mean OD value in each segment. Relative *zif268*-mRNA expression levels are shown as OD-values averaged over the binocular zone Bz and the medial monocular zone Mmz for supra- and granular layers (**f-h**, left panel) and infragranular layers (**f-h**, right panel). Bz comprises V2Lb-V1b (dark gray marking), Mmz includes V1 m-V2M (light gray marking) as illustrated in **e**. Comparison of the OD-values of saline-injected (light gray bars) and WAY-100635-injected 7wME mice (orange bars) indicates decreased reactivation levels in the upper layers of the Bz (**f**, left panel). Comparison of the OD-values of saline-injected (light-gray bars) and ketanserin-treated 7wME mice (green bars) indicates decreased reactivation levels across all layers of the Mmz (**g**). Comparison of the OD-values of saline-injected (light-gray bars) and ondansetron-treated 7wME mice (blue bars) indicates decreased reactivation in the upper layers of the Mmz (**h**, left panel). The number of animals (n) is shown in the bars. *$P < 0.05$

analyzed with High-Performance Liquid Chromatography (HPLC) on whole tissue homogenates of the visual cortex and S1BF 7 weeks after performing ME in adult mice (7wME) (Fig. 2a, b). At this 7wME endpoint, when the cross-modal recruitment of the initially deprived visual cortex is completed [15], we observed a decreased 5-HT concentration in the visual cortex (mean ± SEM, AMC: 82.54 ± 4.77; 7wME: 65.50 ± 4.77, Mann-Whitney test, $p = 0.018$, Fig. 2c). In S1BF, the cortical area in which compensatory plasticity is triggered by vision loss, no significant difference was reached (AMC: 113.40 ± 8.06; 7wME: 86.41 ± 10.49; Mann-Whitney test, $p = 0.114$, Fig. 2d). These results suggest brain region-specific modulations of total 5-HT content in response to visual deprivation.

ME induces pre- and postsynaptic changes in proteins related to 5-HT signaling

Parallel to the ME-induced decrease in total 5-HT concentration in the visual cortex, the impact of partial vision loss might manifest at the level of 5-HT loading into readily releasable vesicles or at the level of 5-HT receptors. To investigate possible brain region-specific expression changes in these pre- and postsynaptic proteins involved in 5-HT signaling, we performed Western blotting experiments on time-course samples from the visual Mmz and Bz separately and from S1BF. Post-ME recovery periods of respectively 1 week (1wME: ongoing open-eye potentiation phase), 3 weeks (3wME: end of the open-eye potentiation phase) and 5 weeks (5wME: ongoing cross-modal phase) were chosen as intermediate time points towards the time point of maximal visual cortex reactivation (7wME) for the evaluation of possible post-ME recovery time-dependent modulations in protein expression in addition to endpoint evaluation (Fig. 1) [15].

We chose to analyze vMAT2 protein expression levels since they provide information on the presynaptic loading of vesicles with 5-HT and because vMAT2 expression levels positively correlate with the total 5-HT

concentration present in a given brain region of interest [60–62]. vMAT2 expression levels were significantly decreased in the Mmz in 1wME, 5wME and 7wME mice (represented as * within the bar, bar graphs in Figs. 3 and 4) compared to AMC (represented as a dashed line in Figs. 3 and 4, mean ± SEM, 1wME: 0.34 ± 0.08, $p = 0.0159$; 3wME: 0.80 ± 0.56, $p = 0.4127$; 5wME: 0.45 ± 0.02, $p = 0.0159$; 7wME: 0.53 ± 0.28, $p = 0.0317$, Mann-Whitney test). No statistically significant modulations occurred as a function of post-ME recovery time (Kruskal-Wallis test: $p = 0.0159$, with no statistical difference in the Dunn's post-hoc test for pairwise comparison) (Fig. 3a). Western analysis of the vMAT2 expression in the Bz indicated increased vMAT2 expression in 1wME and 3wME mice compared to AMC mice (mean ± SEM, 1wME: 1.87 ± 0.19, $p = 0.0317$; 3wME: 1.45 ± 0.06, $p = 0.0159$; 5wME: 1.07 ± 0.07, $p = 0.4127$; 7wME: 1.01 ± 0.04, $p = 0.7302$, Mann-Whitney test). As for the Mmz, also for the Bz no significant recovery time-dependent changes were observed (Kruskal-Wallis test: $p = 0.0095$, with no statistical differences in the Dunn's post-hoc test for pairwise comparison). In this case, however, a trend of decreasing vMAT2 expression was observed over the 1w to 7w post-ME time course (Fig. 3b). In S1BF, vMAT2 expression was significantly increased in 1wME mice compared to AMC (mean ± SEM, 1wME: 1.58 ± 0.11, $p = 0.0317$; 3wME: 1.50 ± 0.10, $p = 0.0635$; 5wME: 0.77 ± 0.09, $p = 0.1905$; 7wME: 1.29 ± 0.11, $p = 0.4127$, Mann-Whitney test, Fig. 3c). Furthermore, in 1wME and 3wME mice, the vMAT2 expression levels were higher compared to 5wME mice (Kruskal-Wallis test: $p = 0.0081$). These results point towards a return to baseline vMAT2 expression levels specifically at the time when the cross-modal whisker take-over of the deprived visual cortex starts to occur [15].

To define the impact of ME on the serotonergic modulation of cortical inhibition through specific 5-HT receptors, we performed Western blotting experiments for 5-HTR$_{1A}$ and 5-HTR$_{3A}$. Besides their role in different types of visual cortex plasticity, reasons supporting these

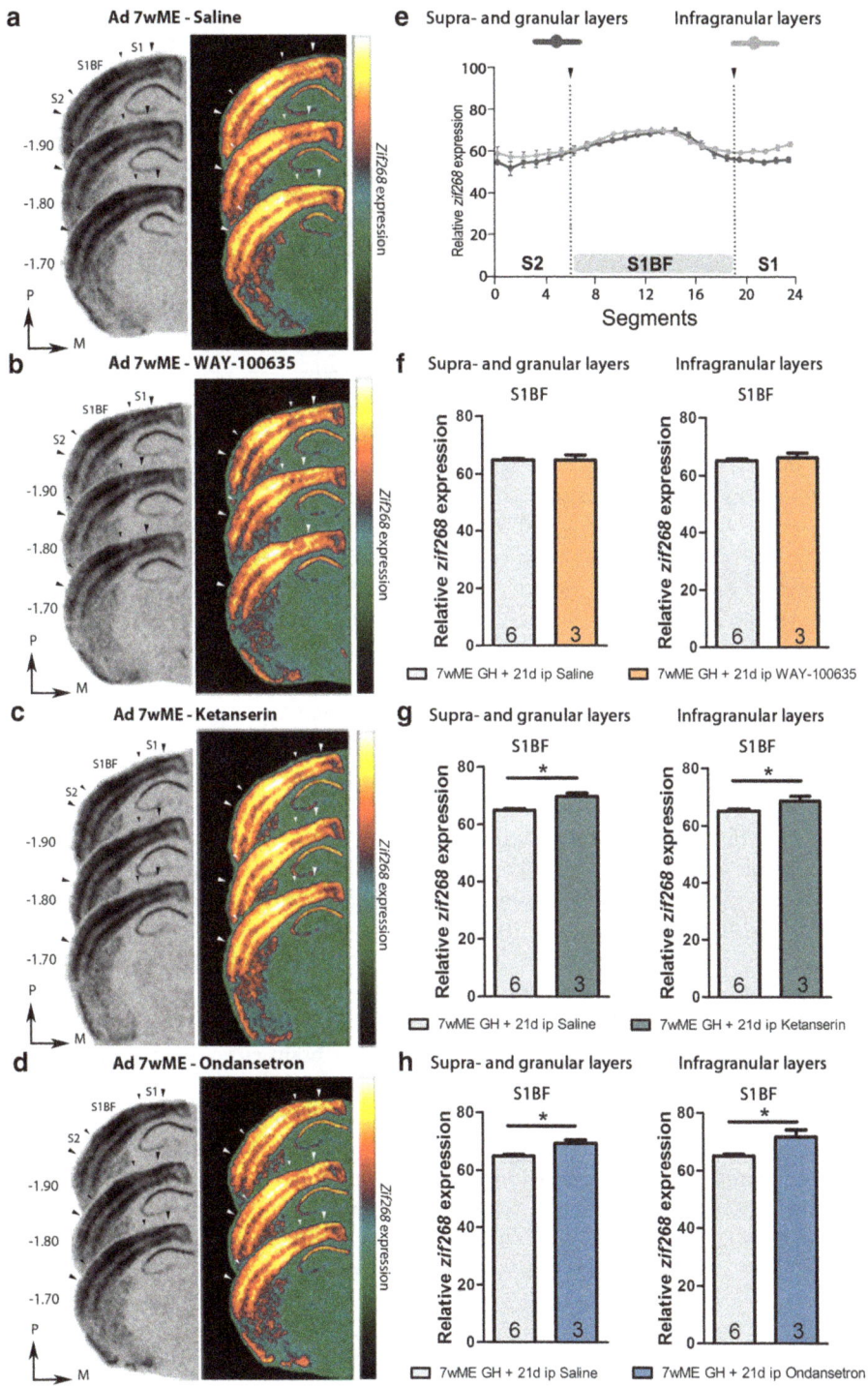

Fig. 6 (See legend on next page.)

Fig. 6 5-HTR antagonist treatment from week 5–7 post-ME affects neuronal activity levels in S1BF. **a-d** Images of 3 adjacent sections (− 1.7-(− 1.9); 2.5–4; 1, relative to Bregma) from adult 7wME mice, injected during the last 3 weeks of the 7wME recovery period with (**a**) saline, (**b**) 5-HTR$_{1A}$ antagonist WAY-100635, (**c**) 5-HTR$_{2A}$ antagonist ketanserin, (**d**) 5-HTR$_{3A}$ antagonist ondansetron. Corresponding pseudocolor representations are displayed next to their respective ISH sections. **e** Line graphs illustrating the relative zif268-mRNA expression level, measured as the average OD-value/segment, for saline-injected 7wME mice. For supra- and granular layers II/III-IV (e, left panel, dark gray line) and for infragranular layers V-VI (e, right panel, light gray line) the expression levels are displayed along the 3 predefined somatosensory subdivisions (black arrowheads are in accordance with the small arrowheads in a-d). Error bars represent the SEM of the mean OD value in each segment. Relative zif268-mRNA expression levels are shown as OD-values averaged over the primary somatosensory barrel cortex (S1BF) for supra- and granular layers (**f-h**, left panel) and infragranular layers (**f-h**, right panel). Comparison of the OD-values of saline-injected (light gray bars) and WAY-100635-injected 7wME mice (orange bars) indicates no post-ME changes in neuronal activity in S1BF due to long-term i.p. injection of 5-HTR$_{1A}$ antagonist (**f**). Comparison of the OD-values of saline-injected (light-gray bars) and ketanserin-treated 7wME mice (green bars) indicates increased neuronal activity across all layers of the S1BF (**g**). Comparison of the OD-values of saline-injected (light-gray bars) and ondansetron-treated 7wME mice (blue bars) indicates increased neuronal activity across all layers of the S1BF (**h**). The number of animals (n) is represented in the bars. *P < 0.05

receptor choices, are the fact that the 5-HTR$_{1A}$ receptor is expressed both on pre-and postsynaptic neurons, respectively acting as an autoreceptor and a Gi-coupled GPCR mediating inhibitory neurotransmission upon ligand binding [90], while 5-HTR$_{3A}$ is a Na$^+$/K$^+$/Ca^{2+} permeable ion channel exclusively expressed on the 5-HTR$_{3A}$ expressing inhibitory interneurons [91]. We did not observe any ME-induced or recovery time-dependent changes in the expression of 5-HTR$_{1A}$ or 5-HTR$_{3A}$ in the Mmz (mean ± SEM, 5-HTR$_{1A}$, 1wME: 1.48 ± 0.21, $p = 0.2857$; 3wME: 0.93 ± 0.15, $p = 0.7302$; 5wME: 1.00 ± 0.07, $p = 0.7302$; 7wME: 0.83 ± 0.06, $p = 0.7302$, 5-HTR$_{3A}$, 1wME: 1.29 ± 0.17, $p = 0.2857$; 3wME: 1.03 ± 0.13, $p = 0.9048$; 5wME: 0.98 ± 0.08, $p = 1.000$; 7wME: 0.78 ± 0.06, $p = 0.1905$, Mann-Whitney test; Kruskal-Wallis test; 5-HTR$_{1A}$: $p = 0.2493$; 5-HTR$_{3A}$: $p = 0.1395$, Fig. 4a, b). In the Bz on the other hand, 1wME and 3wME mice showed increased 5-HTR$_{1A}$ expression levels (mean ± SEM, 5-HTR$_{1A}$, 1wME: 1.69 ± 0.12, $p = 0.0317$; 3wME: 1.44 ± 0.06, $p = 0.0317$; 5wME: 1.12 ± 0.06, $p = 0.2857$; 7wME: 0.99 ± 0.02, $p = 0.9048$, Mann-Whitney test, Fig. 4c) and a gradual decrease in 5-HTR$_{1A}$ expression between 1wME and 7wME mice (Kruskal-Wallis test: $p = 0.0039$). In addition, 5-HTR$_{3A}$ expression levels were significantly increased in the Bz of the 3wME mice compared to the AMCs (mean ± SEM, 5-HTR$_{3A}$, 1wME: 1.59 ± 0.17, $p = 0.1111$; 3wME: 2.10 ± 0.13, $p = 0.0159$; 5wME: 1.45 ± 0.13, $p = 0.1111$; 7wME: 0.87 ± 0.08, $p = 0.5556$, Mann-Whitney test, Fig. 4d) and decreased over time to reach the AMC level at 7 weeks post-ME (Kruskal-Wallis test: $p = 0.0038$). In S1BF, 5-HTR$_{1A}$ expression was increased in 1wME and 3wME mice, gradually decreased to reach the AMC level at 5 weeks post-ME (Kruskal-Wallis test: $p = 0.0039$), and was again increased at 7 weeks post-ME (mean ± SEM, 5-HTR$_{1A}$, 1wME: 1.84 ± 0.09, $p = 0.0159$; 3wME: 1.56 ± 0.08, $p = 0.0159$; 5wME: 1.17 ± 0.07, $p = 0.4127$; 7wME: 1.60 ± 0.12, $p = 0.0317$, Mann-Whitney test, Fig. 4e). We did not observe significant modulations of 5-HTR$_{3A}$ protein expression in S1BF (mean ± SEM, 5-HTR$_{3A}$, 1wME: 1.88 ± 0.19, $p = 0.1905$; 3wME: 2.13 ± 0.34, $p = 0.1111$;

5wME: 1.28 ± 0.13, $p = 0.5556$; 7wME: 2.26 ± 0.43, $p = 0.1111$, Mann-Whitney test; Kruskal-Wallis test: $p = 0.1325$, Fig. 4f). Taken together, these observations indicate brain region-specific alterations in vMAT2-mediated presynaptic monoamine vesicle loading, as well as post-ME recovery time-dependent modulations in 5-HTR$_{1A}$ and 5-HTR$_{3A}$ expression levels specifically in the Bz and in S1BF but not in the Mmz.

5-HTR$_{2A}$ and 5-HTR$_{3A}$ but not 5-HTR$_{1A}$ antagonists suppress ME-induced cross-modal plasticity

We hypothesized that, in case 5-HT receptor function is involved in the whisker-mediated reactivation of the deprived visual cortex, the ME-induced cross-modal recruitment could be suppressed by systemic administration of the 5-HTR$_{1A}$ antagonist WAY-100635 maleate, the 5-HTR$_{2A}$ antagonist ketanserin tartrate, or the 5-HTR$_{3A}$ antagonist ondansetron hydrochloride during the last 3 weeks of recovery of the Mmz in ME mice (Fig. 5a-e). As the 5-HT receptors influence the excitability of brain circuits by modulating excitatory and inhibitory neurotransmission and thus by mediating the cortical E/I balance, we expected to observe effects of these drugs on cortical activity, and ultimately on cortical plasticity [36, 54, 55]. Because it was previously established that the most pronounced impact of whisker inputs on neuronal activity involves the infragranular layers of the visual cortex, as based on the expression of neuronal activity reporter gene zif268, these layers were interrogated separately from the supra- and granular layers.

Suppression of the 5-HTR$_{1A}$ receptor function by long-term administration of WAY-100635 from week 5 to 7 post-ME did not alter the neuronal activity levels reached throughout the Mmz of 7wME mice, compared to saline-injected age-matched control ME mice (Mmz, supra- and granular layers: $p = 0.9048$, infragranular layers: $p = 0.9048$, Bz, supra- and granular layers: $p = 0.0476$, infragranular layers: $p = 0.2619$, Mann-Whitney test, Fig. 5f). However, it did decrease the neuronal activity in the supra- and granular layers of the Bz (Mean ± SEM, supra- and granular layers, saline, Bz: 71.58 ± 1.26; Mmz: 60.14 ± 1.48, WAY-100635, Bz: 65.73 ± 1.58; Mmz: 57.95 ± 3.77, infragranular layers, saline, Bz: 71.31 ± 1.57, Mmz: 56.97 ± 1.84, WAY-100635, Bz: 67.72 ± 3.35; Mmz: 55.96 ± 2.12, Fig. 5f), indicative of Bz-specific 5-HTR$_{1A}$ expression changes during the preceding open-eye potentiation phase.

Blocking 5-HTR$_{2A}$ receptor function by ketanserin administration from week 5 to 7 post-ME significantly decreased the neuronal activity across all layers of the Mmz (Mmz, supra- and granular layers: $p = 0.0476$, infragranular layers: $p = 0.0238$; Bz, supra- and granular layers: $p = 0.0952$, infragranular layers: $p = 0.2619$, Mann-Whitney test, Fig. 5g) but did not induce any change in neuronal activity in the Bz (Mean ± SEM, supra- and granular layers, saline, Bz: 71.58 ± 1.26; Mmz: 60.14 ± 1.48, ketanserin, Bz: 66.15 ± 2.83, Mmz: 51.18 ± 3.25, infragranular layers, saline, Bz: 71.31 ± 1.57; Mmz: 56.97 ± 1.84, ketanserin, Bz: 66.18 ± 3.05; Mmz: 48.85 ± 1.46, Fig. 5g). Suppression of the 5-HTR$_{3A}$ receptor function by administration of ondansetron only reduced the neuronal activity specifically in the supra- and granular layers of the Mmz (Mmz, supra- and granular layers: $p = 0.0476$, infragranular: $p = 0.5476$; Bz, supra- and granular layers: $p = 0.7143$, infragranular layers: $p = 0.5476$, Mann-Whitney test; Mean ± SEM, supra- and granular layers, saline, Bz: 71.58 ± 1.26; Mmz: 60.14 ± 1.48, ondansetron, Bz: 71.63 ± 1.40, Mmz: 51.95 ± 2.04, infragranular layers, saline, Bz: 71.31 ± 1.57; Mmz: 56.97 ± 1.84, ondansetron, Bz: 72.64 ± 0.94; Mmz: 54.70 ± 0.40, Fig. 5h). Taken together, these results point out that modulation of the 5-HTR$_{2A}$ and 5-HTR$_{3A}$ receptor function, influences the late cortical response to ME, suggesting that these receptors play an important role in the cross-modal reactivation phase of the visual cortex following ME.

Previous work has shown that ME induces increased neuronal activity in the spared sensory brain areas adjacent to the deprived visual cortex. For somatosensory cortex, the zif268-mRNA expression levels were found to be significantly higher in adult 7wME mice compared to AMC mice [16, 53]. In order to assess the impact of pharmacological modulation of serotonergic neurotransmission on S1BF neuronal activity, next to mapping the extent of visual cortex reactivation, we compared S1BF activity levels between saline-injected 7wME mice and 7wME mice that were treated with the specific 5-HTR$_{1A}$, 5-HTR$_{2A}$ or 5-HTR$_{3A}$ antagonists.

Analysis of the zif268-mRNA expression levels (– 1.7-(– 1.9); 2.5–4; 1, relative to Bregma) (Fig. 6a-e) indicated that the neuronal activity levels in S1BF of WAY-100635 treated 7wME mice remained unaltered across all cortical layers compared to the saline-injected 7wME mice (S1BF, supra- and granular layers: $p = 0.9048$, infragranular layers: $p = 0.7143$, Mann-Whitney test, Fig. 6f). The mice thus

displayed the expected ME-induced increase in S1BF activity, despite a suppressed 5-HTR$_{1A}$ receptor function (Mean ± SEM, supra- and granular layers, saline: 64.94 ± 0.49; WAY-100635: 64.90 ± 1.76, infragranular layers, saline: 65.17 ± 0.66; WAY-100635: 66.19 ± 1.67, Fig. 6f). Treatment of 7wME mice with ketanserin (Mean ± SEM, supra- and granular layers, saline: 64.94 ± 0.49; ketanserin: 69.77 ± 1.13, infragranular layers, saline: 65.17 ± 0.66; ketanserin: 68.68 ± 1.63, Fig. 6g) and similarly, with ondansetron (Mean ± SEM, supra- and granular layers, saline: 64.94 ± 0.49; ondansetron: 69.35 ± 1.11, infragranular layers, saline: 65.17 ± 0.66; ondansetron: 71.78 ± 2.38, Fig. 6h), also did not prevent the normal ME-induced increase in S1BF activity. On the contrary, it even induced higher neuronal activity across all cortical layers of S1BF, as the zif268-mRNA expression levels were significantly higher in ketanserin and ondansetron treated 7wME mice compared to the saline-injected control group (ketanserin, supra- and granular layers: $p = 0.0238$, infragranular layers: $p = 0.0476$; ondansetron, supra- and granular layers: $p = 0.0238$, infragranular layers: $p = 0.0476$, Mann-Whitney test). Thus, S1BF activation seems preserved in the drug-treated mice, and even intensified as visualized with 5-HTR$_{2A}$ antagonist ketanserin and 5-HT$_{3A}$ antagonist ondansetron.

Discussion

In humans, dysfunction of 5-HT signaling in the brain, is best described in mental illnesses such as depression and anxiety disorders [30, 92]. Drugs that target the serotonergic system, for instance the selective serotonin reuptake inhibitors (SSRIs), are amongst the most-often prescribed first-line treatments, predominantly because low 5-HT levels in the brain were considered to be the main cause of such diseases [93]. However, the observed low efficacy and only very late-onset mood and behavioral improvements suggest large scale, functional and structural neuroplastic changes in the brain, rather than immediate, direct effects of those drugs on their targets [94–98]. Neuropsychological illnesses thus seem more complex than first considered and may in fact be neurological disorders with an underlying plasticity deficit. From research using sensory deprivation models, it is known that monoamine system-targeting drugs like SSRIs elicit plastic adaptations in the mammalian cortex [26, 99, 100]. Evidence for such cortical plasticity brought about by long-term treatment with an SSRI was already provided ten years ago and is based upon the discovery that fluoxetine can reinstate juvenile-like ocular dominance plasticity in the rodent adult visual cortex [26]. Genes involved in synaptic plasticity and chromatin structure remodeling, excitatory/inhibitory neurotransmission, transcription factors and proteolytic enzymes that degrade the extracellular matrix were found to underlie this type of plasticity [101]. It is likely that similar plastic changes occur in human patients in order to be relieved from their neuropsychological illness and to again express a positive mood and behavior.

Late-onset ME modulates 5-HT and vMAT2 levels in adult visual cortex

Our HPLC data imply a lowered whole tissue 5-HT concentration specifically in the visual cortex of long-term ME mice. Since 5-HT release is triggered by neuronal activity in the sensory cortex, the observed decrease in 5-HT concentration in the visual cortex of 7wME mice is possibly due to the ME-induced loss of visual input in the Mmz [102]. A similar decrease in total 5-HT levels was also observed in the deprived visual cortex of adult cats in response to retinal lesions, an animal model for age-related macular degeneration [59]. For more in depth interpretation of brain region-specific alterations in 5-HT signaling, we still depend on new methodological developments that would allow reliable longitudinal analysis of the true local 5-HT release from only 1 mm thick cortical tissue, such as the Bz or the Mmz in our mouse model. For now, predictions based on longitudinal vMAT2 expression changes allow to formulate some possibilities. Tong et al., (2011) indeed already showed that vMAT2 levels are positively correlated with the tissue concentrations of total monoamines (5-HT, dopamine and noradrenaline), as measured in human tissue by means of HPLC analysis [62]. By deduction, the significantly decreased vMAT2 protein expression already shortly after the introduction of ME, may indicate decreased 5-HT concentrations in the Mmz immediately upon the loss of all its visual input. Opposite to the Mmz, the Bz displayed only a temporary increase in vMAT2 expression from week 1 to 3 weeks post-ME, at a time when its remaining open-eye inputs become potentiated. Spared cortical territory seems to share such an early 5-HT mediated response, in relation to compensating for the sensory deficit. Indeed, a similar pattern of early increased vMAT2 expression in S1BF, could go hand in hand with a fast, initial increase in 5-HT concentration and might indicate a compensatory, cortical plasticity mechanism similar to the one described by Jitsuki et al., (2011) after only 2 days of visual deprivation in S1BF of young rats [32]. Once a new functional cortical balance is established for the spared sense, it may be able to subsequently recruit nearby sensory deprived cortical territory. In our model of acquired blindness, somatosensation indeed seems to be capable of recruiting the Mmz once

fine-tuned whisker-information processing has been established in S1BF.

5-HTR$_{1A}$ mediates unimodal open-eye potentiation in the Bz of the visual cortex

Cortical plasticity depends on both excitation and inhibition levels, which is determined by the distribution of excitatory and inhibitory receptors. An established E/I balance defines the stability and efficacy of neuronal circuits and is therefore required for proper processing of sensory information [36, 43, 103, 104]. A study, investigating the serotonergic regulation of the two predominant types of inhibition, respectively the short intermittent bursts of phasic inhibition and the constant long-lasting tonic inhibition, aside from its effect on the pyramidal neurons in the rat visual cortex, showed that 5-HT suppressed tonic inhibition through the 5-HTR$_{1A}$ receptor and Protein Kinase A signaling while phasic inhibition was enhanced through 5-HTR$_{2A}$ receptor function and CaM Kinase II [105, 106]. Clearly, alterations in 5-HT receptor expression and function can exert a major impact on the excitability of brain circuits involved in brain plasticity, as this would influence the inhibitory neurotransmission and the regulation of the cortical E/I balance [36, 54, 55].

Our observations indicate ME-induced increases in 5-HTR$_{1A}$ receptor expression in the spared cortices, the Bz and S1BF, confirming a regionally restricted and modulatory role in maintaining cortical excitability immediately upon insult. In the Bz, the increase in 5-HTR$_{1A}$ expression occurred at the start of the open-eye potentiation phase, pointing towards an early involvement of 5-HTR$_{1A}$-mediated tonic inhibition, which implies the consistent activation of extra- and perisynaptic GABA$_A$R$_{\delta 1}$ receptors on pyramidal and inhibitory neurons by ambient GABA, to regulate the overall cortical excitability during this thalamocortical plasticity process [107]. Of note, such enhanced tonic inhibition also triggers ocular dominance plasticity in the mouse visual cortex during the critical period early in life [108].

Many studies previously reported on 5-HT-mediated induction of unimodal brain plasticity in adulthood. For example, adult rats were again susceptible for monocular deprivation-induced ocular dominance plasticity after cortical infusion of 5-HT directly into the visual cortex [37]. Also in rodents, treatment with the SSRI fluoxetine, was found to induce both hippocampal synaptic plasticity and unimodal ocular dominance plasticity in the visual cortex [26, 37, 109, 110]. In line with this, in the human visual system, long-term systemic treatment with the SSRI sertraline was shown to induce synaptic plasticity by increasing the amplitude of stimulus-induced visually evoked potentials [111]. Fluoxetine even emerged as a possible treatment for persistent amblyopia, or lazy eye, in adult humans [112, 113]. Maya-Vetencourt et al., (2011) could previously also show that the ocular dominance shift, normally occurring in the Bz shortly after monocular deprivation, can be prevented by blocking this receptor with WAY-100635 [37]. Furthermore, local application of this same selective 5-HTR$_{1A}$ antagonist in V1 by means of reverse-phase microdialysis was found to facilitate long-term potentiation (LTP) after theta-burst stimulation (TBS) in adult rats, while LTP was inhibited in juvenile rats, confirming an age-dependent role for 5-HTR$_{1A}$ in gating V1 plasticity [27].

We were not surprised by the observation that 5-HTR$_{1A}$ expression levels remained close to the AMC level in the Mmz, as our lab previously described that well-defined levels of GABA$_A$R$_{\alpha1}$-mediated phasic inhibition, but not GABA$_A$R$_{\delta1}$-mediated tonic inhibition, are crucial for the establishment of the cross-modal reactivation of the Mmz in adult ME mice [53]. Our interpretation, that 5-HTR$_{1A}$ is of central importance to ME-induced open-eye potentiation in the Bz but not to the late cross-modal plasticity phase in the Mmz, is further supported by the observed downregulation of 5-HTR$_{1A}$ receptors in the Bz from the moment that open-eye potentiation is completed, and by the absence of suppressive drug-effects in the Mmz itself during the cross-modal phase. Indeed, the normal zif268-mRNA expression levels observed across the upper and lower cortical layers of the Mmz argue against a substantial contribution of this receptor subtype to the cross-modal take-over of the deprived cortical territory.

Antagonism of 5-HTR$_{2A}$ and 5-HTR$_{3A}$ to spatiotemporally control cross-modal brain plasticity

In this study, next to WAY-100635, we also chronically injected ketanserin or ondansetron to respectively block 5-HTR$_{2A}$ and 5-HTR$_{3A}$ receptor function during the entire time window of cross-modal plasticity, and following a normal period of open-eye potentiation. Although applying a local slow drug-release approach might have allowed a better discrimination of true cortical events from for example subcortical contributions to the observed plasticity phenomena, we still chose the i.p. injection approach because this systemic approach holds a greater prediction value with regards to human clinical trials than an invasive cortical infusion system. Also, long-term cannula implantation may have led to cortical tissue damage and glial scar formation. Such side-effects would have influenced the local neuromodulator levels [63] hampering the read-out as well as the interpretation of the results.

By blocking the 5-HTR$_{2A}$ receptor with ketanserin, we successfully suppressed adult cross-modal visual cortex

reactivation across all layers of the Mmz. This observation accords with literature describing a role for 5-HTR$_{2A}$ in compensatory cross-modal plasticity [32] and with our previous observations, that post-ME cross-modal reactivation of the Mmz only occurs under well-defined levels of GABA$_A$R$_{\alpha1}$-mediated phasic inhibition [53], which is considered to be strictly regulated by upstream 5-HTR$_{2A}$ function [105].

5-HTR$_{3A}$ interneurons constitute a heterogenous population. One type of interneurons dependent on 5-HT signaling are the Vasoactive Intestinal Peptide (VIP)-expressing 5-HTR$_{3A}$ interneurons. VIP-mediated disinhibition is a well-described mechanism in which VIP interneurons inhibit somatostatin and parvalbumin expressing interneurons and may underlie ME-induced cortical plasticity [44, 46–48, 114, 115]. VIP interneurons exert an important function in controlling sensory processing and are target cells of long-range projections that integrate sensory information originating from different brain regions [116, 117]. This interneuron type thus constitutes an ideal candidate for 5-HT to shape cross-modal brain circuits and plasticity patterns via the 5-HTR$_{3A}$ receptor. In a recent study [4], convergence of sensory and neuromodulatory information onto 5-HTR$_{3A}$ cells was shown to vastly contribute to the shaping of critical period plasticity in the primary auditory cortex of the mouse. This research group discovered that a topographic map is formed already early in life, regulated by the non-VIP expressing 5-HTR$_{3A}$ cell population in cortical layer I. As predicted based on the 5-HTR$_{3A}$ cortical distribution pattern, which is predominantly in L1 of the cortex [4], our results indeed indicate that 5-HTR$_{3A}$ receptor antagonism with ondansetron during the cross-modal reactivation phase, specifically suppressed the neuronal activity in the upper layers of the Mmz. It will be interesting to further investigate how and to what extent both the VIP and non-VIP 5-HTR$_{3A}$ cells can spatiotemporally regulate adult cross-modal plasticity as this may enable steering brain plasticity towards the desired outcome as a future therapy, being complete functional recovery of the lost primary sense. Ex-vivo and in vivo electrophysiology and fast-scan voltammetry, should allow dissecting the local molecular cascade and cellular circuit involved in the different cortical plasticity phenomena.

A possible strategy to improve the success rate of bionic implants

The success of bionic implants in restoring sensory function depends on our understanding of how the brain responds to sensory loss. Often, by the time the neuro-electric device is implanted, the brain has already compensated for the loss of sensory input through mechanisms of cross-modal plasticity, thereby possibly impairing the cortical translation of inputs, transmitted by the device, into meaningful sensory information [118]. During the last decades, the attempt to fully restore primary sensory function received much attention, giving rise to very promising neurobionics such as the cochlear implants to restore auditory function [119–121], visual prostheses [122–126] and brain-computer interfaces [127–129]. In addition, patients suffering from progressive vision loss, as caused by the neurodegenerative diseases *Retinitis pigmentosa* or age-related macular degeneration, can nowadays benefit from the recently developed, fully organic, subretinal prosthesis [130], which tackles some of the common mechanical, manufacturing and technical difficulties generally occurring in epiretinal [131], subretinal [132] and suprachoroidal [133] prosthetics.

Given the fact that 5-HT modulates sensory information processing and integration [134] and based on our findings that chronic, systemic administration of the 5-HTR$_{2A}$ antagonist ketanserin and 5-HTR$_{3A}$ antagonist ondansetron can suppress the cross-modal reorganization after partial vision loss in a cortical brain region- and layer-specific manner, we predict that a pharmacological monoamine-oriented strategy in combination with a bionic implant may significantly increase their success rate, as this approach would better allow to spatiotemporally control different forms of cortical plasticity that precede and co-occur with its functional integration.

Conclusions

We report ME-induced molecular and functional adaptations in the visual and somatosensory cortex of adult mice. We observed brain region-specific changes in 5-HT levels, presynaptic vMAT2 expression and postsynaptic 5-HT receptor levels in function of post-ME recovery time. We showed that 5-HTR$_{2A}$ and 5-HTR$_{3A}$ are involved in the cross-modal reactivation of the deprived visual cortex, as pharmacological antagonism of the 5-HTR$_{2A}$ and 5-HTR$_{3A}$ but not 5-HTR$_{1A}$ receptor function hampered this plasticity process, specifically at the time when whiskers normally recruit the Mmz in adult ME mice. Our findings significantly add to the current understanding of the brain plasticity phenomena, occurring in response to chronic treatment with 5-HT-system targeting drugs. In future, promising strategies to restore primary sensory functions, might become spatiotemporally controllable through 5-HT-assisted neurobionics.

Abbreviations

5-HT: 5-Hydroxytryptamine, serotonin; 5-HTR: serotonin receptor; 7wME: 7 weeks post-ME; AMC: age-matched control; AMPAR1: alpha-amino-3-hydroxy-5-methyl-4-isoxazolepropionic acid receptor; BDNF: brain derived neurotrophic factor; Bz: binocular zone; E/I: excitation/inhibition balance; GABA$_A$R$_{α1}$: Gamma-aminobutyric acid receptor subunit alpha 1; HPLC: high performance liquid chromatography; i.p.: intraperitoneal; ISH: in situ hybridization; LTP: long-term potentiation; ME: monocular enucleation; Mmz: medial monocular zone; S1BF: primary somatosensory barrel field; SSRI: selective serotonin reuptake inhibitor; TBS: theta-burst stimulation; TPS: total protein stain; VIP: vasoactive intestinal peptide; vMAT2: vesicular monoamine transporter 2; WB: Western blotting

Acknowledgements

We would like to thank Marijke Christiaens for helping with the creation of the figures, and prof. dr. Roger Huybrechts and drs. Jolien Van Houcke for careful reading of the manuscript during revision and especially for their helpful comments and suggestions. The syringe icon in Fig. 1 was designed by Freepik and adapted from https://www.flaticon.com.

Funding

This work was supported by the KU Leuven Research Council (C14/16/048) and the Research Foundation Flanders (FWO)-Vlaanderen, Belgium (Research Project and PhD fellowship to SG).

Authors' contributions

Study concept and design: NL, JN and LA*. Study supervision: LA*. HPLC, WB and ISH sample preparation: NL, JN, RV, LG, LA and GS. HPLC analysis: AV and IS. Analysis and interpretation of data: NL, JN, LA, GS, SG, MH and LA*. Statistical analysis: NL, JN, LA and GS. Drafting of the manuscript: NL and LA*. Critical revision of the manuscript: JN, AV, IS, SG, MH and LA*. All authors read and approved the final manuscript.

Competing interests

The authors declare that they have no competing interests.

Author details

[1]Laboratory of Neuroplasticity and Neuroproteomics, Katholieke Universiteit Leuven, Naamsestraat 59, Box 2467, B-3000 Leuven, Belgium. [2]Department of Pharmaceutical Chemistry, Drug Analysis and Drug Information, Center for Neurosciences (C4N), Vrije Universiteit Brussel, Laarbeeklaan 103, 1090 Brussels, Belgium. [3]Present Address: Laboratory of Synapse Biology, VIB-KU Leuven Center for Brain and Disease Research, O&N IV, Herestraat 49, box 602, B-3000 Leuven, Belgium.

References

1. Hensch TK. Critical period plasticity in local cortical circuits. Nat Rev Neurosci. 2005;6:877–88.
2. Levelt CN, Hübener M. Critical-period plasticity in the visual cortex. Annu Rev Neurosci. 2012;35:309–30. https://doi.org/10.1146/annurev-neuro-061010-113813.
3. Tucker DM, Poulsen C, Luu P. Critical periods for the neurodevelopmental processes of externalizing and internalizing. Dev Psychopathol. 2015;27:321–46. https://doi.org/10.1017/S0954579415000024.
4. Takesian AE, Bogart LJ, Lichtman JW, Hensch TK. Inhibitory circuit gating of auditory critical-period plasticity. Nat Neurosci. 2018;21:218–27.
5. Bavelier D, Levi DM, Li RW, Dan Y, Hensch TK. Removing brakes on adult brain plasticity: from molecular to behavioral interventions. J Neurosci. 2010; 30:14964–71. https://doi.org/10.1523/JNEUROSCI.4812-10.2010.

6. Mataga N, Fujishima S, Condie BG, Hensch TK. Experience-dependent plasticity of mouse visual cortex in the absence of the neuronal activity-dependent marker egr1/zif268. J Neurosci. 2001;21:9724–32.

7. Hübener M, Bonhoeffer T. Neuronal plasticity: beyond the critical period. Cell. 2014;159:727–37.

8. Keck T, Mrsic-Flogel TD, Vaz Afonso M, Eysel UT, Bonhoeffer T, Hübener M. Massive restructuring of neuronal circuits during functional reorganization of adult visual cortex. Nat Neurosci. 2008;11(10):1162–7.

9. Voss P, Lassonde M, Gougoux F, Fortin M, Guillemot JP, Lepore F. Early- and late-onset blind individuals show supra-normal auditory abilities in far-space. Curr Biol. 2004;14:1734–8.

10. Fieger A, Röder B, Teder-Sälejärvi W, Hillyard SA, Neville HJ. Auditory spatial tuning in late-onset blindness in humans. J Cogn Neurosci. 2006; 18(2):149–57.

11. Norman JF, Bartholomew AN. Blindness enhances tactile acuity and haptic 3-D shape discrimination. Attention Perception Psychophys. 2011;73(7): 2323–31.

12. Burton H. Visual cortex activity in early and late blind people. J Neurosci. 2003;23:4005.

13. Cohen LG, Celnik P, Pascual-Leone A, Corwell B, Faiz L, Dambrosia J, et al. Functional relevance of cross-modal plasticity in blind humans. Nature. 1997;389:180–3.

14. Aerts J, Nys J, Arckens L. A highly reproducible and straightforward method to perform in vivo ocular enucleation in the mouse after eye opening. J Vis Exp. 2014;92:e51936. https://doi.org/10.3791/51936.

15. Van Brussel L, Gerits A, Arckens L. Evidence for cross-modal plasticity in adult mouse visual cortex following monocular enucleation. Cereb Cortex. 2011;21:2133–46. https://doi.org/10.1093/cercor/bhq286.

16. Nys J, Aerts J, Ytebrouck E, Vreysen S, Laeremans A, Arckens L. The cross-modal aspect of mouse visual cortex plasticity induced by monocular enucleation is age dependent. J Comp Neurol. 2014;522:950–70. https://doi.org/10.1002/cne.23455.

17. Gilbert CD, Li W. Adult visual cortical plasticity. Neuron. 2012;75:250–64.

18. Bavelier D, Neville HJ. Cross-modal plasticity: where and how? Nat Rev Neurosci. 2002;3:443–52.

19. Gu Q. Neuromodulatory transmitter systems in the cortex and their role in cortical plasticity. Neuroscience. 2002;111:815–35.

20. Kondo M. Molecular mechanisms of experience-dependent structural and functional plasticity in the brain. Anat Sci Int. 2017;92:1.

21. Berardi N, Pizzorusso T, Ratto GM, Maffei L. Molecular basis of plasticity in the visual cortex. Trends Neurosci. 2003;26:369–78.

22. Rabinowitch I, Bai J. The foundations of cross-modal plasticity. Commun Integr Biol. 2016;9:1–3.

23. Morishita H, Miwa JM, Heintz N, Hensch TK. Lynx1, a cholinergic brake, limits plasticity in adult visual cortex. Science. 2010;330:1238–40. https://doi.org/10.1126/science.1195320.

24. Bear M, Singer W. Modulation of visual cortical plasticity by acetylcholine and noradrenaline. Nature. 1986;320:172–6. https://doi.org/10.1038/320172a0.

25. Kasamatsu T, Pettigrew JD, Ary M. Restoration of visual cortical plasticity by local microperfusion of norepinephrine. J Comp Neurol. 1979;185:163–81.

26. Maya-Vetencourt JF, Sale A, Viegi A, Baroncelli L, De Pasquale R, O'Leary OF, et al. The antidepressant fluoxetine restores plasticity in the adult visual cortex. Science. 2008;320:385–8.

27. Gagolewicz PJ, Dringenberg HC. Age-dependent switch of the role of serotonergic 5-HT1A receptors in gating long-term potentiation in rat visual cortex in vivo. Neural Plast. 2016;2016:6404082.

28. Dahlström A, Fuxe K. Localization of monoamines in the lower brain stem. Experientia. 1964;20:398–9.

29. Lidov HGW, Grzanna R, Molliver ME. The serotonin innervation of the cerebral cortex in the rat—an immunohistochemical analysis. Neuroscience. 1980;5:207–27. https://doi.org/10.1016/0306-4522(80)90099-8.

30. Juckel G, Gallinat J, Riedel M, Sokullu S, Schulz C, Möller HJ, et al. Serotonergic dysfunction in schizophrenia assessed by the loudness dependence measure of primary auditory cortex evoked activity. Schizophr Res. 2003;64:115–24.

31. Ji W, Suga N. Serotonergic modulation of plasticity of the auditory cortex elicited by fear conditioning. J Neurosci. 2007;27:4910–8.

32. Jitsuki S, Takemoto K, Kawasaki T, Tada H, Takahashi A, Becamel C, et al. Serotonin mediates cross-modal reorganization of cortical circuits. Neuron. 2011;69:780–92. https://doi.org/10.1016/j.neuron.2011.01.016.

33. Stutzmann GE, McEwen BS, LeDoux JE. Serotonin modulation of sensory inputs to the lateral amygdala: dependency on corticosterone. J Neurosci. 1998;18:9529–38.

34. Dugué GP, Mainen ZF. How serotonin gates olfactory information flow. Nat Neurosci. 2009;12:673–5.

35. Palacios JM. Serotonin receptors in brain revisited. Brain Res. 1645;2016:46–9.

36. Moreau AW, Amar M, Callebert J, Fossier P. Serotonergic modulation of LTP at excitatory and inhibitory synapses in the developing rat visual cortex. Neuroscience. 2013;238:148–58.

37. Maya-Vetencourt JF, Tiraboschi E, Spolidoro M, Castrén E, Maffei L. Serotonin triggers a transient epigenetic mechanism that reinstates adult visual cortex plasticity in rats. Eur J Neurosci. 2011;33:49–57.

38. Baroncelli L, Sale A, Viegi A, Maya-Vetencourt JF, De Pasquale R, Baldini S, et al. Experience-dependent reactivation of ocular dominance plasticity in the adult visual cortex. Exp Neurol. 2010;226:100–9.

39. Takahashi TT. Serotonin as a mediator of cross-modal cortical reorganization. Commun Integr Biol. 2011;4:459–61. https://doi.org/10.4161/cib.4.4.15470.

40. Lee H, Whitt J. Cross-modal synaptic plasticity in adult primary sensory cortices. Curr Opin Neurobiol. 2015;35:119–26.

41. Petrus E, Isaiah A, Jones AP, Li D, Wang H, Lee HK, et al. Crossmodal induction of Thalamocortical potentiation leads to enhanced information processing in the auditory cortex. Neuron. 2014;81:664–73.

42. Jang H-J, Cho K-H, Park S-W, Kim M-J, Yoon SH, Rhie D-J. Effects of serotonin on the induction of long-term depression in the rat visual cortex. Korean J Physiol Pharmacol. 2010;14:337–43. https://doi.org/10.4196/kjpp.2010.14.5.337.

43. Maya-Vetencourt JF, Pizzorusso T. Molecular mechanisms at the basis of plasticity in the developing visual cortex: epigenetic processes and gene programs. J Exp Neurosci. 2013;7:75–83.

44. Kuhlman SJ, Olivas ND, Tring E, Ikrar T, Xu X, Trachtenberg JT. A disinhibitory microcircuit initiates critical-period plasticity in the visual cortex. Nature. 2013;501:543–6. https://doi.org/10.1038/nature12485.

45. Fu Y, Kaneko M, Tang Y, Alvarez-Buylla A, Stryker MP. A cortical disinhibitory circuit for enhancing adult plasticity. elife. 2015;4:1–12. https://doi.org/10.7554/eLife.05558.

46. Li L, Gainey MA, Goldbeck JE, Feldman DE. Rapid homeostasis by disinhibition during whisker map plasticity. Proc Natl Acad Sci. 2014;111:1616–21. https://doi.org/10.1073/pnas.1312455111.

47. Lee S, Kruglikov I, Huang ZJ, Fishell G, Rudy B. A disinhibitory circuit mediates motor integration in the somatosensory cortex. Nat Neurosci. 2013;16:1662–70. https://doi.org/10.1038/nn.3544.

48. Pfeffer CK. Inhibitory neurons: Vip cells hit the brake on inhibition. Curr Biol. 2014;24:R18–20. https://doi.org/10.1016/j.cub.2013.11.001Dispatch.

49. Jiang X, Wang G, Lee AJ, Stornetta RL, Zhu JJ. The organization of two new cortical interneuronal circuits. Nat Neurosci. 2013;16:210–8.

50. Lee S, Hjerling-Leffler J, Zagha E, Fishell G, Rudy B. The largest group of superficial neocortical GABAergic interneurons expresses ionotropic serotonin receptors. J Neurosci. 2010;30:16796–808. https://doi.org/10.1523/JNEUROSCI.1869-10.2010.

51. Scheyltjens I, Vreysen S, van Den Haute C, Sabanov V, Balschun D, Baekelandt V, et al. Transient and localized optogenetic activation of somatostatin-interneurons in mouse visual cortex abolishes long-term cortical plasticity due to vision loss. Brain Structure and Function. 2018;223:1–23.

52. Rudy B, Fishell G, Lee S, Hjerling-Leffler J. Three groups of interneurons account for nearly 100% of neocortical GABAergic neurons. Dev Neurobiol. 2011;71:45–61. https://doi.org/10.1002/dneu.20853.

53. Nys J, Smolders K, Laramée M-E, Hofman I, Hu T-T, Arckens L. Regional specificity of GABAergic regulation of cross-modal plasticity in mouse visual cortex after unilateral enucleation. J Neurosci. 2015;35:11174–89.

54. Lambe EK, Fillman SG, Webster MJ, Shannon WC. Serotonin receptor expression in human prefrontal cortex: balancing excitation and inhibition across postnatal development. PLoS One. 2011;6:e22799. https://doi.org/10.1371/journal.pone.0022799.

55. Moreau WA, Amar M, Le Roux N, Morel N, Fossier P. Serotoninergic fine-tuning of the excitation-inhibition balance in rat visual cortical networks. Cereb Cortex. 2010;20:456–67.

56. Van Brussel L, Gerits A, Arckens L. Identification and localization of functional subdivisions in the visual cortex of the adult mouse. J Comp Neurol. 2009;514:107–16.

57. El Arfani A, Bentea E, Aourz N, Ampe B, De Deurwaerdère P, Van Eeckhaut A, et al. NMDA receptor antagonism potentiates the l-DOPA-induced

57. extracellular dopamine release in the subthalamic nucleus of hemi-parkinson rats. Neuropharmacology. 2014;85:198–205.

58. Jardí F, Laurent MR, Kim N, Khalil R, De Bundel D, Van Eeckhaut A, et al. Testosterone boosts physical activity in male mice via dopaminergic pathways. Sci Rep. 2018;8:957.

59. Qu Y, Eysel UT, Vandesande F, Arckens L. Effect of partial sensory deprivation on monoaminergic neuromodulators in striate cortex of adult cat. Neuroscience. 2000;101:863–8.

60. Cliburn RA, Dunn AR, Stout KA, Hoffman CA, Lohr KM, Bernstein AI, et al. Immunochemical localization of vesicular monoamine transporter 2 (VMAT2) in mouse brain. J Chem Neuroanat. 2017;83–84:82–90.

61. Schafer MKH, Weihe E, Eiden LE. Localization and expression of vmat2 aross mammalian species. A translational guide for its visualization and targeting in health and disease. Adv Pharmacol. 2013;68:319–34.

62. Tong J, Boileau I, Furukawa Y, Chang L-J, Wilson AA, Houle S, et al. Distribution of vesicular monoamine transporter 2 protein in human brain: implications for brain imaging studies. J Cereb Blood Flow Metab. 2011;31: 2065–75. https://doi.org/10.1038/jcbfm.2011.63.

63. Paxinos, G and Franklin KBJ. Paxinos and Franklin's the mouse brain in stereotaxic coordinates. 2012. https://www.elsevier.com/books/paxinos-and-franklins-the-mouse-brain-in-stereotaxic-coordinates/paxinos/978-0-12-391057-8.

64. Wakabayashi K, Narisawa-Saito M, Iwakura Y, Arai T, Ikeda K, Takahashi H, et al. Phenotypic down-regulation of glutamate receptor subunit GluR1 in Alzheimer's disease. Neurobiol Aging. 1999;20:287–95.

65. Van Damme K, Massie A, Vandesande F, Arckens L. Distribution of the AMPA2 glutamate receptor subunit in adult cat visual cortex. Brain Res. 2003;960:1–8.

66. Aldridge GM, Podrebarac DM, Greenough WT, Weiler IJ. The use of total protein stains as loading controls: an alternative to high-abundance single-protein controls in semi-quantitative immunoblotting. J Neurosci Methods. 2008;172:250–4.

67. Hu TT, Van Den Bergh G, Thorrez L, Heylen K, Eysel UT, Arckens L. Recovery from retinal lesions: molecular plasticity mechanisms in visual cortex far beyond the deprived zone. Cereb Cortex. 2011;21:2883–92.

68. Kasamatsu T, Schmidt EK. Continuous and direct infusion of drug solutions in the brain of awake animals: implementation, strengths and pitfalls. Brain Res Protocol. 1997;1(1):57–69.

69. Dawson LA, Nguyen HQ, Smith DL, Schechter LE. Effect of chronic fluoxetine and WAY-100635 treatment on serotonergic neurotransmission in the frontal cortex. J Psychopharmacol. 2002;16:145–52. https://doi.org/10.1177/026988110201600205.

70. Abbas SY, Nogueira MI, Azmitia EC. Antagonist-induced increase in 5-HT1A-receptor expression in adult rat hippocampus and cortex. Synapse. 2007;61:531–9.

71. Persson B, Heykants J, Hedner T. Clinical pharmacokinetics of Ketanserin. Clin Pharmacokinet. 1991;20:263–79.

72. Gu Q, Singer W. Involvement of serotonin in developmental plasticity of kitten visual cortex. Eur J Neurosci. 1995;7:1146–53.

73. Lakoski JM, Aghajanian GK. Effects of ketanserin on neuronal responses to serotonin in the prefrontal cortex, lateral geniculate and dorsal raphe nucleus. Neuropharmacology. 1985;24:265–73.

74. Jha S, Rajendran R, Fernandes KA, Vaidya VA. 5-HT2A/2C receptor blockade regulates progenitor cell proliferation in the adult rat hippocampus. Neurosci Lett. 2008;441:210–4.

75. Ye J-H, Ponnudurai R, Schaefer R. Ondansetron: a selective 5-HT3 receptor antagonist and its applications in CNS-related disorders. CNS Drug Rev. 2006;7:199–213. https://doi.org/10.1111/j.1527-3458.2001.tb00195.x.

76. Woolley DG, Laeremans A, Gantois I, Mantini D, Vermaercke B, Op de Beeck HP, et al. Homologous involvement of striatum and prefrontal cortex in rodent and human water maze learning. Proc Natl Acad Sci. 2013;110:3131–6. https://doi.org/10.1073/pnas.1217832110.

77. Smolders K, Vreysen S, Laramée ME, Cuyvers A, Hu TT, Van Brussel L, et al. Retinal lesions induce fast intrinsic cortical plasticity in adult mouse visual system. Eur J Neurosci. 2016;44:2165–75.

78. Imbrosci B, Wang Y, Arckens L, Mittmann T. Neuronal mechanisms underlying transhemispheric diaschisis following focal cortical injuries. Brain Struct Funct. 2015;220:1649–64.

79. Arckens L, Van Der GE, Eysel UT, Orban GA, Vandesande F. Investigation of cortical reorganization in area 17 and nine extrastriate visual areas through the detection of changes in immediate early gene expression as induced by retinal lesions. JComp Neurol. 2000;425:531–44.

80. Qu Y, Massie A, Van Der Gucht E, Cnops L, Vandenbussche E, Eysel UT, et al. Retinal lesions affect extracellular glutamate levels in sensory-deprived and remote non-deprived regions of cat area 17 as revealed by in vivo microdialysis. Brain Res. 2003;962:199–206.

81. Massie A, Cnops L, Jacobs S, Van Damme K, Vandenbussche E, Eysel UT, et al. Glutamate levels and transport in cat (Felis catus) area 17 during cortical reorganization following binocular retinal lesions. J Neurochem. 2003;84: 1387–97.

82. Leysen I, Van Der Gucht E, Eysel UT, Huybrechts R, Vandesande F, Arckens L. Time-dependent changes in the expression of the MEF2 transcription factor family during topographic map reorganization in mammalian visual cortex. Eur J Neurosci. 2004;20:769–80.

83. Saffen DW, Cole AJ, Worley PF, Christy BA, Ryder K, Baraban JM. Convulsant-induced increase in transcription factor messenger RNAs in rat brain. Proc Natl Acad Sci U S A. 1988;85:7795–9. https://doi.org/10.1073/pnas.85.20.7795.

84. Worley PF, Christy BA, Nakabeppu Y, Bhat RV, Cole AJ, Baraban JM. Constitutive expression of zif268 in neocortex is regulated by synaptic activity. Proc Natl Acad Sci. 1991;88:5106–10. https://doi.org/10.1073/pnas.88.12.5106.

85. Cole AJ, Saffen DW, Baraban JM, Worley PF. Rapid increase of an immediate early gene messenger RNA in hippocampal neurons by synaptic NMDA receptor activation. Nature. 1989;340:474–6. https://doi.org/10.1038/340474a0.

86. Chaudhuri A, Matsubara JA, Cynader MS. Neuronal activity in primate visual cortex assessed by immunostaining for the transcription factor Zif268. Vis Neurosci. 1995;12:35–50. https://doi.org/10.1017/S095252380000729X.

87. Kaczmarek L, Chaudhuri A. Sensory regulation of immediate-early gene expression in mammalian visual cortex: implications for functional mapping and neural plasticity. Brain Res Brain Res Rev. 1997;23:237–56.

88. Arckens L, Zhang F, Vanduffel W, Mailleux P, Vanderhaeghen JJ, Orban GA, et al. Localization of the two protein kinase C beta-mRNA subtypes in cat visual system. J Chem Neuroanat. 1995;8:117–24. 7598812.

89. Van Der Gucht E, Hof PR, Van Brussel L, Burnat K, Arckens L. Neurofilament protein and neuronal activity markers define regional architectonic parcellation in the mouse visual cortex. Cereb Cortex. 2007;17:2805–19.

90. Giulietti M, Vivenzio V, Piva F, Principato G, Bellantuono C, Nardi B. How much do we know about the coupling of G-proteins to serotonin receptors? Molecular Brain. 2014;7:49.

91. Derkach V, Surprenant A, North RA. 5-HT3 receptors are membrane ion channels. Nature. 1989;339:706–9.

92. Albert PR, Vahid-Ansari F, Luckhart C. Serotonin-prefrontal cortical circuitry in anxiety and depression phenotypes: pivotal role of pre- and post-synaptic 5-HT1A receptor expression. Front Behav Neurosci. 2014;8. https://doi.org/10.3389/fnbeh.2014.00199.

93. Leonard BE. Serotonin receptors and their function in sleep, anxiety disorders and depression. Psychother Psychosom. 1996;65:66–75.

94. Andrews PW, Bharwani A, Lee KR, Fox M, Thomson JA. Is serotonin an upper or a downer? The evolution of the serotonergic system and its role in depression and the antidepressant response. Neurosci Biobehav Rev. 2015;51:164–88.

95. Wainwright SR, Galea LAM. The neural plasticity theory of depression: assessing the roles of adult neurogenesis and psa-ncam within the hippocampus. Neural Plasticity. 2013;2013:805497.

96. Liu W, Ge T, Leng Y, Pan Z, Fan J, Yang W, et al. The role of neural plasticity in depression: from Hippocampus to prefrontal cortex. Neural Plasticity. 2017;2017:6871089.

97. Castrén E. Is mood chemistry? Nat Rev Neurosci. 2005;6:241–6. https://doi.org/10.1038/nrn1629.

98. Krishnan V, Nestler EJ. The molecular neurobiology of depression. Nature. 2008;455:894–902.

99. Ruiz-Perera L, Muniz M, Vierci G, Bornia N, Baroncelli L, Sale A, et al. Fluoxetine increases plasticity and modulates the proteomic profile in the adult mouse visual cortex. Sci Rep. 2015;5:12517.

100. Guirado R, Perez-Rando M, Sanchez-Matarredona D, Castrén E, Nacher J. Chronic fluoxetine treatment alters the structure, connectivity and plasticity of cortical interneurons. Int J Neuropsychopharmacol. 2014;17:1635–46. https://doi.org/10.1017/S1461145714000406.

101. Tiraboschi E, Guirado R, Greco D, Auvinen P, Maya-Vetencourt JF, Maffei L, et al. Gene expression patterns underlying the reinstatement of plasticity in the adult visual system. Neural Plast. 2013;2013:605079.

102. Héry F, Ternaux JP. Regulation of release processes in central serotoninergic neurons. J Physiol Paris. 1981;77:287–301.

103. Fagiolini M, Hensch TK. Inhibitory threshold for critical-period activation in primary visual cortex. Nature. 2000;404:183–6.

104. Turrigiano GG. The self-tuning neuron: synaptic scaling of excitatory synapses. Cell. 2008;135:422–35. https://doi.org/10.1016/j.cell.2008.10.008.

105. Jang HJ, Cho KH, Joo K, Kim MJ, Rhie DJ. Differential modulation of phasic and tonic inhibition underlies serotonergic suppression of long-term potentiation in the rat visual cortex. Neuroscience. 2015;301:351–62.

106. Joo K, Yoon SH, Rhie DJ, Jang HJ. Phasic and tonic inhibition are maintained respectively by CaMKII and PKA in the rat visual cortex. Korean J Physiol Pharmacol. 2014;18:517–24.

107. Connelly WM, Fyson SJ, Errington AC, McCafferty CP, Cope DW, Di Giovanni G, et al. GABAB Receptors Regulate Extrasynaptic GABAA Receptors. J Neurosci. 2013;33:3780–5.

108. Iwai Y, Fagiolini M, Obata K, Hensch TK. Rapid critical period induction by tonic inhibition in visual cortex. J Neurosci. 2003;23:6695–702.

109. Wang J-W, David DJ, Monckton JE, Battaglia F, Hen R. Chronic fluoxetine stimulates maturation and synaptic plasticity of adult-born hippocampal granule cells. J Neurosci. 2008;28:1374–84. https://doi.org/10.1523/JNEUROSCI.3632-07.2008.

110. Mcavoy K, Russo C, Kim S, Rankin G, Sahay A. Fluoxetine induces input-specific hippocampal dendritic spine remodeling along the septotemporal axis in adulthood and middle age. Hippocampus. 2015;25:1429–46.

111. Normann C, Schmitz D, Fürmaier A, Döing C, Bach M. Long-term plasticity of visually evoked potentials in humans is altered in major depression. Biol Psychiatry. 2007;62:373–80.

112. Gore C, Wu C. Medical therapies of amblyopia: translational research to expand our treatment armamentarium. Semin Ophthalmol. 2016;31:155–8. https://doi.org/10.3109/08820538.2015.1114851.

113. Beshara S, Beston BR, Pinto JGA, Murphy KM. Effects of fluoxetine and visual experience on glutamatergic and GABAergic synaptic proteins in adult rat visual cortex. eNeuro. 2016;2. https://doi.org/10.1523/ENEURO.0126-15.2015.

114. Fu Y, Kaneko M, Tang Y, Alvarez-Buylla A, Stryker MP. A cortical disinhibitory circuit for enhancing adult plasticity. elife. 2015;2015:e05558.

115. Pi H-J, Hangya B, Kvitsiani D, Sanders JI, Huang ZJ, Kepecs A. Cortical interneurons that specialize in disinhibitory control. Nature. 2013;503:521–4. https://doi.org/10.1038/nature12676.

116. Acsády L, Görcs TJ, Freund TF. Different populations of vasoactive intestinal polypeptide-immunoreactive interneurons are specialized to control pyramidal cells or interneurons in the hippocampus. Neuroscience. 1996;73:317–34.

117. Dávid C, Schleicher A, Zuschratter W, Staiger JF. The innervation of parvalbumin-containing interneurons by VIP-immunopositive interneurons in the primary somatosensory cortex of the adult rat. Eur J Neurosci. 2007;25:2329–40.

118. Heimler B, Weisz N, Collignon O. Revisiting the adaptive and maladaptive effects of crossmodal plasticity. Neuroscience. 2014;283:44–63.

119. Lee DS, Lee JS, Oh SH, Kim SK, Kim JW, Chung JK, et al. Cross-modal plasticity and cochlear implants. Nature. 2001;409:149–50. https://doi.org/10.1038/35051653.

120. Stropahl M, Debener S. Auditory cross-modal reorganization in cochlear implant users indicates audio-visual integration. NeuroImage Clin. 2017;16:514–23.

121. Lee HJ, Giraud AL, Kang E, Oh SH, Kang H, Kim CS, et al. Cortical activity at rest predicts cochlear implantation outcome. Cereb Cortex. 2007;17(4):909–17.

122. Lewis PM, Ackland HM, Lowery AJ, Rosenfeld JV. Restoration of vision in blind individuals using bionic devices: a review with a focus on cortical visual prostheses. Brain Res. 2014;1595:51–73. https://doi.org/10.1016/j.brainres.2014.11.020.

123. Dobelle WH, Mladejovsky MG, Girvin JP. Artificial Vision for the Blind: Electrical Stimulation of Visual Cortex Offers Hope for a Functional Prosthesis. Science. 1974;183:440–4. https://doi.org/10.1126/science.183.4123.440.

124. Walter P. Visual prostheses. Ophthalmologe. 2016;113:175–89. https://doi.org/10.1007/s00347-015-0202-8.

125. Shepherd RK, Shivdasani MN, Nayagam DAX, Williams CE, Blamey PJ. Visual prostheses for the blind. Trends Biotechnol. 2013;31:562–71.

126. Margalit E, Maia M, Weiland JD, Greenberg RJ, Fujii GY, Torres G, et al. Retinal prosthesis for the blind. Surv Ophthalmol. 2002;47:335–56.

127. Dobkin BH. Brain-computer interface technology as a tool to augment plasticity and outcomes for neurological rehabilitation. In: J Physiol. 2007;579:p. 637–642.

128. Grosse-Wentrup M, Mattia D, Oweiss K. Using brain-computer interfaces to induce neural plasticity and restore function. In: J Neural Eng. 2011;8(2):025004.

129. Rossini PM, Noris Ferilli MA, Ferreri F. Cortical plasticity and brain computer interface. Eur J Phys Rehabil Med. 2012;48:307–12.

130. Maya-Vetencourt JF, Ghezzi D, Antognazza MR, Colombo E, Mete M, Feyen P, et al. A fully organic retinal prosthesis restores vision in a rat model of degenerative blindness. Nat Mater. 2017;16(6):681–9.

131. Gerding H, Benner FP, Taneri S. Experimental implantation of epiretinal retina implants (EPI-RET) with an IOL-type receiver unit. J Neural Eng. 2007;4(1):S38–49.

132. Mathieson K, Loudin J, Goetz G, Huie P, Wang L, Kamins TI, et al. Photovoltaic retinal prosthesis with high pixel density. Nat Photonics. 2012;6(6):391–7.

133. Ayton LN, Blamey PJ, Guymer RH, Luu CD, Nayagam DAX, Sinclair NC, et al. First-in-human trial of a novel suprachoroidal retinal prosthesis. PLoS One. 2014;9(12):e115239.

134. Jacob SN, Nienborg H. Monoaminergic Neuromodulation of Sensory Processing. Front Neural Circuits. 2018;12:51.

13

Vitamin A bio-modulates apoptosis via the mitochondrial pathway after hypoxic-ischemic brain damage

Wei Jiang[1,2,3,4,5†], Min Guo[1,2,3,4,5†], Min Gong[1,2,3,4], Li Chen[1,2,3,4], Yang Bi[1,2,3,4], Yun Zhang[1,2,3,4], Yuan Shi[1,2,3,4], Ping Qu[1,2,3,4], Youxue Liu[1,2,3,4], Jie Chen[1,2,3,4*] and Tingyu Li[1,2,3,4*] (iD)

Abstract

Our previous studies demonstrated that vitamin A deficiency (VAD) can impair the postnatal cognitive function of rats by damaging the hippocampus. The present study examined the effects of retinoic acid (RA) on apoptosis induced by hypoxic-ischemic damage in vivo and in vitro, and investigated the possible signaling pathway involved in the neuroprotective anti-apoptotic effects of RA. Flow cytometry, immunofluorescence staining and behavioral tests were used to evaluate the neuroprotective and anti-apoptotic effects of RA. The protein and mRNA levels of RARα, PI3K, Akt, Bad, caspase-3, caspase-8, Bcl-2, Bax, and Bid were measured with western blotting and real-time PCR, respectively. We found impairments in learning and spatial memory in VAD group compared with vitamin A normal (VAN) and vitamin A supplemented (VAS) group. Additionally, we showed that hippocampal apoptosis was weaker in the VAN group than that in VAD group. Relative to the VAD group, the VAN group also had increased mRNA and protein levels of RARα and PI3K, and upregulated phosphorylated Akt/Bad levels in vivo. In vitro, excessively low or high RA signaling promoted apoptosis. Furthermore, the effects on apoptosis involved the mitochondrial membrane potential (MMP). These data support the idea that sustained VAD following hypoxic-ischemic brain damage (HIBD) inhibits RARα, which downregulates the PI3K/Akt/Bad and Bcl-2/Bax pathways and upregulates the caspase-8/Bid pathway to influence the MMP, ultimately producing deficits in learning and spatial memory in adolescence. This suggests that clinical interventions for HIBD should include suitable doses of VA.

Keywords: Vitamin A (VA), Hypoxic-ischemic brain damage (HIBD), Retinoic acid (RA), Apoptosis, Mitochondrial membrane potential (MMP), PI3K/Akt

Introduction

Hypoxic-ischemic brain damage (HIBD) is the most common central nervous system diseases in the neonatal period and has a poor prognosis. A large number of children have residual nerve damage, which is manifested as mental developmental delay, intellectual disability, or even death [1–3]. Meanwhile, pediatric vitamin A deficiency (VAD) is a global public health problem. A preclinical investigation found that neonates with HIBD suffered from more severe VAD than those who had pneumonia or those who were healthy, and the vitamin A (VA) levels did not significantly increase with advancing age (Additional file 1: Figure S1). It has previously been found that VA could affect neural development after birth [4]. Therefore, it was hypothesized that VA can affect neural tissue and functional outcome after HIBD.

The hippocampus is crucial for learning and memory [5] and is susceptible to HIBD injury [6]. VA is an important fat-soluble vitamin that carries out physiological functions similar to those of hormones via its main derivative, retinoic acid (RA). The hippocampus and its surrounding meninges synthesize and metabolize RA, promoting the expression of retinol-binding protein (RBP) [7]. Apoptosis is the important mechanism of pathological damage in the acute stage of HIBD. Therefore, apoptosis in the hippocampus was the target of the present study.

* Correspondence: jchen010@foxmail.com; tyli@vip.sina.com
†Equal contributors
[1]Children Nutrition Research Center, Children's Hospital of Chongqing Medical University, Chongqing 400014, China
Full list of author information is available at the end of the article

VA plays a pivotal role in a suite of essential biologic processes as a powerful regulator of vision, reproduction, immunity, apoptosis, growth and development. RA is associated with cell proliferation and differentiation, and additionally contributes to the proper development of the vertebrate central nervous system [8, 9]. RA can modulate the transcription or nontranscription of downstream target genes or functional proteins through retinoic acid receptor (RAR)-mediated signal transduction. RAR heterodimers attach to specific DNA sequences or RA response elements (RAREs), which are typically composed of two direct repeats of a core hexameric motif. RA interacts with two major families of nuclear receptors: retinoic acid receptors (RAR) and retinoid X receptors (RXR). Each family is composed of three isotypes: α, β, and γ. The RARα isoform has an essential role in brain development and modulates adult brain function [10, 11].

RA can promote carcinoma cell apoptosis, and larger doses of all-trans retinoic acid are currently used for the therapy of certain cancers [12]. VAD causes apoptosis of pancreatic beta-cell masses [13]. Paradoxically, RA has been reported to have protective effects against the neuronal apoptosis caused by injury, and it enhances proliferation and survival. These effects all depend on transcriptional signaling that involves RA and anti-apoptosis pathways [14]. A previous study found that RARα was primarily a nuclear receptor present in the rat cerebral cortex and white matter during postnatal development [4]. VAD in pregnancy can attenuate the expression of RARα, causing concomitant deficits in active learning and spatial memory function in adolescence [4, 15]. It has been demonstrated that treatment with appropriate concentrations of RA can influence the mitochondrial membrane potential (MMP) to reduce the apoptosis of oxygen-glucose deprivation (OGD)-injured PC12 cells, possibly through the regulation of RARα signaling [16, 17]. It is speculated that the bidirectional regulation of apoptosis depends on the concentration of RA and the types of target cells and tissues. Accordingly, it is hypothesized that a suitable concentration of RA will have an anti-apoptotic effect on neurons in HIBD. Numerous studies have been devoted to investigating the mechanism of apoptosis and the pathway to antagonize hippocampal cell apoptosis after hypoxic-ischemic injury. However, these studies on hypoxic-ischemic damage and the potential mechanism of anti-apoptotic effects involved in RA are still inconclusive.

The present study examined the effects of RA on apoptosis produced by hypoxic-ischemic damage in vivo and in vitro. In addition, adenovirus-transfected primary neurons were used to investigate the possible signaling pathway involved in the neuroprotective anti-apoptotic effects of RA.

Methods

Animals

All animal experiments were approved by the Animal Experimentation Ethical Committee of the Zoology Center at Chongqing Medical University (Chongqing, China) and in accordance with the National Institutes of Health Guide for the Care and Use of Laboratory Animals (NIH Publication No. 8023, revised 1978). Sprague Dawley (SD) rats were procured from the Experimental Animal Center of Chongqing Medical University [SCXK (Yu) 2012–0015]. The rats were randomly assigned into four groups: control (sham), VA normal (VAN), VAD and vitamin A supplemented (VAS). Random number was generated with SPSS 17. The Animal Care Committee of Chongqing Medical University approved the experimental protocol.

Diets

The female breeder rats in the VAD and VAN groups were fed with 300 IU and 7000 IU retinol/kg diet per day, respectively, for 4 weeks, then throughout pregnancy, and the pups were nursed from the VAD or VAN mother rats until the end of the experiment [18]. The VAS rats were VAD rats fed by VAN dams from HIBD P1 until the end of the experiment. The diets were the same except for VA content (Additional file 1: Figure S1).

Hypoxic-ischemic animal model

The hypoxic-ischemic animal model was established using the Rice-Vannucci method [19]. The ligation of left common carotid artery was performed on 7-day-postnatal rats. One hour after the surgical procedure, the rats were put in a hypoxic tank and received hypoxic treatment (8% oxygen and 92% nitrogen) at a flow rate of 0.5 L/min for 2.5 h. The control group received the same treatment as the other groups except for the ligation and hypoxic treatment.

HPLC testing of serum VA

The serum VA concentrations were estimated using HPLC in accordance with our previously described methods with slight modifications [20]. Two hundred microliters of serum was dissolved in 200 μL of dehydrated alcohol; 1000 μL of hexane was added and fully mixed, and the solution was centrifuged at 13,200rpm for 8 min. Then, 500 μL of the supernatant was carefully transferred and dried with nitrogen. The residue was dissolved in the mobile phase (methanol: water = 97:3). Finally, an HPLC apparatus (DGU-20As, Shimadzu Corporation, Japan) was then used to detect the prepared sample (C18, 315 nm).

Measurement of apoptosis by TUNEL immunofluorescence staining

Rats from VAN and VAD groups were killed on post-HIBD days 3 and 7. Additionally, serial hippocampal sections were prepared, and the nuclei were stained with Hoechst 33,258 (Beyotime, China). Imaging was performed using an inverted fluorescence microscope system (NikonTE2000-S, Japan). We counted the number of TUNEL-positive cells in corresponding square regions.

Morris water maze test

A Morris water maze test system [21] (MWM SLY-WMS 2.0, China) was used to evaluate the spatial learning and memory functions of rats, as previously described. Briefly, a visible platform was used to evaluate the rats' vision on the first training day. Animals were exposed to an invisible platform to raise their ability of learning and memory from the second to the fifth day. In the whole 5 days, the average escape latency and path length in locating the platform were recorded. We conducted a probe trial with no escape platform and recorded the number of times that the rats swam across the former platform location in 60 s on the sixth day.

Shuttle box test

A shuttle box test [4] (KE KE ZH-DSX2, China) was performed on post-HIBD day 30. The rats were placed in the shuttle box for 1 min to adapt to the environment and then placed in the shock zone for training on the first day. The formal test was conducted from the second to the fifth day. If the rats ran into the safe chamber within 10 s after the sound, the response was recorded as an active avoidance response; if the rats did not run into the safe chamber when given electric shock, the response was recorded as a passive avoidance response; if there was no response, the result was recorded as a no avoidance response.

Isolation and culture of primary neurons

Zero-day-old rat pups were killed and hippocampal neurons were isolated and cultured according to previous procedures with some modifications [22]. The hippocampus of each rat was removed and digested by treatment with TrypLE (Gibco, USA) at 37°C for 30 min, and then centrifuged at 1000 rpm for 5 min to obtain the precipitate. Finally, the cells were seeded in a 6-well plate with 10% fetal bovine serum (FBS) (Gibco, USA) in DMEM/F12 medium (Gibco, USA). The medium was changed to Neurobasal medium (Gibco, USA) involving 2% B27 supplement (Gibco, USA) and 0. 5 mM L-glutamine (Gibco, USA) the next day.

Oxygen and glucose deprivation

On the day of the experiment, the culture medium was replaced with Earle's balanced salt solution [17] (EBSS; HyClone, USA). OGD was induced by placing the neurons in a humidified incubator (Thermo, USA) containing a mixture of 5% oxygen and 95% nitrogen for 1.5 h to simulate ischemic injury.

RA treatment

RA (Sigma, USA) was added to the Neurobasal medium at final concentrations of 0, 1, 5, 10, 20, or 40 μmol/L for 24 h. Next, the neurons that had been treated with each concentration of RA were injured by OGD.

Detection of apoptosis by annexin V-PI staining and flow cytometry

Each well was washed twice with D-Hank's solution after OGD. The cells were collected and digested with TrypLE for 1 min, and centrifuged at 1000 rpm at 4°C for 5 min. The cells were measured sequentially with a flow cytometer (BD FACSAria, USA).

Measurement of mitochondrial membrane potential by JC-1 staining and flow cytometry

Each well was washed twice with D-Hank's solution after OGD. The cells were collected and digested with 0.5 mL TrypLE for 1 min, and centrifuged at 1000 rpm at 4°C for 5 min. The cells were measured sequentially using a flow cytometer (BD FACSAria, USA).

Measurement of caspase-3 and caspase-8 protein activity by ELISA

Hippocampal tissue homogenates (20~40 mg) and 100 μL/100 million primary neurons were subjected to lysis on ice for 15 min. The lysates were centrifuged at 12,000 rpm at 4°C for 5 min. The caspase-3 and caspase-8 activity levels were measured at 405 nm using an automatic microplate reader ELx800 (BioTek, USA).

RNA interference of RARα

Recombinant adenoviruses carrying the rat RARα (over-RARα) or RNA interference virus RARα-siRNA (siR-ARα) were used to infect neurons [18]. The recombinant adenovirus was allowed to infect the neurons for 24 h to test the mRNA levels and 48 h to explore the protein levels. Red fluorescent protein (RFP) was used to label the nonspecific siRNA (siRARγ) and acted as the negative control.

Real-time PCR RARα and other signaling pathway molecules in the hippocampus and primary neurons

Extraction of the hippocampal and primary neuronal RNA was performed using a total RNA isolation system, EZgenoTM (Genemega, USA). The purified mRNA was reverse transcribed into cDNA using the PrimeScript RT Reagent Kit (TaKaRa, Japan). cDNA quantification by real-time PCR was performed using a StepOne v2.1 Real-Time PCR instrument (ABI, USA) and RealMasterMix (SYBR Green; Tiangen Biotech, China). The cycles were performed as follows: denaturation at 95°C for 10 min, followed by 45 cycles of 95°C for 15 s, 60°C for 60 s, and 72°C for 30 s. Data were standardized to the endogenous expression of β-actin.

RARα	Fwd: 5'CAGGAGGGAGAAGGCAGTGAC3' Rev: 5'ATGGCTTGAGTTCGGAGGACAG3'
caspase-8	Fwd: 5'GGCAGCCAGTTCTTCGTT3' Rev: 5'CTCGGCGACAGGTTACAG3'
caspase-3	Fwd: 5'GGGTGCGGTAGAGTAAGC3' Rev: 5'CTGGACTGCGGTATTGAG3'
Bid	Fwd: 5'CCTGGAAATAGGGAGACG3' Rev: 5'GATACGGCAAGAATTGTGAA3'
Bax	Fwd: 5'AAGTAGAAGAGGGCAACCAC3' Rev: 5'GATGGCAACTTCAACTGGG3'
Bcl-2	Fwd: 5'CGGGAGAACAGGGTATGA3' Rev: 5'CAGGCTGGAAGGAGAAGAT3'
PI3K	Fwd: 5'CTGGAAGCCATTGAGAAG3' Rev: 5'CAGGATTTGGTAAGTCGG3'
Akt	Fwd: 5'CTCTTCTTCCACCTGTCTCG3' Rev: 5'CTTGATGTGCCCGTCCTT3'
Bad	Fwd: 5'CAGGCAGCCAATAACAGT3' Rev: 5'CCTCCATCCCTTCATCTT3'
β-actin	Fwd: 5'GCATAGCCACGCTTGTTCTTGAAG3' Rev: 5'GAACCGCTCATTGCCGATAGTG3'

Western blotting of RARα and other signaling pathway molecules in the hippocampus and primary neurons

The protein extracted from hippocampus or primary neuron homogenates was used for western blotting. The membranes were incubated in primary antibodies including anti-RARα (1:250, Abcam, USA), anti-β-actin (1:150, Santa Cruz, USA), anti-PI3K (1:200, Abcam, USA), anti-p-Akt (1:250, Abcam, USA), anti-Akt(1:250, Cell Signaling, USA), anti-p-Bad(1:100, Santa Cruz, USA), anti-Bad (1:200, Cell Signaling, USA), anti-caspase-3(1:100, Santa Cruz, USA), anti-caspase-8(1:100, Santa Cruz, USA), anti-Bcl-2 (1:150, Santa Cruz, USA), anti-Bax(1:100, Santa Cruz, USA), and anti-Bid(1:200, Abcam, USA) at 4 °C overnight, respectively. The blot was probed with an enzyme-linked secondary antibody (typically horseradish peroxidase) for 1h at room temperature. Then, the blot was stained with 3,3′-diaminobenzidine (DAB) (Tiangen, China) and the signals from the chemiluminescent detection reagents were photographed using an ECL Imaging System (BioRad, USA). The samples were normalized to β-actin.

Statistical analysis

The statistical analyses were performed using one-way analysis of variance (ANOVA), repeated-measures ANOVA, the chi-squared test, and the Student-Newman-Keuls (SNK-q) test. All statistical analyses were computed in SPSS17 software by professional staff. The results are expressed as the means ± SEM. $P \leq 0.05$ was considered significant.

Results

VA levels of the VAN, VAD, and VAS groups (Additional file 2: Figure S2)

The VA level assessment of VAD rats was in accordance with the standards for humans. The serum VA levels of rats were conformed to the WHO standards (1996) concerning VAN (≥ 1.05 μmol/L), marginal VAD (MVAD) (0.7~1.05 μmol/L), VAD (<0.7 μmol/L), and severe VAD (SVAD) (<0.35 μmol/L) status [23]. As shown in Additional file 2: Figure S2, the VAD group showed significantly decreased serum VA level relative to VAN group at every post-HIBD stage. The VAS group showed significantly higher VA level than VAD group on P7~40. The VA levels of all the groups showed increasing trends from P1 to P40, and the trends were in accordance with normal human physiological process.

Learning ability and spatial memory of VAN, VAD, and VAS groups after HIBD (Fig. 1)

Figure 1 (panels a, b) shows that the escape latency and path length of all the groups gradually decreased during the test period. The VAD group showed longer escape latency and path length than VAN and VAS groups on second, third, fourth, and fifth test days. Moreover, the VAD group spent less time than VAN or VAS group in the target quadrant during the probe trial test (panel c). No significant difference of the swimming speed levels between the four experimental groups (panel d). Further, learning ability was examined through the shuttle box test. It was found that the VAD group showed a decreased active avoidance response rate (AARR) from the second to fifth test day (panel i), an increased passive avoidance response rate (PARR) from the third to fifth test days (panel j), and an increased no-avoidance response rate (NARR) on all the test days (panel k). Taken together, these data indicate that VAD group showed impaired learning ability and spatial memory relative to VAN group in the later post-HIBD period, and VA supplement could alleviate the impairment induced by VAD.

Cell apoptosis in the DG, CA3, and CA1 regions of the hippocampus after HIBD (Fig. 2)

To explain why VAN group had a better neurological prognosis than VAD group after HIBD injury, apoptosis

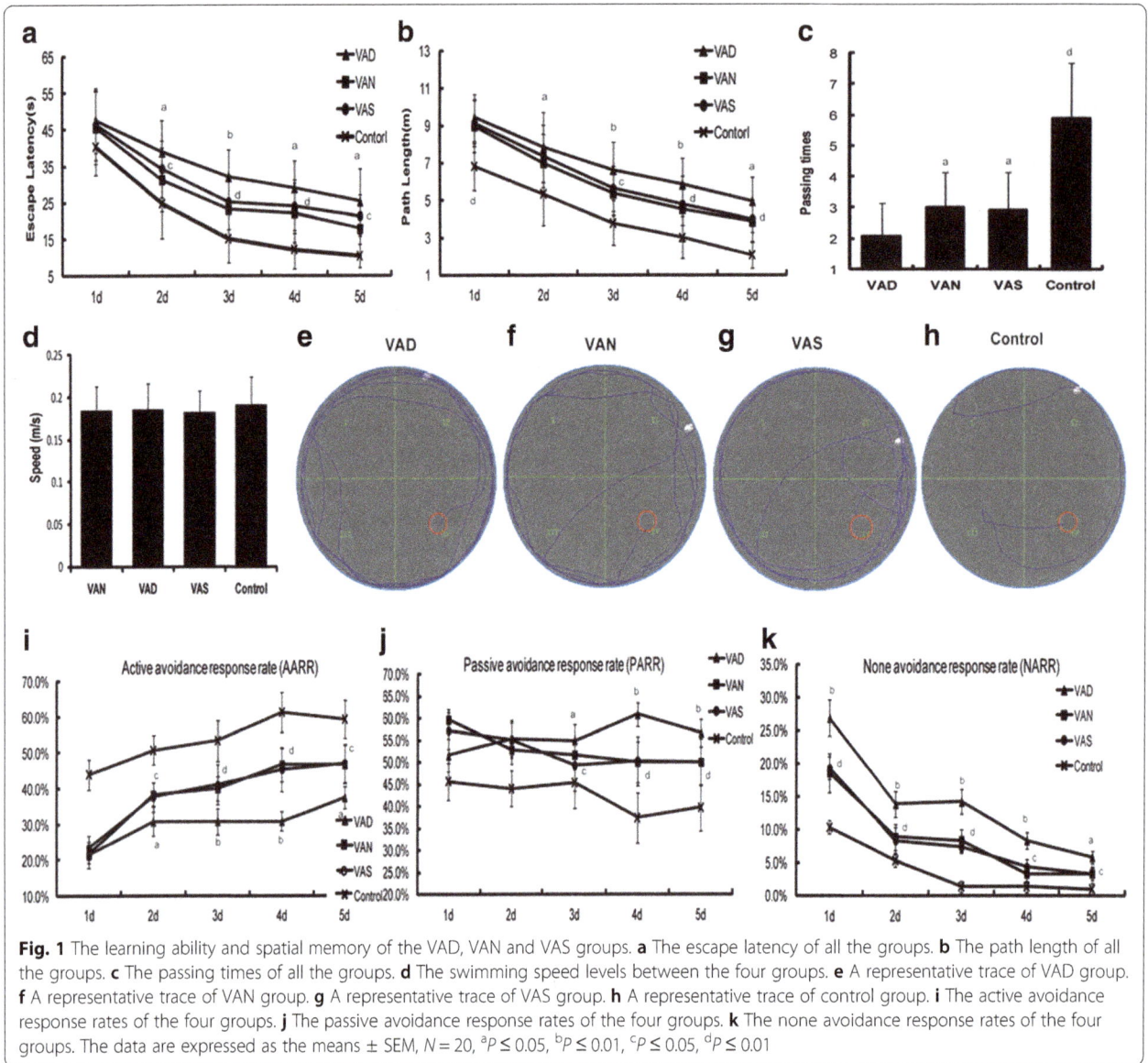

Fig. 1 The learning ability and spatial memory of the VAD, VAN and VAS groups. **a** The escape latency of all the groups. **b** The path length of all the groups. **c** The passing times of all the groups. **d** The swimming speed levels between the four groups. **e** A representative trace of VAD group. **f** A representative trace of VAN group. **g** A representative trace of VAS group. **h** A representative trace of control group. **i** The active avoidance response rates of the four groups. **j** The passive avoidance response rates of the four groups. **k** The none avoidance response rates of the four groups. The data are expressed as the means ± SEM, $N = 20$, $^{a}P \leq 0.05$, $^{b}P \leq 0.01$, $^{c}P \leq 0.05$, $^{d}P \leq 0.01$

in hippocampal sections during the acute stage of HIBD was analyzed by TUNEL staining. As shown in Fig. 2, the numbers of apoptotic cells in the hippocampal DG, CA3, and CA1 regions of VAD group were significantly higher than those of VAN group (yellow arrow) on post-HIBD day 3 and day 7. The apoptotic cells were mainly located in the hippocampal pyramidal layer. The apoptosis also became more severe and began to spread from the pyramidal layer to the molecular layer. The results suggested that VAD can significantly aggravate the apoptosis of hippocampus cells in HIBD.

RA modulates the PI3K/Akt pathway via RARα signaling to influence apoptosis in vivo (Fig. 3)

Then we tested the hypothesis that the RA signaling pathway influenced apoptosis via the PI3K/Akt pathway.

As shown in Fig. 3, the RARα mRNA levels of VAN group were inecreased relative to VAD group on P3~14 (panel **a**). The RARα protein expression level of VAN group was higher than that of VAD group on P14 (panel **e**). The PI3K mRNA and protein expression levels of VAN group were higher than those of VAD group on P3~7 (panels **b, e**). Similarly, the Akt mRNA expression level in VAN group was higher than that in VAD group on P3 (panel **c**), and the Akt protein expression levels in VAN group were higher than those in VAD group on P7~14 (panel **e**). In addition, the protein levels of phosphorylated Akt (a downstream signaling molecule of PI3K) were elevated in VAN group relative to VAD group on P3~7 (panel **e**). However, the mRNA levels of Bad (a molecule downstream of p-Akt) were not significantly different between two groups on P3~14 (panel

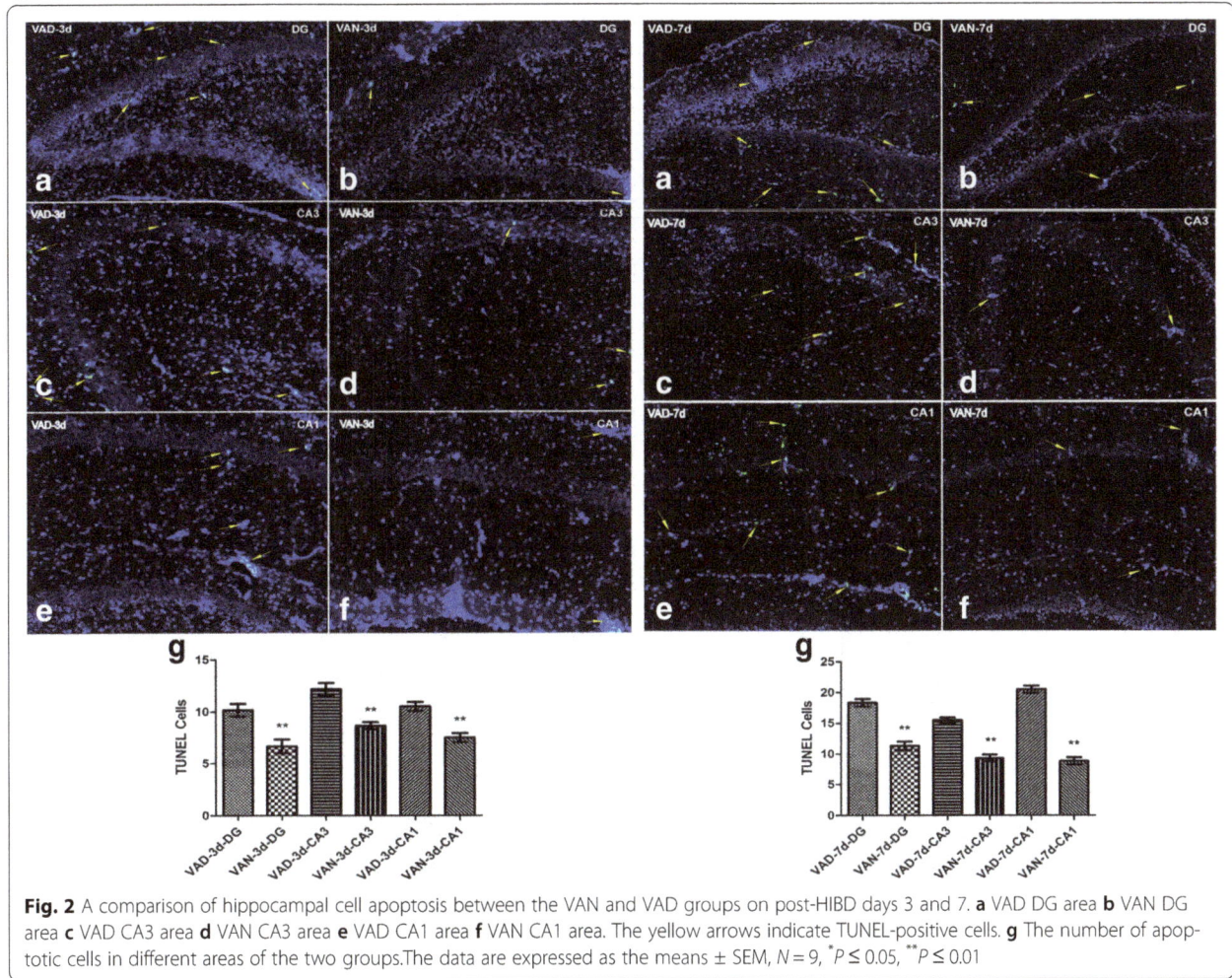

Fig. 2 A comparison of hippocampal cell apoptosis between the VAN and VAD groups on post-HIBD days 3 and 7. **a** VAD DG area **b** VAN DG area **c** VAD CA3 area **d** VAN CA3 area **e** VAD CA1 area **f** VAN CA1 area. The yellow arrows indicate TUNEL-positive cells. **g** The number of apoptotic cells in different areas of the two groups. The data are expressed as the means ± SEM, $N = 9$, $^{*}P \leq 0.05$, $^{**}P \leq 0.01$

d), but the phosphorylated Bad protein expression levels in VAN group were significantly higher than that in VAD group on P3~14 (panel **e**). These results showed that VA could activate the RARα receptor and PI3K through its active metabolite RA, and then further promote the phosphorylation of Akt and Bad.

RA modulates Bcl-2/Bax, Bid/caspase-8, and caspase-3 to influence apoptosis in vivo (Fig. 4)

To understand the effect of RA signaling in detail, we further analyzed several mitochondrial apoptosis-associated molecules. As shown in Fig. 4, the Bcl-2 mRNA and protein expression levels in VAN group were higher than those in VAD group on P7~14 (panels **a, f**). The Bax mRNA levels of VAN group were lower than that of VAD group on P3~7 (panel **b**), and the Bax protein expression level of VAN group was lower than that of VAD group on P14 (panel **f**). In addition, the mRNA and protein expression levels of caspase-8 in VAN group were lower than those in VAD group on P3~7 (panels **c, f**). Similarly, the mRNA and protein expression levels of Bid (a signaling molecule downstream of caspase-8) in VAN group were lower than those

in VAD group on P7~14 (panels **d, f**). Furthermore, it was found that the caspase-3 mRNA and protein levels of VAN group were significantly lower than those of VAD group on P3~7 (panels **e, f**), Finally, the differences in the protein activities of caspase-3 and caspase-8 were analyzed. The protein activities of caspase-3 and caspase-8 in VAN group were significantly lower than those in VAD group on P3~7 (panels **g, h**). These findings revealed that normal VA levels could affect the caspase-8/Bid and caspase-3 pathways through RA signaling and inhibit hippocampal apoptosis.

The apoptosis rate of primary neurons injured by OGD with different concentrations of RA (Fig. 5)

The in vivo tests revealed that normal VA levels can inhibit apoptosis. Attempts were made to discover whether appropriate concentrations of RA could affect neural cell apoptosis after HIBD injury. A concentration range of 0~40 μmol/L of RA were used. As shown in Fig. 5, the apoptosis rates in 1~5 μmol/L concentration range were significantly lower than those of the other concentration groups. However, the apoptosis rates were

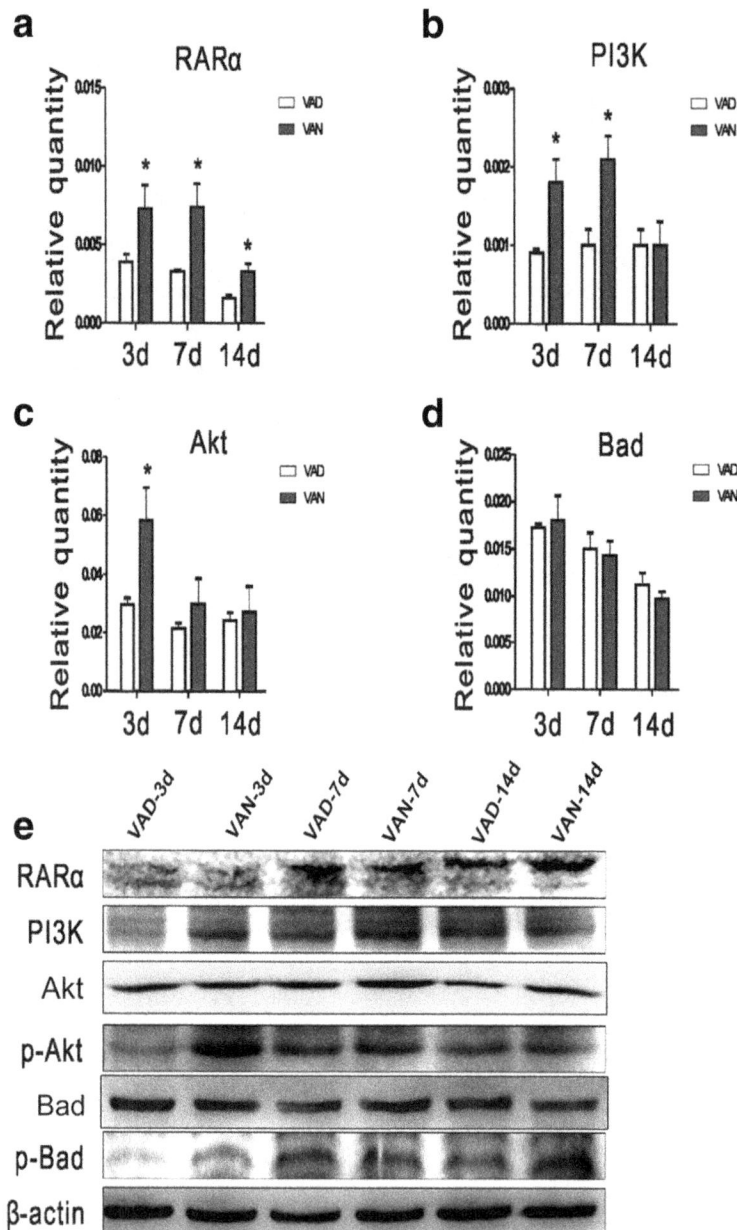

Fig. 3 RA modulates the PI3K/Akt pathway to influence apoptosis via RARα signaling in vivo. **a** The mRNA expressions of RARα in the VAN and VAD groups on P3~14. **b** The mRNA expressions of PI3K in the two groups. **c** The mRNA expressions of Akt in the two groups. **d** The mRNA expression levels of Bad in the two groups. **e** The protein expression levels of RARα, PI3K, Akt, p-Akt, Bad and p-Bad between the two groups in different stages. The data are expressed as the means ± SEM, $N = 9$, $^*P \leq 0.05$, $^{**}P \leq 0.01$

highest at 20~40 μmol/L concentration range. This revealed that neuronal apoptotic protection could be modulated within a physiologically appropriate RA concentration range.

The apoptosis rate of primary neurons injured by OGD at different RA receptor levels (Fig. 6)

The aforementioned findings showed that RA within a suitable concentration range (1~5 μmol/L) protected the neurons from apoptosis. As shown in Fig. 6, the

apoptosis rate of 1 μmol/L RA + OGD group was lower than that of OGD group. And the apoptosis rates in overRARα + 1 μmol/L RA + OGD and siRARα + 1 μmol/L RA + OGD were significantly higer than those of siRARγ + 1 μmol/L RA + OGD group (negative transfection group), which suggest that overexpression and silencing of RARα significantly promoted apoptosis in primary neurons after OGD injury. These results revealed that a moderate level of the RA signal is required to produce an anti-apoptotic effect at the ligand and receptor levels.

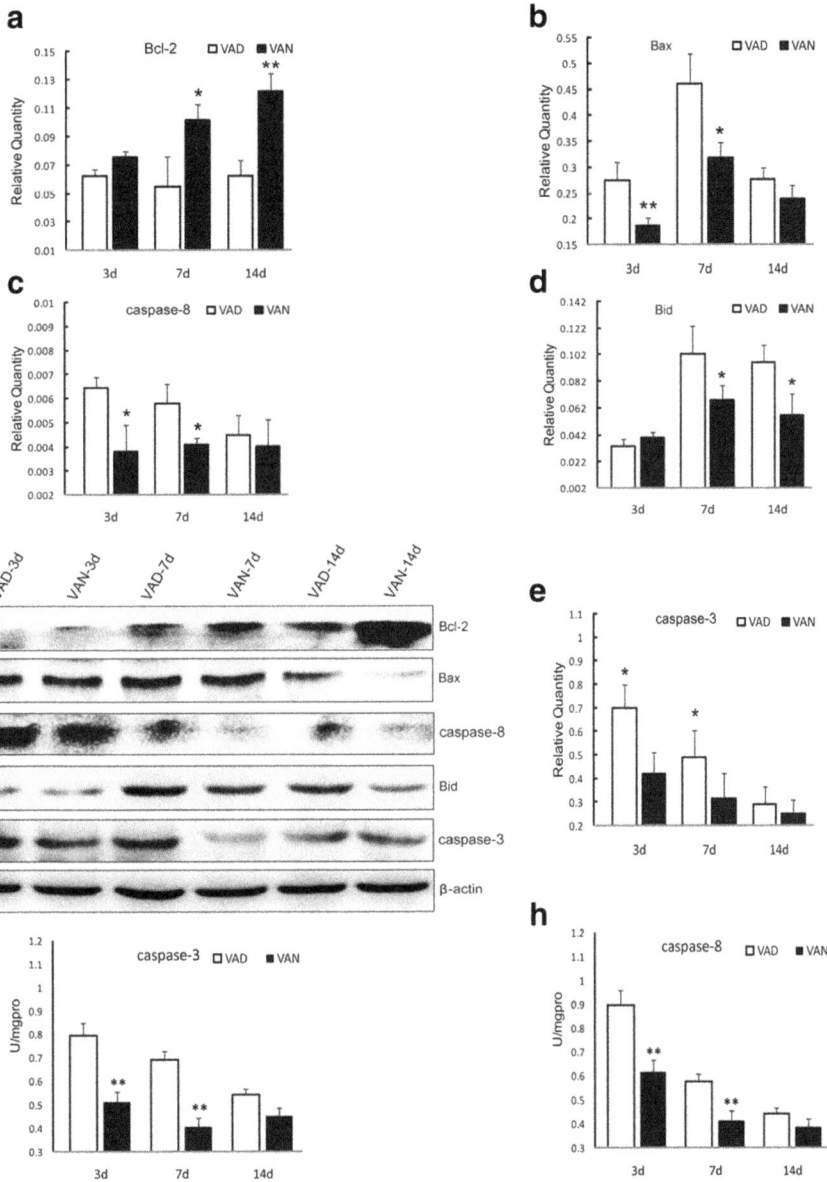

Fig. 4 Hippocampal mRNA and protein levels of the apoptosis pathway in the VAD and VAN groups. **a** The mRNA expression levels of Bcl-2 in the VAN and VAD groups on P3~ 14. **b** The mRNA expression levels of Bax in the two groups. **c** The mRNA expression levels of caspase-8 in in the two groups. **d** The mRNA expression levels of Bid in the two groups. **e** The mRNA expression levels of caspase-3 in the two groups. **f** The protein expression levels of Bcl-2, Bax, caspase-8, Bid, and caspase-3 between the two groups in different stages. **g** The caspase-3 protein activities in the cytoplasm of the VAD and VAN groups. **h** The caspase-8 protein activities in the cytoplasm of the two groups. The data are expressed as the means ± SEM, $N = 9$, $^*P \leq 0.05$, $^{**}P \leq 0.01$

The rate of abnormal mitochondrial membrane potential (MMP) in primary neurons injured by OGD at different RA receptor levels (Fig. 7)

In vivo tests have shown that RA signals can affect multiple signaling pathways, and these signaling pathways are related to mitochondrial apoptosis pathways, such as through MMP. As shown in Fig. 7, the rate of abnormal MMP in overRARα + 1 μmol/L RA + OGD group was the highest of all groups. And abnormal MMP rate in 1 μmol/L RA + OGD group was significantly lower than that in OGD

group or other damage groups. This result revealed that a suitable level of RA signal mitigated MMP abnormalities.

RA modulates the PI3K/Akt pathway to influence apoptosis via RARα signaling in vitro(Fig. 8)

As shown in Fig. 8, different RARα expression levels were used to simulate different levels of RA signaling. The mRNA and protein expression levels of RARα and PI3K in overRARα + 1 μmol/L RA + OGD group and siRARα + 1 μmol/L RA + OGD group were, respectively,

Molecular Neuroscience

a

0μmol/LRA+OGD

Quad	% Gated
UL	0.53
UR	39.42
LL	45.55
LR	14.51

10μmol/LRA+OGD

Quad	% Gated
UL	1.45
UR	28.91
LL	39.21
LR	30.44

1μmol/LRA+OGD

Quad	% Gated
UL	0.60
UR	23.26
LL	63.85
LR	12.30

20μmol/LRA+OGD

Quad	% Gated
UL	0.92
UR	30.06
LL	19.98
LR	49.04

5μmol/LRA+OGD

Quad	% Gated
UL	1.92
UR	18.35
LL	73.07
LR	6.66

40μmol/LRA+OGD

Quad	% Gated
UL	1.14
UR	26.14
LL	26.86
LR	45.87

b

■ Apoptosis Rate

(Bar chart, y-axis 0.0%–90.0%; x-axis: 0μmol/L, 1μmol/L, 5μmol/L, 10μmol/L, 20μmol/L, 40μmol/L; OGD. Significance markers: 1μmol/L ** , 5μmol/L ** , 20μmol/L ** , 40μmol/L *)

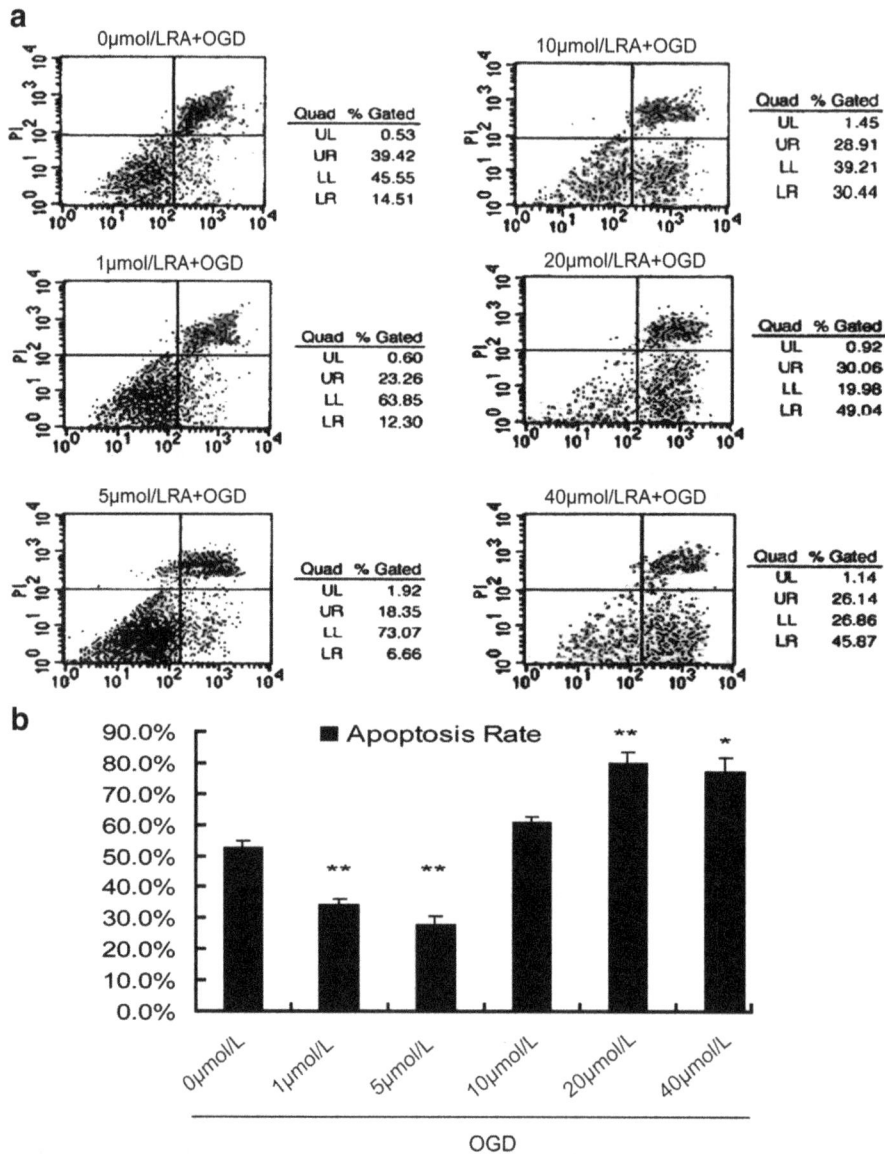

Fig. 5 The apoptosis rate of primary neurons injured by OGD at different concentrations of RA. **a** Flow cytometry for apoptosis in primary hippocampal neurons after 0~ 40 μmol/L RA treatment. **b** A comparison of apoptosis rates for different concentrations of RA. The data are expressed as the means ± SEM, $N = 5$, $^*P \le 0.05$, $^{**}P \le 0.01$

significantly higer and lower than those in siRARγ + 1 μmol/L RA + OGD group. The mRNA and protein expression levels of RARα and PI3K in 1 μmol/L RA + OGD group were higher than those in OGD group (panels **a, c**). The mRNA and protein expression levels of Akt and p-Akt, which are downstream of PI3K, were also similar (panels **b, c**). In addition, no significant difference was noted in mRNA expression of Bad (the p-Akt downstream molecule) among the injury groups, but the protein level of p-Bad, which is activated by p-Akt, was similar to that of PI3K and p-Akt (panels **b, d**). This demonstrated that activation of PI3K via RA signaling can promote the phosphorylation of Akt and further

upregulate phosphorylation of Bad. Finally, Bad was retained in the cytoplasm and inhibited the activation of the mitochondrial apoptotic pathway. Overexpression of RARα yielded the highest PI3K/Akt activation, but this contrasted with the change found in the apoptosis rate of primary neurons.

RA modulates Bcl-2/Bax, Bid/caspase-8, and caspase-3 to influence apoptosis in vitro (Fig. 9)

Interestingly, Fig. 8 shows that a very high RA signal significantly upregulated the PI3K/Akt pathway but did not have a strong anti-apoptotic effect, suggesting that a very high RA signal may significantly activate the other

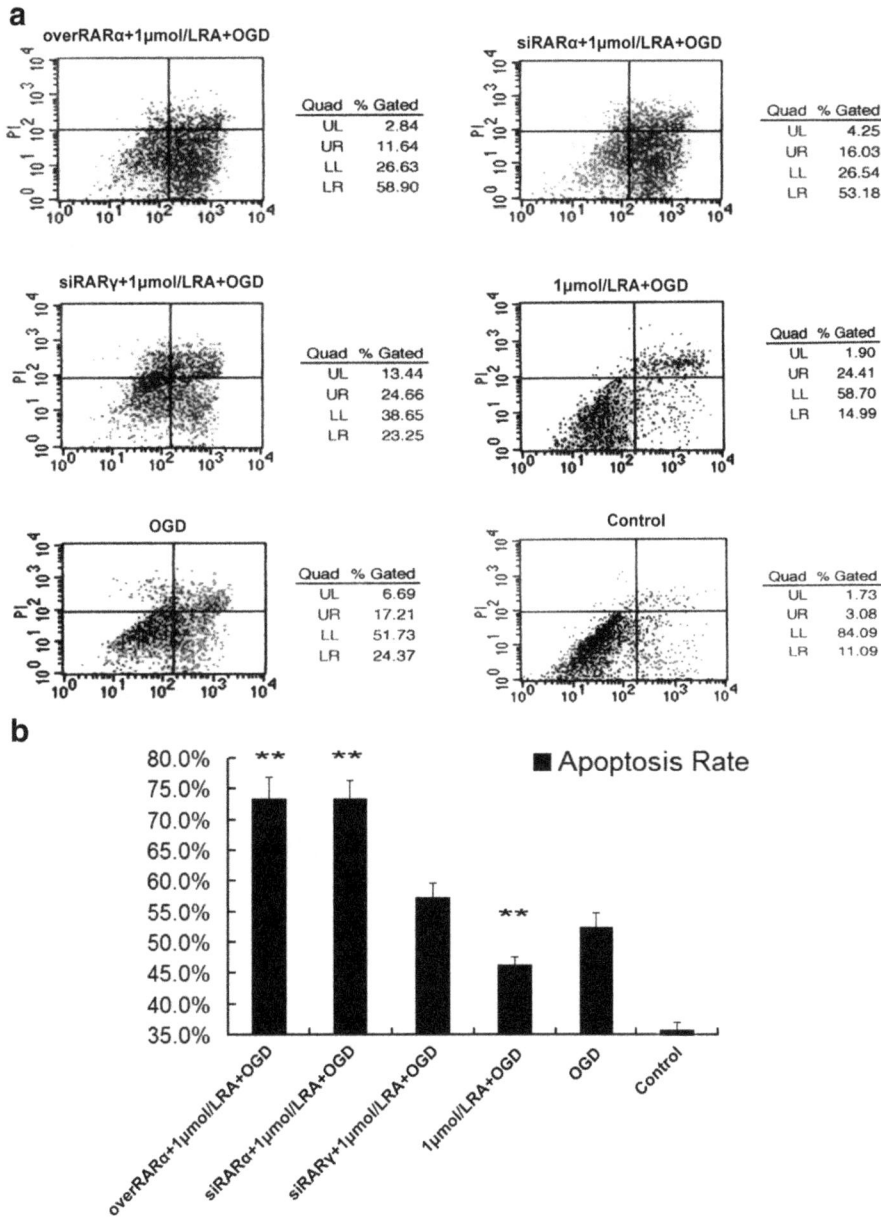

Fig. 6 The apoptosis rate of primary neurons injured by OGD at different RA receptor levels. **a** Flow cytometry for apoptosis in primary hippocampal neurons at different RA receptor levels. The UR (upper right) and LR (lower right) quadrants represent apoptotic cells. **b** A comparison of apoptosis rates for the different RA receptor levels. The data are expressed as the means ± SEM, $N = 5$, $^{*}P \leq 0.05$, $^{**}P \leq 0.01$

apoptotic signaling pathways. As shown in Fig. 9, The mRNA and protein expressions of caspase-3 in over-RARα + 1 μmol/L RA + OGD group and siRARα + 1 μmol/L RA + OGD group were higher than those in siRARγ + 1 μmol/L RA + OGD group. Caspase-8, Bid, Bax were also similar. No differences between the 1 μmol/L RA + OGD and OGD groups were found for the mRNA caspase-3, caspase-8 and Bid. However, the protein expressions of caspase-3, Bid, Bax were lower in 1 μmol/L RA + OGD than those in OGD group. The 1 μmol/L RA + OGD group had higher Bcl-2 mRNA and

protein expressions than those of OGD group. And the protein activities of caspase-3 and caspase-8 in 1 μmol/L RA + OGD group were significantly weaker than those in OGD group. This suggests that RA could directly affect Bcl-2/Bax expression but did not directly affect caspase-3, caspase-8 or Bid expression. Instead, it impacted the activities of caspase-3 and caspase-8, which affected cleavage of Bid and its translocation from the cytoplasm to the mitochondrial membrane. This explains why low and high RA signals can significantly promote apoptosis and why the effect of overexpression

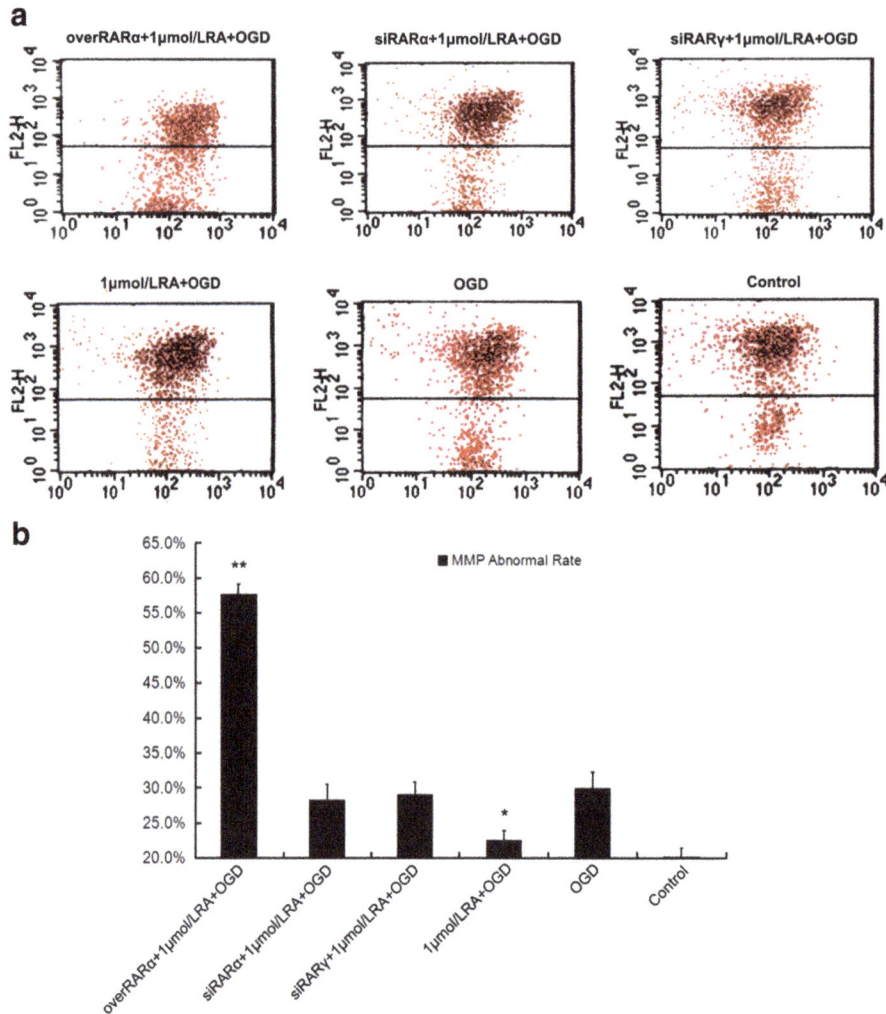

Fig. 7 The rate of abnormal mitochondrial membrane potential in primary neurons injured by OGD at different RA receptor levels. **a** Flow cytometric measurement of the rate of abnormal MMP at different RA receptor levels. The lower quadrants represent cells with abnormal MMP. **b** A comparison of the rates of abnormal MMP for the different RA receptor levels. The data are expressed as the means ± SEM, $N = 5$, $^{*}P \leq 0.05$, $^{**}P \leq 0.01$

was the strongest. Although the overexpression group had the highest activation of anti-apoptotic PI3K/Akt signaling, we noted that Bax, Bid/caspase-8, and caspase-3 expression and activation were also highly promoted. Therefore, the result was a strong pro-apoptotic effect.

Discussion

VA affects long-term neurological function and hippocampal apoptosis after the acute stage of HIBD

HIBD is a brain lesion in perinatal newborns that is caused by hypoxia and decreased cerebral blood perfusion due to neonatal intrauterine asphyxia and anoxia. The global incidence rate is approximately 1/1000 to 3/1000 in full-term infants, with 15–20% mortality. Approximately 25–30% of the survivors have permanent neural defects such as cerebral palsy, epilepsy, memory deficiency, and hypophrenia. No treatment is

currently available, and the pathogenesis of this condition is still not clear [24–26]. The main outcome of HIBD involves neuronal apoptotic processes that spread beyond the immediate ischemic regions [27, 28].

Sufficient VA is required for normal embryonic development and postnatal tissue homeostasis, including cell proliferation, tissue differentiation, immunoregulation, and organogenesis. VAD can modify the structure of the macromolecular components of extracellular matrix, and such alterations potentially leads to organ dysfunction and diseases [29]. Moreover, VAD in gestation and early life leads to spatial learning and memory lesions in adolescence: this process involves the molecular interactions of retinoid acid nuclear receptor α (RARα) [18]. RA acts as a ligand to integrate with RA receptors and receptor-specific nuclear receptor response elements, switching transcription factors from potential repressors to

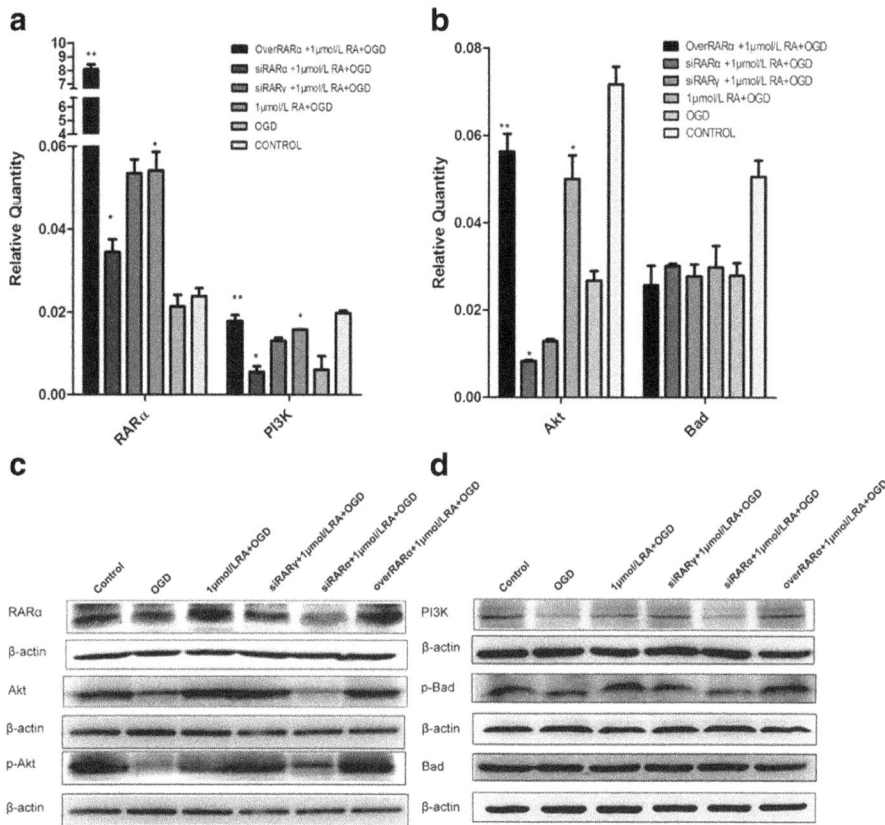

Fig. 8 mRNA and protein levels of the PI3K/Akt signaling pathway in primary hippocampal neurons after OGD injury. **a** With different RA receptor levels, the mRNA expressions of RARα and PI3K in the different groups. **b** With different RA receptor levels, the mRNA expressions of Akt and Bad in the different groups. **c**, **d** With different RA receptor levels, the protein expression levels of RARα, PI3K, Akt, p-Akt, p-Bad and Bad among all the intervention groups. The data are expressed as the means ± SEM, $N = 5$, $^{*}P \leq 0.05$, $^{**}P \leq 0.01$

transcriptional stimulators. RA plays a pivotal role in early phases of neurogenesis, neuronal survival, and synaptic plasticity, and is an essential contributor during development that enables proper cognitive function in adolescence [30–32].

A previous study elucidated that VAD could inhibit learning and spatial memory retrieval via the RARα signaling pathway in the early stage following HIBD [4]. Our results showed that the VAN and VAS groups had advantages in learning and spatial memory after HIBD (Fig. 1). The findings indicate that suitable VA nutritional status is beneficial for the neurological function of newborns with HIBD, and perhaps VA should be included as part of the standard HIBD clinical intervention. Zhu found that RA reduced infarct size and cardiomyocyte apoptosis in myocardial ischemia/reperfusion (I/R) injury [33]. Kong suggested that RA may serve as a new therapeutic approach to prevent blood brain barrier (BBB) dysfunction and tPA-induced rat ICH in ischemic stroke, and the protective effect of RA on the BBB was dependent on RARα [34]. The hippocampal TUNEL test demonstrated that VAN

decreased the apoptosis in the CA1, CA3, and DG regions at the acute stage of HIBD. This finding confirmed the histological results (Fig. 2).

RA signal mediates mitochondrial apoptosis depending on signaling intensity

The in vivo experiment showed that rats with normal physiological levels of VA had better learning and spatial memory than rats with VAD, and the advantage was associated with lower levels of apoptosis in the hippocampus. A number of studies have suggested that an excess of VA can affect neurological development. RA can promote carcinoma cell apoptosis, and large doses of RA are currently applied therapeutically for certain types of cancer [12]. However, RA inhibits the apoptosis of neural cells in rat ischemic stroke [34]. Wang revealed that all-trans retinoic acid (1~10 μmol/L) inhibited cobalt chloride-induced apoptosis in PC12 cells [35]. Upon in depth analysis, it was found that higher doses of RA caused the apoptosis of immune cells and tumors, whereas a smaller dose was

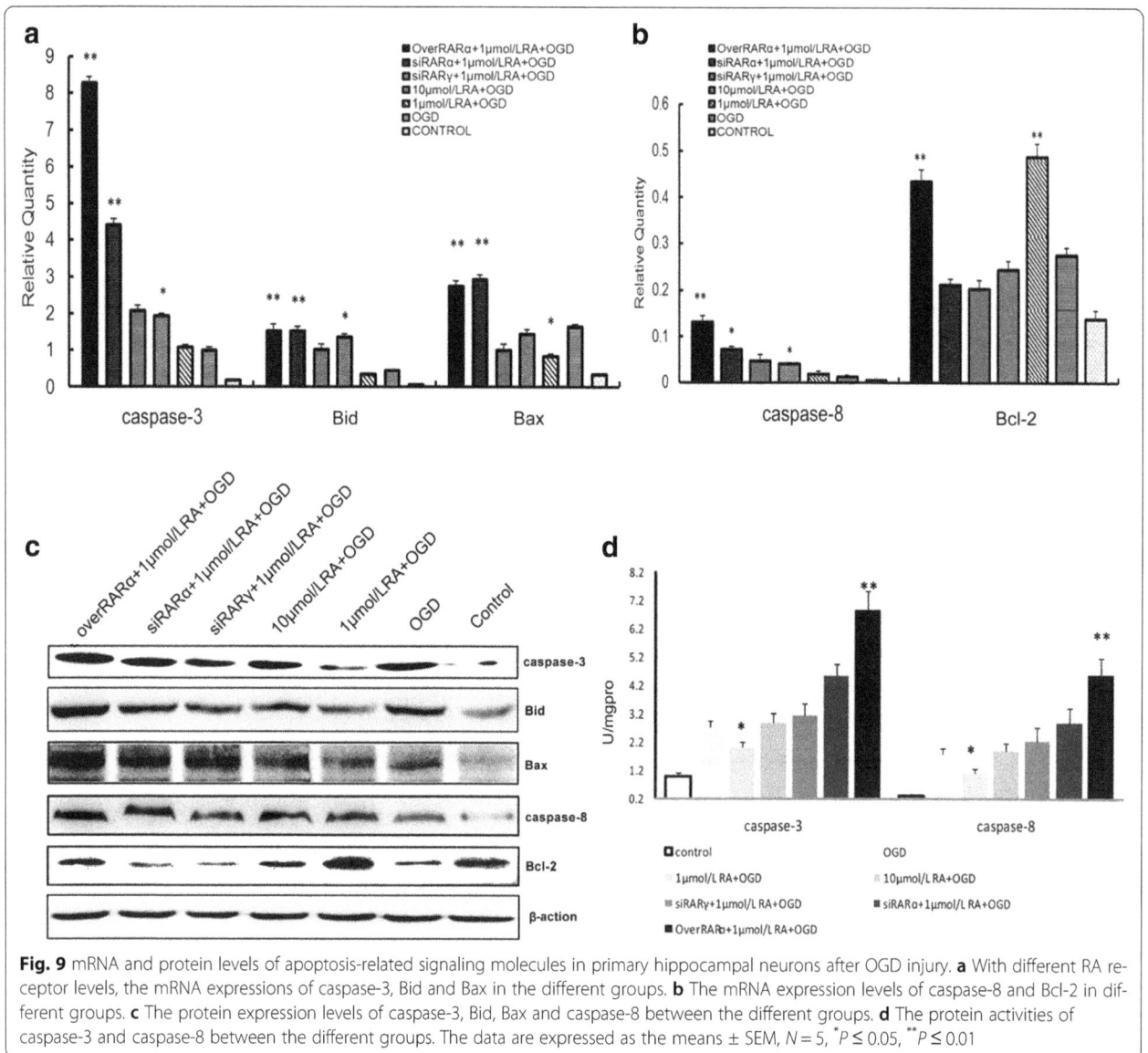

Fig. 9 mRNA and protein levels of apoptosis-related signaling molecules in primary hippocampal neurons after OGD injury. **a** With different RA receptor levels, the mRNA expressions of caspase-3, Bid and Bax in the different groups. **b** The mRNA expression levels of caspase-8 and Bcl-2 in different groups. **c** The protein expression levels of caspase-3, Bid, Bax and caspase-8 between the different groups. **d** The protein activities of caspase-3 and caspase-8 between the different groups. The data are expressed as the means ± SEM, $N = 5$, $^*P \leq 0.05$, $^{**}P \leq 0.01$

required for protection from ischemia in the nerves and myocardial tissue. It is speculated that appropriate RA signaling could inhibit the apoptosis of hippocampal neurons in HIBD. In vitro tests supported the hypothesis that $1\sim5$ μmol/L was the optimal concentration range for anti-apoptotic effects; excessively high or low dose were pro-apoptotic (Fig. 5). Moreover, it was demonstrated through overexpression and silencing of RARα that suitable RA signaling is necessary for the anti-apoptotic effect (Fig. 6). Furthermore, it was found that RA can affect the initial events of mitochondrial apoptosis (MMP). Appropriate RA signaling showed the lowest rate of an abnormal MMP, which was consistent with previous findings [16, 17].

Suitable RA signaling upregulated the PI3K/Akt/Bad and Bcl-2/Bax pathways and downregulated the caspase-8/Bid pathway to protect MMP and thereby inhibit mitochondrial apoptosis

The molecular mechanisms that underlie the effect of RA on hippocampal neuronal apoptosis in HIBD are not clear. Currently, activation of the PI3K/Akt signaling pathway is known to be related to neuronal survival and anti-apoptotic effects after ischemic damage. Zhang et al. and Huang et al. found that increased production and activation of PI3K/Akt can antagonize the apoptosis induced by OGD injury [36, 37]. The neuroprotective mechanisms of Ginsenoside Rb1 and the defense of mesenchymal stromal cells against neuronal apoptosis produced by an ischemic insult occurred through the activation of PI3K/Akt signaling [38, 39]. Accumulating evidence has revealed that PI3K/Akt plays a principal role in the resistance against neural injury. However, a number of studies have shown that RA regulates the PI3K/Akt signaling pathway in some types of cells. Uruno et al. demonstrated that RA played an important role in vascular endothelial cells through RAR-mediated PI3K/Akt pathway activation, in which nitricoxide was produced to resist vascular disease in the event of an endothelial insult [40]. This has been demonstrated in vivo (Fig. 3) and in vitro (Fig. 8).

Bad (Bcl-associated death protein) is a recognized pro-apoptotic protein, and the active form is phosphorylated on its serine residues. Free Bad may cause a decrease in MMP via translocation from the cytosol to the mitochondrial membrane to displace pro-apoptotic Bax (Bcl-2-associated X protein) from the anti-apoptotic Bcl-XL, and Bax subsequently translocates to the mitochondrion and induces cytochrome c release and caspase activation. Bad loses this pro-apoptotic effect after it is phosphorylated and combines with the cytosolic protein 14–3-3 [1, 2]. The phosphorylation of Bad is the target of the PI3K/Akt pathway. Neuregulin-1 upregulates p-Bad through activation of the PI3K/Akt signaling pathway to restrain neuronal apoptosis after transient focal cerebral ischemia [41]. Additionally, astaxanthin upregulates the phosphorylation of Akt/Bad, thus activating the Akt/Bad signaling pathway to dramatically decrease neuronal apoptosis in the early stages of brain damage [42]. In the present study, the expression of PI3K/p-Akt/p-Bad was significantly enhanced in RA-treated primary neurons (Fig. 8) and VAN rats (Fig. 3). Interestingly, the effects on the trends in the PI3K, p-Akt, and p-Bad expression levels were consistent with the changes in the expression level of RARα after infection of OGD-injured neurons with adenovirus (Fig. 8). However, this process depends on the phosphorylation of Bad protein and cannot impact the transcription of the Bad gene. The preliminary results demonstrated that RA regulated the downstream PI3K/Akt signaling cascade via RARα signaling to accelerate the survival of cultured primary neuronal cells and prevent apoptosis, and the effect was dependent on the signal intensity.

Interactions between the Bcl-2 family proteins determine whether cells live or die. The expression levels of Bcl-2 and Bax and the ratio of Bcl-2 to Bax are important factors in mitochondrial apoptosis [43]. Meanwhile, the expression of Bcl-2 and CCND1 was enhanced. In contrast, URG4/URGCP and Bax gene expression declined significantly [44]. The in vivo results demonstrated that the VAN rats had higher Bcl-2 and lower Bax expression than the VAD rats (Fig. 4). The in vitro data showed that suitable RA signal intensity promoted Bcl-2 and inhibits Bax expression, thereby increasing the ratio of Bcl-2 to Bax (Fig. 9). Thus, it suppresses the decrease of MMP (Fig. 7).

The caspase-8/Bid pathway is also an important signaling cascade that impacts MMP in mitochondrial apoptosis [45]. Caspase-3 is the pivotal signal of the apoptotic pathway in neuronal cells [46]. The in vivo results of the present study revealed that the VAN group had lower caspase-8/Bid and caspase-3 expression or activity than the VAD group (Fig. 4). In addition, the in vitro data showed that a suitable RA signal intensity restrained the expression and activity of caspase-8 and caspase-3 (Fig. 9). Interestingly, only a certain optimal range of RA signals significantly inhibited the expression or activity of caspase-8/Bid and caspase-3. Although the overexpression of RARα activates the PI3K/Akt/Bad pathway and Bcl-2, upregulation of caspase-8/Bid and caspase-3 leads to pro-apoptotic signals. Therefore, the balance of these signals is very important in the control of hippocampal apoptosis after HIBD.

Conclusions

In conclusion, after HIBD, sustained VAD caused underexpression of RARα, which downregulated PI3K/Akt/Bad and Bcl-2 signaling. The Bax, caspase-8/Bid, and caspase-3 pathways were also upregulated to reduce MMP and activate mitochondrial apoptosis, ultimately producing deficits in active learning and spatial memory in adolescence. VAS can partly repair the deficit. Meanwhile, excessively high or low RA signals can promote mitochondrial apoptosis. RA signaling bio-modulates mitochondrial apoptosis depending on the signal intensity. A high RA signal activated the PI3K/Akt/Bad pathway which failed to produce anti-apoptotic signals because caspase-8/Bid and caspase-3 signaling was upregulated. These findings suggest that clinical interventions for newborns with HIBD should include a suitable dosage of VA.

Additional files

Additional file 1 Figure S1. (A) HIBD newborns (50 cases): serum VA is 0.474 μmol/L; newborns with neonatal pneumonia (65 cases): 0.761 μmol/L; normal newborns (15 cases): 0.844 μmol/L ($^{**}P \leq 0.01$, $^{*}P \leq$ 0.05, one-way ANOVA). (B) HIBD children with VAD: The incidence of VAD (87.8%) was significantly higher than that in children with pneumonia (40%) ($^{**}P \leq 0.01$, $^{*}P \leq 0.05$, chi-squared test). (C) Newborns over 7 days old had no significant difference in VA level compared with newborns under 7 days old, but the VA level was significantly higher in neonatal pneumonia cases and in normal newborns ($^{**}P \leq 0.01$, $^{*}P \leq 0.05$, one-way ANOVA).

Additional file 2 Figure S2. (A) The experimental flow chart. (B) The special feed formulations for the vitamin A deficiency (VAD) and normal (VAN) groups. (C) The vitamin A level of the VAD, VAN, VA supplement (VAS), and control groups during the course of the study. The VA level of VAN rats ($N = 50$) was significantly higher than that of VAD rats ($N = 50$) at every stage after HIBD ($^{**}P \leq 0.01$, $^{*}P \leq 0.05$, SNK). The VA level of VAS rats ($N = 50$) was significantly higher than that of VAD rats ($N = 50$) on post-HIBD days 7–40(P7–P40) ($^{**}P \leq 0.01$, $^{*}P \leq 0.05$, SNK). The VA levels of all the groups had an increasing trend from P1 to P40. The data are expressed as the means ± SEM.

Abbreviations
HIBD: Hypoxic-ischemic brain damage; MMP: Mitochondrial membrane potential; RARE: Retinoic acid response element; OGD: Oxygen-glucose deprivation; RA: Retinoic acid; RARα: Retinoid acid nuclear receptor α; VA: Vitamin A; VAD: Vitamin A deficiency; VAN: Vitamin A normal; VAS: Vitamin A supplemented

Acknowledgements
This work was supported by grants from the National Natural Science Foundation of China (No. 81571091), National Youth Foundation of China (No. 81100454), and the Key Project of the National Natural Science Foundation of China (No. 30830106).

Funding
This work was supported by the National Natural Science Foundation of China (No. 81571091 and No. 30830106), and National Youth Foundation of China (No. 81100454).

Authors' contributions
WJ, YB, JC and TL designed the research. WJ and MG performed experiments. MG, LC, YZ and PQ helped in experiments. YS, YL and JC analyzed the data. WJ, MG, JC and TL wrote the paper. All authors read and approved the final manuscript

Competing interests
The authors declare that they have no competing interests.

Author details
[1]Children Nutrition Research Center, Children's Hospital of Chongqing Medical University, Chongqing 400014, China. [2]Ministry of Education Key Laboratory of Child Development and Disorders, Chongqing 400014, China. [3]China International Science and Technology Cooperation Base of Child Development and Critical Disorders, Chongqing 400014, China. [4]Chongqing Key Laboratory of Translational Medical Research in Cognitive Development and Learning and Memory Disorders, Chongqing 400014, China. [5]Children Rehabilitation Center, Children's Hospital of Chongqing Medical University, Chongqing, China.

References
1. Yu C, et al. JNK suppresses apoptosis via phosphorylation of the proapoptotic Bcl-2 family protein BAD. Mol Cell. 2004;13(3):329–40.
2. Deng H, et al. Phosphorylation of bad at Thr-201 by JNK1 promotes glycolysis through activation of phosphofructokinase-1. J Biol Chem. 2008; 283(30):20754–60.
3. Kim JJ, et al. Cost-effective therapeutic hypothermia treatment device for hypoxic ischemic encephalopathy. Med Devices (Auckl). 2013;6:1–10.
4. Jiang W, et al. Vitamin A deficiency impairs postnatal cognitive function via inhibition of neuronal calcium excitability in hippocampus. J Neurochem. 2012;121(6):932–43.
5. Squire LR. Memory and the hippocampus: a synthesis from findings with rats, monkeys, and humans. Psychol Rev. 1992;99(2):195–231.
6. Sun Y, et al. Apoptosis-inducing factor downregulation increased neuronal progenitor, but not stem cell, survival in the neonatal hippocampus after cerebral hypoxia-ischemia. Mol Neurodegener. 2012;7:17.
7. Misner DL, et al. Vitamin A deprivation results in reversible loss of hippocampal long-term synaptic plasticity. Proc Natl Acad Sci U S A. 2001; 98(20):11714–9.
8. Gutierrez-Mazariegos J, et al. Vitamin A: a multifunctional tool for development. Semin Cell Dev Biol. 2011;22(6):603–10.
9. Das BC, et al. Retinoic acid signaling pathways in development and diseases. Bioorg Med Chem. 2014;22(2):673–83.
10. Duong V, Rochette-Egly C. The molecular physiology of nuclear retinoic acid receptors. From health to disease. Biochim Biophys Acta. 2011; 1812(8):1023–31.
11. Samarut E, Rochette-Egly C. Nuclear retinoic acid receptors: conductors of the retinoic acid symphony during development. Mol Cell Endocrinol. 2012; 348(2):348–60.
12. Alvarez R, et al. Functions, therapeutic applications, and synthesis of retinoids and carotenoids. Chem Rev. 2014;114(1):1–125.
13. Trasino SE, Benoit YD, Gudas LJ. Vitamin A deficiency causes hyperglycemia and loss of pancreatic beta-cell mass. J Biol Chem. 2015;290(3):1456–73.
14. Noy N. Between death and survival: retinoic acid in regulation of apoptosis. Annu Rev Nutr. 2010;30:201–17.
15. Zhang X, et al. Effect of marginal vitamin A deficiency during pregnancy on retinoic acid receptors and N-methyl-D-aspartate receptor expression in the offspring of rats. J Nutr Biochem. 2011; 22(12):1112–20.
16. Cheng O, et al. Baicalin improved the spatial learning ability of global ischemia/reperfusion rats by reducing hippocampal apoptosis. Brain Res. 2012;1470:111–8.
17. Zhang X, et al. All-trans retinoic acid suppresses apoptosis in PC12 cells injured by oxygen and glucose deprivation via the retinoic acid receptor alpha signaling pathway. Mol Med Rep. 2014;10(5):2549–55.
18. Hou N, et al. Vitamin A deficiency impairs spatial learning and memory: the mechanism of abnormal CBP-dependent histone acetylation regulated by retinoic acid receptor alpha. Mol Neurobiol. 2015;51(2):633–47.
19. Rice JE 3rd, Vannucci RC, Brierley JB. The influence of immaturity on hypoxic-ischemic brain damage in the rat. Ann Neurol. 1981;9(2):131–41.
20. Chen K, et al. Effects of vitamin A, vitamin A plus iron and multiple micronutrient-fortified seasoning powder on preschool children in a suburb of Chongqing, China. J Nutr Sci Vitaminol (Tokyo). 2008;54(6):440–7.
21. Morris R. Developments of a water-maze procedure for studying spatial learning in the rat. J Neurosci Methods. 1984;11(1):47–60.
22. Das A, et al. Post-treatment with voltage-gated Na(+) channel blocker attenuates kainic acid-induced apoptosis in rat primary hippocampal neurons. Neurochem Res. 2010;35(12):2175–83.
23. WHO. Indicators for Assessing Vitamin A Deficiency and their Application in Monitoring and Evaluating Intervention Programmes. Geneva: WHO; 1996.
24. Kurinczuk JJ, White-Koning M, Badawi N. Epidemiology of neonatal encephalopathy and hypoxic-ischaemic encephalopathy. Early Hum Dev. 2010;86(6):329–38.
25. Frisch D, Msall ME. Health, functioning, and participation of adolescents and adults with cerebral palsy: a review of outcomes research. Dev Disabil Res Rev. 2013;18(1):84–94.
26. van Laerhoven H, et al. Prognostic tests in term neonates with hypoxic-ischemic encephalopathy: a systematic review. Pediatrics. 2013;131(1):88–98.
27. Busl KM, Greer DM. Hypoxic-ischemic brain injury: pathophysiology, neuropathology and mechanisms. NeuroRehabilitation. 2010;26(1):5–13.
28. Distefano G, Pratico AD. Actualities on molecular pathogenesis and repairing processes of cerebral damage in perinatal hypoxic-ischemic encephalopathy. Ital J Pediatr. 2010;36:63.
29. Barber T, et al. Vitamin a deficiency and alterations in the extracellular matrix. Nutrients. 2014;6(11):4984–5017.
30. Jacobs S, et al. Retinoic acid is required early during adult neurogenesis in the dentate gyrus. Proc Natl Acad Sci U S A. 2006;103(10):3902–7.
31. Olson CR, Mello CV. Significance of vitamin a to brain function, behavior and learning. Mol Nutr Food Res. 2010;54(4):489–95.
32. Rhinn M, Dolle P. Retinoic acid signalling during development. Development. 2012;139(5):843–58.
33. Zhu Z, et al. All-trans retinoic acid ameliorates myocardial ischemia/ reperfusion injury by reducing cardiomyocyte apoptosis. PLoS One. 2015; 10(7):e0133414.

34. Kong L, et al. Retinoic acid ameliorates blood-brain barrier disruption following ischemic stroke in rats. Pharmacol Res. 2015;99:125–36.

35. Wang S, et al. All-trans retinoic acid inhibits cobalt chloride-induced apoptosis in PC12 cells: role of the dimethylarginine dimethylaminohydrolase/asymmetric dimethylarginine pathway. J Neurosci Res. 2009;87(8):1938–46.

36. Zhang Q, et al. Puerarin protects differentiated PC12 cells from H(2)O(2)-induced apoptosis through the PI3K/Akt signalling pathway. Cell Biol Int. 2012;36(5):419–26.

37. Huang Y, et al. Panaxatriol saponins attenuated oxygen-glucose deprivation injury in PC12 cells via activation of PI3K/Akt and Nrf2 signaling pathway. Oxidative Med Cell Longev. 2014;2014:978034.

38. Schcibe F, et al. Mesenchymal stromal cells rescue cortical neurons from apoptotic cell death in an in vitro model of cerebral ischemia. Cell Mol Neurobiol. 2012;32(4):567–76.

39. Luo T, et al. Inhibition of autophagy via activation of PI3K/Akt pathway contributes to the protection of ginsenoside Rb1 against neuronal death caused by ischemic insults. Int J Mol Sci. 2014;15(9):15426–42.

40. Uruno A, et al. Upregulation of nitric oxide production in vascular endothelial cells by all-trans retinoic acid through the phosphoinositide 3-kinase/Akt pathway. Circulation. 2005;112(5):727–36.

41. Guo WP, et al. Neuregulin-1 regulates the expression of Akt, Bcl-2, and bad signaling after focal cerebral ischemia in rats. Biochem Cell Biol. 2010;88(4):649–54.

42. Zhang XS, et al. Astaxanthin alleviates early brain injury following subarachnoid hemorrhage in rats: possible involvement of Akt/bad signaling. Mar Drugs. 2014;12(8):4291–310.

43. Ku B, et al. Evidence that inhibition of BAX activation by BCL-2 involves its tight and preferential interaction with the BH3 domain of BAX. Cell Res. 2011;21(4):627–41.

44. Dodurga Y, et al. Expression of URG4/URGCP, cyclin D1, Bcl-2, and Bax genes in retinoic acid treated SH-SY5Y human neuroblastoma cells. Contemp Oncol (Pozn). 2013;17(4):346–9.

45. Schug ZT, et al. BID is cleaved by caspase-8 within a native complex on the mitochondrial membrane. Cell Death Differ. 2011;18(3):538–48.

46. D'Amelio M, Cavallucci V, Cecconi F. Neuronal caspase-3 signaling: not only cell death. Cell Death Differ. 2010;17(7):1104–14.

14

Tanshinone I alleviates motor and cognitive impairments via suppressing oxidative stress in the neonatal rats after hypoxic-ischemic brain damage

Chunfang Dai[1,2,3], Yannan Liu[1,2,3] and Zhifang Dong[1,2,3]*

Abstract

Neonatal hypoxia-ischemia is one of the main reasons that cause neuronal damage and neonatal death. Several studies have shown that tanshinone I (TsI), one of the major ingredients of Danshen, exerts potential neuroprotective effect in adult mice exposed to permanent left cerebral ischemia. However, it is unclear whether administration of TsI has neuroprotective effect on neonatal hypoxic-ischemic brain damage (HIBD), and if so, the potential mechanisms also remain unclear. Here, we reported that treatment with TsI (5 mg/kg, i.p.) significantly alleviated the deficits of myodynamia and motor functions as well as the spatial learning and memory in the rat model of HIBD. These behavioral changes were accompanied by a significant decrease in the number of neuronal loss in the CA1 area of hippocampus. Moreover, ELISA assay showed that TsI significantly increased the production of antioxidants including total antioxidant capacity (T-AOC), glutathione (GSH), total superoxide dismutase (T-SOD) and catalase (CAT), and reduced the production of pro-oxidants including hydrogen peroxide (H_2O_2), total nitric oxide synthase (T-NOS) and inducible nitric oxide synthase (iNOS). Taken together, these results indicate that TsI presents potential neuroprotection against neuronal damage via exerting significantly antioxidative activity and against pro-oxidant challenge, thereby ameliorating hypoxia-ischemia-induced motor and cognitive impairments in the neonatal rats, suggesting that TsI may be a potential therapeutic agent against HIBD.

Keywords: Hypoxic-ischemic brain damage, Tanshinone I, Learning and memory, Oxidative stress

Introduction

Neonatal hypoxic-ischemic encephalopathy (HIE), which is caused by perinatal hypoxia-ischemia, is one of the major reasons that lead to neuronal damage and neonatal death. The incidence of HIE is about 1 to 3 per 1000 term births [1, 2], and up to 40,000 to 50,000 infants are affected each year in China. The survivor exhibits motor disability or a variety of serious neurological sequela, such as cerebral palsy, epilepsy, severe learning impairment or intellectual deficiency [3–5], which diminish the quality of life of HIE children and increase the enormous burden of economic and spirit on their families and society. Therefore, the research for a potential neuroprotective therapy in order to guide the clinical treatment for HIE is particularly important.

Recent studies have proposed that oxidative injury to vital cellular structures contributes to the pathogenesis of HIE [6]. The potential mechanism underlying oxidative injury in HIE is that the neonatal brain is selectively vulnerable to oxidative stress, which results in altered reactive oxygen species metabolism [7] including the increased accumulation of hydrogen peroxide and subsequent neurotoxicity [8]. In addition, the brain of neonatal is immature and the nervous system exerts immature antioxidant defenses, which display less activity in antioxidant enzyme systems including superoxide

* Correspondence: zfdong@aliyun.com
[1]Ministry of Education Key Laboratory of Child Development and Disorders, Children's Hospital of Chongqing Medical University, 136 Zhongshan Er Road, Yuzhong District, Chongqing 400014, People's Republic of China
[2]Chongqing Key Laboratory of Translational Medical Research in Cognitive Development and Learning and Memory Disorders, Children's Hospital of Chongqing Medical University, 136 Zhongshan Er Road, Yuzhong District, Chongqing 400014, People's Republic of China
Full list of author information is available at the end of the article

dismutase (SOD) and glutathione peroxides [9, 10]. There is a growing body of evidence has shown that oxidative stress results in calcium mobilization and cell damage via providing the link between activation of glutamate receptors and the intracellular cascade of events. Those findings explain the appearance of delayed cell death and secondary energy failure, suggesting that the inhibition of oxidative stress may be a potential therapeutic for HIE [11].

Danshen (Radix salvia miltiorrhiza root), an annual sage plant, is among the most popular medicinal herbs used in China, whose extract as an antihypertensive and a sedative is widely used for the treatment of cardiovascular and cerebrovascular diseases in recent years [12–14]. The water-soluble Danshen extracts contain several diterpene quinine analogs including tanshinone I (TsI), tanshinone II (TsII), cryptotanshinone (CTs) and dihydrotanshinone I (DTsI) [15], which are able to penetrate the blood-brain barrier [16]. Given its antioxidantive and anti-inflammatory effects both in vitro [17–19] and in vivo [19–21], tanshinone is of particular therapeutic interest in hypoxic-ischemic brain damage (HIBD). Indeed, both TsI and TsII including TsIIA and TsIIB, have obvious potential for neuroprotection against hypoxia-ischemia injury in adult mice and rat [22–24]. In addition, treatment with TsIIA significantly reduced the severity of brain injury induced by hypoxia-ischemia in the immature rat [25, 26]. However, there is no any report on the influence of TsI on motor and cognitive functions in neonatal rat after HIBD.

As aforementioned, TsI has potential anti-oxidative activity. We therefore hypothesize that TsI may present neuroprotective effects through suppressing oxidative stress, and subsequently improve motor function and learning and memory ability in neonatal rat model of HIBD. In the present study, we investigated this hypothesis using a combination of behavioral test, immunohistochemical and anti-oxidative activity analysis in the neonatal rat model of HIBD.

Methods
Experimental animals
Unsexed 7-day-old Sprague-Dawley (SD) rats were used to establish the HIBD model as previously described, with modification [27]. Briefly, the left carotid artery of 7-day postnatal rats was ligated and 2 h later the pups were exposed to hypoxic conditions (8% O_2 + 92% N_2) for 2.5 h at 37 °C. The sham animals were only separated out the left carotid artery without ligation and no exposure to hypoxic conditions. Immediately after hypoxic treatment, pups were transferred back to the nest with their dam until weaning on postnatal day 21, and they were housed in plastic cages with unlimited access to

food and water and maintained in a temperature-controlled colony room (21 °C) under a cycle of 12-h light/12-h dark (8:00 am - 8:00 pm).

TsI treatment
To illustrate the neuroprotective effects of TsI against HIBD, all pups were divided into four groups: sham, sham + TsI, HIBD + saline, HIBD + TsI. TsI was purchased from selleck (Shanghai, China) and dissolved in sterile saline containing 0.5% dimethyl sulfoxide (DMSO). The rats in sham + TsI and HIBD + TsI groups received intraperitoneal (i.p.) injection of TsI at a dose of 5 mg/kg/day from 1 day before hypoxic-ischemic surgery (postnatal day 6) for 7 days, and the second injection was conducted 6 h before the surgery (Fig. 1a), as reported previously [23, 26].

To further examine the therapeutic effects of TsI against HIBD, some rats received 7-day treatment of TsI (5 mg/kg/day, i.p.) from postnatal day 7 to 13, and the first injection was conducted immediately after HIBD (Fig. 3a).

Grasping test
Grasping test was used to evaluate myodynamia according to the instruction (Chatillon, USA). Briefly, 3 weeks after HIBD model established, the left and right forelimbs of each rat were placed on the grasping force sensor, respectively. Gently pulled the trail and recorded the last maximum tensile force until the rat cannot hold on. The myodynamia of left or right forelimb was measured 5 times and mean value was calculated to illustrate the myodynamia of the rats. The Grip Strength Meter was cleaned with 70% ethanol and water between tests.

Rotarod test
Rotarod test was used to evaluate motor performance as previously described, with modifications [28]. Briefly, after grasping test, each rat received 2 rounds of pre-training trials (one trial at 0 rpm and the other trial at 20 rpm) on the rotarod (Stoelting Co.). Twenty-four hours after the pre-training, rats were received formal rotarod test in ten consecutive trials (20-min intervals) with an initial rotation of 5 rpm to last rotation 50 rpm (increasing by 5 rpm each time). The time that the animals remained on the rotarod during each test was monitored, and maximum test time (cut-off limit) was 180 s. The latency to fall off the rotarod was used to express the motor performance. The rotarod was cleaned with 70% ethanol and water between tests.

The Morris water maze test
Four weeks after HIBD, the Morris water maze test was performed to measure spatial learning and memory as

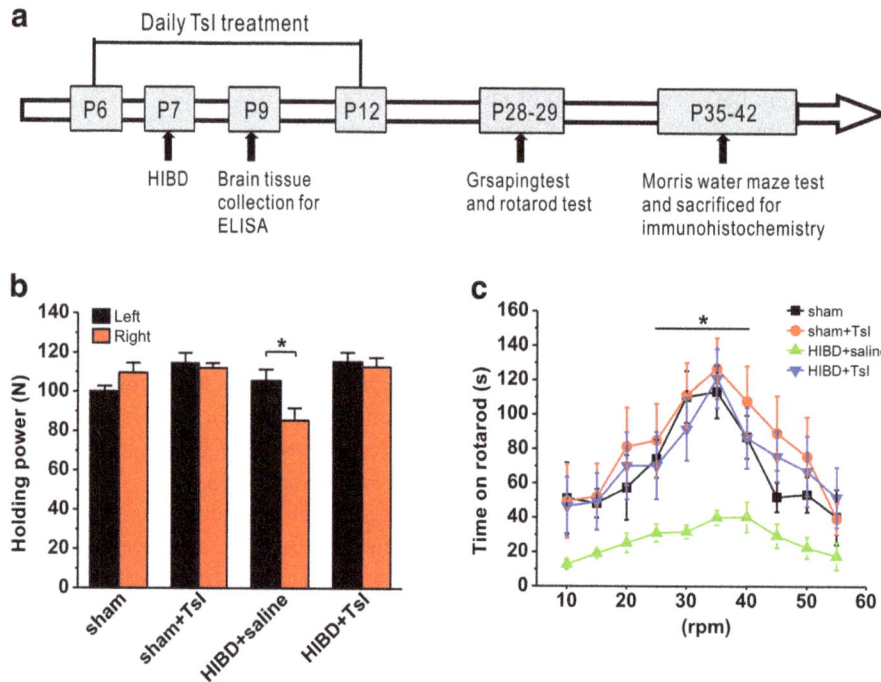

Fig. 1 Pretreatment of TsI rescues the deficits of myodynamia and motor functions in neonatal HIBD rats. **a** The flowchart illustrates the experimental protocols of TsI treatments and behavioral tests. Rats received TsI treatment (5 mg/kg per day, i.p.) twice before and five times after HIBD model establish, and the second treatment of TsI was 6 h before the surgery. Two days after HIBD, brain tissue was collected for oxidative stress analysis. Grasping test and rotarod test were performed on postnatal day 28 and 29 (P28–29), and the Morris water maze test was performed from postnatal day 35 to 42 (P35–42). After behavioral tests, brain tissues were collected for immunohistochemistry. **b** The left and right forelimb myodynamia during the grasping test. **c** The latency to fall off the rod during the rotarod test. The data was presented as mean ± SEM. *$p < 0.05$

described previously [29, 30]. In brief, rats were allowed to adapt to the water maze, which consists of a circular pool (180-cm diameter, 60-cm at the side), for 60 s 24 h before the first spatial learning trial. During training period, rats were trained in the pool over 4 trials per day for 5 consecutive days to find a submerged platform (1-cm below the surface of the water). During each trial, the rats failed to reach the hidden platform within 60 s were guided to the platform where they remained for 30 s. A 60-s probe test was performed without the hidden platform to assess the memory retrieval ability, 24 h after the last training trial. All trials were recorded by using Any-maze tracking system (Stoelting, USA).

Immunohistochemistry

After behavioral tests, the rats were deeply anesthetized with urethane (1.5 g/kg, i.p.) and then transcardially perfused with 0.9% saline followed by 4% paraformaldehyde in 100 mM phosphate-buffered saline (PBS, PH 7.4). Brains were transferred to 30% sucrose in 100 mM PBS for several days before they sunk to the bottom of sucrose solution. Then they were serially sectioned into 30-μm coronal sections using Leica cryostat and every sixth slice with the same reference position was stained.

After blocking and permeabilization, the slices were incubated with diluted anti-NeuN (1:100 dilution, Millipore, MAB377) for overnight at 4 °C. Thereafter, the positive neurons were visualized with anti-mouse Ig HRP detection kit according to the manufacturer's instruction. The number of NeuN-positive cells was quantified in brain sections with typical morphology of the pyramidal neuron in the CA1 area of hippocampus. Briefly, the number of NeuN-immunoreactive neurons was counted manually at five-section intervals throughout the CA1 area of hippocampus by bright-field microscopy using ImageJ software. To quantify changes of the number of NeuN-immunoreactive neurons in the CA1, the number of NeuN-immunoreactive neurons in sham rat was normalized to 100%, and the number of NeuN-immunoreactive neurons in other groups was expressed as a percentage of the sham.

Oxidative stress analysis

Brain tissues of hippocampus and cortex were homogenized with saline (tissue weight: saline volume = 1: 9) on ice, followed by centrifugation at 2500 g for 10 min at 4 °C. The supernatant was used to test the antioxidant activity including total antioxidant capacity (T-AOC), glutathione (GSH), superoxide dismutase (SOD) and catalase (CAT), and pro-oxidants including hydrogen peroxide (H_2O_2), total nitric oxide synthase (TNOS) and inducible nitric oxide synthase (iNOS), by using ELISA kit (Nanjing Jiancheng Bioengineering Institute, Nanjing, China). Briefly, the supernatant of brain tissue homogenate was mixed with Reagent 1 (the volume of supernatant: Reagent 1 = 1: 1) by vortex, and then centrifuged at 3500 g at 4 °C for 10 min. Then, 100 μl mixed tissue sample was pipetted into a well of microplate, and 100 μl Reagent 2 and 25 μl Reagent 3 were added to each well and incubated at room temperature for 5 min. The absorbance was determined at 405 nm by microplate reader (Bio Tek Insruments). Finally, the standard curve was used to determine the concentration of each sample.

Statistical analysis

All data were expressed as means ± standard error (mean ± SEM). The differences of rotarod test and spatial learning in water maze test among different groups were analyzed by two-way AVOVA with treatment (group) as the between-subjects factor and training trials in rotarod test or learning day in water maze test as the within-subjects factor. The data of all other experiments were analyzed by one-way ANOVA followed by Tukey's post hoc test. Significance level was set as at $p < 0.05$.

Results

TsI ameliorates myodynamia and motor deficit in HIBD rat

To determine whether TsI can rescue HIBD-induced motor deficits, two different behavioral tests were introduced: grasping test and rotarod test. In grasping test, myodynamia of the right forelimb was significantly decreased compared to that of the left in HIBD rats (HIBD + saline: $n = 10$, Fig. 1b). Importantly, treatment with TsI (5 mg/kg, i.p.) fully rescued the HIBD-induced myodynamia deficit, as reflected by similar myodynamia in both left and right forelimbs (HIBD + TsI: $n = 11$, Fig. 1b). Notably, myodynamia was not affected with or without TsI treatment in sham groups (sham: n = 10; sham + TsI: n = 10, Fig. 1b).

In rotarod test, the rats in HIBD group spent much less time on the rod compared with those treated with sham surgery (sham: $n = 8$; HIBD + saline: n = 8, $p < 0.05$ vs. sham; Fig. 1c), indicating a significant impairment of motor balance and coordination. Treatment with TsI fully rescued the HIBD-induced motor deficit, as reflected by a dramatic increase in the time spent on the

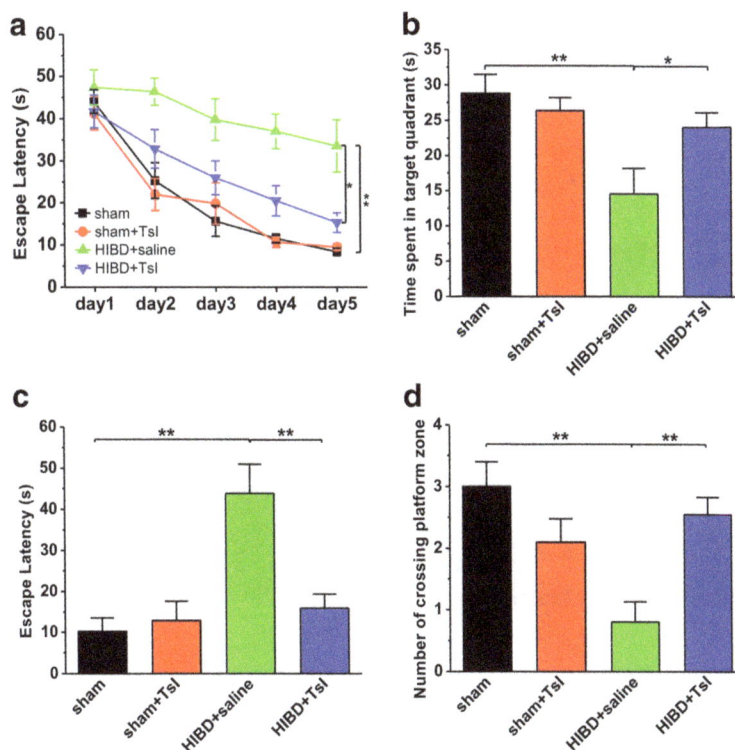

Fig. 2 Pretreatment of TsI alleviates spatial learning and memory deficits in neonatal HIBD rats. **a** The average escape latency to the hidden platform location is plotted for each spatial learning day in the Morris water maze task. **b-d** Bar graph showed the time spent in the hidden platform-located quadrant **b**, the latency of first time to the hidden platform location (**c**) and the number of entries into the platform zone (**d**) during the probe test with absence of the hidden platform, which is conducted 24 h after the last learning trial. Data was expressed as mean ± SEM. *$p < 0.05$, **$p < 0.01$

rod (HIBD + TsI: $n = 9$, $p > 0.05$ vs. sham, p < 0.05 vs. HIBD + saline; Fig. 1c), whereas TsI treatment have no effect on motor function in the sham group (sham + TsI: n = 8, p > 0.05 vs. sham; Fig. 1c). Taken together, these results indicate that TsI treatment alleviates the deficits of myodynamia and motor function in the neonatal rat after HIBD.

TsI ameliorates spatial learning and memory in HIBD rats
It has been well documented that the impairment of learning and memory is the major sequelae of HIBD in human and a variety of animal models [31, 32]. To

identify the effects of TsI treatment on spatial learning and memory deficits induced by hypoxia-ischemia in neonatal rats, the Morris water maze test, a hippocampus-dependent task, was conducted. As shown in Fig. 2, although the escape latency decreased progressively in all groups, the latency in the HIBD group was much longer than that in the sham groups during spatial training period (sham: $n = 10$; sham + TsI: $n = 10$, $p > 0.05$ vs. sham; HIBD + saline: n = 10, $p < 0.01$ vs. sham; Fig. 2a), indicating an impairment of learning after HIBD. Importantly, daily TsI treatment (5 mg/kg, i.p.) significantly ameliorated the impairment, as reflected

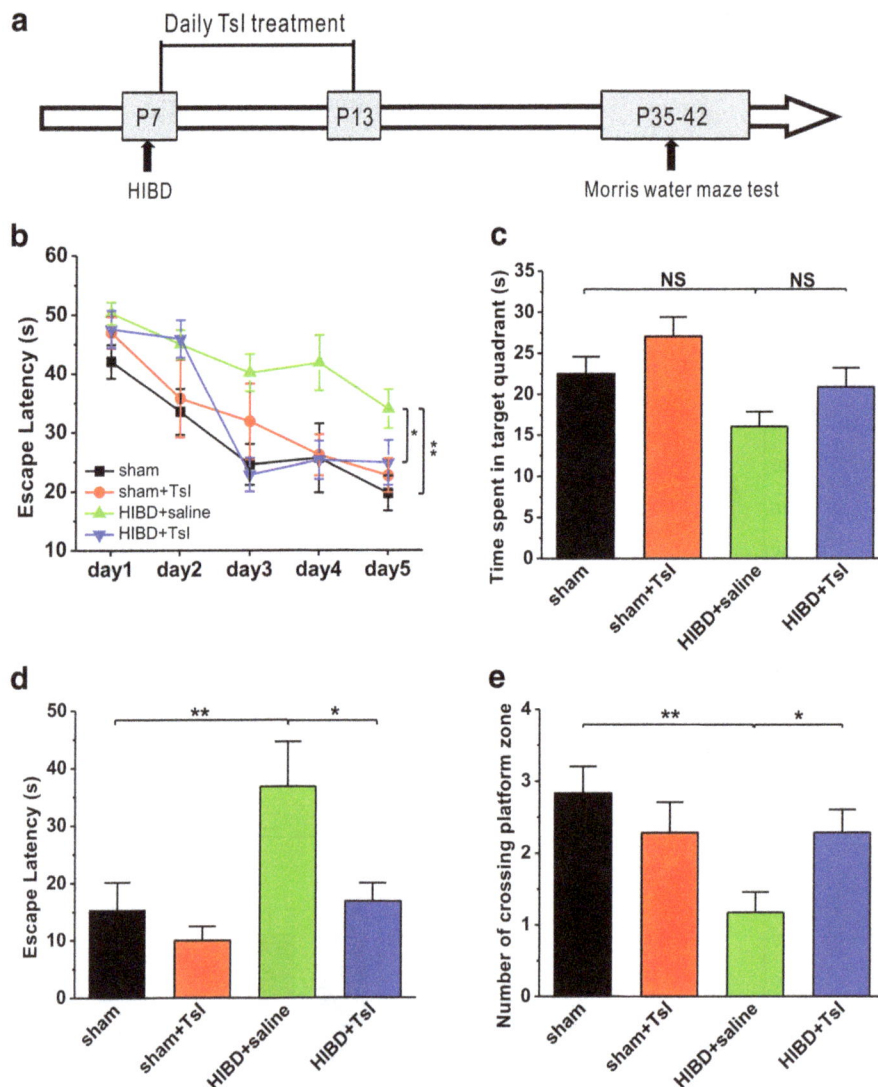

Fig. 3 TsI treatment immediately after HIBD alleviates spatial learning and memory deficits in neonatal HIBD rats. **a** The flowchart illustrates the experimental protocols of TsI treatments and water maze test. Rats received TsI treatment (5 mg/kg per day, i.p.) seven times after HIBD model established, and the first treatment of TsI was conducted immediately after HIBD. The Morris water maze test was performed from postnatal day 35 to 42 (P35–42). **b** The average escape latency to the hidden platform location is plotted for each spatial learning day in the Morris water maze task. **c-e** Bar graph showed the time spent in the hidden platform-located quadrant **c**, the latency of first time to the hidden platform location (**d**) and the number of entries into the platform zone (**e**) during the probe test with absence of the hidden platform, which is conducted 24 h after the last learning trial. Data was expressed as mean ± SEM. *$p < 0.05$, **$p < 0.01$

by an obvious decrease in the latency to the platform, compared with saline treatment (HIBD + TsI: $n = 11$, $p < 0.05$ vs. HIBD + saline; Fig. 2a).

The results from probe test showed that spatial memory retrieval was obviously impaired in HIBD rats since they spent much less time in the quadrant where the hidden platform was previously located (sham: $n = 10$, 28.8 ± 2.7 s; sham + TsI: $n = 10$, 26.4 ± 1.8 s, $p > 0.05$ vs. sham; HIBD + saline: $n = 10$, 14.5 ± 3.6 s, $p < 0.01$ vs. sham; Fig. 2b). As expected, TsI treatment significantly increased the time spent in the target quadrant compared with the HIBD group (HIBD + TsI: $n = 11$, 24.0 ± 2.1 s, $p < 0.05$ vs. HIBD + saline, $p > 0.05$ vs. sham; Fig. 2b). Additionally, the results of latency to cross the location of hidden platform (sham: $n = 10$, 10.2 ± 3.3 s; sham + TsI: n = 10, 12.8 ± 4.8 s, $p > 0.05$ vs. sham; HIBD + saline: $n = 10$, 43.8 ± 7.0 s, $p < 0.01$ vs. sham; HIBD + TsI: $n = 11$, 15.8 ± 3.4 s, $p > 0.05$ vs. sham, $p < 0.01$ vs. HIBD + saline; Fig. 2c) and the number of crossing the location of hidden platform (sham: $n = 10$, 3.0 ± 0.4; sham + TsI: $n = 10$, 2.1 ± 0.4, $p > 0.05$ vs. sham; HIBD + saline: $n = 10$, 0.8 ± 0.3, $p < 0.01$ vs. sham; HIBD + TsI: $n = 11$, 2.5 ± 0.3, $p > 0.05$ vs. sham, $p < 0.01$ vs. HIBD + saline; Fig. 2d) further confirmed that spatial memory retrieval was impaired after HIBD, and TsI treatment succeeded in preventing this impairment.

To further determine the therapeutic effects of TsI on HIBD, we treated the rats with TsI daily for 7 days and the first injection was carried out immediately after HIBD. Four weeks after HIBD, the Morris water maze test was performed. As shown in Fig. 3, the protective effects of TsI on spatial learning and memory in HIBD rats were similar to those that found in pretreatment of TsI, as reflected by an obvious decrease in the latency to the platform, compared with saline treatment (HIBD + TsI: $n = 7$, $p < 0.05$ vs. HIBD + saline; Fig. 3b) during spatial training period. Although the time spent in the target quadrant among these groups was no significant difference (sham: $n = 6$, 22.5 ± 2.1 s; sham + TsI: $n = 7$, 27.1 ± 2.4 s, $p > 0.05$ vs. sham; HIBD + saline: $n = 6$, 16.1 ± 1.8 s, $p > 0.05$ vs. sham; HIBD + TsI: $n = 7$, 20.9 ± 2.3 s, $p > 0.05$ vs. sham, $p > 0.05$ vs. HIBD + saline; Fig. 3c), the latency to cross the location of hidden platform (sham: $n = 6$, 15.3 ± 4.9 s; sham + TsI: $n = 7$, 10.1 ± 2.4 s, $p > 0.05$ vs. sham; HIBD + saline: $n = 6$, 36.8 ± 7.8 s, $p < 0.01$ vs. sham; HIBD + TsI: $n = 7$, 16.8 ± 3.2 s, $p > 0.05$ vs. sham, $p < 0.05$ vs. HIBD + saline; Fig. 3d) and the number of crossing the location of hidden platform (sham: $n = 6$, 2.8 ± 0.4; sham + TsI: n = 7, 2.3 ± 0.4, $p > 0.05$ vs. sham; HIBD + saline: $n = 6$, 1.2 ± 0.3, $p < 0.01$ vs. sham; HIBD + TsI: $n = 7$, 2.3 ± 0.3, $p > 0.05$ vs. sham, $p < 0.05$ vs. HIBD + saline; Fig. 3e) showed that spatial memory retrieval was impaired after HIBD, and TsI treatment succeeded in preventing this impairment.

Taken together, these results suggest that systemic administration of TsI either pretreatment or immediately after HIBD is able to prevent the HIBD-induced impairment of spatial learning and memory.

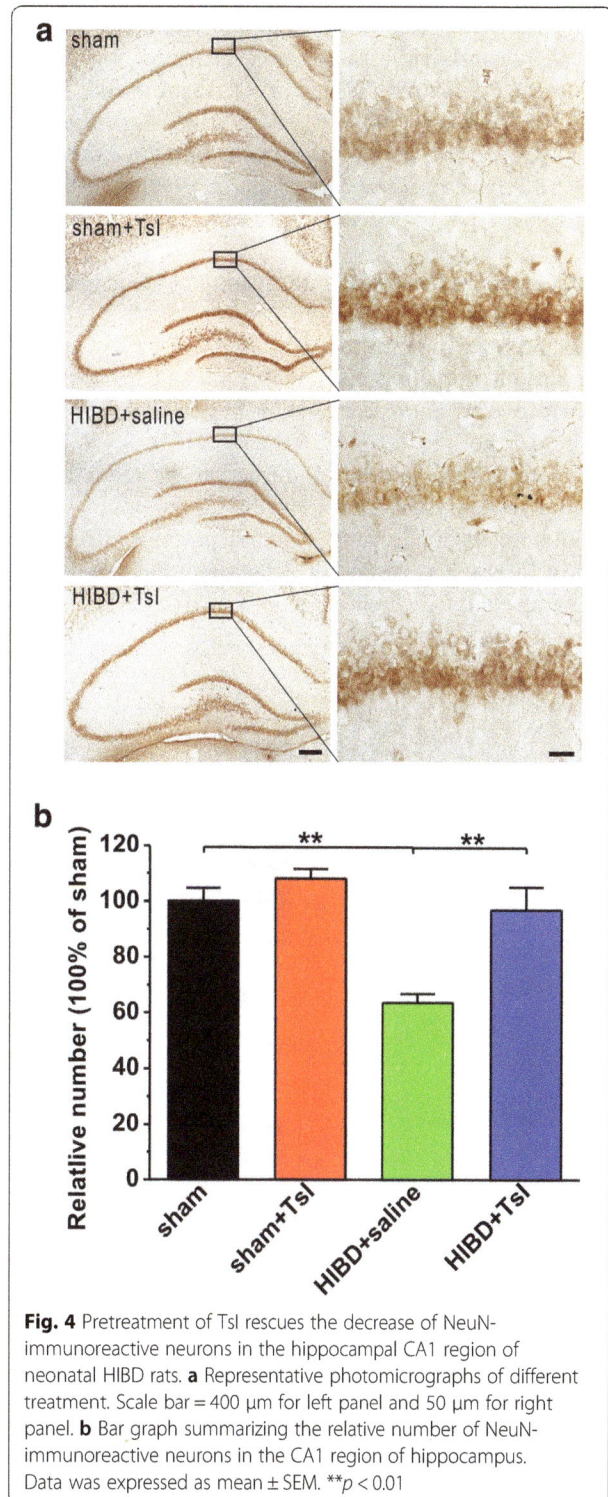

Fig. 4 Pretreatment of TsI rescues the decrease of NeuN-immunoreactive neurons in the hippocampal CA1 region of neonatal HIBD rats. **a** Representative photomicrographs of different treatment. Scale bar = 400 μm for left panel and 50 μm for right panel. **b** Bar graph summarizing the relative number of NeuN-immunoreactive neurons in the CA1 region of hippocampus. Data was expressed as mean ± SEM. **$p < 0.01$

TsI reduces HIBD-induced neuron loss

The number of NeuN-immunoreactive neurons was examined to confirm the neuroprotective effects of TsI on pyramidal neurons after hypoxic-ischemic insult in the CA1 area of hippocampus. The results showed that the number of NeuN-immunoreactive neurons in the CA1 area dramatically decreased in the HIBD group compared with the sham group, and administration of TsI significantly suppressed the decrease of NeuN-immunoreactive neurons (sham: $n = 4$; sham + TsI: $n = 4$, $108.0 \pm 3.5\%$ sham, $p > 0.05$ vs. sham; HIBD + saline: $n = 6$, $63.5 \pm 3.2\%$ sham, $p < 0.01$ vs. sham; HIBD + TsI: $n = 5$, $96.9 \pm 8.1\%$ sham, $p > 0.05$ vs. sham, $p < 0.01$ vs. HIBD + saline; Fig. 4).

TsI reverses the decreased antioxidant and the increased pro-oxidant in HIBD rats

It has been well known that oxidative injury plays an important role in pathogenesis of HIE [6], and TsI has been shown to exert antioxidant action in various experimental models both in vitro [33, 34] and in vivo [35, 36]. We therefore wanted to determine whether the reduction of neuron loss in HIBD rats treated with TsI could be attributed to its suppressing effect on oxidative stress. As shown in Fig. 5, a significant decrease in the production of antioxidants including T-AOC, GSH, CAT and T-

SOD was observed in HIBD group. However, compared with saline treatment, TsI dramatically rescued the T-AOC (sham: $n = 11$, sham + TsI: $n = 11$, $99.5 \pm 2.3\%$ sham, $p > 0.05$ vs. sham; HIBD + saline: $n = 12$, $86.9 \pm 2.1\%$ sham, $p < 0.05$ vs. sham; HIBD + TsI: $n = 13$, $99.4 \pm 2.5\%$ sham, $p > 0.05$ vs. sham, $p < 0.05$ vs. HIBD + saline; Fig. 5a), GSH (sham: $n = 8$, sham + TsI: $n = 8$, $110.2 \pm 13.3\%$ sham, $p > 0.05$ vs. sham; HIBD + saline: $n = 8$, $55.8 \pm 5.2\%$ sham, $p < 0.01$ vs. sham; HIBD + TsI: $n = 8$, $90.1 \pm 6.3\%$ sham, $p > 0.05$ vs. sham, $p < 0.01$ vs. HIBD + saline; Fig. 5b), CAT (sham: $n = 9$, sham + TsI: $n = 10$, $105.1 \pm 9.8\%$ sham, $p > 0.05$ vs. sham; HIBD + saline: $n = 10$, $74.4 \pm 3.7\%$ sham, $p < 0.01$ vs. sham; HIBD + TsI: $n = 12$, $94.0 \pm 3.5\%$ sham, $p > 0.05$ vs. sham, $p < 0.05$ vs. HIBD + saline; Fig. 5c) and T-SOD (sham: $n = 8$, sham + TsI: $n = 7$, $101.8 \pm 3.1\%$ sham, $p > 0.05$ vs. sham; HIBD + saline: $n = 8$, $85.4 \pm 5.2\%$ sham, $p < 0.01$ vs. sham; HIBD + TsI: $n = 7$, $107.0 \pm 4.6\%$ sham, $p > 0.05$ vs. sham, $p < 0.01$ vs. HIBD + saline; Fig. 5d) activity following HIBD in the brain.

Meanwhile, as shown in Fig. 6, a significant increase in the production of pro-oxidants including H_2O_2, TNOS and iNOS was observed in HIBD group. As expected, TsI dramatically suppressed the increase of H_2O_2 (sham: $n = 10$, sham + TsI: $n = 10$, $90.9 \pm 7.9\%$ sham, $p > 0.05$ vs. sham; HIBD + saline: $n = 12$, 132.7

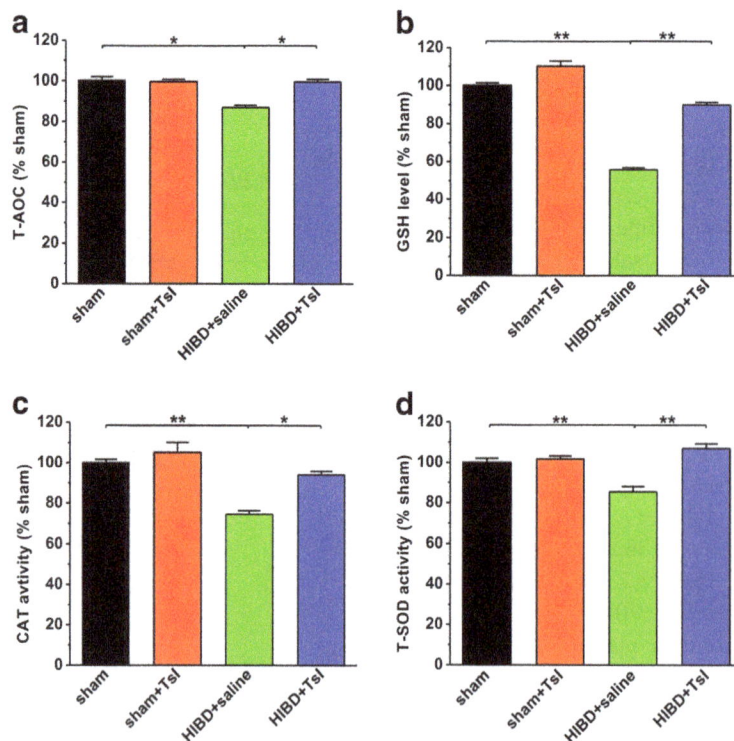

Fig. 5 Pretreatment of TsI restores the decreased antioxidants in the brain of HIBD rats. HIBD results in a significant reduction in antioxidants including T-AOC **a**, GSH **b**, CAT **c** and T-SOD **d**, whereas TsI treatment restores these antioxidants to control level. The results were presented as the mean ± SEM. *$p < 0.05$, **$p < 0.01$

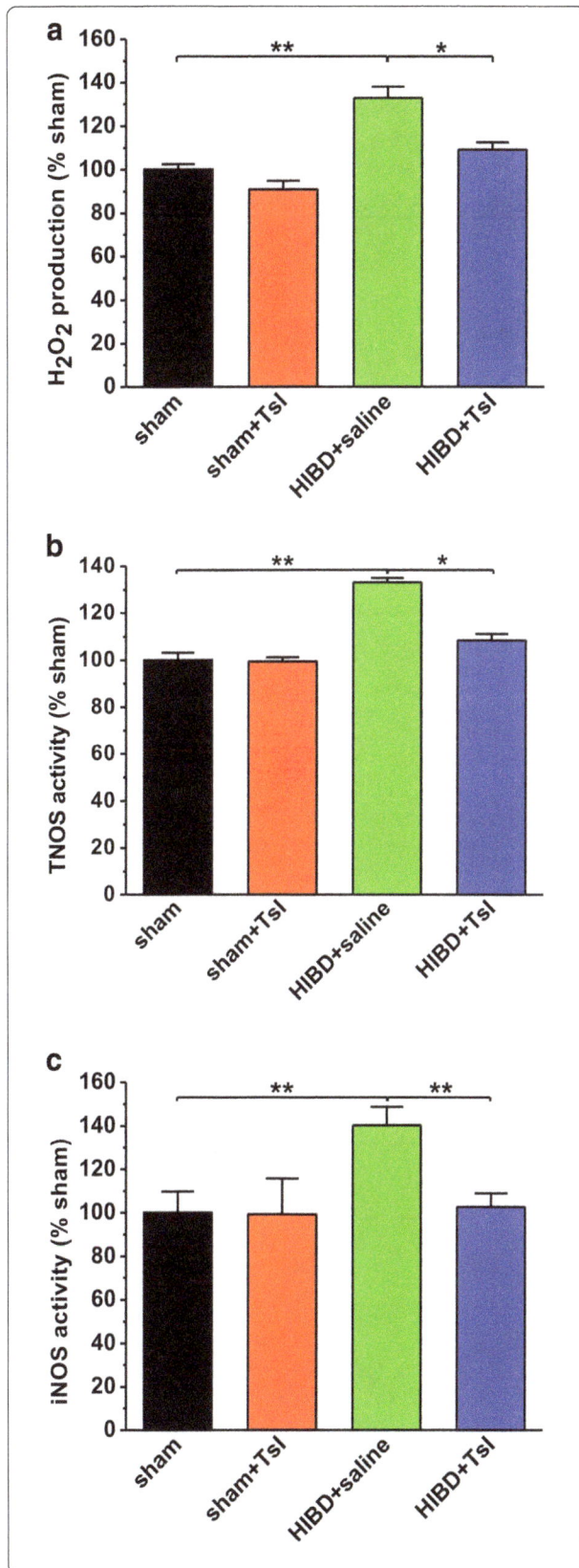

a

b

c

Fig. 6 Pretreatment of TsI restores the increased pro-oxidants in the brain of HIBD rats. HIBD results in a significant increase in pro-oxidants including H_2O_2 **a**, TNOS **b** and iNOS **c**, whereas TsI treatment restores these pro-oxidants to control level. The results were presented as the mean ± SEM. *$p < 0.05$, **$p < 0.01$

± 10.5% sham, $p < 0.01$ vs. sham; HIBD + TsI: n = 12, 109.0 ± 6.8% sham, p > 0.05 vs. sham, p < 0.05 vs. HIBD + saline; Fig. 6a), TNOS (sham: $n = 11$, sham + TsI: n = 9, 99.4 ± 3.6% sham, p > 0.05 vs. sham; HIBD + saline: n = 11, 133.0 ± 3.7% sham, p < 0.01 vs. sham; HIBD + TsI: $n = 13$, 108.3 ± 5.6% sham, p > 0.05 vs. sham, p < 0.05 vs. HIBD + saline; Fig. 6b) and iNOS (sham: n = 10, sham + TsI: n = 10, 99.4 ± 16.3% sham, p > 0.05 vs. sham; HIBD + saline: n = 12, 140.3 ± 8.4% sham, p < 0.01 vs. sham; HIBD + TsI: $n = 14$, 102.7 ± 6.3% sham, p > 0.05 vs. sham, $P < 0.01$ vs. HIBD + saline; Fig. 6c) following HIBD in the brain, compared with saline treatment. These results indicate a powerful antioxidative capacity of TsI in HIBD rats.

Discussion

In the present study, we demonstrate that TsI, a compound purified from the Chinese herb Danshen, suppresses the decrease of pyramidal neurons in the CA1 area of hippocampus, and alleviates the impairment of motor and spatial learning and memory functions in the neonatal rats subjected to HIBD. We further confirm that the beneficial effects of TsI on HIBD rats are associated with the increase of antioxidant activity. We have therefore provided evidence that TsI may suppress HIBD-induced oxidative stress and subsequently block the loss of pyramidal neurons in the CA1 area of hippocampus, thereby ameliorating motor and cognitive decline.

The dried root of Salvia miltiorrhiza, called Danshen in China, has been used effectively for the treatment of many diseases, especially ischemic cardiovascular disease in aging people for over 1000 years [12]. Previous study has indicated that Danshen is able to dilate cerebral arteries, increase cerebral blood flow, inhibit oxidative stress and reduce neuronal death induced by ischemia [14]. In addition, a growing body of evidence has shown that the major lipophilic diterpenes derived from Danshen extract, such as CTs, DTsI, TsI, TsIIA and TsIIB, have neuroprotective effects against transient ischemic damage in different adult animal models including gerbils [35], rats [24] and mice [22, 23]. Recent studies have reported that TsIIA treatment is significantly protective for hypoxia-ischemia in the immature rat [25, 26]. Similar to TsIIA, we here found that treatment with TsI markedly suppressed the loss of pyramidal neurons induced by hypoxia-ischemia in the CA1 region of hippocampus (Fig. 4). However, the dose of TsI we used in the present study was 5 mg/kg/day, which is much lower than TsIIA (10 mg/kg/day) used in previous study [26], suggesting that TsI may be more effective than TsII for treating HIBD.

The neuronal loss induced by hypoxia-ischemia is usually associated with the deficits of motor and cognitive functions both in animal models and in patients [37–39]. Excitedly, recent study has revealed that TsI is able to ameliorate the learning and memory impairments induced by a $GABA_A$ receptor agonist diazepam, or an NMDA receptor antagonist MK-801, in adult mice [40]. However, so far no study to examine the influence of TsI on motor and learning and memory functions in immature animals after hypoxia-ischemia. In the current study, we found that TsI could rescue myodynamia and motor deficits (Fig. 1), and alleviate the spatial learning and memory impairments (Figs. 2 and 3) in neonatal HIBD model rats. Combined with previous report [40], we can therefore conclude that TsI has the ability to ameliorate the learning and memory impairments in both adult and neonatal animals.

Although HIBD is a complex multifactorial disease, a growing body of evidence has shown that oxidative damage to vital cellular structures plays a critical role in the pathogenesis of brain damage in both the immature and mature nervous system [6, 41, 42]. Several studies have indicated that TsI is able to exert antioxidative and antiapoptotic effects in cellular and mouse model of Parkinson's disease (PD) [18, 19, 43]. In full agreement with these findings, we here found that treatment with TsI markedly reversed the decrease of antioxidants and the increase of pro-oxidants induced by HIBD in neonatal rats (Figs. 5 and 6). The exact underlying cellular and molecular mechanisms remain to be determined, but may be at least in part due to the up-regulating effects of TsI on nuclear factor erythroid-2-related factor 2 (Nrf2), since previous studies have supported that the antioxidation of TsI is involved in Nrf2 signaling pathway both in vitro and in mouse model of PD [43, 44]. Thus, future experiments examining Nrf2 signaling pathway in neonatal HIBD animals with or without TsI treatment will help determine whether the therapeutic effects of TsI in neonatal HIBD rats can be attributed to its up-regulation of Nrf2. Furthermore, some studies have reported that the activation of nuclear factor kappa B (NF-κB) promotes cell survival via attenuating reactive oxygen species (ROS), such as NOS, H_2O_2, et al. [45, 46], and increasing the expression of antioxidant proteins, such as GSH, SOD, catalase, and so on [47–49]. Here, we found that TsI significantly promoted the expression of antioxidant proteins and suppressed the expression of pro-oxidants (Figs. 5 and 6). However, further studies would be necessary to elucidate the full mechanism whether TsI produces neuroprotection via activating NF-κB signaling pathway.

Conclusions

In summary, these data provide the first evidence that TsI treatment suppresses HIBD-induced neuronal death and oxidative stress, thereby ameliorating myodynamia and motor abilities as well as spatial learning and memory in neonatal rats after HIBD, an animal model of HIE in patient, suggesting that TsI may represent a potentially effective therapeutic drug for HIE.

Abbreviations
CAT: Catalase; CTs: Cryptotanshinone; DMSO: Dimethyl sulfoxide; DTsI: Dihydrotanshinone I; GST: Glutathione; H_2O_2: Hydrogen peroxide; HIBD: Hypoxic-ischemic brain damage; HIE: Hypoxic-ischemic encephalopathy; iNOS: Inducible nitric oxide synthase; NF-κB: Nuclear factor kappa B; Nrf2: Nuclear factor erythroid-2-related factor 2; ROS: Reactive oxygen species; T-AOC: Total antioxidant capacity; T-NOS: Total nitric oxide synthase; TsI: Tanshinone I; TsII: Tanshinone II; T-SOD: Total superoxide dismutase

Acknowledgements
We thank Dr. Yu Tian Wang from the University of British Columbia for discussion and support.

Funding
This work was supported by grants from the National Natural Science Foundation of China (Grant No. 81571042 and 81,622,015), the National Basic Research Program of China (Grant No. 2014CB548100) and Graduate student Innovation Project of Chongqing (Grant No. CYB17103).

Authors' contributions
CD carried out the behavioral and immunohistochemical studies, and drafted the manuscript. YL carried out the ELISA assays. ZD conceived of the study, and participated in its design and coordination and helped to draft the manuscript. All authors read and approved the final manuscript.

Competing interests
The authors have declares that they have no competing interests.

Author details
[1]Ministry of Education Key Laboratory of Child Development and Disorders, Children's Hospital of Chongqing Medical University, 136 Zhongshan Er Road, Yuzhong District, Chongqing 400014, People's Republic of China. [2]Chongqing Key Laboratory of Translational Medical Research in Cognitive Development and Learning and Memory Disorders, Children's Hospital of Chongqing Medical University, 136 Zhongshan Er Road, Yuzhong District, Chongqing 400014, People's Republic of China. [3]China International Science and Technology Cooperation base of Child Development and Critical Disorders, Children's Hospital of Chongqing Medical University, 136 Zhongshan Er Road, Yuzhong District, Chongqing 400014, People's Republic of China.

References

1. Kurinczuk JJ, Whitekoning M, Badawi N. Epidemiology of neonatal encephalopathy and hypoxic-ischaemic encephalopathy. Early Hum Dev. 2010;86(6):329–38.
2. Graham EM, Ruis KA, Hartman AL, Northington FJ, Fox HE. A systematic review of the role of intrapartum hypoxia-ischemia in the causation of neonatal encephalopathy. Am J Obstet Gynecol. 2008;199(6):587–95.
3. Jacobs SE, Morley CJ, Inder TE, Stewart MJ, Smith KR, McNamara PJ, Wright IM, Kirpalani HM, Darlow BA, Doyle LW. Infant Cooling Evaluation Collaboration. Whole-body hypothermia for term and near-term newborns with hypoxic-ischemic encephalopathy: a randomized controlled trial. Arch Pediatr Adolesc Med. 2011;165(12):692–700.
4. Martinezbiarge M, Diezsebastian J, Kapellou O, Gindner D, Allsop JM, Rutherford MA, Cowan FM. Predicting motor outcome and death in term hypoxic-ischemic encephalopathy. Neurology. 2011;76(24):2055–61.
5. Shankaran S, Pappas A, McDonald SA, Vohr BR, Hintz SR, Yolton K, Gustafson KE, Leach TM, Green C, Bara R, Petrie Huitema CM, Ehrenkranz RA, Tyson JE, Das A, Hammond J, Peralta-Carcelen M, Evans PW, Heyne RJ, Wilson-Costello DE, Vaucher YE, Bauer CR, Dusick AM, Adams-Chapman I, Goldstein RF, Guillet R, Papile LA, Higgins RD; Eunice Kennedy Shriver NICHD Neonatal Research Network. Childhood outcomes after hypothermia for neonatal encephalopathy. N Engl J Med. 2012;366(22):2085–92.
6. Ferriero DM. Oxidant mechanisms in neonatal hypoxia-ischemia. Dev Neurosci. 2001;23(3):198–202.
7. Halliwell B. Reactive oxygen species and the central nervous system. J Neurochem. 1992;120(5):1609–23.
8. Lafemina MJ, Sheldon RA, Ferriero DM. Acute hypoxia-ischemia results in hydrogen peroxide accumulation in neonatal but not adult mouse brain. Pediatr Res. 2006;59(5):680–3.
9. Wallin C, Puka-Sundvall M, Hagberg H, Weber SG, Sandberg M. Alterations in glutathione and amino acid concentrations after hypoxia-ischemia in the immature rat brain. Brain Res Dev Brain Res. 2000;125(1–2):51–60.
10. Khan JY, Black SM. Developmental changes in murine brain antioxidant enzymes. Pediatr Res. 2003;54(1):77–82.
11. Guan J, Gunn AJ, Sirimanne ES, Tuffin J, Gunning MI, Clark R, Gluckman PD. The window of opportunity for neuronal rescue with insulin-like growth factor-1 after hypoxia-ischemia in rats is critically modulated by cerebral temperature during recovery. J Cereb Blood Flow Metab. 2000;20(3):513–9.
12. Ji XY, Tan KH, Zhu YZ. Salvia miltiorrhiza and ischemic diseases. Acta Pharmacol Sin. 2000;21(12):1089–94.
13. Wu B, Liu M. Cochrane systematic review: Danshen agents for acute Ischaemic stroke. J Evid Based Med. 2005;5(2):101–5.
14. Han JY, Fan JY, Horie Y, Miura S, Cui DH, Ishii H, Hibi T, Tsuneki H, Kimura I. Ameliorating effects of compounds derived from salvia miltiorrhiza root extract on microcirculatory disturbance and target organ injury by ischemia and reperfusion. Pharmacol Ther. 2008;117(2):280–95.
15. Gu M, Zhang S, Su Z, Chen Y, Ouyang F. Fingerprinting of salvia miltiorrhiza Bunge by non-aqueous capillary electrophoresis compared with high-speed counter-current chromatography. J Chromatogr A. 2004;1057(1):133–40.
16. Ren Y, Houghton PJ, Hider RC, Howes MJ. Novel diterpenoid acetylcholinesterase inhibitors from salvia miltiorhiza. Planta Med. 2004;70(03):201–4.
17. Zhang XS, Ha S, Wang XL, Shi YL, Duan SS, Li ZA. Tanshinone IIA protects dopaminergic neurons against 6-hydroxydopamine-induced neurotoxicity through miR-153/NF-E2-related factor 2/antioxidant response element signaling pathway. Neuroscience. 2015;303:489–502.
18. de Oliveira MR, Fürstenau CR, de Souza IC, da Costa Ferreira G. Tanshinone I attenuates the effects of a challenge with H2O2 on the functions of tricarboxylic acid cycle and respiratory chain in SH-SY5Y cells. Mol Neurobiol. 2016; [Epub ahead of print].
19. Xu J, Wei X, Ren M, Wang L, Zhang X, Lou H. Neuroprotective effects of Tanshinone I against 6-OHDA-induced oxidative stress in cellular and mouse model of Parkinson's disease through upregulating Nrf2. Neurochem Res. 2015;41(4):779–86.
20. Qiao Z, Ma J, Liu H. Evaluation of the antioxidant potential of salvia miltiorrhiza ethanol extract in a rat model of ischemia-reperfusion injury. Molecules. 2011;16(12):10002–12.
21. Wang S, Jing H, Yang H, Liu Z, Guo H, Chai L, Hu L. Tanshinone I selectively suppresses pro-inflammatory genes expression in activated microglia and prevents nigrostriatal dopaminergic neurodegeneration in a mouse model of Parkinson's disease. J Ethnopharmacol. 2015;164:247–55.
22. Lam BY, Lo AC, Sun X, Luo HW, Chung SK, Sucher NJ. Neuroprotective effects of tanshinones in transient focal cerebral ischemia in mice. Phytomedicine. 2003;10(4):286–91.
23. Lee JC, Park JH, Park OK, Kim IH, Yan BC, Ahn JH, Kwon SH, Choi JH, Kim JD, Won MH. Neuroprotective effects of tanshinone I from Danshen extract in a mouse model of hypoxia-ischemia. Anat Cell Biol. 2013;46(3):183–90.
24. Liu L, Zhang XL, Yang R, Cui L, Li M, Du W, Wang S. The neuroprotective effects of Tanshinone IIA are associated with induced nuclear translocation of TORC1 and upregulated expression of TORC1, pCREB and BDNF in the acute stage of ischemic stroke. Brain Res Bull. 2010;82(3):228–33.
25. Hei M, Luo Y, Zhang X, Liu F. Tanshinone IIa alleviates the biochemical changes associated with hypoxic ischemic brain damage in a rat model. Phytother Res. 2011;25(12):1865–9.
26. Xia WJ, Yang M, Fok TF, Li K, Chan WY, Ng PC, Ng HK, Chik KW, Wang CC, Gu GJ, Woo KS, Fung KP. Partial neuroprotective effect of pretreatment with tanshinone IIA on neonatal hypoxia-ischemia brain damage. Pediatr Res. 2005;58(4):784–90.
27. Rice JE 3rd, Vannucci RC, Brierley JB. The influence of immaturity on hypoxic-ischemic brain damage in the rat. Ann Neurol. 1981;9(2):131–41.
28. Heldermon CD, Hennig AK, Ohlemiller KK, Ogilvie JM, Herzog ED, Breidenbach A, Vogler C, Wozniak DF, Sands S. M: development of sensory, motor and behavioral deficits in the murine model of Sanfilippo syndrome type B. PLoS One. 2007;2(8):e772.
29. Ge Y, Dong Z, Bagot R, Howland J, Phillips A, Wong T, Wang Y. Hippocampal long-term depression is required for the consolidation of spatial memory. Proc Natl Acad Sci U S A. 2010;107(38):16697–702.
30. Dong Z, Han H, Li H, Bai Y, Wang W, Tu M, Peng Y, Zhou L, He W, Wu X, Tan T, Liu M, Wu X, Zhou W, Jin W, Zhang S, Sacktor TC, Li T, Song W, Wang YT. Long-term potentiation decay and memory loss are mediated by AMPAR endocytosis. J Clin Invest. 2015;125(1):234–47.
31. Dilenge ME, Majnemer A, Shevell MI. Long-term developmental outcome of asphyxiated term neonates. J Child Neurol. 2001;16(11):781–92.
32. Golan H, Huleihel M. The effect of prenatal hypoxia on brain development: short- and long-term consequences demonstrated in rodent models. Dev Sci. 2006;9(4):338–49.
33. Ji K, Zhao Y, Yu T, Wang Z, Gong H, Yang X, Liu Y, Huang K. Inhibition effects of tanshinone on the aggregation of α-synuclein. Food Funct. 2016;7(1):409–16.
34. Wang Q, Yu X, Patal K, Hu R, Chuang S, Zhang G, Zheng J. Tanshinones inhibit amyloid aggregation by amyloid-β peptide, disaggregate amyloid fibrils, and protect cultured cells. ACS Chem Neurosci. 2013;4(6):1004–15.
35. Park OK, Choi JH, Park JH, Kim IH, Yan BC, Ahn JH, Kwon SH, Lee JC, Kim YS, Kim M, Kang IJ, Kim JD, Lee YL, Won MH. Comparison of neuroprotective effects of five major lipophilic diterpenoids from Danshen extract against experimentally induced transient cerebral ischemic damage. Fitoterapia. 2012;83(8):1666–74.
36. Kim DH, Jeon SJ, Jung JW, Lee S, Yoon BH, Shin BY, Son KH, Cheong JH, Kim YS, Kang SS, Ko KH, Ryu JH. Tanshinone congeners improve memory impairments induced by scopolamine on passive avoidance tasks in mice. Eur J Pharmacol. 2007;574(2):140–7.
37. Ten VS, Bradley-Moore M, Gingrich JA, Stark RI, Pinsky DJ. Brain injury and neurofunctional deficit in neonatal mice with hypoxic-ischemic encephalopathy. Behav Brain Res. 2003;145(1–2):209–19.
38. Vargha-Khadem F, Gadian DG, Mishkin M. Dissociations in cognitive memory: the syndrome of developmental amnesia. Philos Trans R Soc Lond Ser B Biol Sci. 2001;356(1413):1435–40.
39. Farkas E, Luiten PG, Bari F. Permanent, bilateral common carotid artery occlusion in the rat: a model for chronic cerebral hypoperfusion-related neurodegenerative diseases. Brain Res Rev. 2007;54(1):162–80.
40. Kim DH, Kim S, Jeon SJ, Son KH, Lee S, Yoon BH, Cheong JH, Ko KH, Ryu JH. Tanshinone I enhances learning and memory, and ameliorates memory impairment in mice via the extracellular signal-regulated kinase signalling pathway. Br J Pharmacol. 2009;158(4):1131–42.
41. Vannucci RC, Perlman JM. Interventions for perinatal hypoxic-ischemic encephalopathy. Pediatrics. 1997;100(6):1004–14.
42. Zhao M, Zhu P, Fujino M, Zhuang J, Guo H, Sheikh I, Zhao L, Li XK. Oxidative stress in hypoxic-ischemic encephalopathy: molecular mechanisms and therapeutic strategies. Int J Mol Sci. 2016;17(12):2078.

43. de Oliveira MR, Schuck PF, Bosco SM. Tanshinone I induces mitochondrial protection through an Nrf2-dependent mechanism in Paraquat-TreatedHuman neuroblastoma SH-SY5Y cells. Mol Neurobiol. 2017;54(6):4597–608.

44. Jing X, Wei X, Ren M, Wang L, Zhang X, Lou H. Neuroprotective effects of Tanshinone I against 6-OHDA-induced oxidative stress in cellular and mouse model of Parkinson's disease through upregulating Nrf2. Neurochem Res. 2016;41(4):779–86.

45. Guo Z, Shao L, Du Q, Park KS, Geller DA. Identification of a classic cytokine-induced enhancer upstream in the human iNOS promoter. FASEB J. 2007;21(2):535–42.

46. Morris KR, Lutz RD, Choi HS, Kamitani T, Chmura K, Chan ED. Role of the NF-kappaB signaling pathway and kappaB cis-regulatory elements on the IRF-1 and iNOS promoter regions in mycobacterial lipoarabinomannan induction of nitric oxide. Infect Immun. 2003;71(3):1442–52.

47. Rojo AI, Salinas M, Martin D, Perona R, Cuadrado A. Regulation of cu/Zn-superoxide dismutase expression via the phosphatidylinositol 3 kinase/Akt pathway and nuclear factor-kappaB. J Neurosci. 2004;24(33):7324–34.

48. Xia C, Hu J, Ketterer B, Taylor JB. The organization of the human GSTP1-1 gene promoter and its response to retinoic acid and cellular redox status. Biochem J. 1996;313(Pt 1):155–61.

49. Zhou LZ, Johnson AP, Rando TA. NF kappa B and AP-1 mediate transcriptional responses to oxidative stress in skeletal muscle cells. Free Radic Biol Med. 2001;31(11):1405–16.

15

Interleukin-1 beta promotes neuronal differentiation through the Wnt5a/RhoA/JNK pathway in cortical neural precursor cells

Shin-Young Park, Min-Jeong Kang and Joong-Soo Han*ⓘ

Abstract

Pro-inflammatory cytokine interleukin-1 beta (IL-1β) is a key mediator of inflammation and stress in the central nervous system (CNS), and is highly expressed in the developing brain. In this study, we investigated the possible role of IL-1β in neuronal differentiation of cortical neural precursor cells (NPCs). We showed that stimulation with IL-1β increased expression levels of neurotrophin-3 (NT3) and neurogenin 1 (Ngn1) and promoted neurite outgrowth. We also found that IL-1β increased mRNA and protein levels of Wnt5a. Knockdown of Wnt5a by transfection with Wnt5a siRNA inhibited IL-1β-induced neuronal differentiation. Moreover, IL-1β-induced Wnt5a expression was regulated by nuclear factor kappa B (NF-κB) activation, which is involved in IL-1β-mediated neuronal differentiation. To examine the role of Wnt5a in neuronal differentiation of NPCs, we exogenously added Wnt5a. We found that exogenous Wnt5a promotes neuronal differentiation, and activates the RhoA/Rho-associated kinase (ROCK)/c-jun N-terminal kinase (JNK) pathway. In addition, Wnt5a-induced neuronal differentiation was blocked by RhoA siRNA, as well as by a specific Rho-kinase inhibitor (Y27632) or a SAPK/JNK inhibitor (SP600125). Furthermore, treatment with RhoA siRNA, Y27632, or SP600125 suppressed the IL-1β-induced neuronal differentiation. Therefore, these results suggest that the sequential Wnt5a/RhoA/ROCK/JNK pathway is involved in IL-1β-induced neuronal differentiation of NPCs.

Keywords: Interleukin-1 beta (IL-1β), Neuronal differentiation, Wnt5a, RhoA, C-jun N-terminal kinase (JNK)

Introduction

Interleukin-1 beta (IL-1β) is a pro-inflammatory cytokine, which is produced as an immune response to both injury and infection [1]. Increased production of IL-1β is involved in a variety of cellular activities, including cell proliferation, differentiation, and apoptosis [2]. IL-1β induces an intracellular signaling pathway, leading to altered expression of its target genes and the induction of a pro-inflammatory response [3]. It is considered that inflammatory processes stimulated by IL-1β are associated with an increased risk of neurodevelopmental disorders. Previous studies showed that IL-1β can aggravate the primary damage caused by infection of the central

nervous system (CNS), and IL-1β deficient mice display reduced neuronal loss and infarct volumes after ischemic brain damage in in vivo studies [4, 5]. On the contrary, IL-1β showed beneficial effects on neuronal survival in cultures; it is highly expressed in the developing brain and can directly influence neural precursor cells (NPCs) [6]. In other in vitro models, IL-1β has been shown to stimulate the migration of cultured cortical neurons and promote neurite outgrowth [1, 7]. The findings in various neuronal culture models show that long-term exposure (3–5 days) to high concentrations of IL-1β (500 ng/ml) had neurotoxic effects; however, short-term exposure (1 day) to lower concentrations (10 ng/ml) did not [8]. Thus, it is important to elucidate whether IL-1β mediates neuronal differentiation to understand neural development and the pathogenesis of various neurodevelopmental disorders.

* Correspondence: jshan@hanyang.ac.kr
Biomedical Research Institute and Department of Biochemistry and Molecular Biology, College of Medicine, Hanyang University, 222 Wangsimni-ro, Seongdong-gu, Seoul 04763, Republic of Korea

Wnt signaling plays an important role in embryogenesis and in the late stages of development, by regulating cell survival, growth, and, differentiation via various signaling pathways [9, 10]. Wnt signaling involves a group of pathways, such as the canonical Wnt/β-catenin pathway, the noncanonical Wnt/Ca^{2+} pathway, and the Wnt/planar cell polarity (PCP) pathway [11, 12]. Several Wnt isoforms (Wnt3b, Wnt5a, Wnt7a, and Wnt11) activate various signaling cascades during the maintenance of many organs and tissues [12–14]. A recent report suggested that Wnt5a plays a role in cell differentiation and specialization [15]. Wnt5a promotes the differentiation of mesenchymal stem cells (MSCs) into type II alveolar epithelial cells (AT II cells) [16] and acts as a repulsive guidance cue for cortical axons extending through the corpus callosum in vivo [17]. Wnt5a is also involved in IL-1β-mediated cell migration and differentiation. IL-1β-induced Wnt5a protein enhanced human corneal endothelial cell migration through the regulation of Cdc42 and RhoA [18], and silencing of Wnt5a prevents IL-1β-induced collagen type II degradation in rat chondrocytes [19]. Furthermore, Wnt5a signaling is involved in IL-1β-induced matrix metalloproteinase (MMP)-3-regulated proliferation of ES cell-derived odontoblast-like cells [20]. Although Wnt5a has been associated with the regulation of proliferation and differentiation in different cell types, little is known about the role of Wnt5a signaling in neuronal differentiation of NPCs.

Rho-family GTPases play an important role in regulating intracellular cytoskeletal and signaling pathways that facilitate axonal morphological changes [21, 22]. The most commonly studied Rho-GTPases are RhoA, Cdc42, and Rac1 [23]. Rho family GTPases serve as a molecular switch by converting from an inactive GDP-bound state to an active GTP-bound state and, once activated, they can interact with their specific effectors [24]. The GTP-bound form of RhoA causes Rho-associate kinase (ROCK) activation [25]. The RhoA/ROCK pathway is associated with various neuronal functions, such as migration, dendrite development, and axonal extension [25, 26]. The role of RhoA is complicated in axonal branching and growth cone formation [27]. In some cases, RhoA negatively regulates axon branch that inactivation of intracellular Rho to stimulate axon growth and regeneration [28]. In contrast, other studies indicated that RhoA is involved in the promotion of axon branching [29, 30]. It is, therefore, necessary to determine the distinct physiological functions of RhoA in neuronal differentiation of NPCs.

In the present study, we first investigated the role of IL-1β in neuronal differentiation of NPCs and found that IL-1β activated noncanonical Wnt5a signaling (Wnt5a/RhoA/ROCK/JNK pathway). We also demonstrated that IL-1β-induced noncanonical Wnt5a signaling is required for neuronal differentiation, especially for neurite outgrowth, suggesting that IL-1β can promote the neuronal differentiation of NPCs.

Methods

Materials

Coon's modified Ham's F-12 medium and human insulin were purchased from Sigma Chemical Co (St Louis, MO, USA). Penicillin/streptomycin solution, neurobasal medium, and B27 were purchased from Gibco (Grand Island, NY, USA), and bFGF, recombinant rat IL-1β, and recombinant Wnt5a were purchased from R&D Systems (Minneapolis, MN, USA). The following antibodies were purchased: anti NT3 (#SC-547) and anti Ngn1 (#SC-19231) from Santa Cruz Biotechnology (Santa Cruz, CA, USA); anti p-JNK (#9251S), anti JNK (#9252S), anti p-NF-κB (#3031S) and anti NF-κB (#6956S) from Cell Signaling Technology (Beverly, MA, USA); anti Wnt5a (#MABD136) from Merck (Darmstadt, Germany); anti β-tubulin type III (TUJ1) (#801202) from BioLegend (San Diego, CA, USA); anti calnexin (#ADI-SPA-860-F) from Enzo Life Sciences (Farmingdale, NY, USA). Fluorescein-(DTAF)-conjugated streptavidin (#016–010-084) was purchased from Jackson Immuno Research (Westgrove, PA, USA). Y27632 and SP600125 were purchased from Abcam (Cambridge, UK).

Primary culture of neural precursor cells

Embryonic brain cortices from E14 rat embryos were mechanically triturated in Ca^{2+}/Mg^{2+}-free Hank's balanced salt solution (Gibco), seeded at 2×10^5 cells in 10-cm culture dishes (Corning Life Sciences, Acton, MA, USA), which were precoated with 15 μg/ml poly-L-ornithine (Sigma) and 1 μg/ml fibronectin (Invitrogen, Carlsbad, CA, USA). The cells were then cultured for 5–6 days in serum-free N2 medium supplemented with 20 ng/ml bFGF (R&D Systems Inc.). Cell clusters generated by precursor cell proliferation were dissociated in Hank's balanced salt solution and plated at 2×10^4 cells per well on coated 24-well plates, 2×10^5 cells per well on coated 6-well plates, and 8×10^5 cells per dish on coated 6-cm culture dishes. All experiments were performed using passage 1 (P1) neural precursor cells.

Transient transfection of NSCs

RhoA (Dharmacon, Lafayette, CO, USA, Catalog No. L-095222-02), *Wnt5a* (Dharmacon, Catalog No. L-088203-02), *Control* (Dharmacon, Catalog No. D-001810-10) *or NF-κB p65* siRNA (Bioneer, Daejeon, KOREA, Catalog No. 1783704) were introduced into cells in knockdown experiments using a Nucleofector™ kit (Lonza, Basel, Switzerland, Catalog No. VPG-1003, Program A-031).

Real time PCR and RT (reverse transcription)-PCR

cDNA was prepared using the total mRNA extracted from cells with TRIzol® reagent (Thermo Fisher Scientific); 2 μg samples of RNA were reverse-transcribed using random hexamer mixed primers. The cDNA thus formed was amplified by PCR using the following primers:

Wnt3a (5′-TGCAAATGCCACGGACTATC-3′ and 5′-AGACTCTCGGTGTTTCTCTACC-3′),

Wnt5a (5′-TGCCACTTGTATCAGGACCA-3′ and 5′-GGCTCATGGCATTTACCACT-3′),

Wnt5b (5′-CAAGCTGGAACTGACCAACA-3′ and 5′-AAAGCAACACCAGTGGAACC-3′),

Wnt7a (5′-CACAATTCCGAGAGCTAGGC-3′ and 5′-TAGCCTGAGGGGCTGTCTTA-3′),

Wnt7b (5′-GCTATCAGAAGCCGATGGAG-3′ and 5′-ACGTGTTGCACTTGACGAAG-3′),

Nt3 (5′-GGCACACACACAGGAAGTGTC-3′ and 5′-CTGGACGTCAGGCACGGCCTGT-3′),

Ngn1 (5′-ATGCCTGCCCCTTTGGAGAC-3′ and 5′-TGCATACGGTTGCGCTCGC-3′),

p65 NF-κB (5′-CTAGGAGGACTCGGGCTCTT-3′ and 5′-AGGAGCTCCACAGGACAGAA-3′),

Gapdh (5′-CTCGTCTCATAGACAAGATG-3′ and 5′-AGACTCCACGACATACTCAGCAC-3′).

The PCR conditions for amplification of *Wnt3a*, *Wnt5a*, *Wnt5b*, *Wnt7a*, *Wnt7b*, *Nt3*, *Ngn1*, *p65 NF-κB*, and *Gapdh* were as follows: denaturation at 94 °C for 30 s, annealing at 58 °C for 1 min, and extension at 72 °C for 1 min. 30 cycles were used for amplification of all cDNAs. The PCR products were analyzed on a 1.5% agarose gel. For real-time PCR, 5 μl of RT reaction product was amplified in duplicates at a final volume of 20 μl iQ™ SYBR®-Green Super mix. Thermocycling conditions were 95 °C for 10 min, followed by 40 cycles of 95 °C for 15 s and 60 °C for 1 min. The primer sequences for real-time PCR were same as those used for RT-PCR, and all gene expression values were normalized to those of *Gapdh*.

Western blot analysis

Cells were lysed in 20 mM Tris–HCl (pH 7.5) containing 150 mM NaCl, 1 mM Ethylenediaminetetraacetic acid (EDTA), 1 mM Ethylene glycol-bis(2-aminoethyl ether)-N,N,N′,N′-tetraacetic acid (EGTA), 2.5 mM sodium pyrophosphate, 1% Triton X-100, 1 mM phenylmethylsulfonyl fluoride (PMSF), and 1 mM Na_3VO_4. Protein samples (20–30 μg) were loaded on 10% SDS–polyacrylamide gels, electrophoresed, and transferred to nitrocellulose membranes (Amersham Pharmacia Biotech, Amersharm, UK) after electrophoresis. After blocking with 5% non-fat dried milk for 1 h, membranes were incubated with primary antibodies followed by incubation with HRP-conjugated secondary antibody (Anti-mouse IgG (#7076) and Anti-rabbit IgG (#7074)) (1:2000) (New England Biolabs, Beverly, MA, USA), and specific bands were detected by ECL (Amersham Pharmacia Biotech).

RhoA activation assay

RhoA activity in cells was measured using Rho Activation assay kit (Merck, Catalog No. 17–294), according to the manufacturer's instructions. Briefly, cells were washed with ice-cold PBS, and lysed with Mg^{2+} Lysis/Wash Buffer (MLB). Lysates were collected by centrifugation at 14,000×*g* for 5 min at 4 °C. Equal amounts of protein from cell lysates were incubated for 45 min at 4 °C with 20 μg of Rhotekin-RBD protein agarose beads. Pellets were washed with MLB and subjected to western blotting using the anti-RhoA antibody.

Immunofluorescence staining

Cells were washed with PBS and fixed with 4% paraformaldehyde in PBS, followed by three washes with PBS at room temperature. They were then permeabilized with 0.1% Triton X-100 in PBS for 10 min, followed by three washes with PBS, and then blocked with 10% normal goat serum in PBS containing 0.5% Tween 20 for 1 h at room temperature. Next, the cells were incubated with the mouse monoclonal anti-β-tubulin type III (TUJ1) antibody (1:2000 dilution) primary antibody at 4 °C. Cells were then stained with streptavidin-conjugated secondary antibody (1:400) for 1 h before mounting with Vectashield (Vector Laboratories, Burlingame, CA, USA) containing 4, 6-diamidino-2-phenylindole (DAPI). Immunoreactive cells were detected using a TCS SP5 confocal imaging system (Leica Microsystems, Wetzlar, Germany) at magnification between 40× and 60 ×.

Measurement of neurite outgrowth

Cells were cultured on coverslips coated with fibronectin in 24 well plates, fixed with 0.1% (*w/v*) picric acid/PBS containing 4% (w/v) paraformaldehyde, and incubated overnight at 4 °C with β-tubulin type III (TUJ1) antibody 1:2000. After incubation with Cy3-conjugated secondary antibody (Jackson Immuno Research Laboratories, PA, USA), cells were mounted on slides with Vectashield. TUJ1-positive cells were photographed using the TCS SP5 confocal imaging system (Leica Microsystems) and morphological characteristics were quantitated using Image J software (NIH-http//rsb.Info.nih.gov/ij/). The length of primary neurite was defined as the distance from the soma to the tip of the longest branch. For each graph, data on neurite length were generated from randomly selected areas of at least five independent cultures from three independent experiments and more than 100 cells were counted for each condition in each experiment.

Statistical analysis

Cells were counted in randomly chosen (fractionator) microscope fields. Data are expressed as means ± SDs of three independent experiments. Differences were analyzed using the Student's t test and were considered significant at $p < 0.05$.

Results

IL-1β-induced Wnt5a expression is required for neuronal differentiation

We first established the distribution of IL-1β in neuronal differentiation of NPCs. Nerve growth factors, such as NT3, NT4/5, and BDNF, together with the basic helix-loop-helix transcription factors neuro-D and neurogenin-1 (Ngn1) are closely associated with neuronal differentiation and can be used as markers of this process. Treatment with IL-1β increased the expression levels of NT3 and Ngn1 in a time-dependent manner (0–6 h) (Fig. 1a and b) and enhanced neurite outgrowth (Fig. 1c and d). Several studies suggest that Wnt signaling is involved in cell differentiation [10, 15, 16]; therefore, we examined the role of Wnt signaling in IL-1β-induced neuronal differentiation. As shown in Fig. 1e, stimulation with IL-1β increased mRNA level of Wnt5a, but not of other isoforms, and protein expression of Wnt5a induced by IL-1β gradually increased over 6 h and then decreased (Fig. 1f). We also showed that IL-1β-induced mRNA (Fig. 1g) and protein (Fig. 1h) expression levels of NT3 and Ngn1 were suppressed by Wnt5a knockdown using siRNA. In addition, IL-1β-induced neurite outgrowth was decreased because of knockdown of Wnt5a using siRNA (Fig. 1i and j), suggesting that IL-1β-mediated Wnt5a expression plays a role in neuronal differentiation of NPCs.

Effect of NF-κB on IL-1β-induced Wnt5a expression and neurite outgrowth

The rat Wnt5a promoter contains both conserved and putative nuclear factor kappa B (NF-κB) binding sites [31] and its expression is NF-κB activity dependent [32]. To determine whether NF-κB affects IL-1β-induced Wnt5a expression, we first examined the phosphorylation of p65 NF-κB by IL-1β stimulation. IL-1β increased phosphorylation of NF-κB p65 within 30 min (Fig. 2a). We showed that IL-1β-induced mRNA (Fig. 2b and c) and protein (Fig. 2d) expression levels of Wnt5a were decreased due to knockdown of NF-κB p65 using siRNA, indicating that IL-1β-induced Wnt5a expression is NF-κB dependent. We further showed that IL-1β-induced mRNA (Fig. 2e and f) and protein (Fig. 2g) expression levels of NT3 and Ngn1 were inhibited by NF-κB p65 siRNA, and IL-1β-induced neurite outgrowth was decreased by NF-κB p65 knockdown (Fig. 2h and i).

These results suggest that NF-κB activity is involved in IL-1β-induced Wnt5a expression and in the neurite outgrowth of NPCs.

Wnt5a promotes neurite outgrowth through a RhoA/ROCK/JNK pathway

We tested whether exogenous Wnt5a could enhance neuronal differentiation. As shown in Fig. 3a-c, mRNA (Fig. 3a and b) and protein (Fig. 3c) levels of NT3 and Ngn1 were increased by Wnt5a treatment. Exogenous Wnt5a also markedly increased neurite outgrowth (Fig. 3d and e), indicating the importance of Wnt5a in neuronal differentiation of NPCs. Previous studies suggest that RhoA plays a central role in dendritic development, and that differential activation of Rho-related GTPases contributes to the generation of morphological diversity in the developing cortex [24]. As Wnt5a has recently been found to be involved in the regulation of RhoA [18], we examined the effect of Wnt5a on the activity of RhoA. Treatment with Wnt5a increased RhoA activity (Fig. 3f). Next, we examined the role of RhoA in Wnt5a-induced neuronal differentiation. As shown in Fig. 3g and h, Wnt5a-induced mRNA and Protein levels of NT3 and Ngn1 were decreased by RhoA knockdown with siRNA. Moreover, Wnt5a-induced neurite outgrowth was inhibited by RhoA knockdown (Fig. 3i and j). We further showed that the ROCK inhibitor Y27632 suppressed Wnt5a-induced increase in mRNA (Additional file 1: Figure S1A and B) and protein levels of NT3 and Ngn1 (Additional file 1: Figure S1C), and also Y27632 inhibited neurite outgrowth induced by Wnt5a (Additional file 1: Figure S1D and E), indicating that RhoA/ROCK pathway is implicated in Wnt5a-induced neuronal differentiation.

The JNK (c-Jun N-terminal Kinase), also known as stress-activated protein kinase, has extensive implications in understanding important biological processes, such as cell growth, differentiation, tissue development and regeneration [33, 34]. Previous studies reported that JNK mediates neural differentiation, induction of the neural-specific gene neurofilament light chain (NFLC) and development of embryonic stem cells [35, 36]. Interestingly, Wnt5a/JNK signaling contributed to the differentiation of mesenchymal stem cells [16]. Thus, we examined whether JNK activation is involved in Wnt5a-induced neuronal differentiation of NPCs. As shown in Fig. 4a, Wnt5a treatment increased phosphorylation of JNK. When the cells were pretreated with a JNK inhibitor, SP600125, Wnt5a-induced mRNA (Fig. 4b and c) and protein (Fig. 4d) levels of NT3 and Ngn1 were decreased. Moreover, Wnt5a-induced neurite outgrowth was significantly decreased by SP600125, indicating that JNK

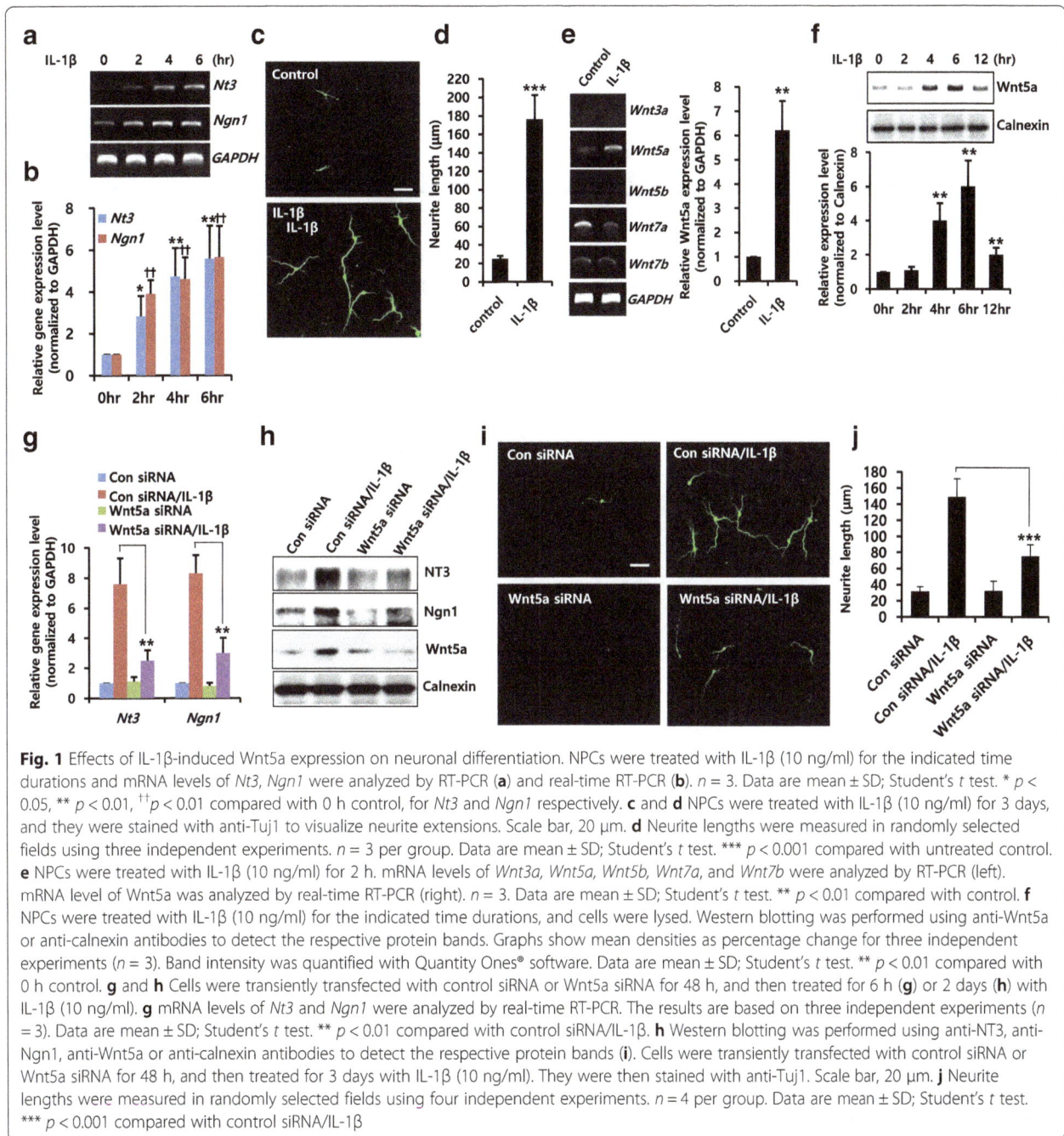

Fig. 1 Effects of IL-1β-induced Wnt5a expression on neuronal differentiation. NPCs were treated with IL-1β (10 ng/ml) for the indicated time durations and mRNA levels of *Nt3*, *Ngn1* were analyzed by RT-PCR (**a**) and real-time RT-PCR (**b**). *n* = 3. Data are mean ± SD; Student's *t* test. * *p* < 0.05, ** *p* < 0.01, ††*p* < 0.01 compared with 0 h control, for *Nt3* and *Ngn1* respectively. **c** and **d** NPCs were treated with IL-1β (10 ng/ml) for 3 days, and they were stained with anti-Tuj1 to visualize neurite extensions. Scale bar, 20 μm. **d** Neurite lengths were measured in randomly selected fields using three independent experiments. *n* = 3 per group. Data are mean ± SD; Student's *t* test. *** *p* < 0.001 compared with untreated control. **e** NPCs were treated with IL-1β (10 ng/ml) for 2 h. mRNA levels of *Wnt3a*, *Wnt5a*, *Wnt5b*, *Wnt7a*, and *Wnt7b* were analyzed by RT-PCR (left). mRNA level of Wnt5a was analyzed by real-time RT-PCR (right). *n* = 3. Data are mean ± SD; Student's *t* test. ** *p* < 0.01 compared with control. **f** NPCs were treated with IL-1β (10 ng/ml) for the indicated time durations, and cells were lysed. Western blotting was performed using anti-Wnt5a or anti-calnexin antibodies to detect the respective protein bands. Graphs show mean densities as percentage change for three independent experiments (*n* = 3). Band intensity was quantified with Quantity Ones® software. Data are mean ± SD; Student's *t* test. ** *p* < 0.01 compared with 0 h control. **g** and **h** Cells were transiently transfected with control siRNA or Wnt5a siRNA for 48 h, and then treated for 6 h (**g**) or 2 days (**h**) with IL-1β (10 ng/ml). **g** mRNA levels of *Nt3* and *Ngn1* were analyzed by real-time RT-PCR. The results are based on three independent experiments (*n* = 3). Data are mean ± SD; Student's *t* test. ** *p* < 0.01 compared with control siRNA/IL-1β. **h** Western blotting was performed using anti-NT3, anti-Ngn1, anti-Wnt5a or anti-calnexin antibodies to detect the respective protein bands (**i**). Cells were transiently transfected with control siRNA or Wnt5a siRNA for 48 h, and then treated for 3 days with IL-1β (10 ng/ml). They were then stained with anti-Tuj1. Scale bar, 20 μm. **j** Neurite lengths were measured in randomly selected fields using four independent experiments. *n* = 4 per group. Data are mean ± SD; Student's *t* test. *** *p* < 0.001 compared with control siRNA/IL-1β

activation is related to Wnt5a-induced neuronal differentiation (Fig. 4e and f). Next, we determined the involvement of the RhoA/ROCK pathway on Wnt5a-mediated JNK activation. As shown in Fig. 4g, Wnt5a-induced phosphorylation of JNK was decreased by RhoA siRNA. Furthermore, pre-treatment with Y27632 reduced Wnt5a-induced phosphorylation of JNK (Fig. 4h). Therefore, these results suggest that Wnt5a-induced neuronal differentiation is regulated by the RhoA/ROCK/JNK pathway.

Evaluation of Wnt5a-mediated pathway on IL-1β-induced neuronal differentiation

We next examined whether the Wnt5a-mediated RhoA/ROCK/JNK pathway is involved in IL-1β-induced neuronal differentiation. We showed that IL-1β-induced RhoA activity was significantly decreased due to knockdown of Wnt5a using siRNA (Fig. 5a). We also found that IL-1β-induced mRNA (Fig. 5b) and protein (Fig. 5c) levels of NT3 and Ngn1 were decreased by RhoA siRNA, and IL-1β-induced neurite outgrowth was

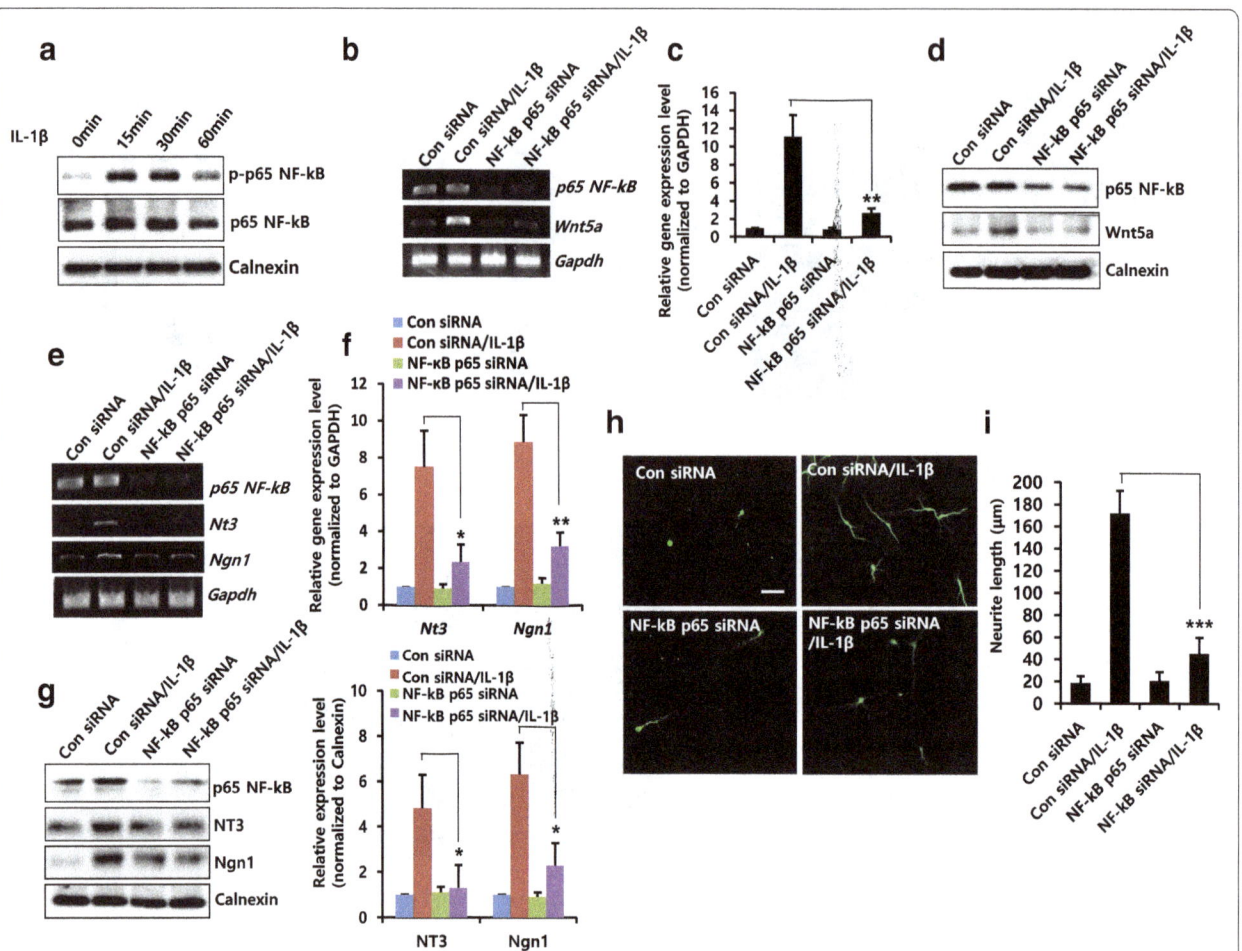

Fig. 2 Effects of NF-κB on IL-1β–induced Wnt5a expression and neuronal differentiation. **a** NPCs were treated with IL-1β (10 ng/ml) for the indicated time durations, lysed, and harvested. Western blotting was performed using anti-p-p65 NF-κB, anti-p65 NF-κB, or anti-calnexin antibodies to detect the respective protein bands. **b-d** Cells were transiently transfected with control siRNA or NF-κB p65 siRNA for 48 h, and then treated for 2 h (**b** and **c**) or 6 h (**d**) with IL-1β (10 ng/ml). mRNA levels of *Wnt5a* were estimated by RT-PCR (**b**) and real-time RT-PCR (**c**). $n = 3$. Data are mean ± SD; Student's *t* test. ** $p < 0.01$ compared with control siRNA/IL-1β. **d** Western blotting was performed using anti-p65 NF-κB, anti-Wnt5a, or anti-calnexin antibodies to detect the respective protein bands. **e** and **f** Cells were transiently transfected with control siRNA or NF-κB p65 siRNA for 48 h, and then treated for 6 h with IL-1β (10 ng/ml). mRNA levels of *Nt3* and *Ngn1* were analyzed by RT-PCR (**e**) and real-time RT-PCR (**f**). $n = 3$. Data are mean ± SD; Student's *t* test. * $p < 0.05$, ** $p < 0.01$ compared with control siRNA/IL-1β. **g** Cells were transiently transfected with control siRNA or NF-κB p65 siRNA for 48 h, and then treated for 2 days with IL-1β (10 ng/ml). Western blotting was performed using anti-p65 NF-κB, anti-NT3, anti-Ngn1, or anti-calnexin antibodies to detect the respective protein bands. Graphs show mean densities as fold change for three independent experiments ($n = 3$). Band intensity was quantified with Quantity Ones® software. Data are mean ± SD; Student's *t* test. $p < 0.05$ compared with control siRNA/IL-1β. **h** and **i** Cells were transiently transfected with control siRNA or NF-κB p65 siRNA for 48 h, and then treated for 3 days with IL-1β (10 ng/ml). They were then stained with anti-Tuj1. Scale bar, 20 μm. **i** Neurite lengths were measured in randomly selected fields using four independent experiments. $n = 4$ per group. Data are mean ± SD; Student's *t* test. *** $p < 0.001$ as compared to control siRNA/IL-1β

significantly inhibited by RhoA siRNA (Fig. 5d and e). In addition, RhoA knockdown with siRNA decreased IL-1β-induced phosphorylation of JNK (Fig. 5f). Furthermore, pre-treatment with Y27632 or SP600125 inhibitors not only suppressed IL-1β-induced mRNA and protein levels of NT3 and Ngn1 (Fig. 5g and h) but also decreased IL-1β-induced neurite outgrowth (Fig. 5i and j). These results suggest that Wnt5a/RhoA/ROCK/JNK pathway is involved in IL-1β-induced neuronal differentiation of NPCs.

Discussion

IL-1β is known to be a key modulator of stress and inflammation in the CNS. Neuroinflammation is implicated in the pathophysiology of many psychiatric and neurodegenerative disorders where cognitive dysfunction and reductions in neurogenesis are evident, including Alzheimer's disease (AD), Parkinson's disease (PD), and depression [2]. IL-1β has been shown to negatively influence the proliferation and differentiation of hippocampal NPCs [37], and that it impairs neurotrophin-induced

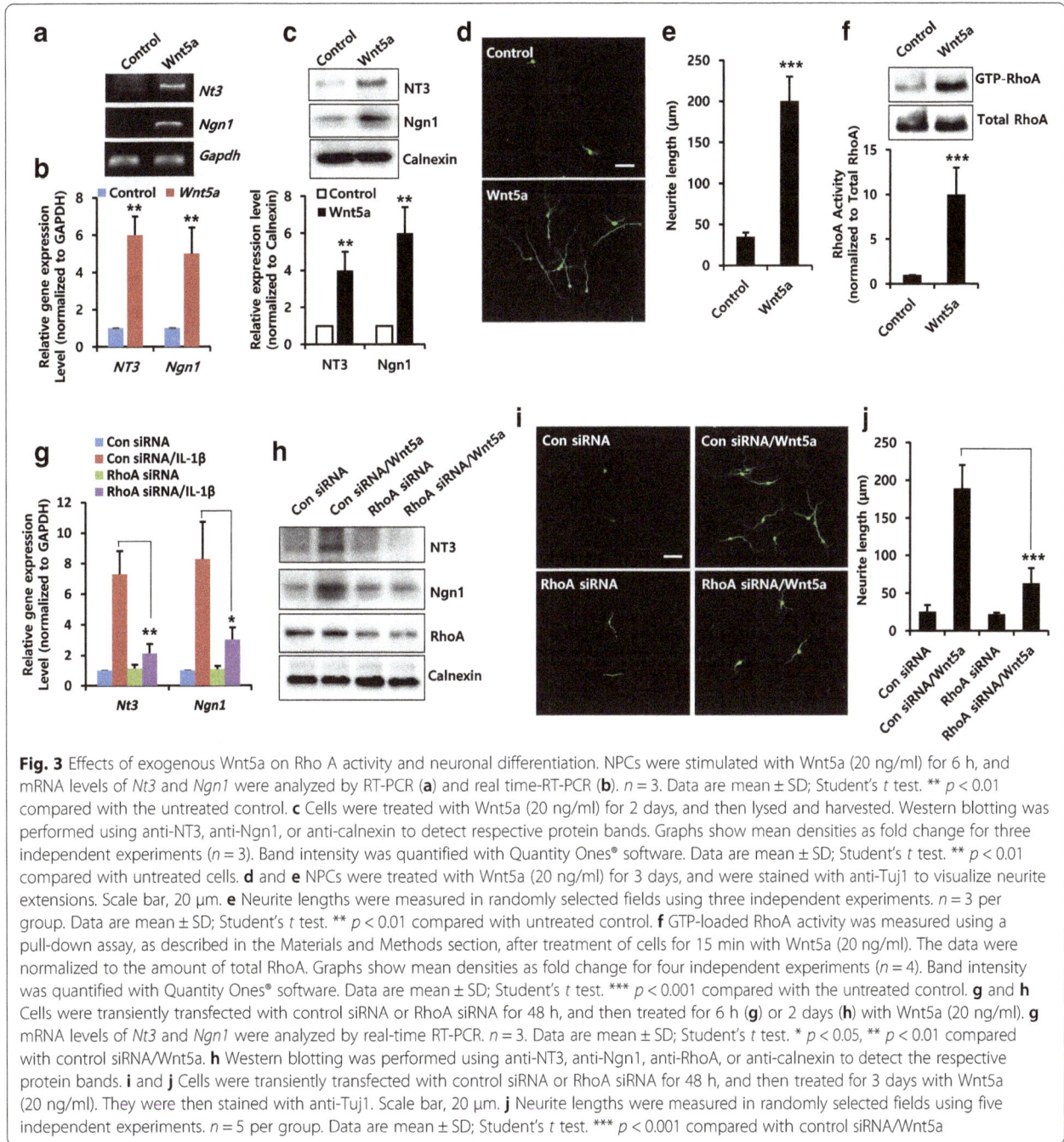

Fig. 3 Effects of exogenous Wnt5a on Rho A activity and neuronal differentiation. NPCs were stimulated with Wnt5a (20 ng/ml) for 6 h, and mRNA levels of *Nt3* and *Ngn1* were analyzed by RT-PCR (**a**) and real time-RT-PCR (**b**). $n = 3$. Data are mean ± SD; Student's *t* test. ** $p < 0.01$ compared with the untreated control. **c** Cells were treated with Wnt5a (20 ng/ml) for 2 days, and then lysed and harvested. Western blotting was performed using anti-NT3, anti-Ngn1, or anti-calnexin to detect respective protein bands. Graphs show mean densities as fold change for three independent experiments ($n = 3$). Band intensity was quantified with Quantity Ones® software. Data are mean ± SD; Student's *t* test. ** $p < 0.01$ compared with untreated cells. **d** and **e** NPCs were treated with Wnt5a (20 ng/ml) for 3 days, and were stained with anti-Tuj1 to visualize neurite extensions. Scale bar, 20 μm. **e** Neurite lengths were measured in randomly selected fields using three independent experiments. $n = 3$ per group. Data are mean ± SD; Student's *t* test. ** $p < 0.01$ compared with untreated control. **f** GTP-loaded RhoA activity was measured using a pull-down assay, as described in the Materials and Methods section, after treatment of cells for 15 min with Wnt5a (20 ng/ml). The data were normalized to the amount of total RhoA. Graphs show mean densities as fold change for four independent experiments ($n = 4$). Band intensity was quantified with Quantity Ones® software. Data are mean ± SD; Student's *t* test. *** $p < 0.001$ compared with the untreated control. **g** and **h** Cells were transiently transfected with control siRNA or RhoA siRNA for 48 h, and then treated for 6 h (**g**) or 2 days (**h**) with Wnt5a (20 ng/ml). **g** mRNA levels of *Nt3* and *Ngn1* were analyzed by real-time RT-PCR. $n = 3$. Data are mean ± SD; Student's *t* test. * $p < 0.05$, ** $p < 0.01$ compared with control siRNA/Wnt5a. **h** Western blotting was performed using anti-NT3, anti-Ngn1, anti-RhoA, or anti-calnexin to detect the respective protein bands. **i** and **j** Cells were transiently transfected with control siRNA or RhoA siRNA for 48 h, and then treated for 3 days with Wnt5a (20 ng/ml). They were then stained with anti-Tuj1. Scale bar, 20 μm. **j** Neurite lengths were measured in randomly selected fields using five independent experiments. $n = 5$ per group. Data are mean ± SD; Student's *t* test. *** $p < 0.001$ compared with control siRNA/Wnt5a

neuronal cell survival [38, 39]. In the spinal cord, IL-1β has been implicated in extensive inflammation and progressive neuro-degeneration after ischemic and traumatic injury [40, 41]. These results indicate that IL-1β might be involved in the pathogenesis of some neurodevelopmental disorders. However, there is increasing evidence that inflammation-associated cytokines can play a key role in stimulating neurite outgrowth and regeneration [42, 43]. Recent studies have provided an indication that IL-1β is able to stimulate the migration of cultured cortical neurons [7], and the potent

neurotropic action of IL-1β leads to rapid neurite growth [44]. In this study, we found that stimulation with IL-1β facilitates neurite outgrowth, as well as increases the expression levels of neuronal factors, such as NT3 and Ngn1. Moreover, IL-1β-induced Wnt5a expression has a critical role in neuronal differentiation of NPCs. These results demonstrate a novel physiological function of IL-1β in neuronal differentiation of cortical NPCs.

Recently, Wnt5a, identified as an axon guidance cue, was shown to activate a non-canonical pathway essential for cortical axonal morphogenesis. In this study, we

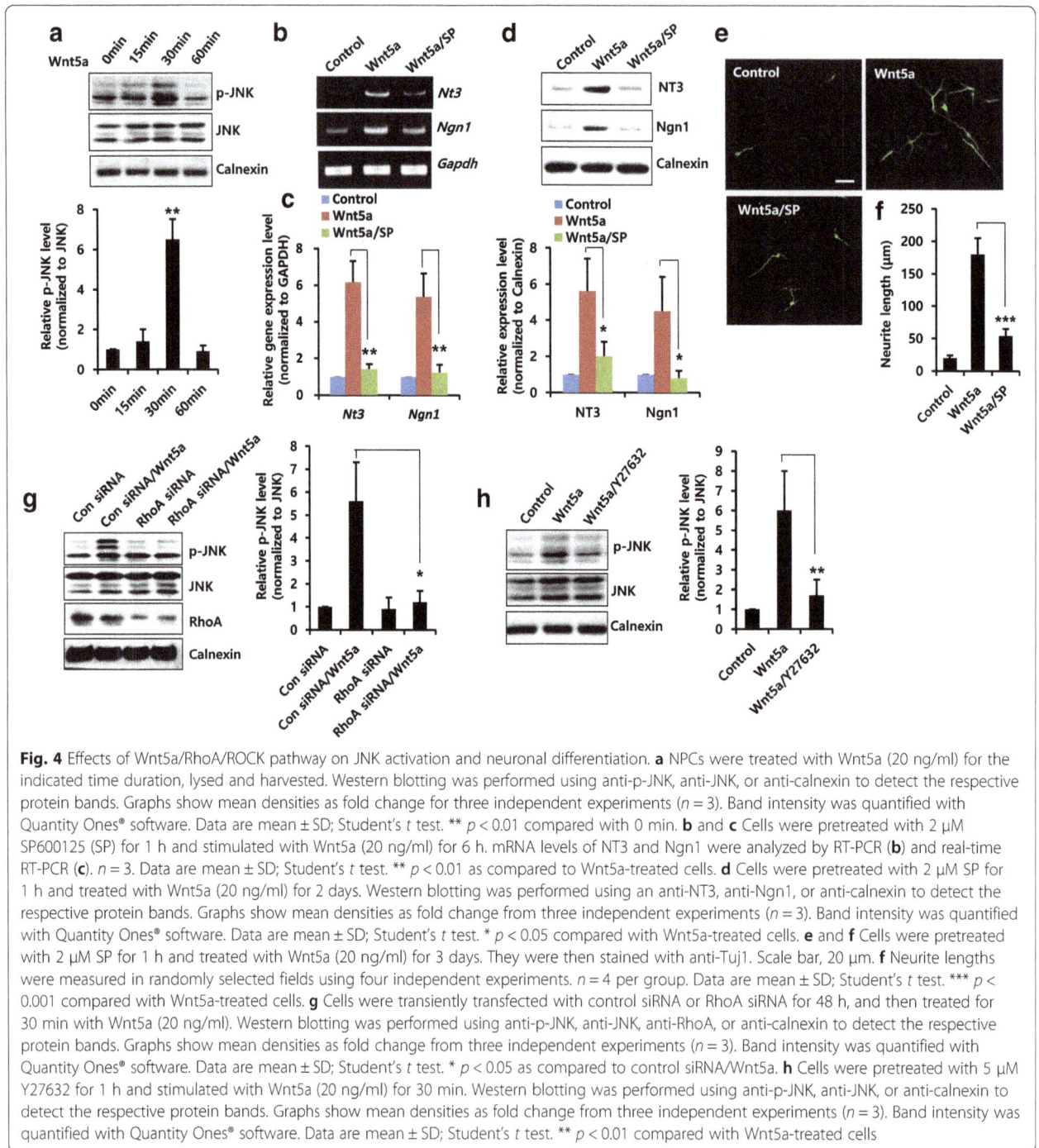

Fig. 4 Effects of Wnt5a/RhoA/ROCK pathway on JNK activation and neuronal differentiation. **a** NPCs were treated with Wnt5a (20 ng/ml) for the indicated time duration, lysed and harvested. Western blotting was performed using anti-p-JNK, anti-JNK, or anti-calnexin to detect the respective protein bands. Graphs show mean densities as fold change for three independent experiments ($n = 3$). Band intensity was quantified with Quantity Ones® software. Data are mean ± SD; Student's t test. ** $p < 0.01$ compared with 0 min. **b** and **c** Cells were pretreated with 2 μM SP600125 (SP) for 1 h and stimulated with Wnt5a (20 ng/ml) for 6 h. mRNA levels of NT3 and Ngn1 were analyzed by RT-PCR (**b**) and real-time RT-PCR (**c**). $n = 3$. Data are mean ± SD; Student's t test. ** $p < 0.01$ as compared to Wnt5a-treated cells. **d** Cells were pretreated with 2 μM SP for 1 h and treated with Wnt5a (20 ng/ml) for 2 days. Western blotting was performed using an anti-NT3, anti-Ngn1, or anti-calnexin to detect the respective protein bands. Graphs show mean densities as fold change from three independent experiments ($n = 3$). Band intensity was quantified with Quantity Ones® software. Data are mean ± SD; Student's t test. * $p < 0.05$ compared with Wnt5a-treated cells. **e** and **f** Cells were pretreated with 2 μM SP for 1 h and treated with Wnt5a (20 ng/ml) for 3 days. They were then stained with anti-Tuj1. Scale bar, 20 μm. **f** Neurite lengths were measured in randomly selected fields using four independent experiments. $n = 4$ per group. Data are mean ± SD; Student's t test. *** $p < 0.001$ compared with Wnt5a-treated cells. **g** Cells were transiently transfected with control siRNA or RhoA siRNA for 48 h, and then treated for 30 min with Wnt5a (20 ng/ml). Western blotting was performed using anti-p-JNK, anti-JNK, anti-RhoA, or anti-calnexin to detect the respective protein bands. Graphs show mean densities as fold change from three independent experiments ($n = 3$). Band intensity was quantified with Quantity Ones® software. Data are mean ± SD; Student's t test. * $p < 0.05$ as compared to control siRNA/Wnt5a. **h** Cells were pretreated with 5 μM Y27632 for 1 h and stimulated with Wnt5a (20 ng/ml) for 30 min. Western blotting was performed using anti-p-JNK, anti-JNK, or anti-calnexin to detect the respective protein bands. Graphs show mean densities as fold change from three independent experiments ($n = 3$). Band intensity was quantified with Quantity Ones® software. Data are mean ± SD; Student's t test. ** $p < 0.01$ compared with Wnt5a-treated cells

found that the Wnt5a/RhoA/ROCK/JNK pathway is required for IL-1β-mediated neurite outgrowth of NPCs. The effect of Wnt5a signaling on axon outgrowth of cortical neurons is consistent with a recent study showing that Wnt5a increases axon length and promotes axon differentiation of dissociated hippocampal neurons [45]. In addition, a recent study suggests that Wnt5a promotes axonal growth through the regulation of calcium signaling during neuronal polarization [46]. In contrast, a previous study has shown that Wnt5a acts via Ryk receptors to inhibit the neurite outgrowth of sensorimotor cortex [47]. The different roles of Wnt5a in neurons are probably related to their activity dependent mechanisms. Therefore, it is necessary to elucidate a more detailed mechanism of Wnt5a signaling in developing neurite outgrowth and axon guidance.

Axon outgrowth and navigation during synapse formation are regulated by extracellular signals. The cytoskeletal

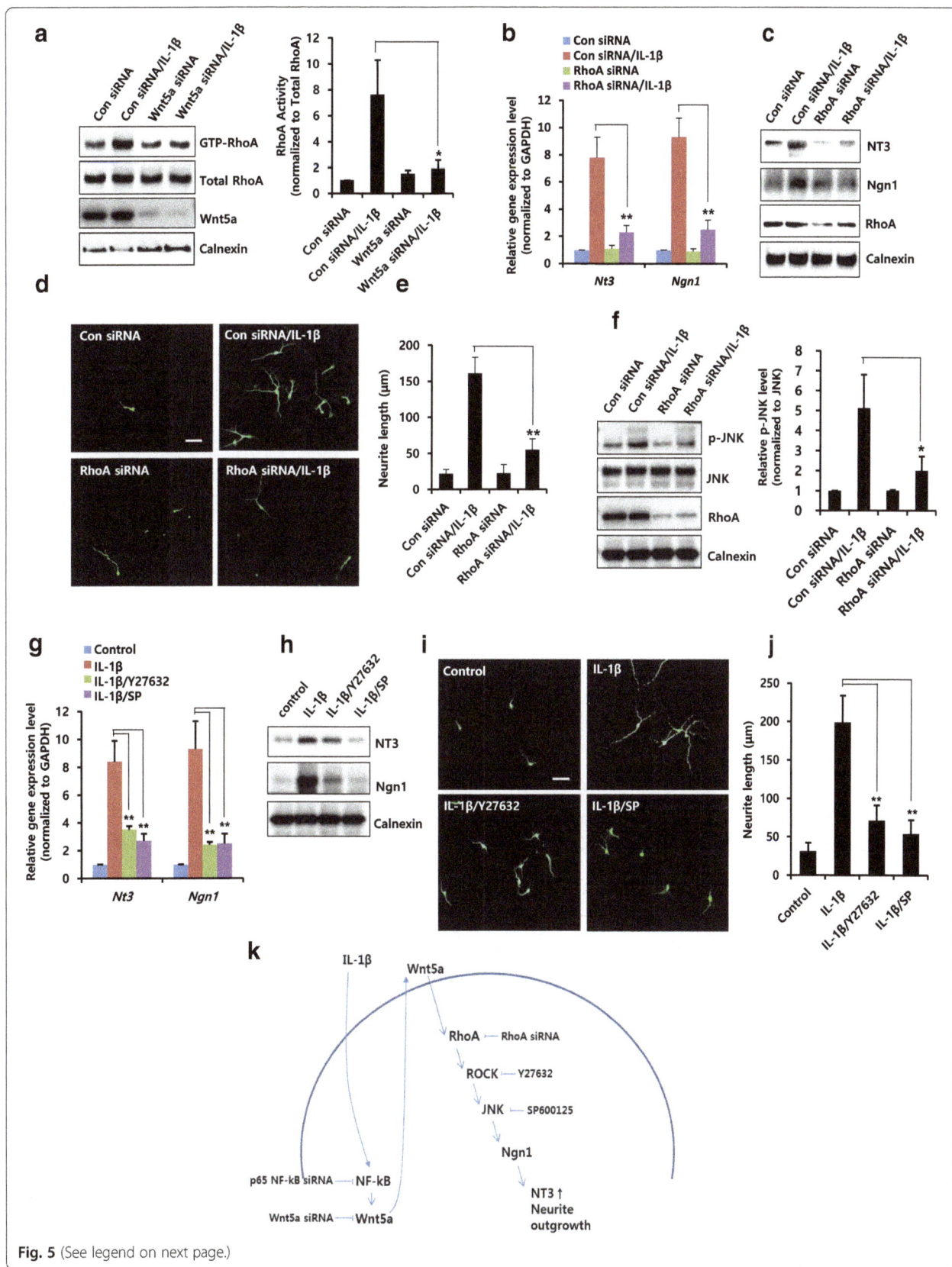

Fig. 5 (See legend on next page.)

(See figure on previous page.)

Fig. 5 Effects of IL-1β on Wnt5a-mediated signaling and neuronal differentiation. **a** NPCs were transiently transfected with control siRNA or Wnt5a siRNA for 48 h, and then incubated for 15 min with IL-1β (10 ng/ml). GTP-loaded RhoA activity was measured using a pull-down assay, as described in the Materials and Methods section. The data were normalized to the amount of total RhoA. Graphs show mean densities as fold change from three independent experiments ($n = 3$). Band intensity was quantified with Quantity Ones® software. Data are mean ± SD; Student's t test. * $p < 0.05$ compared with control siRNA/IL-1β. **b** and **c** Cells were transiently transfected with control siRNA or RhoA siRNA for 48 h, and then incubated for 6 h (B) or 2 days (c) with IL-1β (10 ng/ml). **b** mRNA levels of Nt3 and Ngn1 were analyzed by real-time RT-PCR. $n = 3$. Data are mean ± SD; Student's t test. ** $p < 0.01$ as compared to control siRNA/IL-1β. **c** Cells were transiently transfected with control siRNA or RhoA siRNA for 48 h, and then treated for 2 days with IL-1β (10 ng/ml). Western blotting was performed using anti-NT3, anti-Ngn1, anti-RhoA, or anti-calnexin antibodies to detect the respective protein bands. **d** and **e** Cells were transiently transfected with control siRNA or RhoA siRNA for 48 h, and then incubated for 3 days with IL-1β (10 ng/ml). They were then stained with anti-Tuj1. Scale bar, 20 μm. **e** Neurite lengths were measured in randomly selected fields using three independent experiments. $n = 3$ per group. Data are mean ± SD; Student's t test. ** $p < 0.01$ compared with control siRNA/IL-1β. **f** Cells were transiently transfected with control siRNA or RhoA siRNA for 48 h, and then treated for 30 min with IL-1β (10 ng/ml). Western blotting was performed using anti-p-JNK, anti-JNK, anti-RhoA or anti-calnexin antibodies to detect the respective protein bands. Graphs show mean densities as fold change for three independent experiments ($n = 3$). Band intensity was quantified with Quantity Ones® software. Data are mean ± SD; Student's t test. * $p < 0.05$ compared with control siRNA/IL-1β. **g** and **h** Cells were pretreated with 5 μM Y27632 or 2 μM SP for 1 h, and then treated with IL-1β (10 ng/ml) for 6 h (**g**) or 2 days (**h**). **g** mRNA levels of Nt3 and Ngn1 were analyzed by real-time RT-PCR. $n = 3$. Data are mean ± SD; Student's t test. ** $p < 0.01$ compared with IL-1β-treated cells. **h** Cells were pretreated with 5 μM Y27632 or 2 μM SP for 1 h, and then treated with IL-1β (10 ng/ml) for 2 days. Western blotting was performed using anti-NT3, anti-Ngn1 or anti-calnexin antibodies to detect the respective protein bands. (I and J) Cells were pretreated with 5 μM Y27632 or 2 μM SP for 1 h, and then treated with IL-1β (10 ng/ml) for 3 days. They were then stained with anti-Tuj1. Scale bar, 20 μm. **j** Neurite lengths were measured in randomly selected fields using three independent experiments. $n = 3$ per group. Data are mean ± SD; Student's t test. ** $p < 0.01$ as compared to IL-1β-treated cells. **k** Proposed model for the signaling pathway in IL-1β-mediated neurite outgrowth of cortical NPCs. The model suggests that IL-1β-induced Wnt5a plays a major stimulatory role in neuronal differentiation and that it acts through the RhoA/ROCK/JNK pathway, leading to neurite outgrowth

mechanisms of axonal branching are regulated by Rho GTPases [23]. Recent reports suggest that the Rho GTPases, including RhoA, Rac1, and Cdc42 play a central role in dendritic development, and that differential activation of Rho-related GTPases contributes to the generation of morphological diversity in the developing cortex [24, 48]. Cdc42 and Rac1 facilitate axonal branching and growth cone formation [21]. However, RhoA activity in axonal branch regulation is complex. It has been shown that RhoA negatively regulated axon formation [26]. RhoA/ROCK suppresses axonal protrusive activity by negatively regulating the filopodia from actin patches [27]. In contrast, our present study showed that RhoA/ROCK signaling induced by IL-1β or Wnt5a promotes neurite outgrowth, as well as increases the expression levels of neuronal factors, such as NT3 and Ngn1. In addition, recent studies reported that RhoA/ROCK pathway increased neurite outgrowth in hippocampal immortalized cells [49], and inhibition of RhoA activity reduces axonal branching in hippocampal neurons of embryonic mice [29]. These findings are consistent with our study showing that RhoA/ROCK signaling plays a positive role in neurite outgrowth. Considering that RhoA plays a different role in the regulation of neurite outgrowth depending on the cell environment (culture conditions and type of stimulation) or cell types, it will be necessary to determine the specific contribution of RhoA activity to all components of cytoskeletal mechanics and neurite outgrowth.

Here, we demonstrate a novel function of IL-1β in neuronal differentiation of NPCs. The findings of the present study are summarized in Fig. 5k. First, we found that stimulation with IL-1β promotes neuronal differentiation. Second, IL-1β induces Wnt5a expression through NF-κB activity. Third, IL-1β-induced Wnt5a is required for neuronal differentiation through a RhoA/ROCK/JNK pathway. Taken together, we conclude that IL-1β promotes neuronal differentiation through a Wnt5a/RhoA/ROCK/JNK pathway in cortical NPCs.

Abbreviations
CNS: Central nervous system; IL-1β: Interleukin-1 beta; JNK: c-jun N-terminal kinase; NF-κB: Nuclear factor kappa B; Ngn1: Neurogenin1; NPCs: Neural precursor cells; NT3: Neurotrophin-3; ROCK: Rho-associated kinase

Acknowledgements
We thank Editage (Cactus Communications) for editorial assistance.

Funding
This work was supported by the Basic Science Research Program through the National Research Foundation of Korea (NRF), funded by the Ministry of Science, ICT, & Future Planning (NRF-2015R1C1A1A02037376), and partly supported by (NRF-2018R1A1A1A05022185).

Authors' contributions
SP: Conception and design, manuscript writing, collection and assembly of data, data analysis and interpretation, financial support. MK: Collection and assembly of data. JH: Conception and design, manuscript writing, data analysis and interpretation. All authors read and approved the final manuscript.

Competing interests

The authors declare that they have no competing interests.

References

1. Boato F, Hechler D, Rosenberger K, Ludecke D, Peters EM, Nitsch R, Hendrix S. Interleukin-1 beta and neurotrophin-3 synergistically promote neurite growth in vitro. J Neuroinflammation. 2011;8:183.
2. O'Leime CS, Cryan JF, Nolan YM. Nuclear deterrents: intrinsic regulators of IL-1beta-induced effects on hippocampal neurogenesis. Brain Behav Immun. 2017;66:394–412.
3. Sims JE, Gayle MA, Slack JL, Alderson MR, Bird TA, Giri JG, Colotta F, Re F, Mantovani A, Shanebeck K, et al. Interleukin 1 signaling occurs exclusively via the type I receptor. Proc Natl Acad Sci U S A. 1993;90:6155–9.
4. Loddick SA, Rothwell NJ. Neuroprotective effects of human recombinant interleukin-1 receptor antagonist in focal cerebral ischaemia in the rat. J Cereb Blood Flow Metab. 1996;16:932–40.
5. Huang FP, Wang ZQ, Wu DC, Schielke GP, Sun Y, Yang GY. Early NFkappaB activation is inhibited during focal cerebral ischemia in interleukin-1beta-converting enzyme deficient mice. J Neurosci Res. 2003;73:698–707.
6. Carlson NG, Wieggel WA, Chen J, Bacchi A, Rogers SW, Gahring LC. Inflammatory cytokines IL-1 alpha, IL-1 beta, IL-6, and TNF-alpha impart neuroprotection to an excitotoxin through distinct pathways. J Immunol. 1999;163:3963–8.
7. Ma L, Li XW, Zhang SJ, Yang F, Zhu GM, Yuan XB, Jiang W. Interleukin-1 beta guides the migration of cortical neurons. J Neuroinflammation. 2014; 11:114.
8. Araujo DM, Cotman CW. Differential effects of interleukin-1 beta and interleukin-2 on glia and hippocampal neurons in culture. Int J Dev Neurosci. 1995;13:201–12.
9. Cadigan KM, Nusse R. Wnt signaling: a common theme in animal development. Genes Dev. 1997;11:3286–305.
10. Sassi N, Laadhar L, Allouche M, Achek A, Kallel-Sellami M, Makni S, Sellami S. WNT signaling and chondrocytes: from cell fate determination to osteoarthritis physiopathology. J Recept Signal Transduct Res. 2014;34:73–80.
11. Rao TP, Kuhl M. An updated overview on Wnt signaling pathways: a prelude for more. Circ Res. 2010;106:1798–806.
12. Selvaraj P, Huang JS, Chen A, Skalka N, Rosin-Arbesfeld R, Loh YP. Neurotrophic factor-alpha1 modulates NGF-induced neurite outgrowth through interaction with Wnt-3a and Wnt-5a in PC12 cells and cortical neurons. Mol Cell Neurosci. 2015;68:222–33.
13. Hwang SG, Ryu JH, Kim IC, Jho EH, Jung HC, Kim K, Kim SJ, Chun JS. Wnt-7a causes loss of differentiated phenotype and inhibits apoptosis of articular chondrocytes via different mechanisms. J Biol Chem. 2004;279:26597–604.
14. Ryu JH, Chun JS. Opposing roles of WNT-5A and WNT-11 in interleukin-1beta regulation of type II collagen expression in articular chondrocytes. J Biol Chem. 2006;281:22039–47.
15. Kumawat K, Gosens R. WNT-5A: signaling and functions in health and disease. Cell Mol Life Sci. 2016;73:567–87.
16. Liu A, Chen S, Cai S, Dong L, Liu L, Yang Y, Guo F, Lu X, He H, Chen Q, et al. Wnt5a through noncanonical Wnt/JNK or Wnt/PKC signaling contributes to the differentiation of mesenchymal stem cells into type II alveolar epithelial cells in vitro. PLoS One. 2014;9:e90229.
17. Keeble TR, Halford MM, Seaman C, Kee N, Macheda M, Anderson RB, Stacker SA, Cooper HM. The Wnt receptor Ryk is required for Wnt5a-mediated axon guidance on the contralateral side of the corpus callosum. J Neurosci. 2006; 26:5840–8.
18. Lee JG, Heur M. Interleukin-1beta-induced Wnt5a enhances human corneal endothelial cell migration through regulation of Cdc42 and RhoA. Mol Cell Biol. 2014;34:3535–45.
19. Shi S, Man Z, Li W, Sun S, Zhang W. Silencing of Wnt5a prevents interleukin-1beta-induced collagen type II degradation in rat chondrocytes. Exp Ther Med. 2016;12:3161–6.
20. Ozeki N, Hase N, Hiyama T, Yamaguchi H, Kawai R, Kondo A, Nakata K, Mogi M. IL-1beta-induced, matrix metalloproteinase-3-regulated proliferation of embryonic stem cell-derived odontoblastic cells is mediated by the Wnt5 signaling pathway. Exp Cell Res. 2014;328:69–86.
21. Hall A, Lalli G. Rho and Ras GTPases in axon growth, guidance, and branching. Cold Spring Harb Perspect Biol. 2010;2:a001818.
22. Billuart P, Winter CG, Maresh A, Zhao X, Luo L. Regulating axon branch stability: the role of p190 RhoGAP in repressing a retraction signaling pathway. Cell. 2001;107:195–207.
23. Spillane M, Gallo G. Involvement of rho-family GTPases in axon branching. Small GTPases. 2014;5:e27974.
24. Yoon MS, Cho CH, Lee KS, Han JS. Binding of Cdc42 to phospholipase D1 is important in neurite outgrowth of neural stem cells. Biochem Biophys Res Commun. 2006;347:594–600.
25. Fujita Y, Yamashita T. Axon growth inhibition by RhoA/ROCK in the central nervous system. Front Neurosci. 2014;8:338.
26. Rico B, Beggs HE, Schahin-Reed D, Kimes N, Schmidt A, Reichardt LF. Control of axonal branching and synapse formation by focal adhesion kinase. Nat Neurosci. 2004;7:1059–69.
27. Loudon RP, Silver LD, Yee HF Jr, Gallo G. RhoA-kinase and myosin II are required for the maintenance of growth cone polarity and guidance by nerve growth factor. J Neurobiol. 2006;66:847–67.
28. Bertrand J, Winton MJ, Rodriguez-Hernandez N, Campenot RB, McKerracher L. Application of Rho antagonist to neuronal cell bodies promotes neurite growth in compartmented cultures and regeneration of retinal ganglion cell axons in the optic nerve of adult rats. J Neurosci. 2005;25:1113–21.
29. Ahnert-Hilger G, Holtje M, Grosse G, Pickert G, Mucke C, Nixdorf-Bergweiler B, Boquet P, Hofmann F, Just I. Differential effects of Rho GTPases on axonal and dendritic development in hippocampal neurones. J Neurochem. 2004; 90:9–18.
30. Ohnami S, Endo M, Hirai S, Uesaka N, Hatanaka Y, Yamashita T, Yamamoto N. Role of RhoA in activity-dependent cortical axon branching. J Neurosci. 2008;28:9117–21.
31. Katoh M, Katoh M. Transcriptional mechanisms of WNT5A based on NF-kappaB, hedgehog, TGFbeta, and notch signaling cascades. Int J Mol Med. 2009;23:763–9.
32. Zhao Y, Wang CL, Li RM, Hui TQ, Su YY, Yuan Q, Zhou XD, Ye L. Wnt5a promotes inflammatory responses via nuclear factor kappaB (NF-kappaB) and mitogen-activated protein kinase (MAPK) pathways in human dental pulp cells. J Biol Chem. 2014;289:21028–39.
33. Weston CR, Davis RJ. The JNK signal transduction pathway. Curr Opin Genet Dev. 2002;12:14–21.
34. Lee MH, Koria P, Qu J, Andreadis ST. JNK phosphorylates beta-catenin and regulates adherens junctions. FASEB J. 2009;23:3874–83.
35. Amura CR, Marek L, Winn RA, Heasley LE. Inhibited neurogenesis in JNK1-deficient embryonic stem cells. Mol Cell Biol. 2005;25:10791–802.
36. Zentrich E, Han SY, Pessoa-Brandao L, Butterfield L, Heasley LE. Collaboration of JNKs and ERKs in nerve growth factor regulation of the neurofilament light chain promoter in PC12 cells. J Biol Chem. 2002;277:4110–8.
37. Ryan SM, O'Keeffe GW, O'Connor C, Keeshan K, Nolan YM. Negative regulation of TLX by IL-1beta correlates with an inhibition of adult hippocampal neural precursor cell proliferation. Brain Behav Immun. 2013; 33:7–13.
38. Soiampornkul R, Tong L, Thangnipon W, Balazs R, Cotman CW. Interleukin-1beta interferes with signal transduction induced by neurotrophin-3 in cortical neurons. Brain Res. 2008;1188:189–97.
39. Tong L, Balazs R, Soiampornkul R, Thangnipon W, Cotman CW. Interleukin-1 beta impairs brain derived neurotrophic factor-induced signal transduction. Neurobiol Aging. 2008;29:1380–93.
40. Lu K, Cho CL, Liang CL, Chen SD, Liliang PC, Wang SY, Chen HJ. Inhibition of the MEK/ERK pathway reduces microglial activation and interleukin-1-beta in spinal cord ischemia/reperfusion injury in rats. J Thorac Cardiovasc Surg. 2007;133:934–41.
41. Pineau I, Lacroix S. Proinflammatory cytokine synthesis in the injured mouse spinal cord: multiphasic expression pattern and identification of the cell types involved. J Comp Neurol. 2007;500:267–85.
42. Hendrix S, Peters EM. Neuronal plasticity and neuroregeneration in the skin – the role of inflammation. J Neuroimmunol. 2007;184:113–26.
43. Smorodchenko A, Wuerfel J, Pohl EE, Vogt J, Tysiak E, Glumm R, Hendrix S, Nitsch R, Zipp F, Infante-Duarte C. CNS-irrelevant T-cells enter the brain, cause blood-brain barrier disruption but no glial pathology. Eur J Neurosci. 2007;26:1387–98.
44. Gougeon PY, Lourenssen S, Han TY, Nair DG, Ropeleski MJ, Blennerhassett MG. The pro-inflammatory cytokines IL-1beta and TNFalpha are neurotrophic for enteric neurons. J Neurosci. 2013;33:3339–51.

45. Zhang X, Zhu J, Yang GY, Wang QJ, Qian L, Chen YM, Chen F, Tao Y, Hu HS, Wang T, Luo ZG. Dishevelled promotes axon differentiation by regulating atypical protein kinase C. Nat Cell Biol. 2007;9:743–54.

46. Horigane S, Ageta-Ishihara N, Kamijo S, Fujii H, Okamura M, Kinoshita M, Takemoto-Kimura S, Bito H. Facilitation of axon outgrowth via a Wnt5a-CaMKK-CaMKIalpha pathway during neuronal polarization. Mol Brain. 2016;9:8.

47. Liu Y, Shi J, Lu CC, Wang ZB, Lyuksyutova AI, Song XJ, Zou Y. Ryk-mediated Wnt repulsion regulates posterior-directed growth of corticospinal tract. Nat Neurosci. 2005;8:1151–9.

48. Threadgill R, Bobb K, Ghosh A. Regulation of dendritic growth and remodeling by Rho, Rac, and Cdc42. Neuron. 1997;19:625–34.

49. Choi HJ, Chang BJ, Han JS. Phospholipase D1 is an important regulator of bFGF-induced neurotrophin-3 expression and neurite outgrowth in H19-7 cells. Mol Neurobiol. 2012;45:507–19.

16

Immature morphological properties in subcellular-scale structures in the dentate gyrus of Schnurri-2 knockout mice: a model for schizophrenia and intellectual disability

Akito Nakao[1], Naoyuki Miyazaki[2], Koji Ohira[3], Hideo Hagihara[1], Tsuyoshi Takagi[4,5], Nobuteru Usuda[6], Shunsuke Ishii[5], Kazuyoshi Murata[2] and Tsuyoshi Miyakawa[1*]

Abstract

Accumulating evidence suggests that subcellular-scale structures such as dendritic spine and mitochondria may be involved in the pathogenesis/pathophysiology of schizophrenia and intellectual disability. Previously, we proposed mice lacking Schnurri-2 (Shn2; also called major histocompatibility complex [MHC]-binding protein 2 [MBP-2], or human immunodeficiency virus type I enhancer binding protein 2 [HIVEP2]) as a schizophrenia and intellectual disability model with mild chronic inflammation. In the mutants' brains, there are increases in C4b and C1q genes, which are considered to mediate synapse elimination during postnatal development. However, morphological properties of subcellular-scale structures such as dendritic spine in Shn2 knockout (KO) mice remain unknown. In this study, we conducted three-dimensional morphological analyses in subcellular-scale structures in dentate gyrus granule cells of Shn2 KO mice by serial block-face scanning electron microscopy. Shn2 KO mice showed immature dendritic spine morphology characterized by increases in spine length and decreases in spine diameter. There was a non-significant tendency toward decrease in spine density of Shn2 KO mice over wild-type mice, and spine volume was indistinguishable between genotypes. Shn2 KO mice exhibited a significant reduction in GluR1 expression and a nominally significant decrease in SV2 expression, while PSD95 expression had a non-significant tendency to decrease in Shn2 KO mice. There were significant decreases in dendrite diameter, nuclear volume, and the number of constricted mitochondria in the mutants. Additionally, neuronal density was elevated in Shn2 KO mice. These results suggest that Shn2 KO mice serve as a unique tool for investigating morphological abnormalities of subcellular-scale structures in schizophrenia, intellectual disability, and its related disorders.

Keywords: Mouse model, Schizophrenia, Intellectual disability, 3D electron microscopy

Introduction

Accumulating evidence suggests that abnormalities in subcellular-scale structures such as dendritic spine and mitochondria may be involved in the pathogenesis/pathophysiology of schizophrenia, bipolar disorder, autism spectrum disorder, and intellectual disability [1–4]. Spines are morphologically and biochemically discrete compartments that protrude from dendrites [5]. It has

been reported that spine enlargement parallels long-term potentiation, whereas long-term depression is associated with spine shrinkage [6]. Notably, psychiatric disorders such as schizophrenia, autism spectrum disorder, and intellectual disability have been reported to be accompanied by disruptions in dendritic spine shape, volume, or number [1, 3]. Mitochondria play a central role in various cellular processes that include regulation of ATP production, intracellular Ca^{2+} concentration, and redox homoeostasis [7]. Through these functions, mitochondria control various neural processes [8]. It has been suggested that mitochondrial dysfunction underlies the

---

* Correspondence: miyakawa@fujita-hu.ac.jp
[1]Division of Systems Medical Science, Institute for Comprehensive Medical Science, Fujita Health University, 1-98 Dengakugakubo, Kutsukake-cho, Toyoake, Aichi 470-1192, Japan
Full list of author information is available at the end of the article

pathophysiology of schizophrenia, bipolar disorder, and intellectual disability [2, 9].

Schnurri-2 (Shn2; also called major histocompatibility complex [MHC]-binding protein 2 [MBP-2], human immunodeficiency virus type I enhancer binding protein 2 [HIVEP2], or c-myc intron binding protein 1 [MIBP1]) was originally identified as a nuclear factor-κB (NF-κB) site-binding protein that binds tightly to the enhancers of MHC genes in the MHC regions of chromosome 6 [10]. Recent genome-wide association studies have identified a number of single-nucleotide polymorphisms in the MHC region associated with schizophrenia [11–15]. MHC class I proteins coded in this region are reported to play important roles in neural processes [16]. Genes in the MHC regions often harbor NF-κB-binding sequences in their promoter regions. Shn2 constitutively binds to NF-κB-binding sites to suppress NF-κB-dependent gene expression [17]. To induce an immune response, Shn2 detaches from the NF-κB-binding site, which then leads to the transcription of NF-κB target genes [18, 19]. Accordingly, Shn2 knockout (KO) mice exhibit constitutive NF-κB activation in CD4$^+$ T cells [19]. Shn2 is expressed in several brain regions including the hippocampus, cortex, and cerebellum [10]. We have previously reported that Shn2 KO mice demonstrated mild, widespread brain inflammation characterized by the up-regulation of NF-κB-responsive genes and activation of astrocytes [20]. Shn2 KO mice demonstrated multiple schizophrenia-related phenotypes, including behavioral abnormalities that resemble those of schizophrenics, transcriptome/proteome changes similar to those of postmortem schizophrenia patients, decreased parvalbumin and glutamic acid decarboxylase 67 levels, increased theta power on electroencephalograms, and a thinner cortex [20]. Schizophrenic subjects are reported to have lower mRNA levels for Shn2 [21]. More recently, whole exome sequencing studies demonstrated that nine individuals with intellectual disability have distinct de novo variants in HIVEP2, and they are diagnosed with "HIVEP2 syndrome" [22, 23]. Patients with HIVEP2 syndrome exhibit intellectual disability and behavioral problems that include hyperactivity, attention-deficit disorder, aggression, anxiety, and autism spectrum disorders [22, 23]. Granule cells of the dentate gyrus (DG) failed to mature in Shn2 KO mice, a proposed endophenotype of neuropsychiatric disorders [24, 25]. Thus, the Shn2 KO mouse is an animal model for schizophrenia and intellectual disability that has good concept validity. In the brains of Shn2 KO mice, there are increases in C4b and C1q genes [20], which are thought to mediate synapse elimination during postnatal development [26, 27]. Up-regulation of C1q and C4 genes could be a potential interface between inflammation and synaptic dysfunctions. Taken together, it is of interest that the morphology of neuronal dendritic spines in Shn2 KO mice be investigated.

Serial block-face (SBF) imaging is a novel scanning electron microscopy (SEM) technique that enables much more efficient acquisition of a series of ultrastructural sectional images than previous methods such as high-voltage transmission electron microscopy (TEM) and serial-section TEM [28]. Imaging of neural tissues using SBF-SEM and three-dimensional reconstruction from serial EM images is a powerful technique for analyzing fine subcellular-scale structures [29, 30]. In the present study, we used three-dimensional reconstruction based on SBF images from SBF-SEM to analyze morphology of subcellular-scale structures in DG granule cells in Shn2 KO mice.

Methods
Animals
We used 10-week-old male Shn2 KO mice ($n = 3$) and their male wild-type (WT) littermates ($n = 3$). Mutant and WT mice were group housed in a room with a 12 h light/dark cycle (lights on at 7:00 a.m.), with access to food and water ad libitum. Room temperature was kept at 23 ± 2 °C. All procedures were approved by the Institutional Animal Care and Use Committee of Fujita Health University.

Preparation of DG samples for SBF-SEM
Fixed brain samples were cut into 100-μm-thick slices with a DTK-1000 Microslicer (Dosaka EM, Kyoto, Japan), and the slices were processed largely in accordance with a combinatorial heavy metal staining protocol that has been released on the website of the National Center for Microscopy and Imaging Research (La Jolla, CA) (https://ncmir.ucsd.edu/sbem-protocol). This protocol was designed to enhance signal for backscattered electron imaging at low accelerating voltages. In brief, the tissue slices were further fixed with 2% paraformaldehyde and 2% glutaraldehyde in cacodylate buffer (0.15 M sodium cacodylate containing 2 mM CaCl$_2$, pH 7.4) at 4 °C overnight. The slices were washed three times with cacodylate buffer, and then postfixed with 2% aqueous osmium tetroxide containing 1.5% potassium ferrocyanide in cacodylate buffer for 1 h at 4 °C, filtered 1% thiocarbohydrazide solution for 20 min at room temperature, 2% osmium tetroxide solution for 30 min at room temperature, 1% aqueous uranyl acetate overnight at 4 °C, and Walton's lead aspartate solution [31] for 30 min at 60 °C. The slices were then dehydrated with a graded series of ethanol, and then were infiltrated with durcupan resin and polymerized at 60 °C for 3 days.

SBF-SEM
Small pieces of block including glomerulus were trimmed and mounted on aluminum SBF-SEM specimen pins (Gatan, Pleasanton, CA) using CircuitWorks Conductive Epoxy (Chemtronics, Kennesaw, GA). The entire surface of the specimen was coated with a thin layer (20 nm

thickness) of gold to dissipate the electric charge caused by electron-beam irradiation during SEM imaging. In this study, we used an SBF-SEM system in which an in-chamber ultramicrotome system (3View; Gatan Inc., Pleasanton, CA) was incorporated in a SEM (MERLIN, Carl Zeiss Microscopy, Jena, Germany). SBF-SEM images were acquired as reported previously [32]. Briefly, SBF images were obtained every 50-nm depth with a backscattered electron detector at an acceleration voltage of 1.5 kV. Two different serial SEM images were recorded simultaneously. One is a large field of view image (123 μm × 246 μm) at low resolution (30 nm/pixel), including the granule cell layer used for analyses of nuclear volume and neuronal density. The other is a small field of view image (57 μm × 57 μm) at high resolution (7 nm/pixel) in the middle molecular layer (Additional file 1: Figure S1) used for detailed morphological analyses in dendrites. The contrast of the images was inversed.

Data processing for three-dimensional reconstruction

After 2× binning of the images, the image stack was automatically aligned in a Fiji/ImageJ software package (http://fiji.sc/Fiji) as described previously [33]. Segmentation and three-dimensional reconstruction were carried out in Renovo Neural Inc. (Cleveland, OH) using Reconstruct software (https://synapseweb.clm.utexas.edu). Length and volume were generated using Reconstruct software from tracings of the dendritic shaft, dendritic spine neck, dendritic spine head, or mitochondria. Spine length or volume is the sum of length or volume of the neck and head, respectively. Diameters were calculated geometrically from length and volume assuming that each dendritic shaft, spine, spine neck, or spine head was a simple cylinder. Images and movies for figures were generated using AMIRA 5.6 Software (FEI Visualization Science Group, Burlington, MA) in Maxnet Co., Ltd. (Tokyo, Japan).

Immunohistochemistry

Immunohistochemical analysis was performed essentially the same as previously described [20, 34]. Adult mice were deeply anesthetized and transcardially perfused with 4% paraformaldehyde in phosphate buffered saline (PBS). The brains were dissected, immersed overnight in the same fixative, and transferred to 30% sucrose in PBS for at least 3 days for cryoprotection. Brains were mounted in Tissue-Tek (Miles, Elkhart, IN), frozen, and cut into 8-μm-thick coronal sections using a microtome (CM1850; Leica Microsystems, Wetzlar, Germany). The sections were preincubated for 30 min at room temperature in 5% skim milk in PBS containing 0.05% Tween-20, and then incubated overnight at 4 °C in PBS containing the primary antibodies. We used the following primary antibodies: rabbit polyclonal antibody for GluR1 (AB1504; Millipore, Billerica, MA) and postsynaptic density 95 (PSD95) (51–6900, invitrogen,

Carlsbad, CA), and mouse monoclonal antibody for synaptic vesicle 2 (SV2) (Developmental Studies Hybridoma Bank, Iowa City, IA). The antibody for GluR1 detected a single band of an expected size in Western blotting analysis using mouse brain lysates [34]. Immunoreactivity to the antigen was visualized using Alexa488- or Alexa594-conjugated secondary antibodies (Molecular Probes, Eugene, OR). Nuclear staining was performed with Hoechst 33,258 (Polyscience, Warrington, PA). We used a confocal microscope (LSM 510 META; Zeiss, Göttingen, Germany) to obtain images of the stained sections. Quantification of the immunofluorescence intensities in the DG molecular layer was performed using ZEN software (Zeiss). To quantify the expression levels of synaptic proteins, we calculated average values of immunofluorescence for WT and Shn2 KO mice by using average values of immunofluorescence for each animal. Two or three sections from each animal were processed for quantification.

Data analysis

Statistical analysis was conducted using SAS University Edition (SAS Institute, Cary, NC). Data were analyzed using Student's t-test or Wilcoxon rank sum test.

Results

Immature dendritic spine morphology in DG of Shn2 KO mice

We evaluated the effects of deficiency of Shn2 on the morphology of dendrites in granule cells in the middle molecular layer of the dorsal DG using serial images obtained with SBF-SEM (Additional file 1: Figure S1). Three-dimensional reconstruction of serial SEM images made it possible to visualize EM-quality ultrastructure of subcellular-scale structures. In Shn2 KO mice, thin dendrites with long and thin spines were apparent in granule cells in the middle molecular layer of the dorsal DG (Fig. 1a–d, Additional file 1: Figure S2 and Additional file 1: Figure S3, and Additional file 2: Movie S1 and Additional file 3: Movie S2). We then quantified the diameters of dendritic shaft and spine, spine density, spine length, spine volume, and postsynaptic density (PSD) area using three-dimensional reconstructed images of dendrites. Shn2 KO mice have decreased dendrite diameter compared with that of WT mice ($P = 0.0035$) (Fig. 2a). There was a non-significant tendency toward decrease in spine density per 1 μm of dendritic shaft of Shn2 KO mice ($P = 0.0929$) (Fig. 2b). PSD area was indistinguishable between Shn2 KO and WT mice ($P = 0.3060$) (Fig. 2c). The spine length of Shn2 KO mice increased over WT mice ($P = 0.0004$), which was mainly due to an increase in spine neck length in Shn2 KO mice ($P < 0.0001$) (Fig. 2d–f). Spine diameter and spine neck diameter of Shn2 KO mice were significantly lower than those of WT mice ($P = 0.0050$, and $P < 0.0001$, respectively) (Fig. 2g–i). There

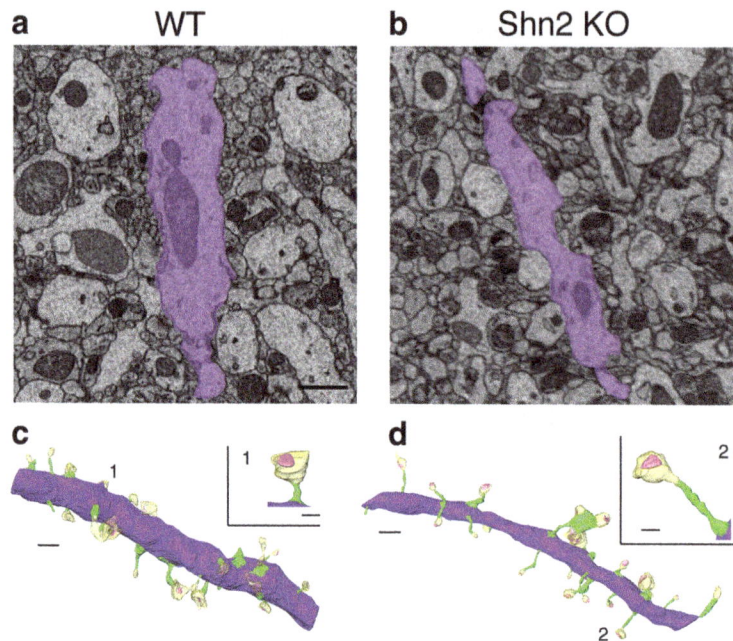

Fig. 1 Three-dimensional reconstruction of dendrites in the DG of Shn2 KO mice. (**a**, **b**) SEM images obtained through SBF-SEM in WT (**a**) and Shn2 KO (**b**) mice. Purple shows a dendritic shaft. (**c**, **d**) Three-dimensional reconstructions of representative dendrites in WT (**a**) and Shn2 KO (**b**) mice. Scale bars: 1 μm. Representative spines are in insets. Numbers indicate the position of spines. Scale bars: 0.3 μm. Purple, green, yellow and pink illustrate the dendritic shaft, spine neck, spine head, and PSD, respectively

was no significant difference between Shn2 KO and WT mice in terms of spine volume (Fig. 2j–l).

Decreased expression levels of synaptic proteins in the DG of Shn2 KO mice

Since Shn2 KO mice showed abnormalities in spine morphology, we then conducted immunofluorescence analyses using laser scanning confocal microscopy to evaluate expression levels of synaptic proteins, such as SV2, GluR1, and PSD95, in hippocampal regions in Shn2 KO mice (Fig. 3 and Additional file 1: Figure S4). In the middle molecular layer of the DG, in which SBF-SEM analyses were conducted, Shn2 KO mice showed decreased expression levels of SV2 ($P = 0.0483$) and GluR1 ($P = 0.0009$) compared with those in WT mice (Fig. 3a and b). PSD95 expression in the middle molecular layer had a non-significant tendency to decrease in Shn2 KO mice ($P = 0.0936$; Fig. 3c). In the inner molecular layer of Shn2 KO mice, expressions of SV2, GluR1, and PSD95 were significantly decreased (Additional file 1: Figure S4a–c; $P = 0.0149$, 0.0015, and 0.0481, respectively). In the outer molecular layer of Shn2 KO mice, GluR1 expression was significantly decreased ($P = 0.0007$; Additional file 1: Figure S4e), while SV2 and PSD95 were not significantly different between Shn2 KO and WT mice (Additional file 1: Figure S4d and f; $P = 0.0573$ and 0.1024, respectively). In the CA1 radiatum layer, there were no significant differences between Shn2 KO and WT mice in the expression levels of SV2,

GluR1, and PSD95 (Additional file 1: Figure S4g–i; $P = 0.7262$, 0.1435, and 0.8364, respectively). To avoid false-positive results caused by the multiple statistical tests performed, Bonferroni correction was applied to these results (the adjusted P-value at the 0.05 significance level for 12 indices was 0.004167). After the correction, the results remained significant for expression levels of GluR1 in the outer, middle, and inner molecular layers of the DG in Shn2 KO mice, while the other expression differences did not survive (Fig. 3 and Additional file 1: Figure S4). These results demonstrated that Shn2 KO mice showed significantly decreased expression levels of GluR1 in the whole molecular layer, whereas there were nominally significant decreases in SV2 and PSD95 in specific regions of the molecular layer in the DG of Shn2 KO mice.

Abnormal mitochondrial morphology in Shn2 KO mice

SEM images show that filamentous mitochondria are found in dendritic shaft (Fig. 4a), which is consistent with previous reports [35, 36]. SEM images and three-dimensional reconstruction of mitochondria suggested that ratios of constricted mitochondria to elongated ones were different between Shn2 KO and WT mice (Fig. 4). We counted the number of constricted and elongated mitochondria whose volumes were greater than 0.1 μm^3, since mitochondria whose volumes were less than 0.1 μm^3 demonstrated a spherical shape. In the mutants, the number of constricted mitochondria was decreased

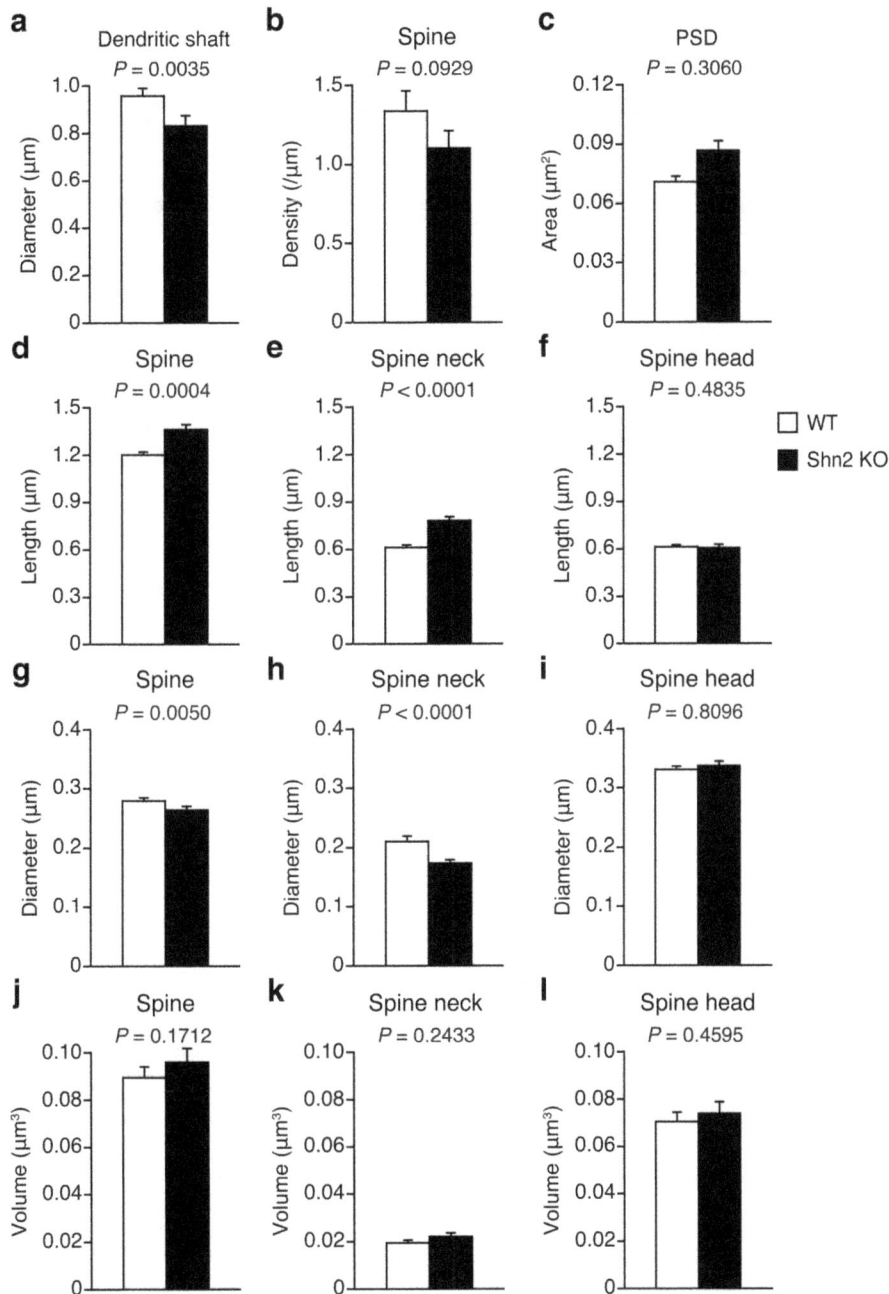

Fig. 2 Immature dendritic spine morphology in the DG in Shn2 KO mice. (**a, b**) Comparison of dendrite diameter (**a**) and spine density (**b**) in WT (n = 24 dendrites, 8 dendrites per each of 3 mice) and Shn2 KO mice (n = 24 dendrites, 8 dendrites per each of 3 mice). (**c–l**) Mean values of PSD area (**c**), spine length (**d**), spine neck length (**e**), spine head length (**f**), spine diameter (**g**), spine neck diameter (**h**), spine head diameter (**i**), spine volume (**j**), spine neck volume (**k**), and spine head volume (**l**) in WT (n = 547 spines from 24 dendrites, 8 dendrites per each of 3 mice) and Shn2 KO mice (n = 386 spines from 24 dendrites, 8 dendrites per each of 3 mice). The P-values were calculated using a Wilcoxon rank sum test

compared with those of WT ($\chi^2 = 6.9873$, $P = 0.0082$) (Table 1). Volumetric comparisons demonstrated that there were no significant differences between Shn2 KO and WT mice in mitochondria volume, mitochondria length, or mitochondria number per 1 μm of dendritic shaft (Additional file 1: Figure S5a–c; $P = 0.7356$, 0.1083, and 0.1703, respectively).

Decreased nuclear volume and increased neuronal density in Shn2 KO mice

SEM images suggest decreased cell body size in the granule cell layer of DG in Shn2 KO mice (Fig. 5a and b). To assess cell body size, nuclei of granule cells were reconstructed in three dimensions (Fig. 5c and d). There was a significant decrease in nuclear volume in the mutants over

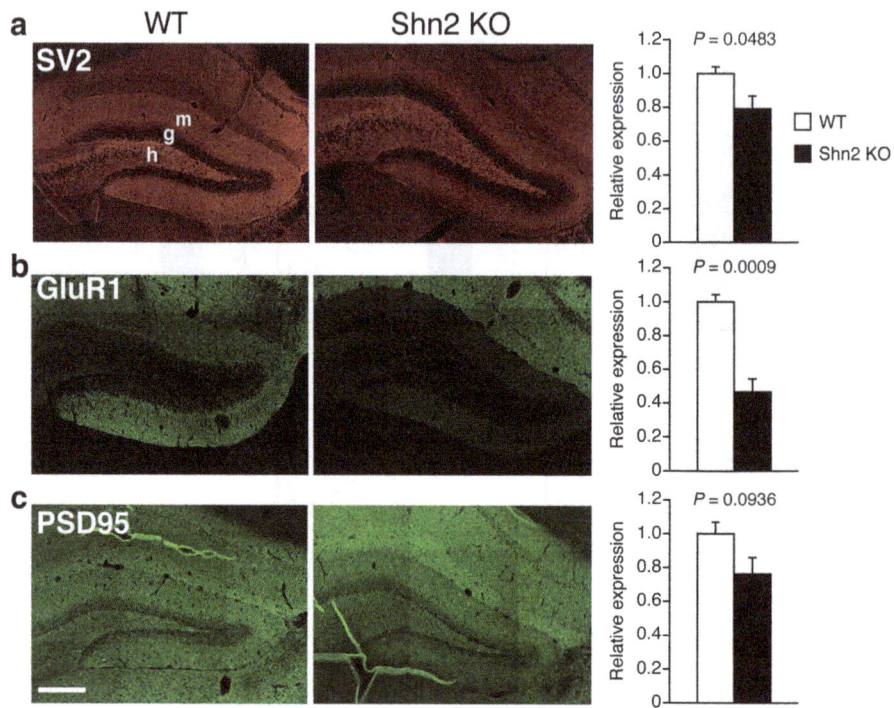

Fig. 3 Decreased expression of GluR1 and a nominally significant decrease in SV2 expression in the middle molecular layer of the DG of Shn2 KO mice. (**a–c**) Representative images of SV2 (**a**), GluR1 (**b**), and PSD95 (**c**) staining in the DG of WT and Shn2 KO mice. Bar graphs represent fluorescence intensity normalized to that in the middle molecular layer in the DG of WT mice, and are presented as the mean ± SEM. For WT, $n = 4$ mice; for Shn2 KO, $n = 4$ mice. The P-values were calculated using Student's t-test. Scale bar, 300 μm; g, granule cell layer; h, hilus; m, molecular layer

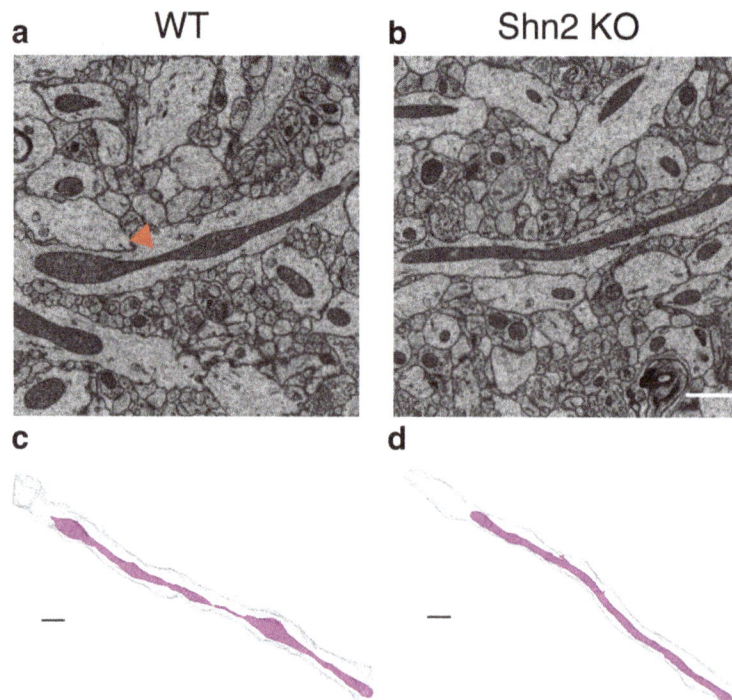

Fig. 4 Abnormal mitochondrial morphology in Shn2 KO mice. (**a**, **b**) SEM images of mitochondria in WT (**a**) and Shn2 KO (**b**) mice. Red triangle indicates constriction in a mitochondrion. Scale bars, 1 μm. (**c**, **d**) Three-dimensional reconstruction of representative constricted mitochondrion in WT (**c**) and elongated mitochondrion in Shn2 KO (**d**) mice. Magenta shows a mitochondrion. Grey indicates dendritic shafts

Table 1 Abnormal mitochondrial morphology in Shn2 KO mice

	Constricted mitochondria	Elongated mitochondria	Total
WT	27	33	60
Shn2 KO	8	33	41
Total	35	66	101

Cross tabulation of the number of constricted and elongated mitochondria in WT ($n = 60$ mitochondria from 24 dendrites, 8 dendrites per each of 3 mice) and Shn2 KO mice ($n = 41$ mitochondria from 24 dendrites, 8 dendrites per each of 3 mice). This cross tabulation yielded a significant chi-square value ($\chi^2 = 6.9873$, $P = 0.0082$)

WT mice ($P < 0.0001$) (Fig. 5e). Neuronal density calculated from the number of nuclei was significantly increased in Shn2 KO mice compared with that in WT mice ($P = 0.0007$) (Fig. 5f), which is consistent with a previous report that cell-packing density was higher in the DG of Shn2 KO mice [20].

Discussion and conclusions

Imaging of neural tissues using SBF-SEM and three-dimensional reconstruction from serial EM images is a powerful technique for analyzing subcellular-scale structures. Using this technique, we identified novel morphological phenotypes in Shn2 KO DG (a schematic is provided in Fig. 6). Shn2 KO mice have long and thin spines resembling immature spine-like structures called filopodia, which may later evolve into dendritic spines [37]. Shn2 KO mice showed a significant reduction in GluR1 expression, and a nominally significant decrease in SV2 expression. PSD95 expression had a non-significant tendency to decrease in Shn2 KO mice, which is consistent with the finding of a non-significant tendency for decreased spine density in Shn2 KO mice compared with that in WT mice. The mutants exhibited decreased numbers of constricted mitochondria, suggesting that a balance between mitochondrial fusion and fission is compromised in Shn2 KO mice. Additionally, there were significant decreases in dendrite diameter and nuclear volume in the mutants. Neuronal density in Shn2 KO mice was increased compared with that in WT mice.

An "immature DG (iDG)" was first discovered in α-CaMKII$^{+/-}$ mice, which display abnormal behaviors related to schizophrenia, bipolar disorder, and other psychiatric disorders [25, 38]. Previously, we have reported that Shn2 KO mice also possessed an iDG phenotype in

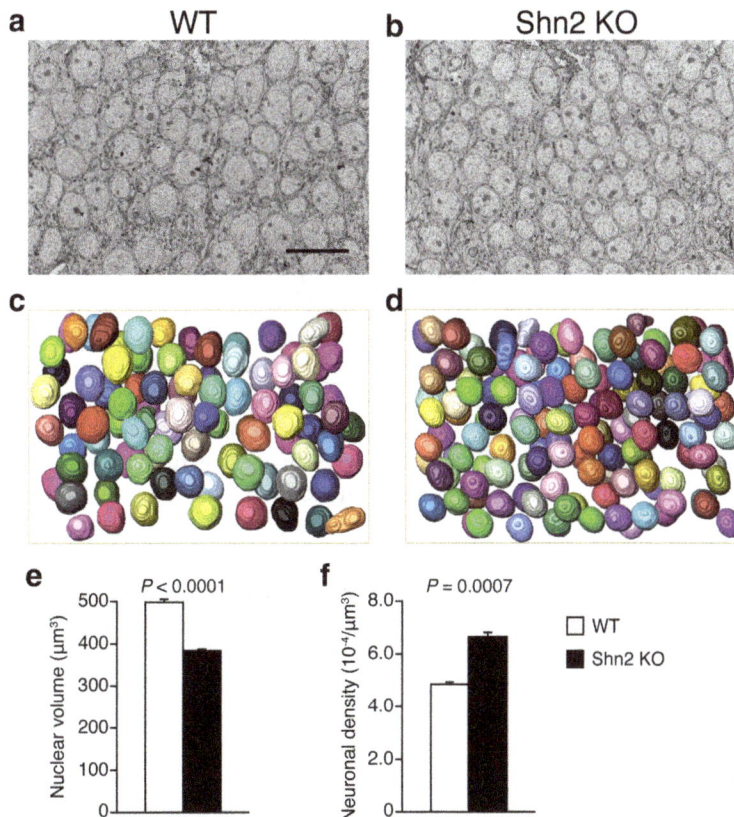

Fig. 5 Decreased nuclear volume and increased neuronal density in Shn2 KO mice. (**a**, **b**) SEM images of cell bodies of granule cells in WT (**a**) and Shn2 KO (**b**) mice. Scale bars, 20 μm (**c**, **d**) Three-dimensional reconstruction of nuclear in granule cells of WT (**c**) and Shn2 KO (**d**) mice. (**e**) Comparison of neuronal density in WT ($n = 3$) and Shn2 KO ($n = 3$) mice. (**f**) Comparison of nuclear volume in WT ($n = 120$ from 3 mice) and Shn2 KO mice ($n = 120$ from 3 mice). The P-values were calculated using Student's t-test (**e**) and Wilcoxon rank sum test (**f**)

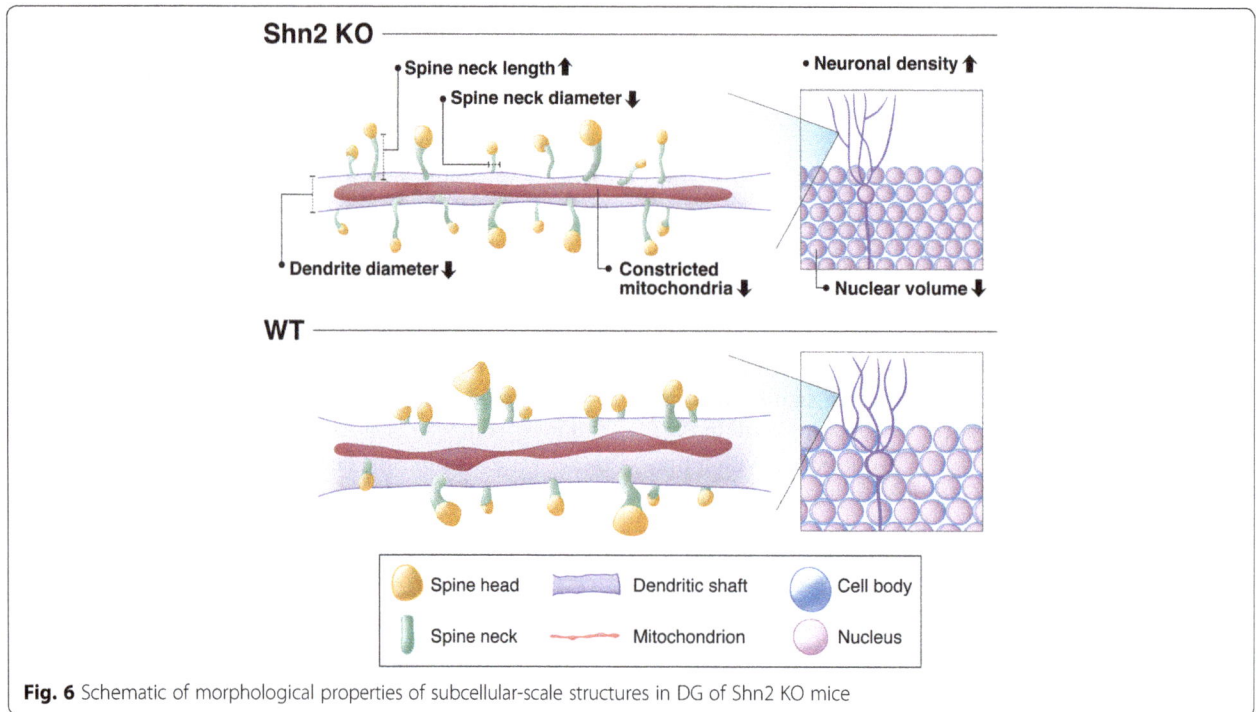

Fig. 6 Schematic of morphological properties of subcellular-scale structures in DG of Shn2 KO mice

terms of gene expression pattern and electrophysiological properties [20]. The present study shows morphological immaturity of the dendritic spine in the DG of Shn2 KO mice, which is consistent with the idea that Shn2 KO mice have iDG phenotypes. Shn2 KO mice showed decreased expression levels of GluR1 in the entire molecular layer of the DG. GluR1 is expressed primarily in mature granule cells, and can be a potential marker for mature granule cells [34]. It has been reported that GluR1 expression is reduced in the DG of α-CaMKII$^{+/-}$ mice [34]. GluR1 reduction may be one of the shared changes among a subgroup of iDG mice. In the inner molecular layers of the DG in Shn2 KO mice, there were statistically significant reductions in GluR1 expression and nominally significant decreases in SV2 and PSD95, suggesting an altered number of synapses. Further SBF-SEM analysis is necessary to clarify the morphological changes in the inner molecular layer of the DG in Shn2 KO mice. Treatment with chronic fluoxetine—a selective serotonin reuptake inhibitor—reverses the neuronal maturation, resulting in the iDG phenotype [39]. Kitahara et al. carried out a morphological analysis of synapses in the molecular layer of the DG after chronic fluoxetine treatment using focused ion beam-SEM [40]. They showed that spine density is indistinguishable between chronic fluoxetine treatment and placebo mice, which is consistent with the result in Shn2 KO mice. While there was no significant difference between Shn2 KO and WT mice in spine volume and PSD area, chronic fluoxetine treatment increased spine and PSD

volume compared with placebo mice. Further studies are required to investigate the effects of shared and unshared morphological changes among iDG mice in dendritic spines on neuronal function.

We previously showed significant increases in expression level of genes involved in immune responses, such as complement genes in Shn2 KO mice [20]. Notably, C1qa, C1qb, C1qc, and C4 were up-regulated in the brains of Shn2 KO mice. Complement proteins are widely expressed in neurons and glia in postnatal brain, and they play an important role in a process critical for establishing precise synaptic circuits [27, 41]. Sekar et al. reported that association of schizophrenia with the MHC locus arises in part from many structurally diverse alleles of C4 genes, and expression of those genes is increased in post-mortem brains of schizophrenic patients [26]. They proposed that excessive complement activity might explain the reduced number of synapses in brains of individuals with schizophrenia. In addition, our previous study showed decreased gene expression of kalirin in the DG of Shn2 KO mice [20]. Kalirin is a schizophrenia-associated gene, and loss of kalirin correlates with decreased spine density in prefrontal cortex neurons [3]. However, spine density was statistically indistinguishable between Shn2 KO and WT mice. It is noteworthy that the level of brain-derived neurotrophic factor (BDNF)—a neurotrophin protein—is increased in the DG of Shn2 KO mice [42]. BDNF stimulation is reported to increase the density of dendritic filopodia and spines [43]. It is possible that Shn2 KO mice have an enhanced turnover of spines due to an increase in expression of BDNF. Interestingly, patients with fragile X syndrome, intellectual disability-related diseases, exhibited an immature dendritic spine morphology and an increased dendritic spine density, suggesting enhanced spine turnover [44]. It has been reported that Fmr1 KO mice, a fragile X syndrome mouse model, displayed enhanced spine turnover [45]. Dendritic spine morphology in Shn2 KO DG neurons recapitulates that seen in fragile X syndrome. Thus, the Shn2 KO mouse may be a good model for investigating spine morphology in intellectual disability.

It is thought that mitochondrial dysfunction may underlie the pathophysiology of schizophrenia, bipolar disorder, and intellectual disability [2, 9]. Shn2 KO mice exhibited a decreased number of constricted mitochondria over WT mice, suggesting that a balance between mitochondrial fusion and fission is compromised in the mutants. Interestingly, Zhao and Li showed that lack of dysbindin, a schizophrenia susceptibility gene [46], increased mitochondrial fission through dynamin-related protein 1 [47]. Mitochondrial fission and fusion play critical roles in maintaining functional mitochondria when cells experience metabolic or environmental stresses [48]. In the DG of Shn2 KO mice, genechip analysis demonstrated altered gene expression related to energy metabolism such as aldo-keto reductase genes *Akr1c18*, ATP-related genes (*Atp2a*, *Atp2b*, *Atp6v*, and *Atp11c*), the cytochrome-related gene *Cyb561*, and the phosphoglycerate-related gene *Phgdh* [20]. Changes in protein amounts were also found in energy metabolism-related molecules, including aldo-keto reductase genes *Akr1b3*, ATP-related genes (*Atp5a*, *Atp5d*, *Atp5f*, *Atp5k*, and *Atp6v*), cytochrome-related genes (*Uqcrfs1*, *Ubcrc2*, *Cox5b*, *Uqcrb*, and *Uchl1*), the NADH dehydrogenase gene *Ndufa10*, and the phosphoglycerate-related gene *Pgk1* in the DG of Shn2 KO mice [20]. These gene/protein expression changes may be related to abnormal mitochondrial morphology in Shn2 KO mice. Further studies are needed to investigate the relationships between morphological abnormality of mitochondria and energy metabolism-related gene/protein expression changes in Shn2 KO mice. Recently, we reported that significantly lower pH and higher lactate levels were observed in brains of mouse models for psychiatric disorders, including Shn2 KO mice, as well as a significant negative correlation between pH and lactate levels [49]. We proposed that elevated glycolysis underlies increases in lactate levels, which is similar to the Warburg effect. Taken together, metabolism in Shn2 KO mice may be compromised due to abnormal mitochondrial morphology and metabolism-related gene/protein expression changes. It is possible that morphological abnormality in mitochondria is one of the shared endophenotypes in subgroups of psychiatric disorders.

Shn2 KO mice showed decreased nuclear volume in DG. In Shn2 KO mice, adult neurogenesis is enhanced

in DG (Hagihara et al., unpublished observation). The present study confirmed that neuronal density in Shn2 KO mice was increased compared with that in WT mice, which is consistent with a previous report [20]. It is possible that decreased nuclear volume in the DG of Shn2 KO mice may be due to increased neuronal density caused by enhanced neurogenesis. Our results are consistent with previous reports that show reduced hippocampal neuronal size in postmortem brains of schizophrenia patients [50].

Taken together, morphological changes in Shn2 KO DG neurons recapitulate some aspects of morphological changes in psychiatric disorders such as schizophrenia and intellectual disability. Thus, Shn2 KO mice serve as a unique tool for investigating morphological abnormalities of subcellular-scale structures in those disorders and their related diseases.

Additional files

Additional file 1: Figure S1. Analysis area of the middle molecular layer of the dorsal DG for SBF-SEM imaging. (a) A schematic of the sampling area (red square) at a distance of approximately 100 μm from the upper blade of the granule cell layer. OML, outer molecular layer; MML, middle molecular layer; IML, inner molecular layer; GCL, granule cell layer. (b) Boxed regions indicate the tissue area sampled used for detailed morphological analyses in the dendrites in three WT mice and three Shn2 KO mice. Scale bar: 100 μm. **Figure S2.** Three-dimensional reconstruction of all dendrites for analysis in WT mice. Dendrite segments (white transparent) are illustrated with mitochondria (blue) and spines (head, orange; neck, green; PSD, magenta). Eight dendrites per each of three WT mice. **Figure S3.** Three-dimensional reconstruction of all dendrites for analysis in Shn2 KO mice. Dendrite segments (white transparent) are illustrated with mitochondria (blue) and spines (head, orange; neck, green; PSD, magenta). Eight dendrites per each of three Shn2 KO mice. **Figure S4.** Decreased expression levels of synaptic proteins in the DG of Shn2 KO mice (a–i) Bar graphs of SV2, GluR1, and PSD95 in the inner (a–c) and outer (d–f) molecular layers of the DG, and CA1 radiatum layer (d–f) represent fluorescence intensity normalized to that of WT mice, and are presented as the mean ± SEM. IML, inner molecular layer; OML, outer molecular layer; Rad, radiatum layer. For WT, n = 4 mice; for Shn2 KO, n = 4 mice. The *P*-values were calculated using Student's *t*-test. **Figure S5.** Volumetric comparisons of mitochondria in WT and Shn2 KO mice. Comparison of mitochondria volume (a), mitochondria length (b), and mitochondria number per 1 μm of dendrite (c) in WT (n = 96 mitochondria from 24 dendrites, 8 dendrites per each of 3 mice) and Shn2 KO mice (n = 57 mitochondria from 24 dendrites, 8 dendrites per each of 3 mice). The *P*-values were calculated using Wilcoxon rank sum test.

Additional file 2: Movie S1. A movie of three-dimensional rendering of an SBF-SEM dataset from DG in WT mouse. Purple, green, yellow, and pink illustrate the dendritic shaft, spine neck, spine head, and PSD, respectively.

Additional file 3: Movie S2. A movie of three-dimensional rendering of an SBF-SEM dataset from DG in Shn2 KO mouse. Purple, green, yellow, and pink illustrate dendritic shaft, spine neck, spine head, and PSD, respectively.

Abbreviations

BDNF: Brain-derived neurotrophic factor; DG: Dentate gyrus; HIVEP2: Human immunodeficiency virus type I enhancer binding protein 2; iDG: Immature dentate gyrus; KO: Knockout; MHC: Major histocompatibility complex; NF-κB: Nuclear factor-κB; PBS: Phosphate buffered saline; PSD: Postsynaptic density 26; PSD95: Postsynaptic density 95; SBF-SEM: serial block-face-

scanning electron microscopy; Shn2: Schnurri-2; SV2: Synaptic vesicle 2;
TEM: Transmission electron microscopy

Acknowledgments
We thank W. Hasegawa, Y. Mobayashi, M. Murai, T. Murakami, M. Takeuchi, Y.
Kagami, H. Mitsuya, A. Miyakawa, and other members of Miyakawa lab for
their support, as well as S. Yamada for specimen preparation for SBF-SEM.

Funding
This research was supported by the Grant-in-Aid for Scientific Research (A)
(25242078) and the Grant-in-Aid for Scientific Research on Innovative Areas
"Unraveling the microendophenotypes of psychiatric disorders at the molecular,
cellular and circuit levels" (15H01297) and "Dynamic regulation of brain function
by Scrap & Build system" (16H06462) from the Ministry of Education, Culture,
Sports, Science, and Technology (MEXT) of Japan, and by Advanced Bioimaging
Support (ABiS) from the Grant-in-Aid for Scientific Research on Innovative Areas,
Japan (to TM).

Authors' contributions
TM was responsible for the original concept and the overall design of the
research. AN, NM, KO, and KM performed SBF-SEM analysis. HH performed
immunohistochemical analysis. TT and SI provided Shn2 KO mice. AN, NU,
and TM wrote the manuscript. All authors read and approved the final
manuscript.

Competing interests
TM received research grants from Astellas Pharma Inc. and Toyama Chemical
Co., Ltd. Other authors have no conflict of interests to declare.

Author details
[1]Division of Systems Medical Science, Institute for Comprehensive Medical
Science, Fujita Health University, 1-98 Dengakugakubo, Kutsukake-cho,
Toyoake, Aichi 470-1192, Japan. [2]National Institute for Physiological Sciences,
National Institutes of Natural Sciences, Okazaki, Japan. [3]Department of Food
Science and Nutrition, Mukogawa Women's University, Nishinomiya, Japan.
[4]Institute for Developmental Research, Aichi Human Service Center, Kasugai,
Japan. [5]RIKEN Tsukuba Institute, Tsukuba, Japan. [6]Department of Anatomy II,
Fujita Health University School of Medicine, Toyoake, Japan.

References
1. Bagni C, Greenough WT. From mRNP trafficking to spine dysmorphogenesis:
   the roots of fragile X syndrome. Nat Rev Neurosci. 2005;6:376–87.
2. Iwamoto K, Bundo M, Kato T. Altered expression of mitochondria-related
   genes in postmortem brains of patients with bipolar disorder or schizophrenia,
   as revealed by large-scale DNA microarray analysis. Hum Mol Genet.
   2005;14:241–53.
3. Penzes P, Cahill ME, Jones KA, VanLeeuwen J-E, Woolfrey KM. Dendritic
   spine pathology in neuropsychiatric disorders. Nat Neurosci. 2011;14:285–93.
4. Prabakaran S, Swatton JE, Ryan MM, Huffaker SJ, Huang JT-J, Griffin JL, et al.
   Mitochondrial dysfunction in schizophrenia: evidence for compromised
   brain metabolism and oxidative stress. Mol Psychiatry. 2004;9:684–97. 643
5. Harris KM, Kater SB. Dendritic spines: cellular specializations imparting both
   stability and flexibility to synaptic function. Annu Rev Neurosci. 1994;17:341–71.

6. Kasai H, Fukuda M, Watanabe S, Hayashi-Takagi A, Noguchi J. Structural
   dynamics of dendritic spines in memory and cognition. Trends Neurosci.
   2010;33:121–9.
7. Kann O, Kovács R. Mitochondria and neuronal activity. Am J Physiol - Cell
   Physiol. 2007;292:C641–57.
8. Cheng A, Hou Y, Mattson MP. Mitochondria and neuroplasticity. ASN Neuro.
   2010;2:AN20100019.
9. Valenti D, de Bari L, De Filippis B, Henrion-Caude A, Vacca RA. Mitochondrial
   dysfunction as a central actor in intellectual disability-related diseases: An
   overview of Down syndrome, autism, Fragile X and Rett syndrome. Neurosci.
   Biobehav. Rev. 2014;46, Part 2:202–217.
10. Fukuda S, Yamasaki Y, Iwaki T, Kawasaki H, Akieda S, Fukuchi N, et al.
    Characterization of the biological functions of a transcription factor, c-myc
    intron binding protein 1 (MIBP1). J Biochem (Tokyo). 2002;131:349–57.
11. Purcell SM, Wray NR, Stone JL, Visscher PM, O'Donovan MC, Sullivan PF, et
    al. Common polygenic variation contributes to risk of schizophrenia and
    bipolar disorder. Nature. 2009;460:748–52.
12. Shi J, Levinson DF, Duan J, Sanders AR, Zheng Y. Pe'er I, et al. common
    variants on chromosome 6p22.1 are associated with schizophrenia. Nature.
    2009;460:753–7.
13. Shi Y, Li Z, Xu Q, Wang T, Li T, Shen J, et al. Common variants on 8p12 and
    1q24.2 confer risk of schizophrenia. Nat Genet. 2011;43:1224–7.
14. Stefansson H, Ophoff RA, Steinberg S, Andreassen OA, Cichon S, Rujescu D, et al.
    Common variants conferring risk of schizophrenia. Nature. 2009;460:744–7.
15. Yue W-H, Wang H-F, Sun L-D, Tang F-L, Liu Z-H, Zhang H-X, et al. Genome-
    wide association study identifies a susceptibility locus for schizophrenia in
    Han Chinese at 11p11.2. Nat Genet. 2011;43:1228–31.
16. Shatz CJMHC. Class I: an unexpected role in neuronal plasticity. Neuron.
    2009;64:40–5.
17. Kumar A, Takada Y, Boriek AM, Aggarwal BB. Nuclear factor-kappaB: its role
    in health and disease. J Mol Med Berl Ger. 2004;82:434–48.
18. Kimura MY, Hosokawa H, Yamashita M, Hasegawa A, Iwamura C, Watarai H,
    et al. Regulation of T helper type 2 cell differentiation by murine Schnurri-2.
    J Exp Med. 2005;201:397–408.
19. Kimura MY, Iwamura C, Suzuki A, Miki T, Hasegawa A, Sugaya K, et al.
    Schnurri-2 controls memory Th1 and Th2 cell numbers in vivo. J. Immunol.
    Baltim. Md 1950. 2007;178:4926–36.
20. Takao K, Kobayashi K, Hagihara H, Ohira K, Shoji H, Hattori S, et al. Deficiency of
    Schnurri-2, an MHC enhancer binding protein, induces mild chronic inflammation
    in the brain and confers molecular, neuronal, and behavioral phenotypes related
    to schizophrenia. Neuropsychopharmacology. 2013;38:1409–25.
21. Volk DW, Chitrapu A, Edelson JR, Roman KM, Moroco AE, Lewis DA.
    Molecular mechanisms and timing of cortical immune activation in
    schizophrenia. Am. J. Psychiatry. 2015;appi.ajp.2015.15010019.
22. Srivastava S, Engels H, Schanze I, Cremer K, Wieland T, Menzel M, et al.
    Loss-of-function variants in HIVEP2 are a cause of intellectual disability.
    Eur J Hum Genet. 2016;24:556–61.
23. Steinfeld H, Cho MT, Retterer K, Person R, Schaefer GB, Danylchuk N, et al.
    Mutations in HIVEP2 are associated with developmental delay, intellectual
    disability and dysmorphic features. Neurogenetics. 2016;17:159–64.
24. Hagihara H, Takao K, Walton NM, Matsumoto M, Miyakawa T. Immature
    dentate gyrus: an endophenotype of neuropsychiatric disorders. Neural
    Plast. 2013;2013:318596.
25. Yamasaki N, Maekawa M, Kobayashi K, Kajii Y, Maeda J, Soma M, et al.
    Alpha-CaMKII deficiency causes immature dentate gyrus, a novel candidate
    endophenotype of psychiatric disorders. Mol Brain. 2008;1:6.
26. Sekar A, Bialas AR, de Rivera H, Davis A, Hammond TR, Kamitaki N, et al.
    Schizophrenia risk from complex variation of complement component 4.
    Nature. 2016;530:177–83.
27. Stevens B, Allen NJ, Vazquez LE, Howell GR, Christopherson KS, Nouri N, et
    al. The classical complement cascade mediates CNS synapse elimination.
    Cell. 2007;131:1164–78.
28. Kremer A, Lippens S, Bartunkova S, Asselbergh B, Blanpain C, Fendrych M, et al.
    Developing 3D SEM in a broad biological context. J Microsc. 2015;259:80–96.
29. Denk W, Horstmann H. Serial block-face scanning electron microscopy to
    reconstruct three-dimensional tissue nanostructure. PLoS Biol. 2004;2:e329.
30. Sai K, Wang S, Kaito A, Fujiwara T, Maruo T, Itoh Y, et al. Multiple roles of
    afadin in the ultrastructural morphogenesis of mouse hippocampal mossy
    fiber synapses. J Comp Neurol. 2017;525:2719–34.
31. Walton J. Lead asparate, an en bloc contrast stain particularly useful for
    ultrastructural enzymology. J Histochem Cytochem. 1979;27:1337–42.

32. Miyazaki N, Esaki M, Ogura T, Murata K. Serial block-face scanning electron microscopy for three-dimensional analysis of morphological changes in mitochondria regulated by Cdc48p/p97 ATPase. J Struct Biol. 2014;187:187–93.

33. Negishi T, Miyazaki N, Murata K, Yasuo H, Ueno N. Physical association between a novel plasma-membrane structure and centrosome orients cell division. elife. 2016;5:e16550.

34. Hagihara H, Ohira K, Toyama K, Miyakawa T. Expression of the AMPA receptor subunits GluR1 and GluR2 is associated with granule cell maturation in the dentate gyrus. Front Neurogenesis. 2011;5:100.

35. Kislin M, Sword J, Fomltcheva IV, Croom D, Pryazhnikov E, Lihavainen E, et al. Reversible disruption of neuronal mitochondria by ischemic and traumatic injury revealed by quantitative two-photon imaging in the neocortex of anesthetized mice. J Neurosci. 2017;37:333–48.

36. Popov V, Medvedev NI, Davies HA, Stewart MG. Mitochondria form a filamentous reticular network in hippocampal dendrites but are present as discrete bodies in axons: a three-dimensional ultrastructural study. J Comp Neurol. 2005;492:50–65.

37. Ziv NE, Smith SJ. Evidence for a role of dendritic filopodia in synaptogenesis and spine formation. Neuron. 1996;17:91–102.

38. Hagihara H, Horikawa T, Nakamura HK, Umemori J, Shoji H, Kamitani Y, et al. Circadian gene circuitry predicts hyperactive behavior in a mood disorder mouse model. Cell Rep. 2016;14:2784–96.

39. Kobayashi K, Ikeda Y, Sakai A, Yamasaki N, Haneda E, Miyakawa T, et al. Reversal of hippocampal neuronal maturation by serotonergic antidepressants. Proc Natl Acad Sci U S A. 2010;107:8434–9.

40. Kitahara Y, Ohta K, Hasuo H, Shuto T, Kuroiwa M, Sotogaku N, et al. Chronic fluoxetine induces the enlargement of perforant path-granule cell synapses in the mouse dentate gyrus. PLoS ONE [Internet]. 2016 [cited 2016 Apr 27]; 11. Available from: http://www.ncbi.nlm.nih.gov/pmc/articles/PMC4720354/

41. Stephan AH, Barres BA, Stevens B. The complement system: an unexpected role in synaptic pruning during development and disease. Annu Rev Neurosci. 2012;35:369–89.

42. Koshimizu H, Ohira K, Hagihara H, Takao K, Takagi T, Kataoka M, et al. Dysregulation of BDNF-MAPK signaling pathway in the hippocampus of mice with "immature dentate gyrus". SfN Meet. Abstr. 2013;

43. Shimada A, Mason CA, Morrison ME. TrkB signaling modulates spine density and morphology independent of dendrite structure in cultured neonatal purkinje cells. J Neurosci. 1998;18:8559–70.

44. Irwin SA, Galvez R, Greenough WT. Dendritic spine structural anomalies in fragile-X mental retardation syndrome. Cereb Cortex. 2000;10:1038–44.

45. Pan F, Aldridge GM, Greenough WT, Gan W-B. Dendritic spine instability and insensitivity to modulation by sensory experience in a mouse model of fragile X syndrome. Proc Natl Acad Sci. 2010;107:17768–73.

46. Guo AY, Sun J, Riley BP, Thiselton DL, Kendler KS, Zhao Z. The dystrobrevin-binding protein 1 gene: features and networks. Mol Psychiatry. 2008;14:18–29.

47. Zhao J, Li Z. Dysbindin regulates mitochondrial fission in hippocampal excitatory neurons through the dynamin-like-protein DLP1. Abstr. SfN Meet; 2016.

48. Youle RJ, Bliek AM. Van der. Mitochondrial fission, fusion, and stress. Science. 2012;337:1062–5.

49. Hagihara H, Catts VS, Katayama Y, Shoji H, Takagi T, Huang FL, et al. Decreased brain pH as a shared endophenotype of psychiatric disorders. Neuropsychopharmacology [Internet]. 2017 [cited 2017 Aug 9]. Available from: http://www.nature.com/npp/journal/vaop/naam/abs/npp2017167a.html.

50. Weinberger D. Cell biology of the hippocampal formation in schizophrenia. Biol Psychiatry. 1999;45:395–402.

17

Exposure to mild blast forces induces neuropathological effects, neurophysiological deficits and biochemical changes

Adan Hernandez[1†], Chunfeng Tan[1†], Florian Plattner[1,2†], Aric F. Logsdon[3], Karine Pozo[1], Mohammad A. Yousuf[1], Tanvir Singh[1], Ryan C. Turner[3], Brandon P. Luke-Wold[3], Jason D. Huber[4], Charles L. Rosen[3†] and James A. Bibb[5*†]

Abstract

Direct or indirect exposure to an explosion can induce traumatic brain injury (TBI) of various severity levels. Primary TBI from blast exposure is commonly characterized by internal injuries, such as vascular damage, neuronal injury, and contusion, without external injuries. Current animal models of blast-induced TBI (bTBI) have helped to understand the deleterious effects of moderate to severe blast forces. However, the neurological effects of mild blast forces remain poorly characterized. Here, we investigated the effects caused by mild blast forces combining neuropathological, histological, biochemical and neurophysiological analysis. For this purpose, we employed a rodent blast TBI model with blast forces below the level that causes macroscopic neuropathological changes. We found that mild blast forces induced neuroinflammation in cerebral cortex, striatum and hippocampus. Moreover, mild blast triggered microvascular damage and axonal injury. Furthermore, mild blast caused deficits in hippocampal short-term plasticity and synaptic excitability, but no impairments in long-term potentiation. Finally, mild blast exposure induced proteolytic cleavage of spectrin and the cyclin-dependent kinase 5 activator, p35 in hippocampus. Together, these findings show that mild blast forces can cause aberrant neurological changes that critically impact neuronal functions. These results are consistent with the idea that mild blast forces may induce subclinical pathophysiological changes that may contribute to neurological and psychiatric disorders.

Keywords: Blast-induced traumatic brain injury, Neuroinflammation, Microvascular damage, Axonal swelling, Short-term plasticity, Calpain, p25

Introduction

Blast-induced traumatic brain injury (bTBI) results from direct or indirect exposure to an explosive event as may occur in domestic or industrial accidents, terrorist attacks, or in military conflicts [1, 2]. Primary bTBI is induced by a blast overpressure wave that penetrates the skull and causes physical damage to neurons, glia and vasculature. Primary bTBI is normally characterized by internal injuries that are difficult to detect and assess for severity. Parameters affecting the severity of primary bTBI include proximity to explosion focus, the force of the explosion, as well as the duration and characteristics of the explosion. While strong blasts may cause severe and acute brain injury or death, exposure to mild blast forces may result in delayed or subclinical neuropathological changes. bTBI is comorbid with an increased incidence of neuropsychiatric disorders and long-term physical, cognitive, behavioral, and emotional changes [3]. Furthermore, bTBI has been suggested to contribute to the pathogenesis of neurodegenerative disorders [4, 5].

Over the past decade various animal models using moderate to severe blast forces have been developed to study the pathophysiological effects of bTBI, [4, 6–10].

* Correspondence: jbibb@uab.edu
†Adan Hernandez, Chunfeng Tan, Florian Plattner, Charles L. Rosen and James A. Bibb contributed equally to this work.
[5]Departments of Surgery, Neurobiology, and Neurology, The University of Alabama at Birmingham Medical Center, 1720 2nd Ave S, THT 1052, Birmingham, AL 35294, USA
Full list of author information is available at the end of the article

These studies report characteristic neuropathological changes, including neuronal injury, neuroinflammation, hematomas, or contusion in rodent models of bTBI. Moreover, induction of common biochemical and molecular mechanisms associated with neuronal injury have been reported [4, 6, 11, 12]. Together, these studies revealed that primary bTBI induced by stronger blasts negatively affects a variety of cerebral structures and neuronal functions. While these more profound effects demonstrate the ability to model moderate to severe bTBI, the physiological impact of mild blast forces remains poorly defined. It is hypothesized that milder blast forces, still may induce neuropathophysiological changes, however a better understanding of the effect of mild bTBI on neuronal functions is needed.

In order to investigate the effects of mild blast forces on neuropathological, histological, biochemical and neurophysiological outcomes in rodents, we used a scaled, bench-top blast tube set-up [6]. We found that mild blast forces do not induce macroscopic neuropathological changes, including tissue damage, hemorrhage, hematoma and contusion. In fact, mild blast induced microvascular damage, axonal injury and neuroinflammation in various brain regions, including cortex, striatum and hippocampus. Consistent with these neuropathological changes, evaluation of hippocampal synaptic plasticity revealed deficits in short-term plasticity and synaptic excitability after mild blast exposure, but no impairment of hippocampal long-term potentiation (LTP). Finally, brains exposed to mild blast forces exhibited biochemical changes, including proteolytic cleavage of spectrin and formation of the aberrant cyclin-dependent kinase 5 (Cdk5) activator, p25, which have been implicated with neuronal injury and excitotoxicity.

Methods
Antibodies and materials
The following antibodies were used, including the phospho-specific neurofilament antibody, SMI-31 (Covance Research Products Inc. Cat # SMI-31, RRID: AB_2314901), glial fibrillary acidic protein (GFAP) antibody (Millipore Cat # AB5804, RRID: AB_2109645), the ionized Ca^{2+}-binding adapter molecule (Iba1) antibody (Wako Cat # 019–19741, RRID: AB_839504), the spectrin (α-Fodrin) antibody (Enzo Life Sciences Cat # BML-FG6090–0500, RRID: AB_11179351), the GAPDH antibody (Sigma-Aldrich Cat # G8795, RRID:AB_1078991), the p35 (C-19) antibody (Santa Cruz Biotechnology Cat # sc-820, RRID: AB_632137), Goat anti-mouse IgG (Thermo Fisher Scientific Cat # 31432, RRID: AB_228302) and goat anti-rabbit IgG peroxidase conjugated secondary antibodies (Thermo Fisher Scientific Cat # 31462, RRID:AB_228338). All materials were obtained from Sigma-Aldrich unless stated otherwise.

Animals
All procedures involving animals were approved by the Institutional Animal Care and Use Committees (IACUC) of West Virginia University and UT Southwestern Medical Center, and were performed according to the principles of the *Guide for the Care and Use of Laboratory Animals*. Male Sprague-Dawley rats were acquired from Hilltop Lab Animals (Hilltop Lab Animals, Inc., Scottsdale, PA, RRID: RGD_734476). At the time of blast exposure the rats were 12 weeks old and weighed ~ 300–350 g. Animals were housed single-caged with a 12 h light/dark cycle and access to food and water ad libitum. Prior to experimental use animals were acclimated for 1 week. The study involved the following numbers of animals: neuropathological/histological analysis (18 rats), neurophysiological analysis (17 rats) and biochemical analysis (26 rats). No animals have been excluded from the analyses.

Blast exposure protocol
Prior to blast exposure, animals were anesthetized with 4% isoflurane (Henry Schein, Cat # NDC 11695–6776-2). The blast was delivered to the left side of the head with the animal's body oriented perpendicular to the compressed gas-driven blast tube (length 15 cm; diameter 7.2 cm), and with the peripheral organs protected by a polyvinyl chloride pipe shield (Fig. 1a). The head was placed 12.5 cm from the blast origin. The animals were exposed to a mild blast (0.076 mm membrane; incident peak overpressure of ~ 15 psi.), which was established to cause neuropathophysiological changes, but no external wounds and mortality in previous work [6]. To reduce distress and pain animals are under isoflurane anesthesia during exposure to the mild blast. Immediately following blast exposure, animals were returned to a holding cage equipped with a heating blanket to maintain body temperature at 37 °C. A rectal thermometer was used to monitor body temperature. Once basic reflexes were restored, animals were returned to their home cage and monitored over the next 24 h for adverse reactions. Neuropathological, neurophysiological and biochemical analyses were conducted in rats that had been subjected to one single mild blast overpressure wave and were subsequently sacrificed at 1, 2, 3, 7 or 21 day(s) post-bTBI (see Experimental timeline (Fig. 1c)). Control subjects were anesthetized and placed in proximity to the blast set-up, but were not subjected to blast forces.

Study design
Animals were randomly assigned to an experimental group (i.e. various post-bTBI delay or control). Neuropathological, neurophysiological and biochemical analyses were performed with the researchers blind to treatment condition. Experimental sample sizes have been based on numbers established in previous experiments (e.g. [13, 14]).

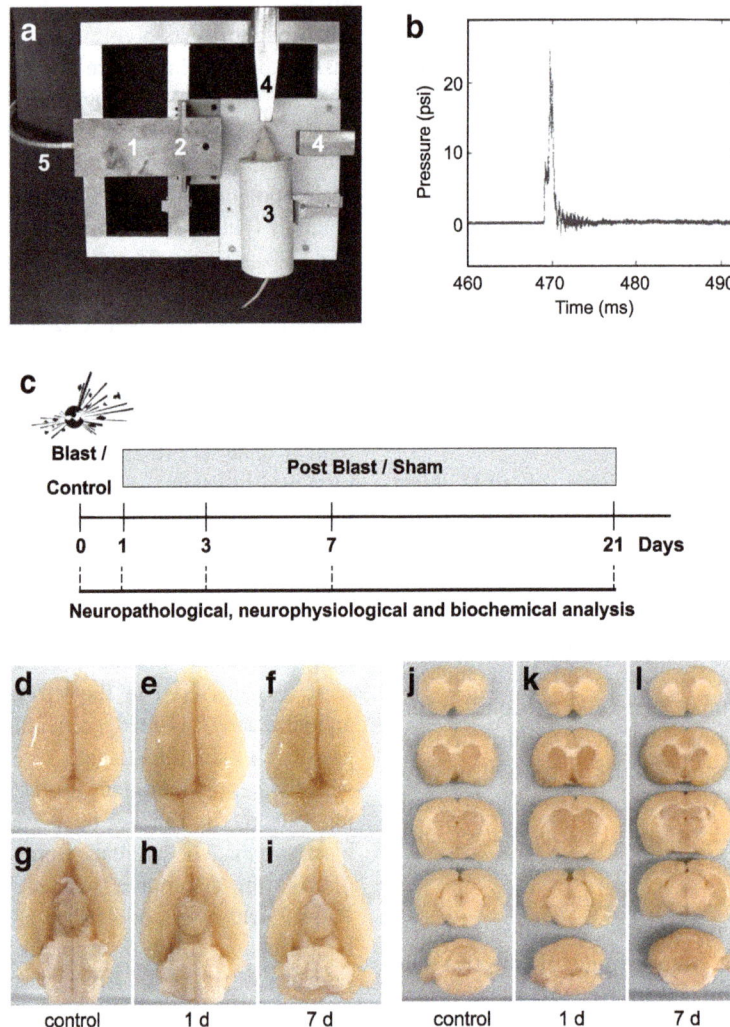

Fig. 1 Absence of macroscopic tissue damage after mild bTBI. **a** Image of compressed gas-driven blast tube set-up. *1*) Blast tube (diameter: 7.2 cm) *2*) Membrane (0.076 mm thickness) *3*) rat holding tube *4*) pressure sensors *5*) connection to nitrogen gas tank. **b** Temporal pressure force plot of blast overpressure wave. **c** Experimental timeline. **d-i** Absence of macroscopic tissue damage at 1 and 7 day(s) post-bTBI as compared to control. Dorsal view of brain (**d-f**); ventral view of brain (**g-i**). **j-l** No macroscopic tissue damage at 1 and 7 day(s) post-bTBI compared to control as tested in anterior-posterior, 4 mm coronal rat brain sections from controls (**j**), 1 day (**k**) and 7 days (**l**) post-bTBI (*n* = 3/number of animals)

No sample size calculation, or power analysis has been performed prior to data collection.

Neuropathological analysis

The neuropathological analysis was conducted in a sham-treated control group and animals at 1, 3, 7 or 21 day(s) post-blast (*n* = 3 for each time point). Animals were euthanized by CO_2 asphyxiation and perfused transcardially with ice-cold 0.9% saline followed by 10% formalin for a total of 10 min. The brains were dissected and placed in fresh 10% formalin for 72 h. Brains were block-sectioned into 5 coronal slabs, paraffin-embedded, and serially sectioned at 5 μm at Bregma level of 2.20, 1.00, − 2.80, − 7.30 and − 11.30 mm. Standard protocols were utilized for staining with hematoxylin and eosin

(H&E; Leica, Cat # 3801570) [15] and Fluoro-Jade B (FJB, Millipore Corporation, Cat # AG310-30MG) [16]. For the immunohistochemical analysis, paraffin-embedded sections were labeled with SMI-31 to detect phosphorylated neurofilaments (1:500; Covance, Emeryville, CA), glial fibrillary acidic protein (GFAP) to detect astrocyte activation (1:1200; Chemicon) and ionized Ca^{2+}-binding adapter molecule (Iba1) to detect microglial activation (1:1000; Wako) and visualized by immunoperoxidase method [17]. Briefly, 5 μm sections were deparaffinized, subjected to microwave antigen retrieval (citrate buffer, pH 6.0; Bio-Genex, Cat # HK086-9 K), permeabilized with 0.3% (vol/vol) Triton, quenched free of endogenous peroxidases, and blocked with a cocktail of normal goat serums (2.5% (vol/vol) each) prior to overnight incubation of primary antibodies at 4 °C. Bound primary antibodies were detected by sequential incubation with biotinylated secondary antisera and streptavidin-peroxidase, diaminobenzidine chromagen was used to detect immunoperoxidase signal (Vector; anti-mouse IgG kit, Cat # MP-7602, anti-rabbit kit, Cat # MP-7601). Quantification of GFAP-positive astrocytes was conducted using semi-stereology and the optical fractionator technique as previously described [6]. GFAP-positive astrocytes were quantitated in brain regions, including cortex (GFAP-positive cells counted in squares of 100×100 μm; $n = 53$–77 squares), striatum ($n = 32$–53 squares) and hippocampus ($n = 19$–34 squares). Semi-quantitative analysis of the immunohistochemical signal of the activated microglia marker, Iba1, and phospho-specific anti-neurofilament antibody, SMI-31 was performed using the open source image processing package FIJI (http://www.fiji.sc). Images were captured on an epifluorescence microscope (Nikon) in TIFF format. Following standardized color deconvolution and thresholding of images, the signal was quantified on 2–3 slides from 3 individual rats for each treatment group. Iba1 was quantified in brain regions, including cortex (% area of signal; $n = 12$–17 regions of interest), striatum ($n = 11$–15 regions of interest) and hippocampus ($n = 8$–12 regions of interest).

Neurophysiological analysis

Neurophysiological studies were conducted in rats at 1, 3, 7 or 21 day(s) post-bTBI and controls ($n = 6$). Following rapid decapitation and dissection, brains were placed in ice-cold artificial cerebrospinal fluid (ACSF; 75 mM sucrose, 87 mM NaCl, 2.5 mM KCl, 1.25 mM NaH_2PO_4, 25 mM $NaHCO_3$, 7 mM $MgCl_2$, 0.5 mM $CaCl_2$ and 10 mM glucose), and transverse hippocampal slices (350 μm) were prepared using a vibratome (Leica Microsystems Inc., VT1000S). Slices were recovered in oxygenated Krebs' buffer (125 mM NaCl, 2.5 mM KCl, 1.25 mM NaH_2PO_4, 25 mM $NaHCO_3$, 1.1 mM $MgCl_2$, 2 mM $CaCl_2$ and 25 mM glucose) at 30 °C for 30 min after slicing. Subsequently slices were moved into oxygenated Krebs' buffer at room temperature (22–25 °C) before recordings. Slices for recordings were transferred into a perfusion chamber on the upright microscope stage (Axioscop 2, Carl Zeiss, Inc). The perfusion bath was maintained at 30 °C during the recordings (TC-324B Automatic Temperature Controller, Warner Instruments Corporation). A Multiclamp 700A amplifier with a Digidata 1322 and pClamp 10 software (Axon, Molecular devices, LLC) was used for electrophysiological recordings and data acquisition. Field excitatory postsynaptic potentials (fEPSP) from CA1 were evoked by square current pulses (0.1 ms) at 0.033 Hz with a bipolar stimulation electrode (FHC, Bowdoinham, ME) placed at the Schaffer collaterals (~ 250–300 μm) from the recording electrode. Results were obtained using a stimulus intensity to induce 50% of the maximal fEPSP slope and the same intensity was used to explore the paired pulse ratio (PPR) at different intervals. The stimulation intensity was established through the input-output curve, the maximal stimulation was considered when a population spike appeared in the fEPSP. A stable baseline was recorded for at least 15 min prior to high frequency stimulation (HFS, 4 trains, 100 Hz, 1 s duration, separated by 20 s). Post-tetanic potentiation (PTP) was analyzed by taking the average of the slopes from the traces recorded during the first 2 min after HFS. LTP was assessed for at least 60 min after HFS. The time-course showing baselines and LTP is expressed as a percent of change from the baseline fEPSP slope. The PPR values were calculated by dividing the second fEPSP slope by the first fEPSP slope (fEPSP2/fEPSP1). For the input-output curve recordings were normalized for each slice, assigning the maximal fiber volley amplitude (obtained with maximal stimulation) to the value of 1.0, and the plots were derived for the respective fEPSP slopes. All recordings were performed in the absence of any drug treatment and only 1 or 2 slices were recorded from each individual rat. Data were analyzed with Clampfit 10 software (Axon, Molecular devices, LLC). Prism 6 (GraphPad Software, Inc.) was used to make graphs and statistical analysis.

Quantitative immunoblot analysis

Brain dissection, tissue removal, lysate preparation, and immunoblotting were performed as previously described [18, 19]. Rats for immunoblotting were sacrificed at 1, 3, 7 and 21 day(s) post-bTBI. Tissue lysates from hippocampal dissections were prepared using protease- and phosphatase inhibitors (Roche Diagnostics GmbH, Cat # 05 892 791 001) and equal amounts of protein were run on 7% acrylamide gels or 10–20% gradient acrylamide gels. The blots were probed with primary antibodies raised against spectrin (1:1000, Enzo Life Sciences), p35/25 (1:500, Santa Cruz Biotechnology) and GAPDH (1:5000, Sigma). Signal was detected with HRP-conjugated secondary antibodies (1:1000–10000, Thermo Fisher Scientific) and enhanced chemiluminescence (Thermo Scientific, Cat # 34580). For quantitative immunoblot analysis, immunoreactivity signals were captured by autoradiography, scanned and quantified using ImageJ software (NIH, Bethesda, MD). The band intensities were normalized to signals from GAPDH.

Statistical analysis

Data are presented as mean $\pm$ SEM. Student's t-test or one-way ANOVA were performed to analyze datasets using GraphPad Prism 6 (GraphPad Software Inc., San Diego, CA, USA) unless stated otherwise. A p-value < 0.05 was considered statistically significant for all data analyzed. $^*p < 0.05$, $^{**}p < 0.01$ and $^{***}p < 0.001$. For all experiments the whole set of data was analyzed and no data points were excluded. No specific assessment of the normality of data was carried out and no specific test for outliers was conducted, as no data points were excluded.

Results

Mild blast forces induce neuroinflammation, but no overt neuropathological effects

Previously, we developed a scaled, bench-top compressed gas-driven blast tube for rodents for the induction of bTBI and characterized the relationship between force intensity and injury severity with regard to general neuropathology using this blast set-up (see Fig. 1a) [6]. These studies defined an incident peak overpressure of approximately 15 psi as a sub-threshold blast force that does not induce overt neuropathological effects, such as tissue damage, hematoma, hemorrhage or contusion. These findings were consistent with those reported in comparable bTBI studies [4, 11, 20, 21].

Here, we first defined the temporal characteristics and the force profile of the blast overpressure wave produced by our bench-top set-up (Fig. 1b). We found that membrane rupture (thickness 0.076 mm) in this system generates a single overpressure pulse lasting a few milliseconds that models the blast waves generated at the start of an explosion. Next, we investigated whether exposure to a single pulse of overpressure in our set-up induced macroscopic neuropathological effects in adult male rats. Gross examination of rat brains at 1, 3, 7 and 21 day(s) following blast exposure revealed no macroscopic evidence of contusion, necrosis, hematoma, hemorrhage, or focal tissue damage of bTBI brains (Fig. 1d-l; data shown for 1 and 7 day(s) post-bTBI, vs. control). In line with our previous observations [6], this result confirms that the blast forces used here to induce bTBI are below the threshold for induction of gross neuropathological effects or damage to the dura.

Previous studies showed that exposure to higher intensity blast forces induce deficits in learning and memory as well as motor performance (e.g. [22]). These functions are dependent upon the hippocampus, cerebral cortex, and striatum. The hippocampus is also highly susceptible to oxidative stress and neuroinflammation, which are acutely increased following TBI [2, 23]. Furthermore, the cerebral cortex is amongst the most susceptible brain areas for neuropathological effects, including neuroinflammation and diffuse axonal injury induced by moderate to strong blast forces [24]. Therefore, we evaluated the ability of mild blast forces to induce subtle neuropathological effects in these brain regions.

First, we analyzed the effects of mild bTBI on markers of neuroinflammation immunohistologically in the hippocampus, cerebral cortex, and striatum. As observed in previous studies that used higher intensity bTBI protocols, we found that mild blast induced neuroinflammation in cerebral cortex, striatum and hippocampus, as evidenced by both astrogliosis (Fig. 2) and microglial activation (Fig. 3). The number of reactive astrocytes detected by immunohistochemical staining for GFAP increased throughout the brain, including the cerebral cortex (Fig. 2a-c), striatum (Fig. 2d-f) and hippocampus (Fig. 2g-i) following bTBI. Astrogliosis was evident at 1, 3 and 7 day(s) post-bTBI, but had receded by 21 days to levels comparable to controls (Fig. 2c, f, i). The levels of reactive astrocytes in the ipsilateral brain hemisphere (side facing the blast tube) and the contralateral hemisphere were comparable (data not shown). Brainstem and cerebellum exhibited low levels of astrogliosis (data not shown). In addition, semi-quantitative analysis of Iba 1 immunohistochemical signal showed that levels of activated microglia were increased in the cerebral cortex (Fig. 3a-c), striatum (Fig. 3d-f) and hippocampus (Fig. 3g-i) post-bTBI as compared to non-treated controls. Significant increases in microglia activation could be appreciated at 1, 3 and 7 days post-bTBI in striatum and on day 1 post-bTBI in cortex and hippocampus. Together, these findings show that the mild bTBI protocol used here induces a robust neuroinflammatory response, without causing gross neuropathological effects, such as tissue damage, hemorrhage, or contusion.

Mild blast forces induce microvascular damage

The presence of a neuroinflammation in absence of macroscopic neuropathological effects, suggests that some microscopic tissue damage may have occurred. Indeed, a detailed microscopic examination of the bTBI brains revealed notable, but sparse alterations to the microvasculature in bTBI brains. Some of the microvascular damage observed included small hemorrhagic foci, which showed the presence of intraparenchymal red blood cells (Fig. 4a) and robust reactive astrogliosis (Fig. 4b) in the striatum of post-bTBI brains. Furthermore, the extravasation of blood plasma was observed in a small number of venule-like (Fig. 4c) and arteriole-like (Fig. 4d) microvessels of the cerebral cortex and striatum post-bTBI. The presence of blood plasma extravasation was confirmed by staining for rat immunoglobulin G (IgG; Fig. 4e). Together, these results show that mild bTBI induced microvascular damage, but this did not lead to hematoma or hemorrhage. Our previous results revealed that higher blast forces correlate with increased damage to the blood vessels, including hematoma and hemorrhage [6]. Our mild blast results may be subtle, but could prove significant, as there is a growing perception that damage to the microvasculature may be an important contributor to the etiology of bTBI [25] and other neurological disorders.

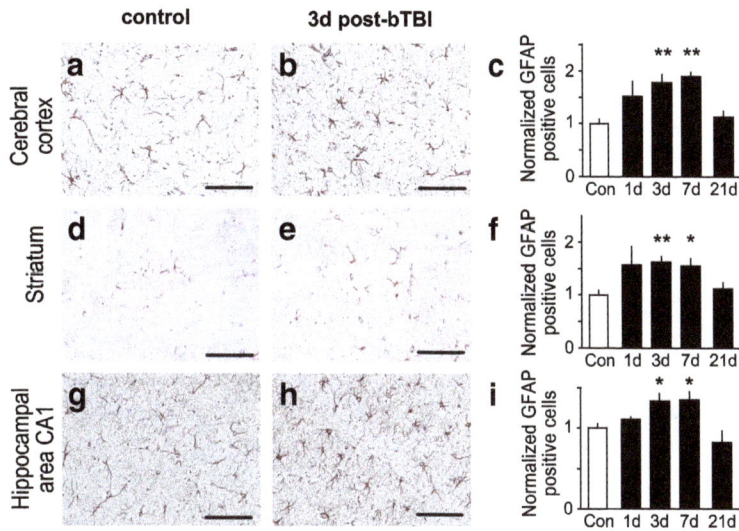

Fig. 2 Astrogliosis induction after mild bTBI. **a-i** Mild blast forces caused increases in reactive astrocytes throughout the brain, including the brain regions: cerebral cortex (**a-c**), striatum (**d-f**) and hippocampal area CA1 (**g-i**). Representative images of brain regions stained for GFAP, a marker for reactive astrocytes, are shown for controls (**a**, **d** and **g**) and rats at 3 days post-bTBI (**b**, **e** and **h**). Quantifications of GFAP-positive cells expressed as normalized mean cell number per 0.01 mm^2 are shown for corresponding brain regions for controls and rats at 1, 3, 7 and 21 day(s) post-bTBI (**c**, **f** and **i**). GFAP-positive cells were counted in $n = 19–77$ squares of 100×100 μm on slides from 3 individual rats for each treatment group (6–32 squares/rat). All scale bars indicate 50 μm. All data are presented as mean ± SEM; *$p < 0.05$, **$p < 0.01$; ANOVA with Bonferroni post hoc

The effect of mild blast forces on hippocampus

The hippocampus is critically involved in memory formation. Dysregulation of the hippocampal circuitry is thought to underlie some of the pathophysiological changes observed in TBI. Therefore, to better understand the impact of mild bTBI on neuronal circuitry associated with learning and memory, we specifically examined the neuropathological changes induced by mild bTBI in the hippocampus. Coronal hippocampal sections of rats subjected to bTBI exhibited no gross signs of neuropathology or tissue damage (Fig. 5a). H&E staining revealed no degenerating or ischemic neurons in the hippocampus following

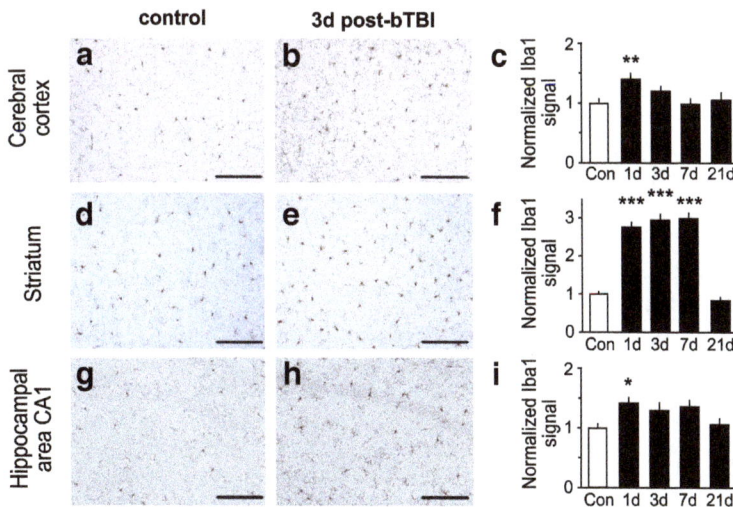

Fig. 3 Induction of activated microglia after mild bTBI. **a-i** Rats subjected to mild bTBI showed increased levels of activated microglia throughout the brain, including the brain regions: cerebral cortex (**a-c**), striatum (**d-f**) and hippocampal area CA1 (**g-i**). Representative images of brain regions stained for the ionized Ca^{2+}-binding adaptor molecule 1 (Iba1), a marker of activated microglia, are shown for controls (**a**, **d** and **g**) and rats at 3 days post-bTBI (**b**, **e** and **h**). Bar graph of the normalized signal of Iba1 for corresponding brain regions for controls and rats at 1, 3, 7 and 21 day(s) post-bTBI is shown (**c**, **f** and **i**). Signal was quantitated on $n = 6–9$ slides from 3 individual rats for each treatment group (2–3 slides/rat). All scale bars indicate 100 μm. All data are presented as mean ± SEM; *$p < 0.05$, **$p < 0.01$, ***$p < 0.001$; ANOVA with Bonferroni post hoc

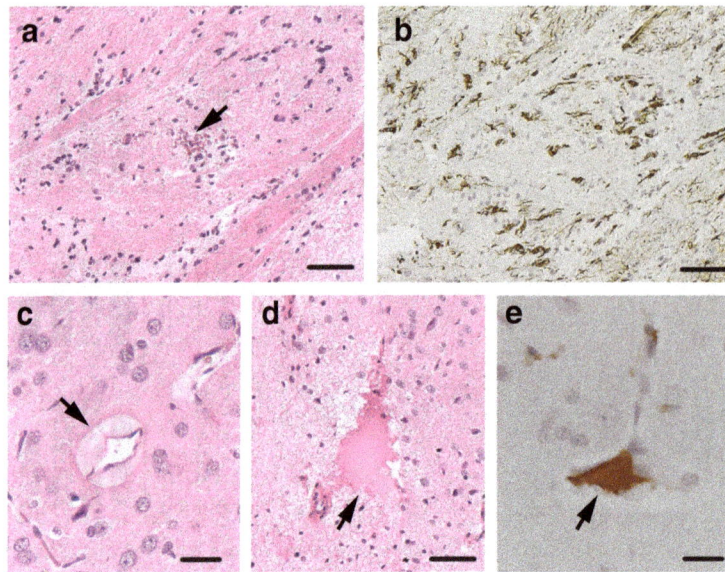

Fig. 4 Induction of microvascular damage after mild bTBI. **a** and **b** Microvascular damage in rat brain 3 days post-bTBI as indicated by small hemorrhagic focus (arrowhead) in the corpus callosum (**a**), in conjunction with reactive astrogliosis in the same area (**b**). **c** Extravasation of blood plasma in a venule-like microvessel in the deep layer of the cerebral cortex at 3 days post-bTBI are indicated by an arrowhead. **d** Extravasation of blood plasma in an arteriole-like microvessel in striatum at 3 days post-bTBI. **e** Immunoreactivity for rat immunoglobulin G (IgG) was detected in the same area as the extravasation of blood plasma in (**d**). Representative microscope pictures of brain regions stained with H&E (**a**, **c** and **d**), anti-GFAP antibody (**b**) and anti-rat IgG antibody (**e**) are shown. Analysis included $n = 3$ rats for each treatment group. Scale bars: 50 μm (**a**, **b** and **d**); 20 μm (**c** and **e**)

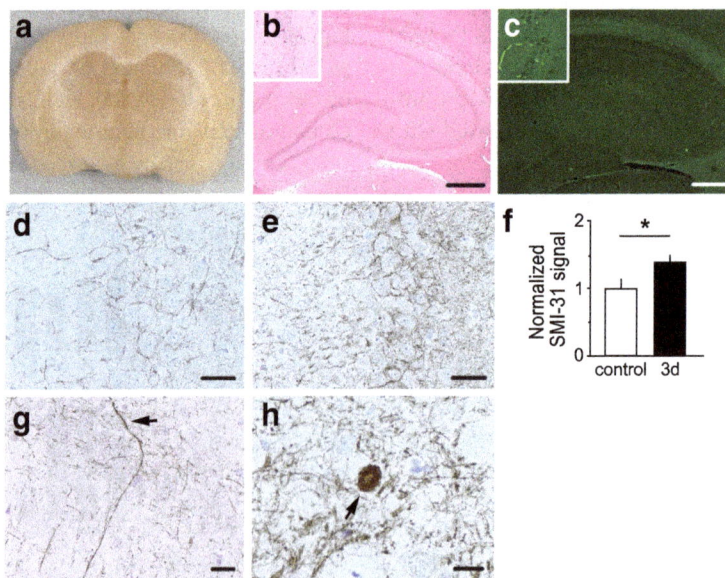

Fig. 5 Mild bTBI caused axonal injury in the hippocampus. Mild blast exposure did not result in macroscopic damage, but induced microscopic pathological effects, such as axonal damage and neuroinflammation in the hippocampus. **a** Absence of macroscopic hippocampal tissue damage at 7 days post-bTBI as tested in anterior-posterior 4 mm coronal rat brain sections. **b** Absence of overt neuronal injury in hippocampus at 7 days post-bTBI as assessed with H&E staining. Insert shows no overt pathology in the CA3 hippocampal subfield. **c** Absence of Fluoro-Jade B-positive neurons in the hippocampus at 7 days post-bTBI. Insert shows no degenerating neurons in CA3. **d** and **e** Increased phosphorylated neurofilament immunostaining in CA3 at 3 days post-bTBI (**e**) compared to control subjects (**d**). **f** Bar graph of normalized signal of phospho-specific anti-neurofilament antibody, SMI-31, staining in hippocampal area CA3 from controls and rats at 3 days post-bTBI is shown. Signal was quantitated on $n = 9$–12 slides from 3 individual rats for each treatment group (3–4 slides/rat). Data are presented as mean ± SEM; *$p < 0.05$; Student's t-test. **g** Swollen dystrophic axon in hippocampal CA1 stratum pyramidale at 3 days post-blast are indicated by arrowhead. **h** Axonal bulb in the hippocampal hilus at 7 days post-bTBI is indicated by arrowhead. Representative microscope pictures of hippocampal sub-regions immunostained with SMI-31 antibody (**d**, **e**, **g**, and **h**). Scale bars: 50 μm (**b-e**); 20 μm (**g** and **h**)

mild bTBI (Fig. 5b). Accordingly, FJB staining did not reveal signs of neurodegeneration in the hippocampus of bTBI-treated rats (Fig. 5c).

One of the primary neuropathological effects observed in most forms of TBI is diffuse axonal injury, which is characterized by distinct axonal pathology including swellings or varicosities along the length of axons, and the presence of axonal bulbs [26]. The axonal swellings contain accumulations of proteins, such as neurofilaments [27]. Previous studies reported that the phosphorylation level of neurofilaments is elevated following axonal injury and bTBI [28, 29]. Therefore, we examined the axonal integrity within the hippocampus from rats subjected to mild bTBI.

To evaluate the impact of mild bTBI on axonal integrity and phosphorylation levels of neurofilaments in the hippocampus, we performed immunohistochemical staining using the phospho-specific neurofilament antibody, SMI-31, followed by a semi-quantitative analysis. We found that immunoreactivity for phosphorylated neurofilaments was significantly increased in the hippocampal subfield CA3 of rats 3 days after exposure to mild bTBI as compared to controls (Fig. 5d-f). Interestingly, neurofilament phosphorylation has been implicated in neurofilament compaction [26], which may underlie axonal pathologies. Hence, we examined the integrity of the axonal architecture after mild bTBI. A detailed evaluation of axonal structures stained by SMI-31 revealed a small number of beaded or irregularly swollen dystrophic axons (Fig. 5g) as well as rare axonal bulbs in the hippocampus of rats exposed to mild bTBI (Fig. 5h). In controls no swollen dystrophic axons or axonal bulbs were observed (data not shown). These indicators of axonal injury observed in hippocampus of bTBI brains were accompanied by increased levels of reactive astrogliosis (Fig. 2g, h) and activated microglia (Fig. 3e, f). Together, these results show that mild blast forces induce neuropathological changes, including axonal injury and neuroinflammation in the hippocampus.

Mild blast forces induce neurophysiological deficits in the hippocampus

Considering the importance of the hippocampus for higher cognitive functions, the effects of the blast-induced neuropathological changes (see above; Fig. 5) on neurophysiological outcomes were interrogated in the hippocampus. For this purpose, we investigated the effects of mild bTBI on basic synaptic properties and synaptic plasticity in acutely prepared rat hippocampal slices. High frequency stimulation (HFS) induced robust LTP at Schaffer collateral-CA1 synapses in bTBI rats, as well as controls (Fig. 6a). In control slices, tetanic stimulation resulted in a $166 \pm 11\%$ potentiation of fEPSP slope compared to baseline at 60 min post-stimulus (*$p < 0.05$, Student's t-test). At 1, 3, 7 and 21 day(s) post-bTBI HFS induced

comparable levels of LTP after 60 min (Fig. 6a), suggesting that bTBI-induced neuropathological changes did not affect LTP expression. In contrast, assessment of short-term synaptic responses revealed that post-tetanic potentiation (PTP) was significantly attenuated in slices from rats at 7 and 21 days post-bTBI (Fig. 6a, b; *$p < 0.05$, **$p < 0.01$, one-way ANOVA, Newman-Keuls post hoc). In order to explore a possible pre-synaptic effect, we employed the paired pulse facilitation paradigm to assess changes on neurotransmitter release. A significant reduction on paired pulse ratio (PPR) was observed in response to HFS in control slices (Fig. 6c; 1.38 ± 0.03 baseline for control to 1.14 ± 0.02 during PTP phase for control; *$p < 0.05$, $n = 8$, Wilcoxon test) indicating an increase in the probability of neurotransmitter release during the PTP phase. In contrast, PPR was attenuated during PTP in slices from rats at 7 days post-bTBI as compared to controls (Fig. 6c; 1.39 ± 0.03 baseline for 7d to 1.27 ± 0.07 PTP for 7d; $p > 0.05$, $n = 8$, Wilcoxon test). Interestingly, slices from rats at 21 days post-bTBI showed a significant increase in PPR at baseline compared to control (Fig. 6c; 1.38 ± 0.03 baseline for control to 1.60 ± 0.06 baseline for 21d; #$p < 0.05$, $n = 8$, Mann-Whitney test), indicating changes in basal synaptic properties at 21 days post-bTBI that are likely to affect physiological neuronal functions. In conjunction with an increased PPR at baseline at 21 days post-bTBI, the PPR in response to HFS was significantly reduced during the PTP phase (Fig. 6c; 1.60 ± 0.06 baseline for 21d to 1.27 ± 0.06 PTP for 21d; **$p < 0.01$, $n = 8$, Wilcoxon test).

To assess hippocampal synaptic excitability, field potential recordings were used to derive input-output curves (Fig. 6d). The input-output curve for rats at 7 days post-bTBI was significantly reduced (Fig. 6d; $p < 0.01$, non-linear regression using a polynomial quadratic function). Consistently, the maximal response for rats at 7 days post-bTBI was significantly decreased (Fig. 6d; *$p < 0.03$, maximal stimulation in control vs. 7 day post-bTBI Mann-Whitney test). To further characterize the effect of bTBI on synaptic responses, paired pulse facilitation (PPF) was assessed at different inter-stimulus intervals (Fig. 6e). Slices from rats at 21 days post-bTBI showed significant increase in PPF at shorter inter-stimulus intervals (Fig. 6e; 20 and 50 ms, **$p < 0.01$, two-way ANOVA, Tukey's post hoc). No difference in PPF was observed in slices from rats at 1, 3 and 7 day(s) post-bTBI as compared to controls.

Together, these results show that mild blast forces induced deficits in hippocampal circuitry basal synaptic properties and short-term plasticity, but did not alter LTP expression. These neurophysiological deficits were not detected prior to 7 days post-bTBI and were more pronounced by 21 days post-bTBI, suggesting that neuronal functions can be critically affected by mild bTBI even after 21 days. Interestingly, the primary injuries, such as microvascular damage and increased phosphorylation levels of

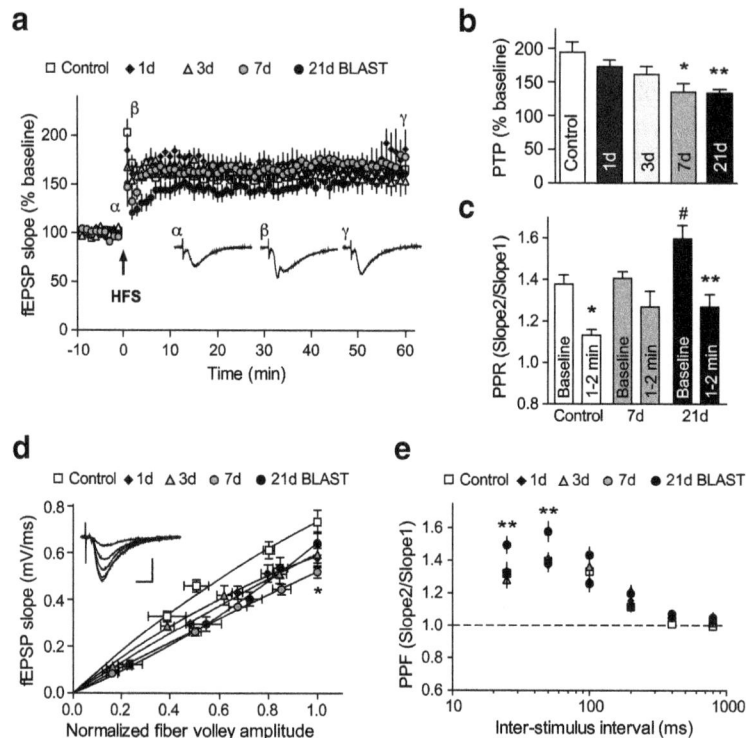

Fig. 6 Mild bTBI caused deficits in basic synaptic properties and short-term plasticity. **a** Assessment of the effect of mild blast forces on long-term potentiation (LTP) in rats at 1, 3, 7 and 21 day(s) after bTBI exposure, as well as in controls. The graph shows the time-course of the field excitatory postsynaptic potential (fEPSP) slopes before and after high frequency stimulation (HSF) in percentage from the baseline. Insets show representative traces of recordings from control slices (α: baseline, β: post-tetanic potentiation (PTP) phase, γ: LTP phase). Arrowhead indicates the time point of HFS. **b** Summary of PTP changes in response to HFS shows a significant reduction at 7 and 21 days post-bTBI (*$p < 0.05$, **$p < 0.01$, vs. control, one-way ANOVA, Newman-Keuls post hoc). **c** Paired pulse ratio (PPR) at baseline and during PTP phase in slices from rats at 7 and 21 days post-bTBI, as well as in controls (*$p < 0.05$, **$p < 0.01$, vs. baseline, Wilcoxon test, #$p < 0.05$, vs. control, Mann-Whitney test). **d** Input-output curves from fEPSP slopes against normalized fiber volley amplitudes. Connecting lines show a non-linear regression using a polynomial quadratic function for each group. Inset shows representative traces of recordings from control slices at different stimulation intensities. **e** Paired pulse facilitation (PPF) at different inter-stimulus intervals shows a significant difference at 21 days post-bTBI (**$p < 0.01$, two-way ANOVA, Tukey's post hoc). All data are presented as mean ± SEM; $n = 7–9$ slices from 2 to 4 individual rats

neurofilament, as well as neuroinflammation had receded by 21 days post-bTBI, when neurophysiological deficits became most apparent.

Mild blast forces induce biochemical changes in the hippocampus

TBI causes neuronal depolarization resulting in a large influx of ions. In response to activation of voltage-gated Ca^{2+} channels, high levels of glutamate are released, triggering excitotoxicity. Swelling of neurons, oxidative stress, and free radical production, all affect neuronal viability, contribute to neuronal death, and are associated with TBI pathology [30]. Following initial trauma, a delayed and spreading process of injury occurs. At the subcellular level, mitochondrial dysfunction and disruption in Ca^{2+}-homeostasis have been implicated in TBI pathogenesis [31]. Over-activation of Ca^{2+}-dependent enzymes such as the protease calpain may contribute to the etiology of TBI [32, 33].

Here, we examined the effects of mild bTBI on calpain activity in hippocampal lysates from blast-exposed rat brains using quantitative immunoblotting. As a marker of calpain activity, the levels of cleaved spectrin were assessed (Fig. 7a). The levels of the 100 kDa fragment of cleaved spectrin were significantly elevated at 1, 3 and 7 day(s) post-bTBI in comparison to controls. Another well-characterized calpain substrate is p35, the activating cofactor of the protein kinase Cdk5. Calpain-dependent cleavage of p35 produces the truncated protein p25. The resulting Cdk5/25 holoenzyme engenders aberrant activity, has been implicated in experimental TBI [14] and can contribute to neuronal cell death [34]. Consistent with an increase in calpain activity, p25 levels were significantly elevated at 3 and 7 days following mild bTBI (Fig. 7b). Taken together, these results demonstrate that effectors of excitotoxicity are invoked by mild bTBI, and may contribute to the etiology of TBI.

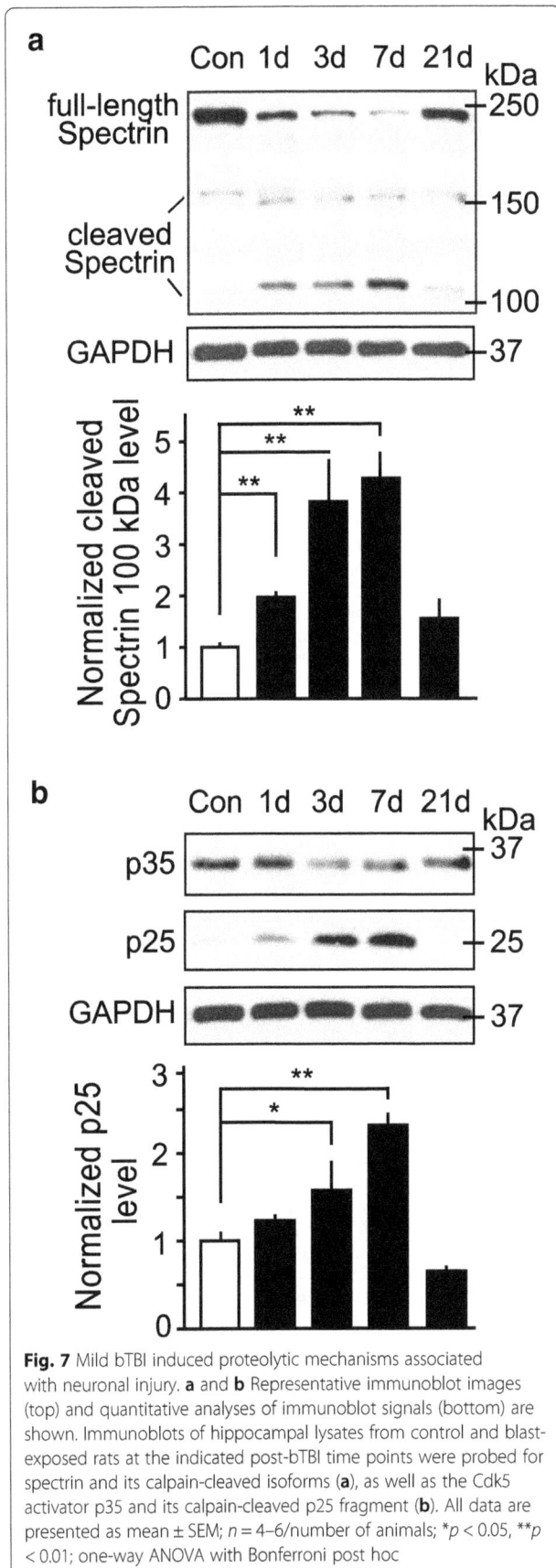

Fig. 7 Mild bTBI induced proteolytic mechanisms associated with neuronal injury. **a** and **b** Representative immunoblot images (top) and quantitative analyses of immunoblot signals (bottom) are shown. Immunoblots of hippocampal lysates from control and blast-exposed rats at the indicated post-bTBI time points were probed for spectrin and its calpain-cleaved isoforms (**a**), as well as the Cdk5 activator p35 and its calpain-cleaved p25 fragment (**b**). All data are presented as mean ± SEM; $n = 4$–6/number of animals; *$p < 0.05$, **$p < 0.01$; one-way ANOVA with Bonferroni post hoc

Discussion

Growing evidence suggests that brain injury from blast exposure is a unique and particularly problematic form of neuropathology that may be linked to severe mental illness and chronic neurodegeneration [24]. Here, we investigated the pathophysiological effects induced by mild blast forces in adult male rats at various time points after bTBI. Consistent with our previous studies [6], the overpressure wave generated by the scaled, bench-top blast tube used here did not cause macroscopic neuropathological changes, such as tissue damage, hemorrhage, hematoma, or contusion to the brain or dura. However, close examination revealed that one single mild overpressure wave induces microvasculature damage and axonal injury accompanied by neuroinflammation in various brain regions including cortex, striatum and hippocampus. These neuropathological changes are correlated with deficits in neurophysiological outcomes, including basic synaptic properties and short-term plasticity in hippocampus. Finally, a biochemical analysis revealed that the Ca^{2+}-dependent protease calpain is overactivated after mild bTBI, indicating that Ca^{2+} homeostasis is disturbed by mild blast forces. Together, these results show that even mild blast forces can cause subtle, but deleterious pathophysiological changes in the absence of major neuropathological injuries.

Numerous studies have demonstrated that basic synaptic properties and synaptic plasticity are affected in rodent models of TBI, including fluid percussion injury (FPI) and controlled cortical impact (CCI) [35–39]. The effect of primary bTBI on neurophysiological outcomes is less explored. One study reported that CA1 LTP was reduced in mouse brains at 2- and 4-weeks after a single sub-lethal blast (167 kPa/msec) [4]. Another study found that low-level primary blast trauma is associated with electrophysiological white matter dysfunction at 2 weeks post-injury [40]. Our results show that mild blast forces induce deficits in basal synaptic properties and short-term plasticity, but do not alter LTP expression. These neurophysiological deficits are not observed prior to 7 days post-bTBI and are more pronounced by 21 days post-bTBI, suggesting that neuronal functions can be critically affected by some process set in motion by mild bTBI. Furthermore, these findings also indicate that primary injuries, such as microvascular damage and neuroinflammation, as well as increased phosphorylation levels of neurofilaments do not directly induce neurophysiological deficits, as the primary injuries are present early on following bTBI but had receded by 21 days post-bTBI, whereas the neurophysiological deficits appear only after 7 days post-bTBI. Thus, our data suggests that mild blast forces can induce long-lasting pathophysiological changes, other than the primary injuries, that lead to deficits in basal synaptic properties and short-term plasticity weeks after the initial injury that may impact brain functions.

Despite the absence of gross neuropathological effects, such as tissue damage, hemorrhage or contusion, we find increased astrogliosis and microglia activation after mild bTBI in cortex, hippocampus and striatum. Consistent with previous TBI studies [41], we observed neuroinflammation during the initial phases of injury, namely at 1, 3 and 7 day(s) after bTBI. By 21 days post-bTBI astrogliosis and microgliosis levels were comparable to controls showing that the acute early activation of gliosis is significant for injury expansion but resolves over time. Moreover, previous research using different blast intensities in rats and organotypic hippocampal slice cultures showed that increasing blast intensity resulted in elevated levels of astrogliosis and microglia activation [6, 42].

Our results show that the Ca^{2+}-dependent protease calpain is overactivated post-bTBI as indicated by increased degradation of its substrates spectrin and the Cdk5 activator p35 (Fig. 7). Compromised microvascular integrity is often related to brain injuries involving excitotoxicity. Activation of Ca^{2+}-dependent proteases, such as calpain, is a predicted outcome of membrane depolarization and loss of Ca^{2+} homeostasis. Spectrin is involved in actin binding and maintaining the shape of synapses thereby regulating synaptic functions, including synaptic plasticity [43]. Thus, calpain activation and cleavage of spectrin is consistent with deficits in axonal architecture and disruption of synaptic plasticity [44]. Indeed, rats exposed to bTBI can exhibit shortened axon initial segments, suggesting such subcellular changes [45]. Moreover, spectrin cleavage in the corpus callosum after bTBI has been suggested to attenuate overall electrophysiological responses [40] and neuronal death [46]. Calpain-dependent conversion of p35 to p25 results in dysregulation of the protein kinase Cdk5, causing relocation of the protein kinase and redirection towards aberrant substrates that mediate neuronal injury [34]. Thus, exposure to moderate blast forces may initiate subtle but still meaningful neuropathological processes.

Taken together, the results presented here demonstrate that even mild blast forces can induce a panoply of pathophysiological effects with long-lasting consequences for neuronal functions. Future studies into the molecular and cellular changes underlying these pathophysiological changes will be needed to advance our understanding of bTBI etiology. Finally, the changes observed in this study, would probably not be detected using structural brain imaging techniques, giving a rational as to why most structural imaging studies of mild TBI in human failed to reveal significant insights. However, our results suggest that even mild bTBI might have significant neuronal/functional consequences that occur long after the actual blast exposure/injury.

Abbreviations
ACSF: Artificial cerebrospinal fluid; bTBI: Blast-induced traumatic brain injury; CCI: Controlled cortical impact; Cdk5: Cyclin-dependent kinase 5; fEPSP: Field excitatory post synaptic potential; FPI: Fluid percussion injury; GFAP: Glial fibrillary acidic protein; H&E: Hematoxylin and eosin; HFS: High frequency stimulation; IACUC: Institutional Animal Care and Use Committees; Iba1: Ionized Ca^{2+}-binding adapter molecule; IgG: Immunoglobulin G; LTP: Long-term potentiation; PPF: Paired pulse facilitation; PPR: Paired pulse ratio; PTP: Post-tetanic potentiation; RRID: Research Resource Identifiers; TBI: Traumatic brain injury

Acknowledgements
We thank G. Mettlach and L. O'Connor for technical assistance. We thank R. Gettens, N. St. Johns, P. Bennet and J. Robson for their contributions to the blast model. We thank K. Phelps for help with the quantitative analysis and Sai Javangula for help with manuscript revision.

Funding
This work was supported by a Discovery Award from the Texas Institute for Brain Injury and Repair and was facilitated by grants to J.A.B. from the National Institute of Mental Health (MH083711), National Institute on Drug Abuse (DA033485) and National Institute of Neurological Disorders and Stroke (NS073855). This research was also supported in part through funding to F.P. from the Friends of the Alzheimer's Center and the Darrell K. Royal Research Fund for Alzheimer's Disease and pre-doctoral fellowships from the American Foundation for Pharmaceutical Education to A.F.L and B.P.L., as well as a pre-doctoral fellowship from the American Association of Pharmaceutical Scientists to B.P.L.

Authors' contributions
AH, AFL, CT, FP, RCT, JDH, CLR and JAB conceived and designed experiments. AH, AFL, CT, TS, MAY, BPL and FP performed the experiments. AH, CT, TS, KP, MAY and FP analyzed the data. FP and JAB wrote the manuscript with help from BPL. All authors read and approved the final manuscript.

Competing interests
The authors declare that they have no competing interests.

Author details
[1]Department of Psychiatry, University of Texas Southwestern Medical Center, Dallas, TX 75390, USA. [2]Center for Translational Neurodegeneration Research, University of Texas Southwestern Medical Center, Dallas, TX 75390, USA. [3]Department of Neurosurgery, West Virginia University School of Medicine, Morgantown, WV 26506-9183, USA. [4]Department of Basic Pharmaceutical Sciences, West Virginia University School of Medicine, Morgantown, WV 26506-9530, USA. [5]Departments of Surgery, Neurobiology, and Neurology, The University of Alabama at Birmingham Medical Center, 1720 2nd Ave S, THT 1052, Birmingham, AL 35294, USA.

References

1. Wolf SJ, Bebarta VS, Bonnett CJ, Pons PT, Cantrill SV. Blast injuries. Lancet. 2009;374:405–15.
2. Huber BR, Meabon JS, Martin TJ, Mourad PD, Bennett R, Kraemer BC, Cernak I, Petrie EC, Emery MJ, Swenson ER, Mayer C, Mehic E, Peskind ER, Cook DG. Blast exposure causes early and persistent aberrant phospho- and cleaved-tau expression in a murine model of mild blast-induced traumatic brain injury. J Alzheimers Dis. 2013;37:309–23.
3. Tompkins P, Tesiram Y, Lerner M, Gonzalez LP, Lightfoot S, Rabb CH, Brackett DJ. Brain injury: neuro-inflammation, cognitive deficit, and magnetic resonance imaging in a model of blast induced traumatic brain injury. J Neurotrauma. 2013;30:1888–97.
4. Goldstein LE, Fisher AM, Tagge CA, Zhang XL, Velisek L, Sullivan JA, Upreti C, Kracht JM, Ericsson M, Wojnarowicz MW, Goletiani CJ, Maglakelidze GM, Casey N, Moncaster JA, Minaeva O, Moir RD, et al. Chronic traumatic encephalopathy in blast-exposed military veterans and a blast neurotrauma mouse model. Sci Transl Med. 2012;4:134ra160.
5. Miller G. Neuropathology. Blast injuries linked to neurodegeneration in veterans. Science. 2012;336:790–1.
6. Turner RC, Naser ZJ, Logsdon AF, DiPasquale KH, Jackson GJ, Robson MJ, Gettens RT, Matsumoto RR, Huber JD, Rosen CL. Modeling clinically relevant blast parameters based on scaling principles produces functional & histological deficits in rats. Exp Neurol. 2013;248:520–9.
7. Rubovitch V, Ten-Bosch M, Zohar O, Harrison CR, Tempel-Brami C, Stein E, Hoffer BJ, Balaban CD, Schreiber S, Chiu WT, Pick CG. A mouse model of blast-induced mild traumatic brain injury. Exp Neurol. 2011;232:280–9.
8. Elder GA, Dorr NP, De Gasperi R, Gama Sosa MA, Shaughness MC, Maudlin-Jeronimo E, Hall AA, McCarron RM, Ahlers ST. Blast exposure induces post-traumatic stress disorder-related traits in a rat model of mild traumatic brain injury. J Neurotrauma. 2012;29:2564–75.
9. de Lanerolle NC, Bandak F, Kang D, Li AY, Du F, Swauger P, Parks S, Ling G, Kim JH. Characteristics of an explosive blast-induced brain injury in an experimental model. J Neuropathol Exp Neurol. 2011;70:1046–57.
10. Abdul-Muneer PM, Schuetz H, Wang F, Skotak M, Jones J, Gorantla S, Zimmerman MC, Chandra N, Haorah J. Induction of oxidative and nitrosative damage leads to cerebrovascular inflammation in an animal model of mild traumatic brain injury induced by primary blast. Free Radic Biol Med. 2013;60:282–91.
11. Sosa MA, De Gasperi R, Paulino AJ, Pricop PE, Shaughness MC, Maudlin-Jeronimo E, Hall AA, Janssen WG, Yuk FJ, Dorr NP, Dickstein DL, McCarron RM, Chavko M, Hof PR, Ahlers ST, Elder GA. Blast overpressure induces shear-related injuries in the brain of rats exposed to a mild traumatic brain injury. Acta Neuropathol Commun. 2013;1:51.
12. Kochanek PM, Dixon CE, Shellington DK, Shin SS, Bayir H, Jackson EK, Kagan VE, Yan HQ, Swauger PV, Parks SA, Ritzel DV, Bauman R, Clark RS, Garman RH, Bandak F, Ling G, et al. Screening of biochemical and molecular mechanisms of secondary injury and repair in the brain after experimental blast-induced traumatic brain injury in rats. J Neurotrauma. 2013;30:920–37.
13. Plattner F, Hernandez A, Kistler TM, Pozo K, Zhong P, Yuen EY, Tan C, Hawasli AH, Cooke SF, Nishi A, Guo A, Wiederhold T, Yan Z, Bibb JA. Memory enhancement by targeting Cdk5 regulation of NR2B. Neuron. 2014; 81:1070–83.
14. Yousuf MA, Tan C, Torres-Altoro MI, Lu FM, Plautz E, Zhang S, Takahashi M, Hernandez A, Kernie SG, Plattner F, Bibb JA. Involvement of aberrant cyclin-dependent kinase 5/p25 activity in experimental traumatic brain injury. J Neurochem. 2016;138:317–27.
15. Fischer AH, Jacobson KA, Rose J, Zeller R. Hematoxylin and eosin staining of tissue and cell sections. CSH Protoc. 2008;2008:pdb prot4986.
16. Schmued LC, Hopkins KJ. Fluoro-jade B: a high affinity fluorescent marker for the localization of neuronal degeneration. Brain Res. 2000;874:123–30.
17. Sinclair RA, Burns J, Dunnill MS. Immunoperoxidase staining of formalin-fixed, paraffin-embedded, human renal biopsies with a comparison of the peroxidase-antiperoxidase (PAP) and indirect methods. J Clin Pathol. 1981; 34:859–65.
18. Sahin B, Kansy JW, Nairn AC, Spychala J, Ealick SE, Fienberg AA, Greene RW, Bibb JA. Molecular characterization of recombinant mouse adenosine kinase and evaluation as a target for protein phosphorylation. Eur J Biochem. 2004;271:3547–55.
19. Plattner F, Angelo M, Giese KP. The roles of cyclin-dependent kinase 5 and glycogen synthase kinase 3 in tau hyperphosphorylation. J Biol Chem. 2006;281:25457–65.

20. Mez J, Stern RA, McKee AC. Chronic traumatic encephalopathy: where are we and where are we going? Curr Neurol Neurosci Rep. 2013;13:407.
21. Mishra V, Skotak M, Schuetz H, Heller A, Haorah J, Chandra N. Primary blast causes mild, moderate, severe and lethal TBI with increasing blast overpressures: experimental rat injury model. Sci Rep. 2016;6:26992.
22. Zuckerman A, Ram O, Ifergane G, Matar MA, Sagi R, Ostfeld I, Hoffman JR, Kaplan Z, Sadot O, Cohen H. Controlled low-pressure blast-wave exposure causes distinct behavioral and morphological responses modelling mild traumatic brain injury, post-traumatic stress disorder, and comorbid mild traumatic brain injury-post-traumatic stress disorder. J Neurotrauma. 2017;34:145–64.
23. Ansari MA, Roberts KN, Scheff SW. A time course of NADPH-oxidase up-regulation and endothelial nitric oxide synthase activation in the hippocampus following neurotrauma. Free Radic Biol Med. 2014;77:21–9.
24. Shively SB, Horkayne-Szakaly I, Jones RV, Kelly JP, Armstrong RC, Perl DP. Characterisation of interface astroglial scarring in the human brain after blast exposure: a post-mortem case series. Lancet Neurol. 2016;15:944–53.
25. Sajja VS, Galloway M, Ghoddoussi F, Kepsel A, VandeVord P. Effects of blast-induced neurotrauma on the nucleus accumbens. J Neurosci Res. 2013;91: 593–601.
26. Blennow K, Hardy J, Zetterberg H. The neuropathology and neurobiology of traumatic brain injury. Neuron. 2012;76:886–99.
27. Siedler DG, Chuah MI, Kirkcaldie MT, Vickers JC, King AE. Diffuse axonal injury in brain trauma: insights from alterations in neurofilaments. Front Cell Neurosci. 2014;8:429.
28. Chung RS, Staal JA, McCormack GH, Dickson TC, Cozens MA, Chuckowree JA, Quilty MC, Vickers JC. Mild axonal stretch injury in vitro induces a progressive series of neurofilament alterations ultimately leading to delayed axotomy. J Neurotrauma. 2005;22:1081–91.
29. Koliatsos VE, Cernak I, Xu L, Song Y, Savonenko A, Crain BJ, Eberhart CG, Frangakis CE, Melnikova T, Kim H, Lee D. A mouse model of blast injury to brain: initial pathological, neuropathological, and behavioral characterization. J Neuropathol Exp Neurol. 2011;70:399–416.
30. Cernak I, Noble-Haeusslein LJ. Traumatic brain injury: an overview of pathobiology with emphasis on military populations. J Cereb Blood Flow Metab. 2010;30:255–66.
31. Wang KK, Larner SF, Robinson G, Hayes RL. Neuroprotection targets after traumatic brain injury. Curr Opin Neurol. 2006;19:514–9.
32. Werner C, Engelhard K. Pathophysiology of traumatic brain injury. Br J Anaesth. 2007;99:4–9.
33. Yang Z, Wang Z, Wei X, Han H, Meng X, Zhang Y, Shi W, Li F, Xin T, Pang Q, Yi F. NLRP3 deficiency ameliorates neurovascular damage in experimental ischemic stroke. J Cereb Blood Flow Metab. 2014;34:660–7.
34. Hisanaga S, Endo R. Regulation and role of cyclin-dependent kinase activity in neuronal survival and death. J Neurochem. 2010;115:1309–21.
35. Miyazaki S, Katayama Y, Lyeth BG, Jenkins LW, DeWitt DS, Goldberg SJ, Newlon PG, Hayes RL. Enduring suppression of hippocampal long-term potentiation following traumatic brain injury in rat. Brain Res. 1992;585:335–9.
36. Reeves TM, Lyeth BG, Povlishock JT. Long-term potentiation deficits and excitability changes following traumatic brain injury. Exp Brain Res. 1995;106:248–56.
37. Albensi BC, Sullivan PG, Thompson MB, Scheff SW, Mattson MP. Cyclosporin ameliorates traumatic brain-injury-induced alterations of hippocampal synaptic plasticity. Exp Neurol. 2000;162:385–9.
38. Albensi BC. Models of brain injury and alterations in synaptic plasticity. J Neurosci Res. 2001;65:279–83.
39. Bach-y-Rita P. Theoretical basis for brain plasticity after a TBI. Brain Inj. 2003;17:643–51.
40. Park E, Eisen R, Kinio A, Baker AJ. Electrophysiological white matter dysfunction and association with neurobehavioral deficits following low-level primary blast trauma. Neurobiol Dis. 2013;52:150–9.
41. Svetlov SI, Prima V, Glushakova O, Svetlov A, Kirk DR, Gutierrez H, Serebruany VL, Curley KC, Wang KK, Hayes RL. Neuro-glial and systemic mechanisms of pathological responses in rat models of primary blast overpressure compared to "composite" blast. Front Neurol. 2012;3:15.
42. Miller AP, Shah AS, Aperi BV, Budde MD, Pintar FA, Tarima S, Kurpad SN, Stemper BD, Glavaski-Joksimovic A. Effects of blast overpressure on neurons and glial cells in rat organotypic hippocampal slice cultures. Front Neurol. 2015;6:20.
43. Greer JE, Hanell A, McGinn MJ, Povlishock JT. Mild traumatic brain injury in the mouse induces axotomy primarily within the axon initial segment. Acta Neuropathol. 2013;126:59–74.

proBDNF is modified by advanced glycation end products in Alzheimer's disease and causes neuronal apoptosis by inducing p75 neurotrophin receptor processing

Catherine Fleitas[1], Gerard Piñol-Ripoll[4], Pau Marfull[1], Daniel Rocandio[1], Isidro Ferrer[2,3], Claire Rampon[5], Joaquim Egea[1,6] and Carme Espinet[6*]

Abstract

Alzheimer disease (AD) is a complex pathology related to multiple causes including oxidative stress. Brain-derived neurotrophic factor (BDNF) is a neutrotrophic factor essential for the survival and differentiation of neurons and is considered a key target in the pathophysiology of various neurodegenerative diseases, as for example AD. Contrarily to BDNF, the precursor form of BDNF (proBDNF) induces apoptosis through the specific interaction with p75 and its co-receptor, Sortilin.

We used hippocampal tissue and cerebrospinal fluid from AD patients and controls. to study the localization and the levels of proBDNF, p75 and Sortilin as well as the post-traduccional modifications of proBDNF induced by Radical Oxygen Species, by immunofluorescence and Western blot. Differentiation and survival were assessed on differentiated mouse hippocampal neurons derived from postnatal neural stem cells from WT animals or from the transgenic AD animal model APP/PS1ΔE9, based on mutations of familiar AD. In AD patients we observe a significative increase of proBDNF and Sortilin expression and a significative increase of the ratio proBDNF/BDNF in their cerebrospinal fluid compared to controls. In addition, the proBDNF of AD patients is modified by ROS-derived advanced glycation end products, which prevent the processing of the proBDNF to the mature BDNF, leading to an increase of pathogenicity and a decrease of trophic effects. The cerebrospinal fluid from AD patients, but not from controls, induces apoptosis in differentiated hippocampal neurons mainly by the action of AGE-modified proBDNF present in the cerebrospinal fluid of the patients. This effect is triggered by the activation and processing of p75 that stimulate the internalization of the intracellular domain (ICD) within the nucleus causing apoptosis. Induction of apoptosis and p75 ICD internalization by AD patients-derived proBDNF is further enhanced in neuron cultures from the AD model expressing the APP/PS1ΔE9 transgene.

Our results indicate the importance of proBDNF neurotoxic signaling in AD pathology essentially by three mechanisms: i) by an increase of proBDNF stability due to ROS-induced post-traductional modifications; ii) by the increase of expression of the p75 co-receptor, Sortilin and iii) by the increase of the basal levels of p75 processing found in AD.

Keywords: Alzheimer's disease, Biomarkers, BDNF, p75, proBDNF, Oxidative stress, Sortilin

* Correspondence: carme.espinet@cmb.udl.cat
[6]Serra Húnter fellow, Associate Professor, Generalitat de Catalunya, Barcelona, Spain
Full list of author information is available at the end of the article

Background

Alzheimer's disease (AD) is a neurodegenerative disorder characterized by episodic memory decline at onset and deficits in multiple cortical functions in later stages. Neuropathology hallmarks are senile plaques and neurofibrillary tangles accompanied by deficits in axonal transport, synaptic dysfunction, and neuronal loss. The exact molecular mechanisms that trigger AD pathogenesis and disease course are not entirely understood. Among them, the increase of oxidative stress related to aging seems to play a central role, not only in AD but also in other neurodegenerative diseases [1]. There has been much research into the possible involvement of neurotrophins in AD pathogenesis, including Nerve Growth factor (NGF) and Brain Derived Neurotrophic Factor (BDNF) [2]. This interest was further supported by studies demonstrating the neuroprotective activity against neurodegeneration in different animal models of several neurodegenerative diseases, including AD, which suggested therefore a promising therapeutic role for neurotrophins [3].

BDNF binds to TrkB tyrosine kinase receptor to trigger the neurotrophic signaling including neuron survival, differentiation and synaptic plasticity of various nerve cell populations during normal development and during tissue repair after injury [4, 5]. BDNF is synthesized as a precursor form (proBDNF) that is processed by the activity of several proteases rendering three main products of 14 kDa (mature BDNF), 28 kDa and 34 kDa [6]. ProBDNF was reported to be biologically active and, unlike BDNF, it was shown to induce apoptosis through its interaction with p75 and its co-receptor, Sortilin [6–11]. p75 belongs to the family of tumor necrosis factor receptors, has not catalytic activity but a conserved non functional death domain [12]. The signaling mechanisms of p75 are complex and involve several intracellular interactors which trigger specific effects including Sc1, NRAGE and Necdine (cell cycle arrest) [13], RhoA (neuritogenesis) [12] and NRIF (apoptosis) [14]. An important signaling event for p75 involved in apoptosis is the processing of the receptor by convertases, in particular by a α-protease (BACE1) followed by a γ-secretase activity (presenilin 1 or PS1), that yield a 20 kDa intracellular domain (p75ICD) that is translocated into the nucleus [15–18]. p75ICD regulates the activity of the transcription factor NRIF inducing apoptosis [19]. Besides all these functions, p75 has also been reported to act as a co-receptor for Trk, indicating that p75 plays a central role in integrating the neurotrophic effects triggered by neurotrophins (as Trk co-receptor) and the pro-apoptotic signaling triggered by pro-neurotrophins (as Sortilin co-receptor).

In normal brains, the pro-apoptotic function of pro-neurotrophins and the neurotrophic effects of mature neurotrophins are tightly controlled by their expression levels as well as by the expression levels of their receptors, in particular p75 which is crucial for the integration of the two effects. It is conceivable therefore that neurodegeneration during AD might be caused by an imbalance of survival and death mechanisms due to changes in the relative levels of these proteins. Accordingly, the cerebral cortex of AD patients showed increased levels of p75 [20, 21] concomitant with decreased levels of Trk receptors which will favor an apoptotic signaling [22–24]. BDNF signaling was also shown to be altered in AD as an splicing form of TrkB, which gives rise to a truncated form of the receptor lacking the tyrosine kinase domain (presumably acting as a dominant negative), is expressed predominantly in hippocampus and frontal cortex in AD [23]. On the other hand, several works have described a reduced concentration of BDNF in the CSF of AD-affected patients [24]. Paradoxically, some authors have shown a decrease of proBDNF expression in AD-affected human brains [25, 26]. However, in the CSF of AD-affected patients, the levels of proBDNF have not been analyzed yet. Moreover, there is no data in the literature about the relative levels of proBDNF and BDNF in the CSF of AD-affected individuals compared to controls.

The relative levels of proBDNF and BDNF are directly regulated by the activity of the proteases involved in their processing. We have previously shown that proNGF extracted from brains of AD patients was more resistant to be processed by convertases in comparison to the proNGF isolated from control brains [27, 28]. We reported that the relative stability of proNGF in AD brains was due to post-traduccional modifications as a consequence of an increase of oxidative stress in the affected tissue [28]. In particular, we observed that Glyoxal (GO) and methylglyoxal (MGO), two highly reactive dicarbonyls that are increased during OS, reacted with free amino groups of Lys, Arg and Cys residues in proNGF, leading to the formation of the AGE/ALE adducts Nε-(carboxymethyl)-lysine (CML), Nε-(carboxyethyl)-lysine (CEL) and intermolecular crosslink and making proNGF in AD patients more resistant to the action of convertases [28].

In the present work we have studied the relative levels of BDNF and proBDNF and their receptors in AD patients and found a significant increase of Sortilin and proBDNF in the hippocampus. We also detected a significant increase of the ratio proBDNF/BDNF in the CSF of the AD patients, which shows a good correlation with the pathogenic effect of the pro-neurotrophin in the brain. Interestingly, the proBDNF in the CSF of AD patients showed an increase of CEL modifications which account for the increase of the proBDNF/BDNF ratio due to the major stability of the modified pro-form. Stimulation of primary cultures of hippocampal neurons with CSF from AD patients increased significantly the apoptotic cell death and the nuclear localization of p75ICD compared with the CSF from controls. Similar effects were observed when neurons were stimulated with a proBDNF that was modified in vitro by MGO. Importantly apoptosis and p75ICD nuclear localization were strongly reduced when the CSF of AD patients was immunodepleted of proBDNF, indicating that these effects were mediated, to a large extent, by the presence of proBDNF in the CSF. Finally, we demonstrated that the modified proBDNF had a stronger effect on apoptosis and p75ICD nuclear localization on primary cultures of hippocampal neurons obtained from a transgenic AD mouse model expressing the APP/PS1ΔE9 transgene. In summary, we propose that in AD, proBDNF-p75/Sortilin signaling has an important contribution to the pathogenesis of the disease, causing an increase of cell death and impairing neuronal differentiation.

Methods

Human brain samples

Brain samples were obtained from the Institute of Neuropathology, Bellvitge University Hospital. Brain tissue was obtained from the Institute of Neuropathology HUB-ICO-IDIBELL Biobank and the Hospital Clinic-IDIBAPS Biobank following the guidelines of Spanish legislation on this matter (Real Decreto de Biobancos 1716/2011) and approval of the local ethics committees. At autopsy, one hemisphere was rapidly cut in coronal sections 1 cm thick and selected areas of the encephalon were dissected, frozen on dry ice, and stored at − 80 °C in labeled plastic bags until use. The other hemisphere was fixed by immersion in 4% buffered formalin for three weeks for morphologic examination. The neuropathological study was carried out on twenty-five regions of the cerebral cortex, diencephalon, thalamus, brainstem, and cerebellum. De-waxed paraffin sections were stained with hematoxylin and eosin and Klüver-Barrera and processed for immunohistochemistry to microglia-specific markers, glial fibrillary acidic protein, β-amyloid, phosphorylated tau, α-synuclein, TDP-43, ubiquitin, and p62. Neuropathological diagnosis of the AD was carried out following the Braak, and Braak stages [29] adapted to paraffin sections [30]. Cases with concomitant pathologies, including Lewy body diseases, tauopathies (particularly argyrophilic grain disease), vascular diseases, TDP-43pathies, and metabolic syndrome were excluded. Control and disease cases were processed in parallel. The anterior hippocampus area was used for further immunohistochemical studies.

Human CSF samples

CSF samples were obtained from control and AD-affected patients and maintained at 4 °C for less than 4 h. All patients have signed informed consent and the study has been approved by the hospital's ethics committee. All patients underwent lumbar puncture between 8:00 and 10:00 in the morning to avoid variations relating to the circadian rhythm. Protein concentration was determined by DC-Protein Assay (Bio-Rad). Samples were collected and frozen in polypropylene tubes. Post-puncture, CSF was centrifuged at 2000 g for 10 min at 4 °C and stored at − 80 °C until the use of the samples. The levels in CSF Aβ42, t-tau and p-tau were determined by a method of enzyme-immuno assay (ELISA) using the kit Innotest Amyliod β (1–42), Innotest htau and phospho-tau 181 (Innogenetics ®) according to the manufacturer's instructions. All samples were measured in duplicate and were expressed as pg/ml. We use cut off points based on the calculation of sensitivity and specificity of our own study population (different from this sample).

Animal model

APPswe/PS1DE9 with a C57Bl/6 background (double transgenic mice expressing a chimeric mouse/human amyloid precursor protein and a mutant human PS1 with deletion in exon 9) were purchased from The Jackson Laboratory and kept in specific pathogen free conditions under standard animal housing conditions in a 12-h dark–light cycle with free access to food and water in the animal house facility of the Universitat de Lleida [31, 32]. Heterozygous males were bred with wild-type C57/Bl6 females. Animal procedures were conducted according to ethical guidelines (European Communities Council Directive 86/609/EEC) and approved by the local ethics committee of the Universitat de Lleida. For experiments, tail biopsies were taken from P0 offsprings for genotyping by PCR according to the PCR conditions suggested by The Jackson Laboratory. Mice not expressing the transgene were used as controls.

Cell culture

Hippocampal Neural Stem Cells (NSCs) were isolated from neonatal pups (P0–P1) from controls and APP/PS1 transgenic mice. Briefly, the brains were dissected in Hanks Medium 1X (Gibco 11,039–021) supplemented with Penicillin-Streptomycin (P/S) (1%) (Sigma-Aldrich P4333). After dissection, the hippocampi were washed with Hanks Medium with P/S (1%) and dissociated in Hanks Medium with Papain (Sigma-Aldrich 1,001,992,754) for 20 min at 37 °C. Papain activity was stopped with two washes with Trypsin inhibitor (10 mg/ml in Hanks medium) (Roche Diagnostics 10,109,886,001) plus three washes with 1 ml of Dulbecco's modified Eagle's medium (DMEM)/F12, supplemented with B27 (2%) (Gibco 12,587–010) and P/S. Mechanical dissociation was performed with a heat-rounded Pasteur pipette tip. Dissociated cells were centrifuged at 600 rpm for 4 min, and the pellet was resuspended in DMEM/F12 (37 °C) supplemented with B27 (2%), P/S(1%), Epidermal Growth Factor (EGF) (20 μg/ml) (Sigma-Aldrich E9644) and Fibroblast Growth Factor (FGF) (20 μg/ml) (Alomone Labs F-170). Cells were platted on bacterial, non-treated, P35 plates and incubated for four days at 37 °C. After four days, the supernatant was centrifuged at 600 rpm for 4 min, the supernatant was removed and the pellet was washed in complete medium DMEM/F12 (37 °C) supplemented with B27 (2%) and P/S (1%), without growth factors. Then the neurospheres were dissociated with a pipette in 500 μl of complete medium and determined the cell concentration by Trypan Blue dye exclusion. Cells were plated at 6000 cells/well concentration in 8-well on a glass slide coated with poly-D-lysine (Sigma-Aldrich P-7886) and laminin (Invitrogen 23,017–015) with complete medium (DMEM/F12, B27 (2%) and P/S (1%)). Neurons were treated at 1 DIV. Treatments were done after two washes with DMEM/F12 without B27. The treatments with neurotrophins and controls are done with DMEM/F12 containing 0,25% B27. For treatments with CSF, all the media is substituted by CSF from controls and AD with P/S (1%). After six days (7 DIV in total), were fixed for 30 min in 4% (w/v) paraformaldehyde (PFA)/PBS for immunofluorescence assays.

Western blotting

CSF samples were obtained as described in 2.2., from control and AD-affected patients and maintained at 4 °C for less than 4 h. Previously to the western blotting, CSF samples were concentrated 20X using Amicon Ultra 10,000 MWCO (Ultracel Low Binding Cellulose) (Millipore). Protein concentration was determined by DC-Protein Assay (Bio-Rad). Proteins were separated by electrophoresis in 12% SDS-PAGE and transferred to Immobilon-P membranes (Millipore). Membranes were blocked for 1 h at room temperature in TBS-T (50 mM Tris, pH 8.0; 133 mM NaCl, 0.2% Tween 20) with 5% skimmed milk and incubated with primary antibodies against the mature BDNF (1:1000 in TBS-T (Alomone) at 4 °C overnight and with HRP-conjugated secondary antibodies (Jackson) (1:5000 in TBS-T) at room temperature for 1 h. Detection was performed using an ECL chemiluminescence system (Amersham-Pharmacia) following the manufacturer's instructions. For densitometry analysis of the immunoreactive bands, we used ImageJ (http://rsbweb.nih.gov/ij/) with local background subtracted. For each sample, the relative abundance of each BDNF isoform was expressed as a ratio of that particular BDNF isoform related to the total BDNF signal (sum of proBDNF and mature BDNF). The data were shown as the mean ± standard deviation (SD).

Differences between groups were calculated using a 2-tailed Student's t-test.

AGE modifications of recombinant proBDNF

Recombinant human proBDNF (Alomone) was modified by the reactive carbonyl specie MGO that react with free amino groups of Lys residues on proteins, leading to the formation of CEL adducts and intermolecular crosslinks [28]. The reactions were performed for 24 h at 37 °C by mixing 500 μg recombinant protein with 250 μl 50 μM GO or MGO and 250 μl 100 mM sodium phosphate. The modified proBDNF was dialyzed using Amicon Ultra-4 Centrifugal Filter Units (Millipore) to remove the excess of MGO and replace the solution with PBS.

Immunohistochemistry

Microtome sections of fixed and paraffin-embedded human hippocampus 30 μm thick were processed free-floating, and collected in slides. Before immunodetection, they were deparaffined, and rehydrated using standard procedures. Epitope retrieval was performed by incubating the slides in 10 mM sodium citrate buffer (pH 6.0) for 20 min at 95-98 °C in a water bath. After washing with PBS at room temperature, sections were permeabilized with PBS with 0, 1% Triton X-100 (PBST) and blocked for 1 h at room temperature with 5% donkey serum in PSBT. Sections were incubated with primary antibodies in blocking solution over night at 4 °C (rabbit anti-proBDNF, 1:100 (Alomone); mouse anti-CEL, 1:100 (Trans Genic Inc); rabbit anti-ECDp75, 1:100 (Abcam); goat anti-Sortilin, 1:100 (R&D System)). After washing the sections were incubated for 2 h at room temperature with the corresponding secondary antibodies in blocking solution containing DAPI 1:2000 (donkey anti-goat Cy3, 1:500; donkey anti-rabbit Alexa488, 1:500; donkey anti-mouse Cy3, 1:500 (all from Jackson Immunoresearch). Blockage of anti-proBDNF antibody immunoreactivity was performed by incubating the antigenic peptide with the antibody in a proportion 10:1, during 2 h at room temperature, before the immunohistochemistry procedure. Fluorescence images were imaged on an Olympus Bx51 fluorescence microscope or under a Fluo View FV-1000 Olympus laser-scanning confocal microscope, and micrographs were uniformly adjusted for levels, brightness, and contrast in Adobe Photoshop.

Immunocytochemistry

Cells were fixed with 4% PFA in PBS for 30 min at room temperature, permeabilized with TBST for 60 min at room temperature and blocked with 5% donkey serum in TBST. Primary antibodies were diluted in blocking solution and incubated overnight at 4 °C (rabbit anti-human p75, 1:100 (Promega) to detect intracellular domain, rabbit anti-ECD p75, 1:100 (Abcam) to detect the extracellular domain of p75NTR, goat anti-Sortilin, 1:100 (R&D System); rabbit anti-TrkB, 1:100 (H-181, Santa Cruz Biotech.); goat anti-SV2,1:100 (DSHB); mouse anti-βIII tubulin, 1:100 (Sigma); mouse anti-doublecortin, 1:100 (Cell Signaling), rabbit anti-calbindin, rabbit anti-calretinin and parvalbumin,1:100 (Swant)). After washing samples were incubated for 2 h at room temperature with the corresponding secondary antibodies diluted in blocking solution containing DAPI 1:2000 (monkey anti-goat Cy3, 1:500; donkey anti-rabbit Alexa488, 1:500; donkey anti-mouse Cy3, 1:500 (all from Jackson Immunoresearch)). Fluorescence images were acquired on a confocal microscopy setup (Olympus FV1000, 60X PlanApo using software Fluoview v.4.3) or on an inverted fluorescence microscope (OlimpusIX71, 20X LCPlanFl).

Quantitative imaging

All microscope settings were set to collect images below saturation and were kept constant for all images taken in one experiment. Statistical significance (p values) was assessed using the two-tailed Student's t-test unless otherwise indicated. Results were shown as the mean +/− standard deviation (SD).

Statistical analysis

Statistical analysis of data was performed using SPSS statistical software (SPSS for Windows, v.16, SPSS, Inc., Chicago, IL). Student's t-test and One-way ANOVA analysis are used to identify significant differences.

Results

proBDNF expression and the ratio Sortilin/p75 are increased in the hippocampus of AD patients

The hippocampus is one of the brain regions most affected in the AD [29, 30]. Particularly vulnerable are a group of neurons located in the hilus, also known as hilear Mossy cells [33, 34]. We obtained brain samples containing this region from AD patients and controls as summarized in Table 1 and using antibodies directed

Table 1 Summary of the patients from whom hippocampal samples were obtained and studied

N	Age	Gender	Diagnostic	Braak Stages	Post-mortem delay /hours
1	46	F	C	0	9
2	47	M	C	0	5
3	24	F	C	0	6
4	79	M	AD	V/B	5
5	82	F	AD	V/B	2
6	79	M	AD	V/C	7
7	85	F	AD	VI/C	12

C control, *AD* Alzheimer's Disease, *A, B and C* Braak and Braak's classification of AD stages depending on amyloid plaques, *0-V* Braak and Braak's classification of AD stages depending on the distribution and amount of neurofibrillary tangles

against the extracellular domain of p75 (p75ECD), Sortilin and the pro-domain of BDNF, we performed immunofluorescence assays to determine the levels of these proteins in the two groups. We observed that fluorescence intensity for p75 in individual hileal cells of AD brains was not significantly different on average compared to control brains (Fig. 1b, f, i). However, Sortilin fluorescence as well as the percentage of double positive cells for Sortilin and p75 increased significantly in AD brains (Fig. 1c, g, i). We also observed an abundant expression of proBDNF in the cytoplasm of the hileal neurons of human hippocampus (Fig. 1k, m).

However, in AD brain samples, fluorescence intensity of proBDNF was significantly higher than in control brains (Fig. 1k, m, n). Next we asked whether proBDNF and BDNF could be detected in the CSF of AD patients and controls since this technique has been traditionally used to study the expression profile of different markers in alive individuals for the diagnostic and/or the prognostic of neurodegenerative diseases. In this case, we analyzed the CSF by western blot and used antibodies against the mature form of BDNF that also detects the proBDNF. Levels of mature BDNF (14 kDa band) in CSF were very low compared to proBDNF (34 kDa band) and required longer exposure times that were shown in a separate panel (Fig. 1o). Densitometric analysis of the two bands in 15 AD-affected patients and 15 control individuals (see Table 2 summarizing the demographic and clinical characteristics of CSF donors) revealed that the total levels of BDNF (proBDNF+BDNF) were similar between the two groups (Fig. 1p). However, in AD patients we observed an increase of proBDNF associated with a decrease of BDNF, compared to controls (Fig. 1o). When we calculated the ratio proBDNF/BDNF in each sample, we observed that the average ratio proBDNF/BDNF was significantly higher in the CSF from AD patients (Fig. 1p). These results indicate that the CSF is a reliable sample that recapitulates the changes in proBDNF/BDNF expression that take place in the brain of AD patients. In summary, we conclude that hileal neurons of AD patients are more susceptible to cell death due to the higher levels of proBDNF and Sortilin expression and the higher proportion of cells expressing both p75 and Sortilin.

AGE modifications in proBDNF are increased in the hippocampus and the CSF of AD patients

The increase of oxidative stress in the brain with aging has been proposed to be a key factor triggering and/or enhancing AD [1, 34]. The molecular mechanisms involved are diverse and include post-traductional modifications of specific proteins. For instance, GO and MGO, two highly reactive dicarbonyls that are increased during OS, react with free amino groups of Lys, Arg and Cys

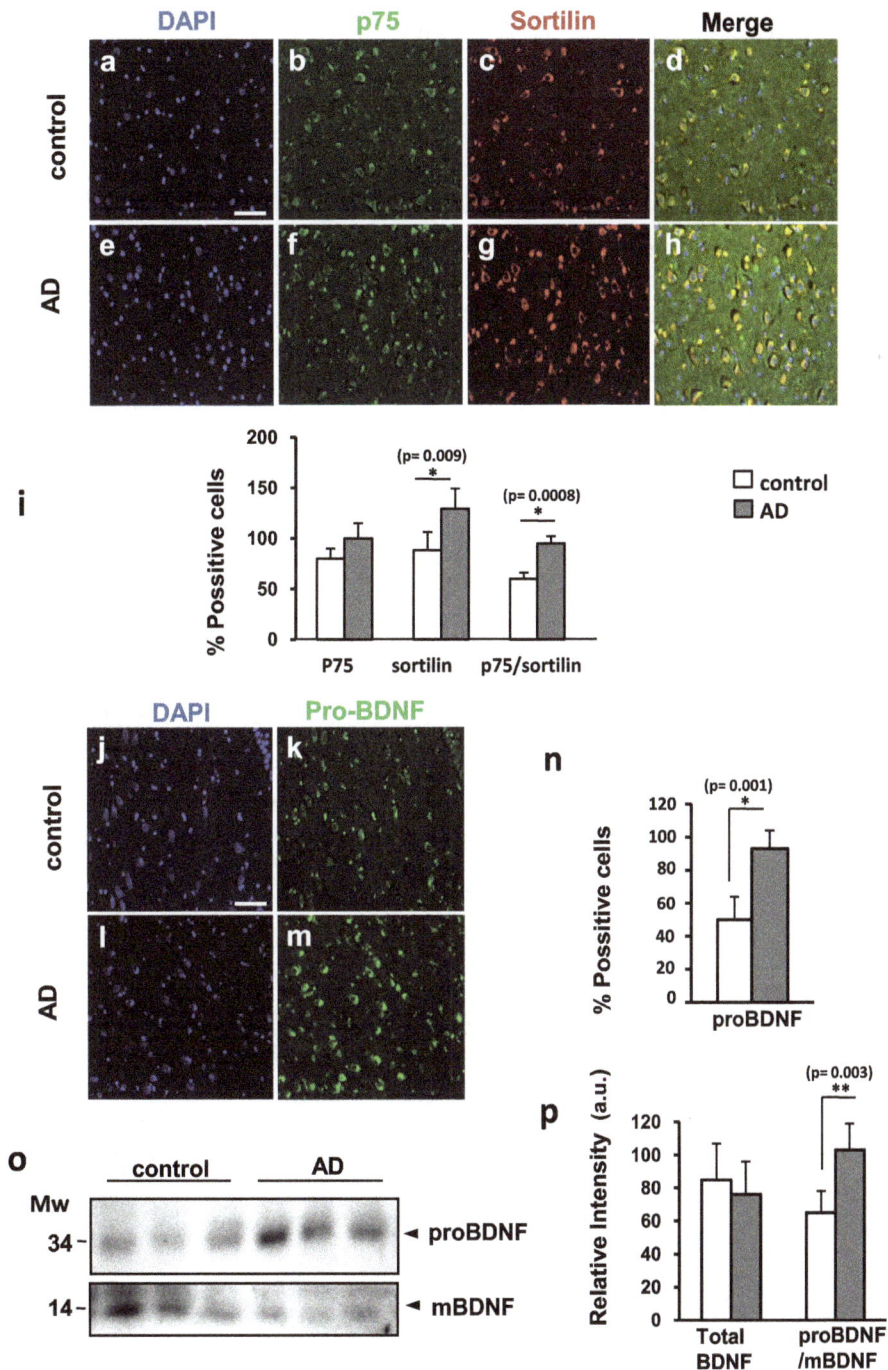

Fig. 1 Sortilin and proBDNF expression is increased in the hippocampal hilus in human control and AD-affected cases. Representative immunofluorescence pictures stained with DAPI (**a, e, j, l**), ECDp75 (**b, f**), Sortilin (**c, g**) and proBDNF (**k, m**) at control and AD cases. **i)** Quantification of Sortilin immunoreactivity and p75/Sortilin co-localization in the AD is significantly increased respect to the controls. **n)** Quantification of proBDNF expression is significantly increased in the AD respect to the controls. Bars represent the mean of % positive cells ± SD. respect to DAPI stained cells. Positive cells are considered those with staining in the whole cell body. 300 total cells from each sample from 5 control and 5 AD-affected cases are counted. **o)** Western blotting analysis of BDNF forms in human CSF samples. The anti mBDNF antibody detect proBDNF (34 kDa) and mBDNF (14 kDa). Both panels correspond to the same WB. Lanes correspond to different representative individuals. **p)** Densitometry analysis of immunodetected bands shows a significant increase proBDNF/mBDNF ratio in AD-affected patients. Bars represent the mean of 9 control and 9 AD samples as the percentage of the highest value in each WB, corrected for the corresponding densitometric values of the Coomassie-stained membrane. Scale bar =50 μm. * $p < 0.05$, ** $p < 0.01$, two tailed Student's "t" test

Table 2 Demographic and clinical characteristics of the patients from whom CSF samples were studied. Case (AD); control (C); p (Student's t-test)

	Case(n = 15)	C(n = 15)	P
Male	4 (26.7%)	5 (33.3%)	0.7
Years	73.5 ± 12,1	70.5 ± 7,1	0.6
Age schooling	11.3 ± 5,0	11.3 ± 2,2	0.2
MMSE	19,1 ± 6,0	28,1 ± 1,8	0
Family history			
Presenilin AD	2(13.3%)	0(0%)	0.14
EA > 65 years	3(20.0%)	5(33.3%)	0.4
Pathological history			
Hypertension	6(40%)	8(53%)	0.46
Diabetes	3(20.0%)	2(13.3%)	0.6
Hypercolesterolemia	2(13.3%)	7(46.7%)	0.04
Depression	2(13.3%)	7(46.7%)	0.04
CSF AD Biomarkers	**pg/ml**	**pg/ml**	
Amyloid β	386,128	856 ± 204	0
Total Tau	615 ± 270	281 ± 103	0.01
PhosphoTau	85 ± 28	55 ± 18	0

residues leading to the formation of the AGE/ALE adducts CML, CEL and intermolecular crosslink [35, 36]. As we have previously reported, these modifications affect proNGF during AD making the pro-neurotrophin form of NGF more stable (as it cannot be converted to mature NGF), which in turn increases cell death [28]. To determine whether proBDNF could be also modified by reactive dicarbonyls in AD, we performed different approaches. First, we studied the co-localization of proBDNF and CEL by immunohistochemistry in the hileal region of human hippocampal samples from controls and AD-affected brains. We observed a remarkable increase of CEL immunoreactivity in AD brains compared to controls (Fig. 2c, g). Interestingly, almost all the cells in the hillial region of AD patients with significant CEL staining, also co-expressed proBDNF, while in control brains very few neurons displayed double immunoreactivity (Fig. 2b-d, f-h, i). These results strongly suggested that proBDNF could be modified by reactive dicarbonyls. In order to address this question directly we performed a more specific assay. We immunoprecipitated proBDNF from the CSF of controls and AD patients and analyzed the precipitates by Western blot with an antibody against CEL. We found that the proBDNF in the CSF from AD patients showed a prominent CEL modification, around 6-fold on average, compared to controls (Fig. 2j, k). Altogether these results indicate that the proBDNF in AD patients displays AGE post-traduccional modifications as consequence of an increase of oxidative stress during neurodegeneration that

might prevent the action of convertases to produce mature BDNF (see below).

proBDNF modified in vitro by MGO induces neuronal apoptosis and decreases neuron differentiation

In order to test the effects of the AGE modifications of proBDNF induced by oxidative stress conditions on neuron survival and differentiation, we treated recombinant proBDNF in vitro with reactive oxygen species that react with Arg and Cys residues, resulting in the formation of intermolecular modifications and crossovers of the protein (see Methods section). This modified proBDNF (MproBDNF) was used to stimulate primary cultures of neurons along with mature BDNF, unmodified proBDNF as well as an unrelated protein, Bovine Serum Albumin (BSA), modified in the same way as the proBDNF (MBSA), as stimulation controls. In these experiments we used differentiated hippocampal neurons obtained from hippocampal NSCs plated on laminin-coated plates (see Methods). At 1 day in vitro (DIV), the neurons started to differentiate but it was between 4 and 7 DIV that the degree of maturation is significative. In longer culture periods, neurons displayed a complex degree of neuritogenesis and differentiation, mainly in the mBDNF treated wells, which was difficult to quantify. Differentiated neurons expressed doublecortin (DCX), βIIItubulin, SV2, p75, Sortilin, TrkB and calretinin (Fig. 3, Additional file 1: Figures S1-S3). These neurons, however, were negative for parvoalbumin and calbindin (Additional file 1: Figure S3), indicating that they are young granular differentiated neurons. In control cultures treated with mature BDNF for 6 DIV, neurons increased significantly their differentiation compared to unstimulated cultures, as demonstrated by β IIItubulin staining (Fig. 3a). Interestingly, control stimulation with proBDNF, without AGE modifications, did not increase apoptotic cell death over basal levels; in contrast, it produced similar effects on neuron differentiation as the mature BDNF (Fig. 3a, b). However, stimulation with MproBDNF, produced a significant increase of apoptosis and impaired neuron differentiation (Fig. 3a, b, c). These effects were specific for the AGE modified form of proBDNF (MproBDNF) since they were not observed upon stimulation with MGO modified BSA (MBSA) (Fig. 3a, b, c). These results suggest that proBDNF is quickly converted into the mature form in culture, inducing nearly the same effects as the BDNF, while the MproBDNF, which is more resistant to the action of convertases, is more stable and triggers the adverse effects associated with its pro-apoptotic activity.

CSF from AD patients induces neuronal apoptosis through proBDNF/p75

Our results have shown so far that in AD patients there is an increase of proBDNF/BDNF expression ratio as well as

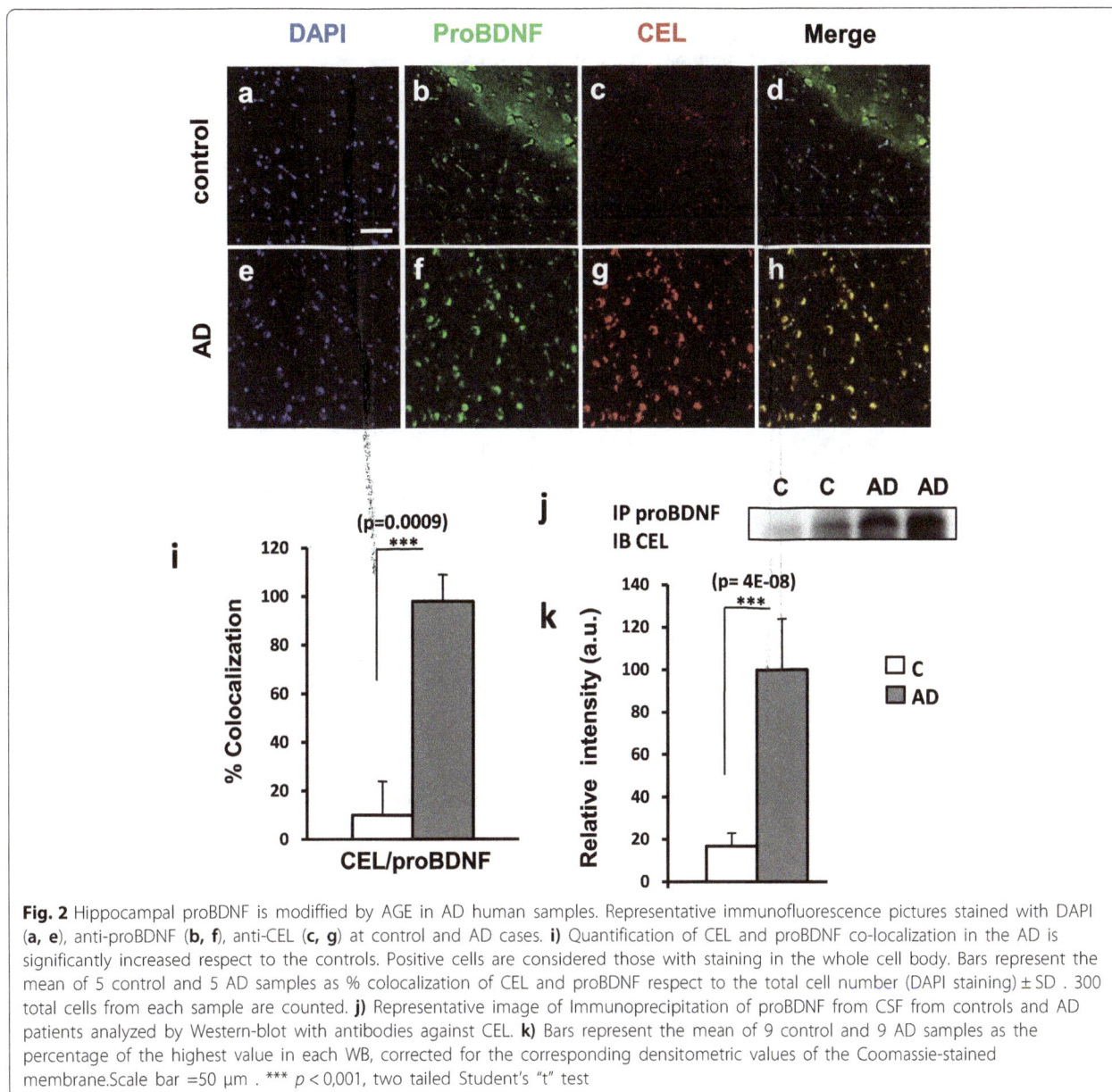

Fig. 2 Hippocampal proBDNF is modified by AGE in AD human samples. Representative immunofluorescence pictures stained with DAPI (**a**, **e**), anti-proBDNF (**b**, **f**), anti-CEL (**c**, **g**) at control and AD cases. **i)** Quantification of CEL and proBDNF co-localization in the AD is significantly increased respect to the controls. Positive cells are considered those with staining in the whole cell body. Bars represent the mean of 5 control and 5 AD samples as % colocalization of CEL and proBDNF respect to the total cell number (DAPI staining) ± SD . 300 total cells from each sample are counted. **j)** Representative image of Immunoprecipitation of proBDNF from CSF from controls and AD patients analyzed by Western-blot with antibodies against CEL. **k)** Bars represent the mean of 9 control and 9 AD samples as the percentage of the highest value in each WB, corrected for the corresponding densitometric values of the Coomassie-stained membrane.Scale bar =50 μm . *** $p < 0,001$, two tailed Student's "t" test

an increase of expression of some of the key signaling elements involved in the pro-apoptotic effects of this pro-neurotrophin. Moreover, we have observed that proBDNF from AD patients displays AGE post-traductional modifications as a consequence of the increase of the oxidative stress during neurodegeneration. Finally, our in vitro experiments on differentiated neurons suggest that these modifications produce a more stable form of proBDNF, a process which can account for 1) the increased levels of proBDNF in AD brains and CSF and 2) the contribution of proBDNF to the cell death associated with the disease. To evaluate further this hypothesis we directly evaluate the effects of the proBDNF contained in the CSF of AD patients and controls on differentiated

primary neurons, as above. Thus, we stimulated the cultures for 6 DIV with CSF (substituting all the culture media, see Methods) from control and AD patients and stained the neurons with antibodies against p75ICD or with DAPI staining, in order to assess the subcellular localization of the protein by confocal microscopy and the apoptotic cell death, respectively (Fig. 4a and Additional file 1: Figure S3). Control CSF-treated neurons survived and differentiated normally showing a basal rate of apoptotic cell death of around 10% (Fig. 4a and c). A high proportion of these neurons displayed a peripheral distribution of p75 in the soma consistent with the presence of the intact receptor in the plasma membrane (Fig. 4a, c). In contrast, cultures treated with ADCSF showed an altered

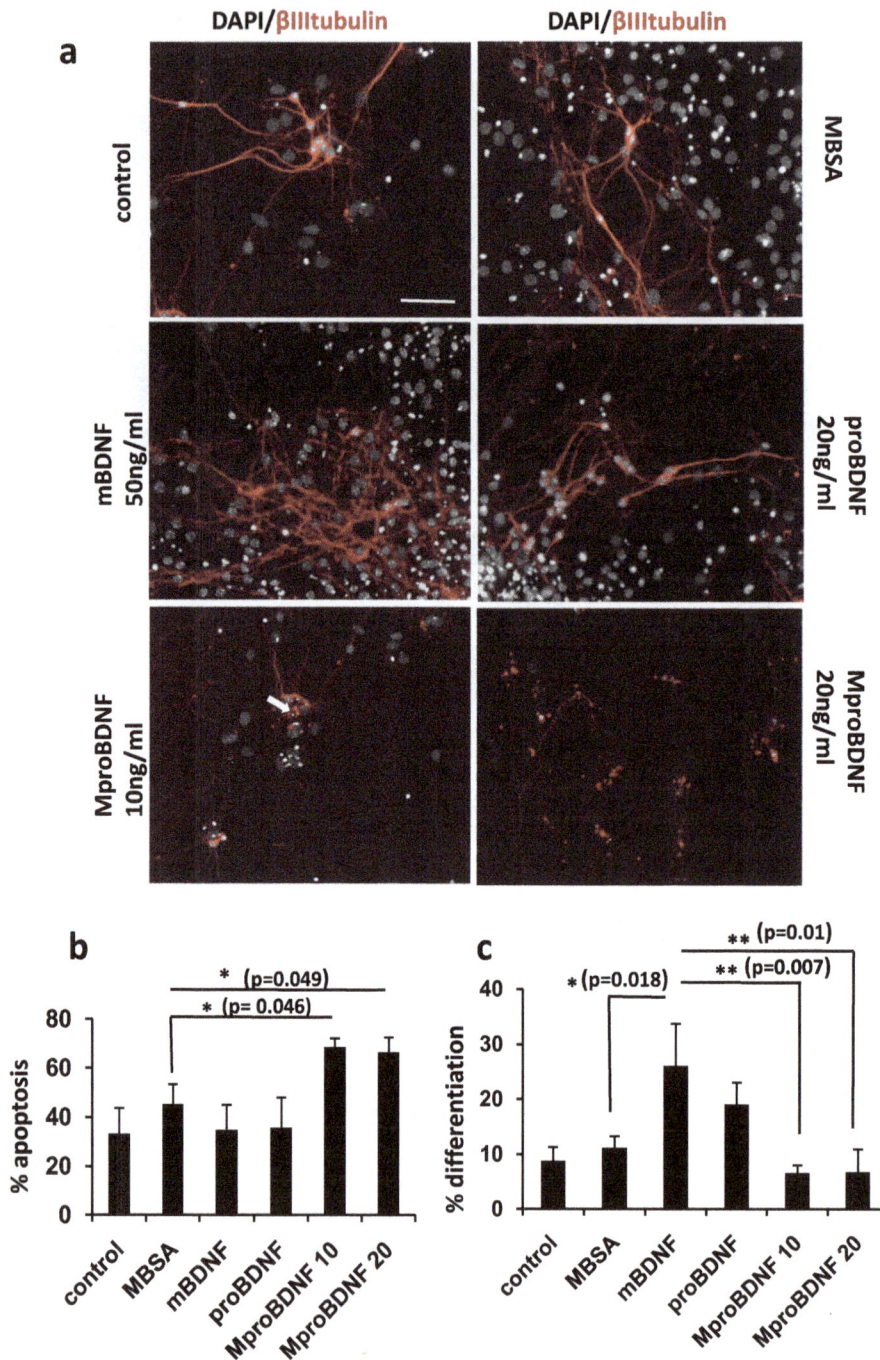

Fig. 3 proBDNF modified by MGO induces apoptosis in control mice differentiated hippocampal neural stem cells . **a)** Representative pictures of neuronal primary culture treated for 6 days (7DIV) with: untreated (control), MGO modified BSA (MBSA), mBDNF, proBDNF and two doses of MGO modified proBDNF (MproBDNF). DAPI staining (white) of nuclei shows apoptotic morphology (white arrow). Immunostaining with anti βIIItubulin (red) show differentiation degree. **b)** Bars represent the quantification of apoptosis (by nuclei morphology), expressed as the mean of % apoptosis ± SD of the total nuclei. **c)** The quantification of differentiation is expressed as the mean of % differentiation (βIIItubulin immunoreactivity quantified by ImageJ, divided by the number of β III tubulin positive cells). Values represent the mean of three independent experiments. Scale bar =25 μm . ** $p < 0,01$, *** $p < 0,001$ two tailed Student's "t" test

morphology with impaired differentiation and a dramatic increase the number of apoptotic nuclei (reaching 60%) (Fig. 4a, c). Moreover, under ADCSF treatment, there was a significant increase in the percentage of neurons with nuclear immunoreacitvity for p75, indicating that the 20 kDa ICD fragment was shed and translocated to the

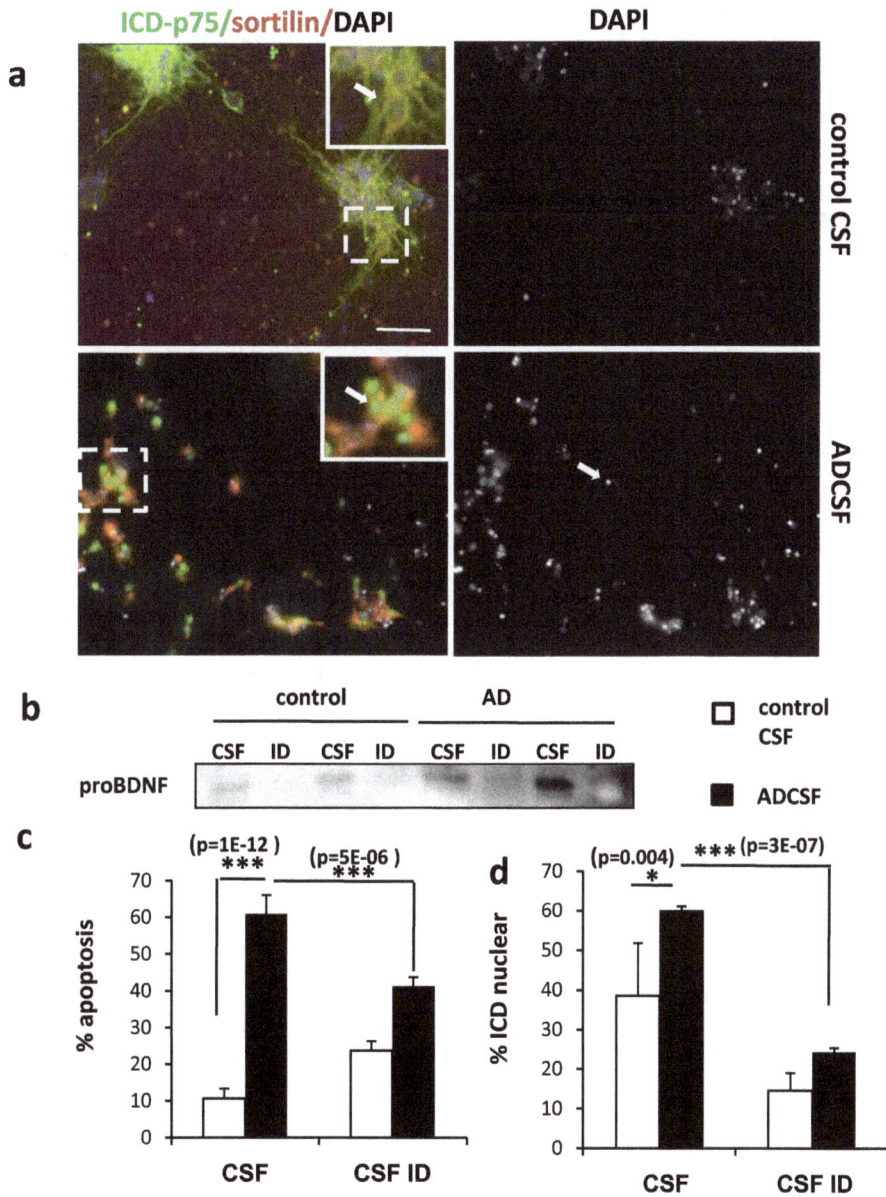

Fig. 4 Human proBDNF from CSF AD patients induces apoptosis in neuronal culture. **a)** Representative pictures of neuronal primary culture from control mice Dentate Gyrus. Cells were treated for 6 days (7DIV) with human CSF from controls (control CSF) and from AD-affected patients (ADCSF). DAPI staining of nuclei shows apoptotic morphology (white arrow). Immunofluorescence with anti p75 ICD domain (green) and anti Sortilin (red). Inset indicate a higher magnification image of the boxed areas. White arrow in control CSF shows neurons with peripheral p75ICD location. White arrows in AD CSF show p75ICD nuclear location. **b)** Representative image of western blot showing the levels of proBDNF in CSF and in CSF immunodepleted with anti proBDNF (ID), from control and AD samples. **c and d)** Cells are treated with human 8 control CSF and 8 ADCSF, in both cases directly (CSF) or proBDNF immunodepleted (SCFID). **c)** Bars represent the quantification of apoptosis (by nuclei morphology), expressed as the mean of % apoptosis ± SD of the positive cells for both p75 and Sortilin. **d)** Bars represent the quantification of the mean of the % ± SD of neurons with the ICDp75 translocated to the nuclei (% ICD nuclear). Scale bar =50 μm . * $p < 0,05$, ** $p < 0,01$, two tailed Student's "t" test

nucleus (Fig. 4a, d). The CSF from AD patients is known to contain several other factors, such as Au, that might be responsible for these neurotoxic effects. To determine whether proBDNF present in the CSF of AD patients we specifically immunodepleted the CSF samples from proBDNF with specific anti-proBDNF antibodies coupled to sepharose AG beads. Successful depletion was demonstrated by Western blot with antibodies against proBDNF (Fig. 4b). We then compared the effects of the immunodepleted CSF (CSFID) and the normal CSF from both, AD patients and controls, in our neuron cultures after 6 DIV. As shown in Fig. 4c and d, depletion of proBDNF produced a remarkable reduction of the percentage of apoptosis as well as the percentage of neurons with nuclear immunoreactivity for p75. Therefore, these results indicate that the proBDNF in the CSF of AD patients is biologically active and that it is the main responsible of the pro-apoptotic effects triggered by AD CSF. Moreover, these results strongly suggest that the effects of proBDNF in AD CSF are mediated by activation of p75 signaling.

APP/PS1 mutations increase p75 processing and apoptosis induction

In the familiar AD, one of the most frequent targets of inherited mutations is the presenilin-gamma secretase complex [37]. Some of these mutations affect mainly presenilin 1 (PS1) including the deletion of exon 9 (u9) or M146 V [38]. These are supposed to be gain of function mutations leading to an increase of protease activity [39]. The study of the pathogenic mechanisms underlying these mutations and the development of AD has been focused on several of the PS1 substrates, mainly Aβ [39]. Since p75 is also a substrate of PS1 activity [18, 40], we hypothesized that the harmful consequences of proBDNF on neuron survival and differentiation in AD, due to its higher stability as a consequence of AGE modifications, could be boosted by the effects of PS1 mutations on p75 signaling. In particular, we were interested in ascertain whether the shedding of p75, which requires PS1 activity, changes during AD and whether these changes can sensitize the effects of pro-neurotrophins. To test this hypothesis we set up primary neuron cultures from NSCs from heterozygous APP/PS1 mice or from wild type littermates as controls (see Methods). This APP/PS1 animal model has been widely used in studies of neurological disorders of the brain, specifically AD, amyloid plaque formation, and aging [41]. After 6 DIV, when all the conditions are considered for the analysis (regardless to the treatment), APP/PS1 cultures does not show a % of apoptosis significantly different than WT (One-way ANOVA $p = 0.1$). However under treatment with MBSA (control), these transgenic APP/PS1 neurons displayed higher percentage of apoptotic nuclei and higher percentage of neurons with nuclear immunoreactivity for p75 (Fig. 5a, b, c and Additional file 1: Figure S3). Interestingly, stimulation with MproBDNF induced a stronger and significant increase in cell death and p75 nuclear immunoreactivity in these transgenic neurons compared to controls (Fig. 5a, b, c). We therefore conclude that PS1 mutations involved in familiar AD potentiate the effects of proBDNF on cell death most probably by increasing p75 signaling and, in particular, p75ICD nuclear translocation.

Discussion

The pathogenic mechanisms underlying the development of AD are complex and yet not fully understood.

Some important research lines have focused on the role of neurotrophins in AD both, as regulating factors of cell survival and cell death, involved in the pathogenesis and/or the course of the disease, and as therapeutic tools [2, 3]. Today, most of our knowledge about the role of neurotrophins in AD comes from the study of the NGF and its precursor form, proNGF. Thus, proNGF has been reported to be increased during aging and AD in vulnerable regions such as the hippocampus [42]. Moreover, the proNGF isolated from AD patients displays higher neurotoxicity than proNGF from controls [27]. More controversial is the role of proBDNF/BDNF alterations in the pathogenicity of the AD. In part, because contradictory evidences were reported regarding the expression and secretion of BDNF in its precursor form [6, 43, 44]. It was suggested that these opposing results reflect a more complex regulation of proBDNF processing that depends on the regulation by third-parties such as glial cells and plasmin inhibitors [45]. Indeed, BDNF is more important for the maintenance and function of central nervous system than NGF and thus, reduced levels of BDNF, due to impairment of proBDNF processing, could be involved in some aspects of the AD disease, such as depression, in addition to the neurotoxic effects of the pro-neurotrophin [46].

In the present work we have addressed the role of proBDNF and its pro-apoptotic signaling mechanisms in AD. We showed that in brains from AD patients there is an increase of the levels of proBDNF are increased, as are also some of the key signaling components involved in its pro-apoptotic effects, such as the co-receptor Sortilin. We were also able to detect an increase of proBDNF in the CSF of AD patients. Interestingly, this increase of proBDNF in the CSF is associated with a decrease of BDNF. Moreover, we have demonstrated that the proBDNF in the CSF from AD patients is highly modified by oxidative stress and that the presence of this AGE modified proBDNF induces apoptosis and impairs differentiation on primary cultures of neurons. Finally, we have shown that the damaging effects of proBDNF can be potentiated by mutations commonly found in familiar forms of AD that affects PS1 protease activity. This synergistic effect is due to the enhancement of p75 signaling, in particular of p75ICD internalization. The present results further reveal the important role of neurotrophin signaling in the development of the AD and, in particular, our results provide evidence for the relevance of the proBDNF/p75 pathway in the pathogenesis and/or the course of AD. Thus, these results highlight the importance of proBDNF/p75 signaling as potential targets to develop novel pharmacological therapies to fight AD.

During aging and especially during neurodegeneration there is an increase of oxidative stress in the tissue that

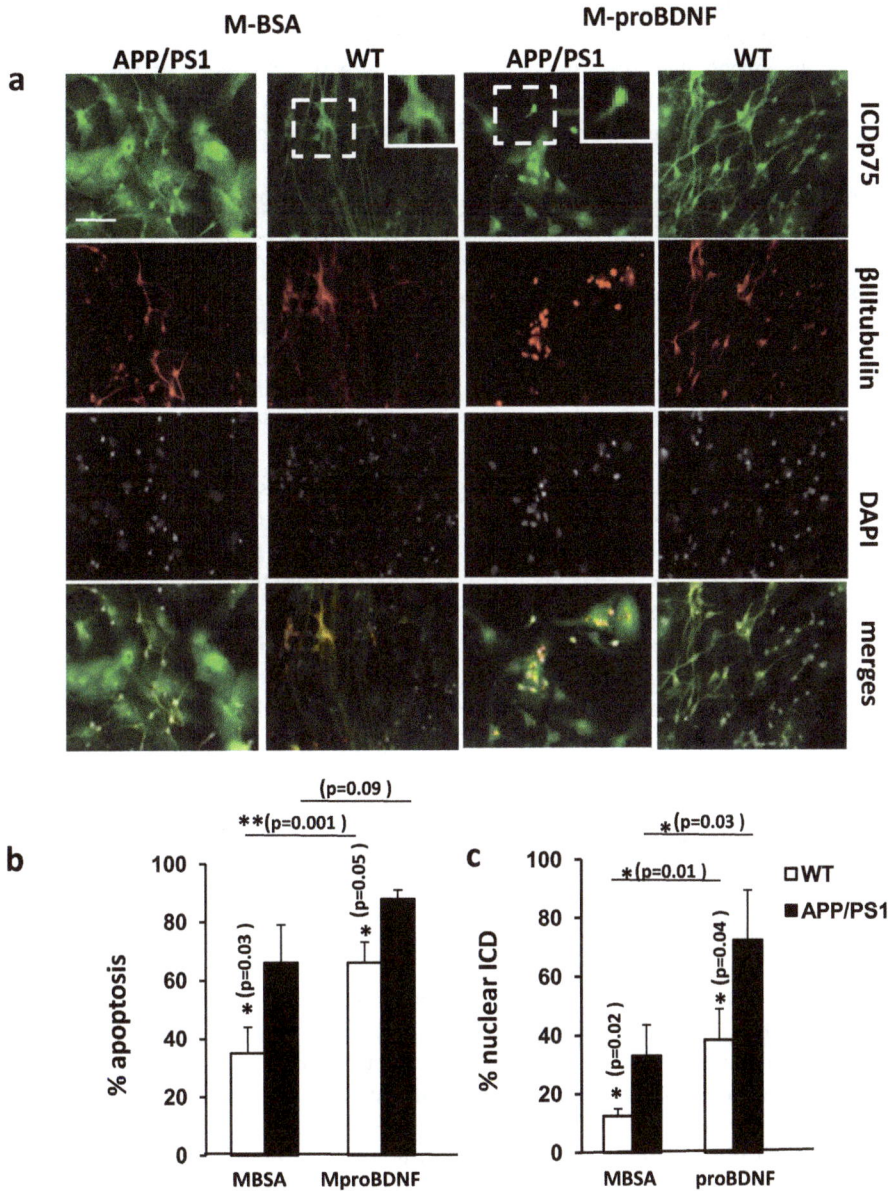

Fig. 5 Apoptosis and p75 processing are increased in neuronal cultures from APP/PS1 animals. Primary cultures of differentiated mouse hippocampal NSCs were treated for 6 days (7DIV) with MGO modified BSA (MBSA) or with MGO modified proBDNF (MproBDNF). **a)** Representative immunofluorescence pictures of cells from WT and APP/P1 mice labeled with ICDp75 (green), βIIItubulin (red) and DAPI (white). Inset represents a higher magnification image of the boxed areas indicating citoplasmatic (WT) and nuclear localization (APP/PS1) of ICDp75. **b)** Bars represent the quantification of apoptosis (by nuclei morphology), expressed as the mean of % apoptosis ± SD of the positive cells for both ICDp75 and βIIItubulin. **c)** Bars represent the mean of the % ± SD of neurons with the ICDp75 translocated to the nuclei (% ICD nuclear). The values represent the mean of three independent experiments Scale bar =50 μm . ** $p < 0,01$, two tailed Student's "t" test

contributes to the pathogenesis of AD [1]. The neurotoxic mechanisms involved, however, are not clearly understood. Glyoxal (GO) and methylglyoxal (MG) are highly reactive dicarbonyl formed during the metabolism that, in excess, can increase ROS production and cause oxidative stress. GO, and MGO can react with free amino groups of Lys, Arg and Cys residues, leading to the formation of the AGE/ALE adducts CML, CEL and intermolecular crosslink [47]. The relationship between protein carbonylation and neurodegeneration (ND) has been widely established. Changes in protein carbonyl samples from both disease experimental animal models and patients with neurodegeneration have been reported [48, 49]. Moreover, mass spectrometry analysis of human brain homogenates has shown that several AGE/ALE adducts, HNEL, CEL, CML and Nε-(malondialdehyde)-lysine (MDAL) increase in ND [1, 35]. Oxidative non-enzymatic modifications can also affect protein structure and function by other means, for example increasing protein crosslinking and thus contributes to protein aggregation during ND [1]. These general effects on protein structure might affect the function of some proteins in a specific manner. In the present work, we found that proBDNF co-localizes almost entirely with CEL in AD samples and that the proBDNF isolated from the CSF of AD patients display higher CEL modifications than controls. We therefore suggest that the increase of proBDNF in AD patients, in brain samples and in CSF, is due to a higher stability of this precursor form resulting from post-traductional modifications triggered by oxidative stress that make this modified pro-neurotrophin more resistant to be processed by convertases into the mature BDNF. The target sequence for Furin and other convertases (plasmin and metalloproteases) contains Lys, Arg, and Cys residues that are indeed suitable sites for AGE/ALEs formation [50]. Similar results were obtained by our group when we analyzed the role of proNGF/NGF in human hippocampal samples from AD patients [16, 27, 28]. We cannot rule out the possibility that AGE modified proBDNF could have acquired gain-of-function effects independent of proBDNF signaling. Nevertheless, since there is a strong correlation between proBDNF levels in AD and p75 signaling (see below) we rather favor the hypothesis these oxidative stress-induced modifications makes the proBDNF more stable and tip the balance in favour of cell death (increase of proBDNF) at expenses of cell survival (decrease of BDNF). Accordingly, we observed in the CSF of AD patients an increase of proBDNF that was associated with a decrease of BDNF. In a more functional approach we demonstrated that the CSF from AD patients, but not the CSF from controls, induces apoptosis in a primary culture of differentiated neurons obtained from NSCs from the Dentate Gyrus. In contrast, CSF from control individuals maintained the survival and differentiation of these neurons up to 6 DIV. Interestingly, depletion of proBDNF from AD CSF samples reduced strongly the apoptotic effect of the original AD CSF (apoptosis reduced from 40 to 20%), suggesting that proBDNF is a main factor that triggers the apoptotic effect of the AD CSF. The remaining 20% apoptosis could be due to other pro-apoptotic inducers such as Aβ or proNGF (references). Finally, we propose that the ratio proBDNF/BDNF measured in the in the CSF could be a potential diagnostic marker for AD. To further validate this approach, it would be interesting to measure the proBDNF/BDNF ratio in the CSF of a larger cohort of patients and controls and analyze this ratio in regard to the different stages of the disease.

BDNF genetic variation may affect the risk of developing AD [51]. One of these variations, proBDNF[Val66Met], impairs the normal processing of proBDNF resulting in higher levels of expression of proBDNF [52]. The Val66-Met polymorphism affects a particular step of proBDNF processing that is sufficient to impair the formation of enough levels of mature BDNF and trigger familiar depression [46]. The mutation blocks proBDNF maturation and affects activity-dependent secretion of BDNF and human memory and hippocampal function [53, 54] and worsens vulnerability to stress and response to antidepressants [55]. Despite the proBDNF[Val66Me] is able to interact with p75 and Sortilin, altering the neuronal morphology [52], a recent meta-analysis did not show an association of the Val66Met polymorphism and the risk of AD [56]. It is possible that the proBDNF[Val66Met] is still partially processed reducing the neurotoxic effects of the full proBDNF form.

Besides the increase of proBDNF levels in AD patients, we provide evidence for the existence of at least two additional mechanisms that could potentiate the neurotoxic action of proBDNF and accelerate the disease. First, we observed that the levels of Sortilin, the co-receptor of p75NTR involved in the pro-apoptotic effect of proBDNF, are increased in the hileal region of the hippocampus of AD patients thus making the neurons of this region more vulnerable to cell death. Sortilin levels seem to be particularly sensitive to ageing and neurodegeneration. For instance, Sortilin immunoreactivity was described to be increased in ageing rodent basal forebrain and sympathetic neurons while the levels of p75NTR were either unchanged or reduced [57]. On the other hand and similarly to our results, Sortilin was shown to be increased in the temporal cortical area of human AD brains as well as in brains of 6-months old PS1delta9 transgenic mice [58]. Interestingly, this increase was suggested to be triggered by amyloid beta$_{1-42}$ (Aβ$_{42}$) through the p75/RhoA signaling pathway suggesting a potential physiological interaction of Aβ$_{42}$, p75NTR and sortilin in AD [57]. From all this data we propose that neurodegeneration in AD patients may be enhanced by an increase of sortilin expression in neurons, probably induced by Aβ$_{42}$, together with elevated levels of proBDNF in specific regions.

Secondly, we found that proBDNF effects in AD can also be enhanced by mutations found in familiar AD that affect the convertase activity of the γ-secretase PS1. We propose that these mutations make neurons more sensitive to the pro-apoptotic effect of proBDNF by increasing the susceptibility of p75 to be processed and induce nuclear translocation of the p75ICD. Although in familiar AD PS1 mutations are described to increase Aß42/40 ratio, the effect of these mutations on its convertase activity as gain or loss of function is controversial [39]. In the present work, we have observed an increase of basal cleavage of p75 and an increase of p75ICD nuclear translocation and apoptosis (further induced by MproBDNF), in neurons from the animal model of AD APP/PS1 bearing the mutation Δ9 in PS1. Therefore we favor the idea that, at least the Δ9 deletion in PS1, behaves as a gain of function mutation.

More than fifty membrane proteins, including APP and p75, are cleaved by the presenilin1- γ-secretase complex [59, 60]. APP processing and Aβ production is one of the hallmarks of AD [29]. On the other hand, the cleavage of p75 and the production of the ICD fragment that is translocated to the nucleus, is considered a key step during the apoptotic signaling pathway triggered by this receptor although the exact physiological effects of p75ICD release depends on the neuronal subtype [18, 40]. Recently, experimental evidence indicates that p75 signaling, including cleavage and release of the ICD, is indeed strongly related to AD, highlighting the central role of p75 during AD pathogenesis [59]. Thus, several mechanisms have been proposed involving p75 signaling in AD. For instance, it was shown that Aβ is able to bind to p75 and trigger activation of the receptor inducing the cleavage of the ICD [60]. Moreover, amyloidogenesis is aggravated by the interaction of beta-site amyloid precursor protein cleaving enzyme-1 (BACE1) with p75 upon the binding of Aβ to p75 [21]. In contrast, it was shown that the p75ECD has a neuroprotective effect against Aβ toxicity [61] and that transmembrane domain of p75, has trophic effects by inducing phosphorylation of TrKB [62]. Our results emphasize the important contribution of p75 signaling, including p75ICD internalization and apoptosis, in AD pathogenesis upon AGE-modified proBDNF stimulation. More importantly, our data provide a novel pro-apoptotic mechanism in AD and involving p75 in which higher levels of cleavage due to mutations in PS1 make these neurons more sensitive to the adverse effects of AGE-modified proBDNF. Moreover, we suggest that this is a general mechanism in AD, also for the non-familiar, spontaneous form of the disease, given the fact that Aβ is able to trigger p75 cleavage and p75ICD release and could therefore prime p75 signaling for AGE modified proBDNF independenty of PS1 mutations.

Abbreviations

AD: Alzheimer disease; AGEs: ROS derived advanced glycation end products; ALEs: Advanced lipooxidation end products; BACE1: α-protease; BDNF: Brain-derived neurotrophic factor; BSA: Bovine Serum Albumin; CEL: Nε-(carboxyethyl)-lysine; CML: Carboxymethyl)-lysine; CSF: Cerebrospinal fluid; CSFID: Immunodepleted CSF; DIV: Day in vitro; DMEM: Dulbecco's modified Eagle's medium; EGF: Epidermal Growth Factor; ELISA: Enzyme-immuno assay; FGF: Fibroblast Growth Factor; GO: Glyoxal; HNEL: 4-hydroxy-2-nonenal-lysine; ICD: Intracellular domain; MBSA: MGO-modified BSA; MDAL: Nε-(malondialdehyde)-lysine; MGO: methylglyoxal; MMSE: Minimental state examination; MproBDNF: MGO-modified proBDNF; ND: Neurodegeneration; NSCs: Hippocampal Neural Stem Cells; OS: Oxidative stress; P/S: Penicylin/Streptomycin; PBS: Phosphate buffered saline; PBS-T: PBS with 0, 1% Triton X-100; PFA: Paraformaldehyde; pH 8.0: 133 mM NaCl, 0.2% Tween 20; proBDNF: Precursor form of BDNF; PS1: Presenilin 1; ROS: Radical Oxygen Species; SD: Standard deviation; TBS-T: 50 mM Tris

Acknowledgements

We thank Ester Aso for caring transgenic mice, Jesus Moreno for helping in the management of human post-mortem samples, and Ricard Curia, and Andrea Rios for helping with different aspects of the experimental work. We thank Montse Ortega, Sonia Rius, Noel Perez and Marc Tarres and the animal house facility staff of the Unversity of Lleida for technical assistance.

Funding

This work was supported by "Fundació La Marató 2015" (C.E.). We thank, IRBLleida Biobank (B.0000682), PLATAFORMA BIOBANCOS PT13/0010/0014, HUB-ICO-IDIBELL Biobank for providing human tissue and UAI IRBLleida for management support.

Authors' contributions

All authors have participated in the work to take public responsibility for appropriate portions of the content; and agreed to be accountable for all aspects of the work in ensuring that questions related to the accuracy or integrity of any part of the work are appropriately investigated and resolved. FC and EC are responsible of the main part of the design of the work and of acquisition, analysis and interpretation of data. MP and RD contributed to the experimental work. PG is responsible of the obtention and analysis of the human CSF samples. FI is responsible of the obtention and analysis of the human brain samples. RC, EJ and EC have been involved in drafting the manuscript and revising it critically. All authors read and approved the final manuscript.

Competing interests

The authors declare that they have no competing interests.

Author details

[1]Molecular Developmental Neurobiology Group, IRBLleida-UDL Rovira Roure 82, 25198 Lleida, Spain. [2]Departament de Patologia i Terapèutica Experimental, Universitat de Barcelona, Barcelona, Spain. [3]Centro de Investigación Biomédica en Red de Enfermedades Neurodegenerativas (CIBERNED), Hospitalet de Llobregat, Barcelona, Spain. [4]Unitat Trastorns Cognitius, IRBLleida-Hospital Universitari Santa Maria Lleida, Lleida, Spain. [5]Centre de Recherches sur la Cognition Animale (CRCA), Centre de Biologie Intégrative (CBI), Université de Toulouse, CNRS, UPS, 31062 Toulouse, France. [6]Serra Húnter fellow, Associate Professor, Generalitat de Catalunya, Barcelona, Spain.

References

1. Pamplona R, Dalfó E, Ayala V, Bellmunt MJ, Prat J, Ferrer I, et al. Proteins in human brain cortex are modified by oxidation, glycoxidation, and lipoxidation. Effects of Alzheimer disease and identification of lipoxidation targets. J Biol Chem. 2005;280:21522–30.
2. Hennigan A, O'Callaghan RM, Kelly AM. Neurotrophins and their receptors: roles in plasticity, neurodegeneration and neuroprotection. Biochem. Soc. Trans. 2007;35:424–7.
3. Pezet S, Malcangio M. Brain-derived neurotrophic factor as a drug target for CNS disorders. Expert Opin Ther Targets. 2004;8:391–9.
4. Barbacid M. Neurotrophic factors and their receptors. Curr Opin Cell Biol. 1995;7:148–55.
5. Lewin GR, Barde YA. Physiology of the neurotrophins. Annu Rev Neurosci. 1996;19:289–317.
6. Lee R, Kermani P, Teng KK, Hempstead BL. Regulation of cell survival by secreted proneurotrophins. Science. 2001;294:1945–8.
7. Beattie MS, Harrington AW, Lee R, Kim JY, Boyce SL, Longo FM, et al. ProNGF induces p75-mediated death of oligodendrocytes following spinal cord injury. Neuron. 2002;36:375–86.
8. Nykjaer A, Lee R, Teng KK, Jansen P, Madsen P, Nielsen MS, et al. Sortilin is essential for proNGF-induced neuronal cell death. Nature. 2004;427:843–8.

9. Teng HK, Teng KK, Lee R, Wright S, Tevar S, Almeida RD, et al. ProBDNF induces neuronal apoptosis via activation of a receptor complex of p75 and Sortilin. J Neurosci. 2005;25:5455–63.

10. Massa SM, Xie Y, Yang T, Harrington AW, Kim ML, Yoon SO, et al. Small, nonpeptide p75 ligands induce survival signaling and inhibit proNGF-induced death. J Neurosci. 2006;26:5288–300.

11. Koshimizu H, Hazama S, Hara T, Ogura A, Kojima M. Distinct signaling pathways of precursor BDNF and mature BDNF in cultured cerebellar granule neurons. Neurosci Lett. 2010;473:229–32.

12. Barker PA. p75NTR is positively promiscuous: novel partners and new insights. Neuron. 2004;42:529–33.

13. López-Sánchez N, Rodríguez JR, Frade JM. Mitochondrial c-Jun NH2-terminal kinase prevents the accumulation of reactive oxygen species and reduces necrotic damage in neural tumor cells that lack trophic support. Mol Cancer Res. 2007;5(1):47–60.

14. Volosin M, Trotter C, Cragnolini A, Kenchappa RS, Light M, Hempstead BL, Carter BD, Friedman WJ. Induction of proneurotrophins and activation of p75-mediated apoptosis via Neurotrophin receptor interacting factor (NRIF) in hippocampal neurons after seizures. J Neurosci. 2008;28(39):9870–9.

15. Frade JM. Nuclear translocation of the p75 neurotrophin receptor cytoplasmic domain in response to neurotrophin binding. J Neurosci. 2005; 25(6):1407–11.

16. Podlesniy P, Kichev A, Pedraza C, Saurat J, Encinas M, Perez B, et al. ProNGF from Alzheimer's disease and normal human brain displays distinctive abilities to induce processing and nuclear translocation of intracellular domain of p75 and apoptosis. Am J Pathol. 2006;169(1):119–31.

17. Kenchappa RS, Tep C, Korade Z, Urra S, Bronfman FC, Yoon SO, et al. p75 neurotrophin receptor-mediated apoptosis in sympathetic neurons involves a biphasic activation of JNK and up-regulation of tumor necrosis factor-alpha-converting enzyme/ADAM17. J Biol Chem. 2010;285(26):20358–68.

18. Parkhurst CN, Zampieri N, Chao MV. Nuclear localization of the p75 neurotrophin receptor intracellular domain. J Biol Chem. 2010;285(8):5361–8.

19. Kenchappa RS, Zampieri N, Chao MV, Barker PA, Teng HK, Hempstead BL, et al. Ligand-dependent cleavage ofthe P75 neurotrophin receptor is necessary for NRIF nuclear translocation and apoptosis in sympathetic neurons. Neuron. 2006;50:219–32.

20. Chakravarthy B, Ménard M, Ito S, Gaudet C, Dal Prà I, Armato U, Whitfield J. Hippocampal membrane-associated p75NTR levels are increased in Alzheimer's disease. J Alzheimers Dis. 2012;30(3):675–84.

21. Saadipour K, Mañucat-Tan NB, Lim Y, Keating DJ, Smith KS, Zhong JH, Liao H, Bobrovskaya L, Wang YJ, Chao MV, Zhou XF. p75 neurotrophin receptor interacts with and promotes BACE1 localization in endosomes aggravating amyloidogenesis. J Neurochem. 2018;144(3):302–17.

22. Allen SJ, Wilcock GK, Dawbarn D. Profound and selective loss of catalytic TrkB immunoreactivity in Alzheimer's disease. Biochem Biophys Res Commun. 1999;264(3):648–51.

23. Ferrer I, Marin C, Rey MJ, Ribalta T, Goutan E, Blanco R, et al. BDNF and full-length and truncated TrkB expression in Alzheimer disease. Implications in therapeutic strategies. J Neuropathol Exp Neurol. 1999;58(7):729–39.

24. Forlenza OV, Diniz BS, Teixeira AL, Radanovic M, Talib LL, Rocha NP, et al. Lower cerebrospinal fluid concentration of brain-derived neurotrophic factor predicts progression from mild cognitive impairment to Alzheimer's disease. NeuroMolecular Med. 2015;17:326–32.

25. Holsinger RM, Schnarr J, Henry P, Castelo VT, Fahnestock M. Quantitation of BDNF mRNA in human parietal cortex by competitive reverse transcription-polymerase chain reaction: decreased levels in Alzheimer's disease. Brain Res Mol Brain Res. 2000;76:347–54.

26. Hock C, Heese K, Hulette C, Rosenberg C, Otten U. Region-specific neurotrophin imbalances in Alzheimer disease: decreased levels of brain-derived neurotrophic factor and increased levels of nerve growth factor in hippocampus and cortical areas. Arch Neurol. 2000;57:846–51.

27. Pedraza CE, Podlesniy P, Vidal N, Arévalo JC, Lee R, Hempstead B, et al. ProNGF isolated from the human brain affected by Alzheimer's disease induces neuronal apoptosis mediated by p75. Am J Pathol. 2005;166(2):533–43.

28. Kichev A, Ilieva EV, Piñol-Ripoll G, Podlesniy P, Ferrer I, Portero-Otín M, et al. Cell death and learning impairment in mice caused by in vitro modified proNGF can be related to its increased oxidative modifications in Alzheimer disease. Am J Pathol. 2009;175:2574–85.

29. Braak H, Alafuzoff I, Arzberger T, Kretzschmar H, Del Tredici K. Staging of Alzheimer disease-associated neurofibrillary pathology using paraffin sections and immunocytochemistry. Acta Neuropathol. 2006;112:389–404.

30. Braak H, Braak E. Demonstration of amyloid deposits and neurofibrillary changes in whole brain sections. Brain Pathol. 1991;1:213–6.

31. Borchelt DR, Thinakaran G, Eckman CB, Lee MK, Davenport F, Ratovitsky T, et al. Familial Alzheimer's disease-linked presenilin 1 variants elevate Abeta1-42/1-40 ratio in vitro and in vivo. Neuron. 1996;17:1005–13.

32. Aso E, Lomoio S, López-González I, Joda L, Carmona M, Fernández-Yagüe N, Moreno J, Juvés S, Pujol A, Pamplona R, Portero-Otin M, Martín V, Díaz M, Ferrer I. Amyloid generation and dysfunctional immunoproteasome activation with disease progression in animal model of familial Alzheimer's disease. Brain Pathol. 2012;22(5):636–53.

33. Carpenter AE, Jones TR, Lamprecht MR, Clarke C, Kang IH, Friman O, et al. CellProfiler: image analysis software for identifying and quantifying cell phenotypes. Genome Biol. 2006;7:R100.

34. Espinet C, Gonzalo H, Fleitas C, Menal MJ, Egea J. Oxidative stress and neurodegenerative diseases: a neurotrophic approach. Curr Drug Targets. 2015;16(1):20–30.

35. Uchida K, Shiraishi M, Naito Y, Torii Y, Nakamura Y, Osawa T. Activation of stress signaling pathways by the end product of lipid peroxidation. 4-hydroxy-2-nonenal is a potential inducer of intracellular peroxide production. J.Biol Chem. 1999;274:2234–42.

36. Stitt AW, Frizzell N, Thorpe SR. Advanced glycation and advanced lipoxidation: possible role in initiation and progression of diabetic retinopathy. Curr Pharm Des. 2004;10(27):3349–60.

37. Lanoiselée HM, Nicolas G, Wallon D, Rovelet-Lecrux A, Lacour M, Rousseau S, et al. APP, PSEN1, and PSEN2 mutations in early-onset Alzheimer disease: A genetic screening study of familial and sporadic cases. PLoS Med. 2017;14(3):e1002270.

38. Pigino G, Pelsman A, Mori H, Busciglio J. Presenilin-1 mutations reduce cytoskeletal association, deregulate neurite growth, and potentiate neuronal dystrophy and tau phosphorylation. J Neurosci. 2001;21(3):834–42.

39. Lessard CB, Wagner SL, Koo EH. And four equals one: presenilin takes the gamma-secretase role by itself. Proc Natl Acad Sci U S A. 2010;107(50):21236–7.

40. Vicario A, Kisiswa L, Tann JY, Kelly CE, Ibanez CF. Neuron-type specific signaling by the p75NTR death receptor is regulated by differential proteoloytic cleavage. J Cell Sci. 2015;128:1507–17.

41. Webster SJ, Bachstetter AD, Nelson PT, Schmitt FA, Van Eldik LJ. Using mice to model Alzheimer's dementia: an overview of the clinical disease and the preclinical behavioral changes in 10 mouse models. Front Genet. 2014;5:88.

42. Fahnestock M, Michalski B, Xu B, Coughlin MD. The precursor pro-nerve growth factor is the predominant form of nerve growth factor in brain and is increased in Alzheimer's disease. Mol Cell Neurosci. 2001;18(2):210–20.

43. Pang PT, Lu B. Regulation of late-phase LTP and long-term memory in normal and aging hippocampus: role of secreted proteins tPA and BDNF. Ageing Res Rev. 2004;3(4):407–30.

44. Matsumoto T, Rauskolb S, Polack M, Klose J, Kolbeck R, Korte M, Barde YA. Biosynthesis and processing of endogenous BDNF: CNS neurons store and secrete BDNF, not proBDNF. Nat Neurosci. 2008;11(2):131–3.

45. Yang J, Siao C-J, Nagappan G, Marinic T, Jing D, McGrath K, et al. Neuronal release of proBDNF. Nat Neurosci. 2009;12:113–5.

46. Chen ZY, Jing D, Bath KG, Ieraci A, Khan T, Siao CJ, Herrera DG, Toth M, Yang C, BS ME, Hempstead BL, Lee FS. Genetic variant BDNF (Val66Met) polymorphism alters anxiety-related behavior. Science. 2006;314(5796):140–3.

47. Zhang Q, Ames JM, Smith RD, Baynes JW, Metz TO. A perspective on the Maillard reaction and the analysis of protein glycation by mass spectrometry: probing the pathogenesis of chronic disease. J Proteome Res. 2009;8:754–69.

48. Smerjac SM, Bizzozero OA. Cytoskeletal protein carbonylation and degradation in experimental autoimmune encephalomyelitis. J Neurochem. 2008;105:763–72.

49. Harris RA, Amor S. Sweet and sour--oxidative and carbonyl stress in neurological disorders. CNS Neurol Disord Drug Targets. 2011;10:82–107.

50. Ullrich A, Gray A, Berman C, Dull TJ. Human beta-nerve growth factor gene sequence highly homologous to that of mouse. Nature. 1983;303:821–5.

51. Voineskos AN, Lerch JP, Felsky D, Shaikh S, Rajji TK, Miranda D, et al. The brain-derived neurotrophic factor Val66Met polymorphism and prediction of neural risk for Alzheimer disease. Arch Gen Psychiatry. 2011;68:198–206.

52. Anastasia A, Deinhardt K, Chao MV, Will NE, Irmady K, Lee FS, et al. Val66Met polymorphism of BDNF alters prodomain structure to induce neuronal growth cone retraction. Nat Commun. 2013;4:2490.

53. Egan MF, Kojima M, Callicott JH, Goldberg TE, Kolachana BS, Bertolino A, et al. The BDNF val66met polymorphism affects activity-dependent secretion of BDNF and human memory and hippocampal function. Cell. 2003;112:257–69.

54. Chen Z-Y. Variant brain-derived neurotrophic factor (BDNF) (Met66) alters the intracellular trafficking and activity-dependent secretion of wild-type BDNF in neurosecretory cells and cortical neurons. J Neurosci. 2004;24:4401–11.

55. Yu H, Wang D-D, Wang Y, Liu T, Lee FS, Chen Z-Y. Variant brain-derived neurotrophic factor Val66Met polymorphism alters vulnerability to stress and response to antidepressants. J Neurosci. 2012;32:4092–101.

56. Ji H, Da D, Wang Y, Jiang D, Zhou X, Lin P, et al. Association of BDNF and BCHE with Alzheimer's disease: Meta-analysis based on 56 genetic case-control studies of 12,563 cases and 12,622 controls. Exp. Ther. Med. 2015;9:1831–40.

57. Al-Shawi R, Hafner A, Chun S, Raza S, Crutcher K, Thrasivoulou C, Simons P, Cowen T. ProNGF, sortilin, and age-related neurodegeneration. Ann N Y Acad Sci. 2007;1119:208–15.

58. Saadipour K, Yang M, Lim Y, Georgiou K, Sun Y, Keating D, et al. Amyloid beta$_{1-42}$ (Aβ_{42}) up-regulates the expression of Sortilin via the p75(NTR)/RhoA signaling pathway. J Neurochem. 2013;127(2):152–62.

59. Chao MV. Cleavage of p75 neurotrophin receptor is linked to Alzheimer's disease. Mol Psychiatry. 2016;21(3):300–1.

60. Sotthibundhu A, Sykes AM, Fox B, Underwood CK, Thangnipon W, Coulson EJ. Beta-amyloid(1–42) induces neuronal death through the p75 neurotrophin. Receptor J Neurosci. 2008;28(15):3941–6.

61. Yao XQ, Jiao SS, Saadipour K, Zeng F, Wang QH, Shen LL, et al. p75NTR ectodomain is a physiological neuroprotective molecule against amyloid-beta toxicity in the brain of Alzheimer's disease. Mol Psychiatry. 2015;20:1301–10.

62. Saadipour K, MacLean M, Pirkle S, Ali S, Lopez-Redondo ML, Stokes DL, Chao MV. The transmembrane domain of the p75 neurotrophin receptor stimulates phosphorylation of the TrkB tyrosine kinase receptor. J Biol Chem. 2017;292(40):16594–604.

Permissions

List of Contributors

Hadhimulya Asmara, Arsalan P. Rizwan, Giriraj Sahu, Brett A. Simms, Jordan D. T. Engbers and Ray W. Turner
Department of Cell Biology and Anatomy, University of Calgary, Calgary, AB T2N 4N1, Canada

Ileana Micu and Peter K. Stys
Department of Clinical Neurosciences, University of Calgary, Calgary, AB T2N 4N1, Canada

Fang-Xiong Zhang
Department of Physiology and Pharmacology, University of Calgary, Calgary, AB T2N 4N1, Canada

Hadhimulya Asmara, Ileana Micu, Arsalan P. Rizwan, Giriraj Sahu, Brett A. Simms, Jordan D. T. Engbers, Peter K. Stys, Gerald W. Zamponis and Ray W. Turner
Hotchkiss Brain Institute, University of Calgary, Calgary, AB T2N 4N1, Canada

Fang-Xiong Zhang and Gerald W. Zamponi
Alberta Children's Hospital Research Institute, Cumming School of Medicine, University of Calgary, Calgary, AB T2N 4N1, Canada

Ray W. Turner
HRIC 1AA14, University of Calgary, 3330 Hospital Dr. N.W, Calgary, AB T2N 4N1, Canada

María Rodríguez-Muñoz, Yara Onetti, Elsa Cortés-Montero, Javier Garzón and Pilar Sánchez-Blázquez
Neuropharmacology. Department of Traslational Neuroscience, Cajal Institute, CSIC, E-28002 Madrid, Spain

Lesly Puspita and Jae-won Shim
Soonchunhyang Institute of Medi-bio Science (SIMS), Soonchunhyang University, 25, Bongjeong-ro, Dongnam-gu, Cheonan-si 31151, South Korea

Sun Young Chung
Center for Stem Cell Biology, Sloan-Kettering Institute, New York, NY 10065, USA

Chun-Kui Zhang, Zhi-Hong Li, Yu Qiao, Ting Zhang, Ya-Cheng Lu, Tao Chen, Yu-Lin Dong, Yun-Qing Li and Jin-Lian Li
Department of Anatomy and K.K. Leung Brain Research Centre, The Fourth Military Medical University, Xi'an, People's Republic of China

Yu Qiao
Student Brigade, Fourth Military Medical University, Xi'an, People's Republic of China

Zoé Husson and Ewan St. John Smith
Department of Pharmacology, University of Cambridge, Tennis Court Road, Cambridge CB2 1PD, UK

Soo-Jin Oh, Junsung Woo and C. Justin Lee
Center for Neuroscience, Korea Institute of Science and Technology, Seoul, Korea

Soo-Jin Oh, Nam-Chul Cho and Ae Nim Pae
Convergence Research Center for Diagnosis, Treatment and Care System of Dementia, Korea Institute of Science and Technology, Seoul, Korea

Soo-Jin Oh, Junsung Woo and C. Justin
Center for Glia-Neuron interaction, Korea Institute of Science and Technology, Seoul, Korea

Minhee Cho
Center for Functional Connectomics, Korea Institute of Science and Technology, Seoul, Korea

C. Justin Lee and Eun Mi Hwang
Neuroscience Program, University of Science and Technology (UST), Daejeon, Korea

Young-Sun Lee
School of Biosystem and Biomedical Science, College of Health Science, Korea University, Seoul, Korea

Shuang Qiu, Min Zhuo and Kohei Koga
Center for Neuron and Disease, Frontier Institute of Science and Technology, Xi'an Jiaotong University, Xi'an 710049, China

Shuang Qiu, Min Zhuo and Kohei Koga
Department of Physiology, Faculty of Medicine, University of Toronto, Medical Science Building, 1 King's College Circle, Toronto, ON M5S 1A8, Canada

Shuang Qiu, Yu Wu and Xinyou Lv
Department of Neurobiology, Key Laboratory of Medical Neurobiology of the Ministry of Health of China, Zhejiang University School of Medicine, Zhejiang 310058, Hangzhou, China

Xia Li
Department of Neurology, The First Affiliated Hospital, Zhejiang University School of Medicine, Zhejiang 310003, Hangzhou, China

Kohei Koga
Department of Neurophysiology, Hyogo College of Medicine, Nishinomiya, Hyogo 663-8501, Japan

Jiali Shao, Jian Wang, Jiangju Huang, Chang Liu, Yundan Pan, Qulian Guo and Wangyuan Zou
Department of Anesthesiology, Xiangya Hospital, Central South University, 87 Xiangya Road, Changsha 410008, Hunan, China

Tzu-Hao Harry Chao and Chen-Tung Yen
Department of Life Science, National Taiwan University, No. 1, Sec. 4, Roosevelt Rd, Taipei 10617, Taiwan

Jyh-Horng Chen
Interdisciplinary MRI/MRS Lab, Department of Electrical Engineering, National Taiwan University, No. 1, Sec. 4, Roosevelt Rd, Taipei 10617, Taiwan

Keunjung Heo, Min-Jung Lee and Seungbok Lee
Department of Brain and Cognitive Sciences, College of Natural Sciences, Seoul National University, Seoul 08826, South Korea

Keunjung Heo and Min-Jung Lee
Department of Cell & Developmental Biology, Dental Research Institute, Seoul National University, Seoul 03080, South Korea.

Seung Hyun Kim and Minyeop Nahm
Department of Neurology, Hanyang University College of Medicine, Seoul 04763, South Korea

Young-Eun Kim and Chang-Seok Ki
Department of Laboratory Medicine and Genetics, Samsung Medical Center, Sungkyunkwan University School of Medicine, Seoul 06351, South Korea

Wei Jen Chang and Bai Chuang Shyu
Institute of Biomedical Sciences, Academia Sinica, Taipei 11529, Taiwan, ROC

Wei Pang Chang
Department of Anesthesiology and Perioperative Medicine, School of Medicine, University of Alabama, Birmingham, AL 35211, USA

Nathalie Lombaert, Maroussia Hennes, Sara Gilissen, Giel Schevenels, Laetitia Aerts, Ria Vanlaer, Lieve Geenen, Julie Nys and Lutgarde Arckens
Laboratory of Neuroplasticity and Neuroproteomics, Katholieke Universiteit Leuven, Naamsestraat 59, Box 2467, B-3000 Leuven, Belgium

Ann Van Eeckhaut and Ilse Smolders
Department of Pharmaceutical Chemistry, Drug Analysis and Drug Information, Center for Neurosciences (C4N), Vrije Universiteit Brussel, Laarbeeklaan 103, 1090 Brussels, Belgium

Julie Nys
Laboratory of Synapse Biology, VIB-KU Leuven Center for Brain and Disease Research, O&N IV, Herestraat 49, box 602, B-3000 Leuven, Belgium

Wei Jiang, Min Guo, Min Gong, Li Chen, Yang Bi, Yun Zhang, Yuan Shi, Ping Qu, Youxue Liu and Jie Chenand Tingyu Li
Children Nutrition Research Center, Children's Hospital of Chongqing Medical University, Chongqing 400014, China
Ministry of Education Key Laboratory of Child Development and Disorders, Chongqing 400014, China
China International Science and Technology Cooperation Base of Child Development and Critical Disorders, Chongqing 400014, China
Chongqing Key Laboratory of Translational Medical Research in Cognitive Development and Learning and Memory Disorders, Chongqing 400014, China

Wei Jiang and Min Guo
Children Rehabilitation Center, Children's Hospital of Chongqing Medical University, Chongqing, China

Chunfang Dai, Yannan Liu and Zhifang Dong
Ministry of Education Key Laboratory of Child Development and Disorders, Children's Hospital of Chongqing Medical University, 136 Zhongshan Er Road, Yuzhong District, Chongqing 400014, People's Republic of China
Chongqing Key Laboratory of Translational Medical Research in Cognitive Development and Learning and Memory Disorders, Children's Hospital of Chongqing Medical University, 136 Zhongshan Er Road, Yuzhong District, Chongqing 400014, People's Republic of China
China International Science and Technology Cooperation base of Child Development and Critical Disorders, Children's Hospital of Chongqing Medical University, 136 Zhongshan Er Road, Yuzhong District, Chongqing 400014, People's Republic of China

Shin-Young Park, Min-Jeong Kang and Joong-Soo Han
Biomedical Research Institute and Department of Biochemistry and Molecular Biology, College of Medicine, Hanyang University, 222 Wangsimni-ro, Seongdong-gu, Seoul 04763, Republic of Korea

Akito Nakao, Hideo Hagihara and Tsuyoshi Miyakawa
Division of Systems Medical Science, Institute for Comprehensive Medical Science, Fujita Health University, 1-98 Dengakugakubo, Kutsukake-cho, Toyoake, Aichi 470-1192, Japan

Naoyuki Miyazaki
National Institute for Physiological Sciences, National Institutes of Natural Sciences, Okazaki, Japan

Koji Ohira
Department of Food Science and Nutrition, Mukogawa Women's University, Nishinomiya, Japan

Tsuyoshi Takagi
Institute for Developmental Research, Aichi Human Service Center, Kasugai, Japan

Tsuyoshi Takagi and Shunsuke Ishii
RIKEN Tsukuba Institute, Tsukuba, Japan

Nobuteru Usuda
Department of Anatomy II, Fujita Health University School of Medicine, Toyoake, Japan

Adan Hernandez, Chunfeng Tan, Florian Plattner, Karine Pozo, Mohammad A. Yousuf and Tanvir Singh
Department of Psychiatry, University of Texas Southwestern Medical Center, Dallas, TX 75390, USA

Florian Plattner
Center for Translational Neurodegeneration Research, University of Texas Southwestern Medical Center, Dallas, TX 75390, USA

Aric F. Logsdon, Ryan C. Turner and Brandon P. Luke-Wold
Department of Neurosurgery, West Virginia University School of Medicine, Morgantown, WV 26506-9183, USA

Jason D. Huber
Department of Basic Pharmaceutical Sciences, West Virginia University School of Medicine, Morgantown, WV 26506-9530, USA

James A. Bibb
Departments of Surgery, Neurobiology, and Neurology, The University of Alabama at Birmingham Medical Center, 1720 2nd Ave S, THT 1052, Birmingham, AL 35294, USA

Catherine Fleitas, Pau Marfull, Daniel Rocandio and Joaquim Egea
Molecular Developmental Neurobiology Group, IRBLleida-UDL Rovira Roure 82, 25198 Lleida, Spain

Isidro Ferrer
Departament de Patologia i Terapèutica Experimental, Universitat de Barcelona, Barcelona, Spain
Centro de Investigación Biomédica en Red de Enfermedades Neurodegenerativas (CIBERNED), Hospitalet de Llobregat, Barcelona, Spain

Gerard Piñol-Ripoll
Unitat Trastorns Cognitius, IRBLleida-Hospital Universitari Santa Maria Lleida, Lleida, Spain

Claire Rampon
Centre de Recherches sur la Cognition Animale (CRCA), Centre de Biologie Intégrative (CBI), Université de Toulouse, CNRS, UPS, 31062 Toulouse, France

Joaquim Egea and Carme Espinet
Serra Húnter fellow, Associate Professor, Generalitat de Catalunya, Barcelona, Spain

Index